Advances in Endocrinology

Advances in Endocrinology

Editor: Donovan Douglas

AMERICAN
MEDICAL PUBLISHERS
www.americanmedicalpublishers.com

AMERICAN
MEDICAL PUBLISHERS
www.americanmedicalpublishers.com

Cataloging-in-Publication Data

Advances in endocrinology / edited by Donovan Douglas.
p. cm.
Includes bibliographical references and index.
ISBN 978-1-63927-109-2
1. Endocrinology. 2. Endocrinology, Comparative. 3. Endocrinology, Experimental.
4. Developmental endocrinology. 5. Hormones. I. Douglas, Donovan.
RC648 .A38 2022
616.4--dc23

American Medical Publishers,
41 Flatbush Avenue,
1st Floor, New York,
NY 11217, USA

ISBN 978-1-63927-109-2 (Hardback)

Contents

Preface

This book aims to highlight the current researches and provides a platform to further the scope of innovations in this area. This book is a product of the combined efforts of many researchers and scientists, after going through thorough studies and analysis from different parts of the world. The objective of this book is to provide the readers with the latest information of the field.

Endocrinology is a domain of biology and medicine that is concerned with the endocrine system and its diseases and hormones. It also deals with psychological activities and the behavioral activities of metabolism, growth and development, tissue function, sleep, digestion, movement and sensory perception, which are caused by hormones. The specializations within this field are behavioral endocrinology and comparative endocrinology. The endocrinal disorders are divided into three groups - endocrine gland hyposecretion, which leads to hormone deficiency, endocrine gland hypersecretion, which leads to hormone excess, and tumors of endocrine glands. Some of the common endocrine disorders are glucose homeostasis disorders, thyroid disorders, calcium homeostasis disorders, pituitary gland disorder, sex hormone disorder, etc. This book provides comprehensive insights into the field of endocrinology. It includes some of the vital pieces of work being conducted across the world, on various topics related to this domain. The book is a vital tool for all researching and studying this field.

I would like to express my sincere thanks to the authors for their dedicated efforts in the completion of this book. I acknowledge the efforts of the publisher for providing constant support. Lastly, I would like to thank my family for their support in all academic endeavors.

Editor

1

The association of hypertriglyceridemia with cardiovascular events and pancreatitis

M Hassan Murad[1,2*], Ahmad Hazem[1,2,3], Fernando Coto-Yglesias[1], Svitlana Dzyubak[1], Shabnum Gupta[1], Irina Bancos[1,5], Melanie A Lane[1], Patricia J Erwin[1], Lars Berglund[4], Tarig Elraiyah[1] and Victor M Montori[1,5]

Abstract

Background: Hypertriglyceridemia may be associated with important complications. The aim of this study is to estimate the magnitude of association and quality of supporting evidence linking hypertriglyceridemia to cardiovascular events and pancreatitis.

Methods: We conducted a systematic review of multiple electronic bibliographic databases and subsequent meta-analysis using a random effects model. Studies eligible for this review followed patients longitudinally and evaluated quantitatively the association of fasting hypertriglyceridemia with the outcomes of interest. Reviewers working independently and in duplicate reviewed studies and extracted data.

Results: 35 studies provided data sufficient for meta-analysis. The quality of these observational studies was moderate to low with fair level of multivariable adjustments and adequate exposure and outcome ascertainment. Fasting hypertriglyceridemia was significantly associated with cardiovascular death (odds ratios (OR) 1.80; 95% confidence interval (CI) 1.31-2.49), cardiovascular events (OR, 1.37; 95% CI, 1.23-1.53), myocardial infarction (OR, 1.31; 95% CI, 1.15-1.49), and pancreatitis (OR, 3.96; 95% CI, 1.27-12.34, in one study only). The association with all-cause mortality was not statistically significant.

Conclusions: The current evidence suggests that fasting hypertriglyceridemia is associated with increased risk of cardiovascular death, MI, cardiovascular events, and possibly acute pancreatitis.
Précis: hypertriglyceridemia is associated with increased risk of cardiovascular death, MI, cardiovascular events, and possibly acute pancreatitis

Keywords: Hypertriglyceridemia, Cardiovascular disease, Pancreatitis, Systematic reviews and meta-analysis

Background

Hypertriglyceridemia is a manifestation of several common metabolic disorders in the western world. A recent cross-sectional study found that over 33% of adults in the United States had hypertriglyceridemia (serum triglyceride levels over 150 mg/dl (1.7 mmol/L)) of whom over 50% had serum triglyceride levels exceeding 200 mg/dl (2.2 mmol/L) [1].

The association of hypertriglyceridemia and clinically important complications such as cardiovascular events and acute pancreatitis has been suggested by several studies. Previous epidemiologic studies demonstrated increase in the risk of cardiovascular events although there has always been significant confounding due to varying levels of adjustments for traditional risk factors and other lipid subfractions [2-4]. As for pancreatitis, case series and uncontrolled studies reported that very severely elevated triglyceride levels are associated with lipemic serum, chylomicronemia syndrome, and increased risk of pancreatitis [5-7]. Serum triglycerides levels of 1000 mg/dl (11.3 mmol/L) and higher have been observed in 12% to 38% of patients presenting with acute pancreatitis [5]. However, the association with pancreatitis has not been evaluated in controlled studies or with less severe hypertriglyceridemia.

* Correspondence: Murad.mohammad@mayo.edu
[1]Knowledge and Evaluation Research Unit, Mayo Clinic, Rochester, MN, USA
Full list of author information is available at the end of the article

To update the evidence base to the present time (last meta-analysis [2] was performed 6 years ago), we conducted this systematic review and meta-analysis. Our goal was to assess the magnitude of association and the quality of supporting evidence linking hypertriglyceridemia with cardiovascular events, mortality and pancreatitis. We specifically aimed at comparing association measures in studies with varying levels of adjustment for cardiovascular risk factors and to search for controlled studies evaluating the risk of pancreatitis.

Methods

This systematic review was conducted according to a priori established protocol that was commissioned and funded by the Endocrine Society and is reported according to the PRISMA statement (Preferred Reporting Items for Systematic Reviews and Meta-analyses) [8].

Eligibility criteria

Eligible studies were randomized and observational studies that enrolled patients with untreated hypertriglyceridemia and reported a relative association measure between fasting serum triglycerides levels and the outcomes of interest: all-cause mortality, cardiovascular death, cardiovascular events and pancreatitis. We excluded uncontrolled studies and studies of nonfasting hypertriglyceridemia.

Study identification and data extraction

An expert reference librarian (P.J.E) created and implemented the electronic search strategy with input from study investigators (V.M.M. & M.H.M). We searched Ovid MEDLINE, Ovid EMBASE, Web of Science and SCOPUS through August of 2010. The detailed search strategy is available in Additional file 1. We also sought recommendations from content expert for potentially relevant studies to be included in the screening process.

Reviewers working independently and in duplicate assessed each abstract for eligibility. Disagreements yielded an automatic inclusion into the following level of screening. Included studied were retrieved and full text screening commenced in duplicate as well. Disagreements in this level were resolved by discussion and consensus. Online reference management system was used to conduct this review and it reported a real-time chance-adjusted agreement (kappa) statistic to evaluate the agreement among reviewers. Kappa averaged 0.80. Two reviewers working independently and in duplicate extracted baseline and outcome data and assessed the quality of included study. A third reviewer compared the reviewer's data and resolved inconsistencies by referring to the full text article.

Quality

Using the Newcastle-Ottawa scale, [9] reviewers assessed the quality of included observational studies (and control arms of RCT, considered as observational cohorts) by determining outcome ascertainment, adjustment for confounders, proportion of patients lost to follow-up as well as sample selection. We used the GRADE approach in evaluating the evidence yielded from included studies [10].

Statistical analysis

We pooled the relative association measures of relevant complications from included studies and analyzed the data using the random-effects model described by DerSimonian and Laird [11]. Heterogeneity in results across studies was measured using the I^2 statistic, which estimates the proportion of variation in results across studies that is not due to chance. An I^2 of 50% or more indicates large inconsistency between studies. Meta-analysis was completed using Comprehensive Meta-analysis (CMA) version 2.2 (Biostat Inc., Englewood, NJ).

Subgroup analyses and publication bias

A priori hypotheses were designed to explain between-study inconsistencies in results. These analyses sought an interaction with whether triglycerides levels were adjusted for other lipid fractions or not; whether the underlying metabolic disorder was diabetes vs. not; and whether the association differed between men and women. Publication bias was evaluated by assessing the symmetry of funnel plots and using Egger's regression test. In this regression, the size of the treatment effect is captured by the slope of the regression line and bias is captured by the intercept [12].

Results

Search results and included studies

Electronic search yielded 760 potentially eligible studies. Following screening, 60 studies met inclusion criteria, of which 35 reported data sufficient for meta-analysis [Figure 1].

Methodological quality and risk of bias

Included studies had a fair methodological quality (Table 2) with follow-up period reported by 85% of studies averaging 114 months; 58% of studies reported loss to follow-up of participants that ranged 0% to 27%. Adjustment for potential confounders was reported in 90% of studies and the outcome ascertainment method was reported in all studies. Cohort selection was random in 18% of the studies.

Meta-analysis

The total number of included studies was 35 enrolling 927,218 patients who suffered 132,460 deaths and 72,654 cardiac events; respectively. Hypertriglyceridemia was significantly associated with cardiovascular death, cardiovascular events, myocardial infarction, and pancreatitis; with odds ratios (95% confidence interval) of

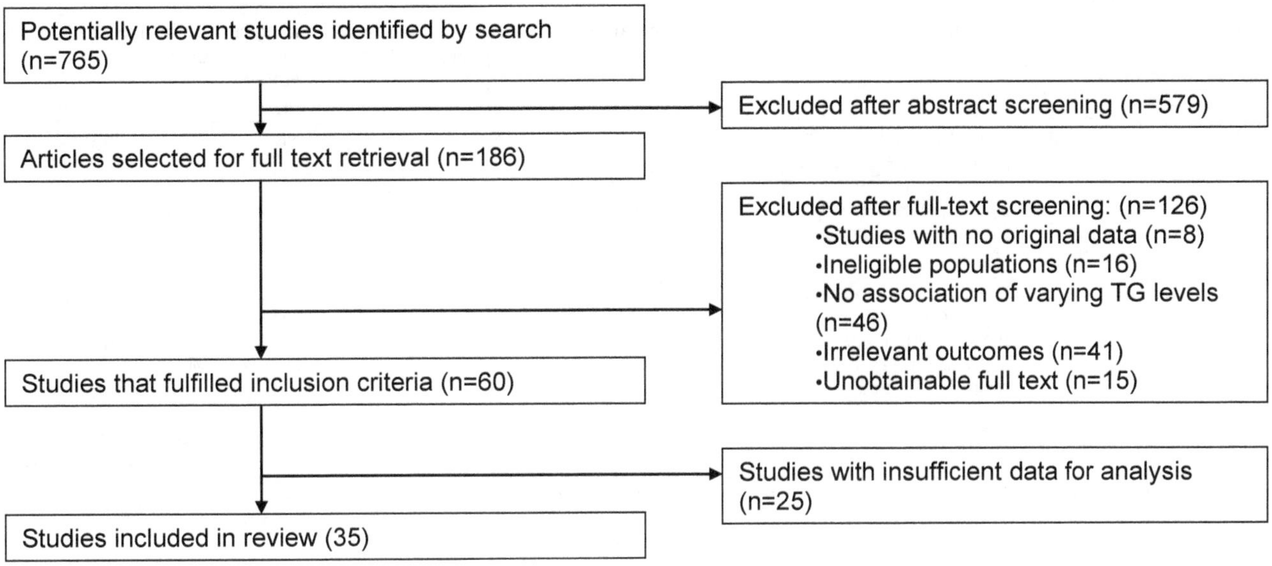

Figure 1 Study selection process.

1.80 (1.31-2.49), 1.37 (1.23-1.53), 1.31 (1.15-1.49) and 3.96 (1.27-12.34); respectively. There was nonsignificant association with all-cause mortality (OR: 1.10; 95% CI: 0.90-1.36). Forest plots depicting the results of random effects meta-analysis are presented in Figures 2, 3, 4 and 5.

It is worth noting that the association with acute pancreatitis was estimated by only one eligible study that included 129 patients with severe hypertriglyceridemia (119 with type IV phenotypes and 10 with type V phenotypes according to Fredrickson's classification) of whom 26 suffered acute pancreatitis [33]. In this study, subjects in the third tertile of TG had a 4.0-fold increased risk (95% confidence interval, 1.3-12.3) compared with the first tertile and those diagnosed with dyslipidemia at a younger age also had increased risk.

All analyses were associated with important heterogeneity (I^2 > 50%) that our planned subgroup analyses could only partially explain (Table 3). The association of hypertriglyceridemia with mortality and cardiovascular mortality seemed to be stronger in women. These findings are consistent with a previous meta-analysis published in 1996. Hokanson and Austin estimated adjusted relative risks for incident cardiovascular events of 1.14 (95% Cl 1.05-1.28) in men and 1.37 (95% Cl 1.13-1.66) in women. The association with cardiovascular events was somewhat stronger in patients with diabetes although this effect was not statistically significant. Hence, there were no other significant subgroup interactions to explain heterogeneity (based on the level of adjustment for lipids subfractions, sex or the presence of diabetes).

There was no evidence of publication bias (P value for Eggers test > 0.05 for all outcomes) although these analyses were underpowered to detect this problem and the presence of heterogeneity further limits the ability to detect publication bias.

Discussion

We conducted a systematic review and meta-analysis and documented an association between fasting hypertriglyceridemia and the risk of several cardiovascular adverse events and with pancreatitis.

Limitations, strengths and comparison with other reports

The main limitation of association studies is the observational nature of the existing evidence. Therefore, confounders (particularly, baseline risk of patients for developing cardiovascular disease and the effect of other lipid subfractions abnormalities) threaten the validity of results. In meta-analyses of observational studies, the ability to adjust for confounding is limited by the level of adjustment conducted in the original studies. We attempted to evaluate confounding by conducting subgroup analysis; however, this analysis was underpowered. Other limitations pertain to heterogeneity of the meta-analytic estimates, publication bias (which remains likely in the context of observational studies that do not require prospective registration) and reporting bias (which is also likely considering that several studies met the eligibility criteria for this review but did not report the outcomes of interest) [48]. It was unclear in most studies if enrolled patients did not have some of the outcomes pre-existent at baseline and it was also unclear if patients were treated with drugs that can affect TG level (both of these elements lower the confidence in the observed associations). We only found one controlled study that evaluated the association with acute pancreatitis.

Table 1 Baseline Characteristics of Included Studies

Study Label	Design	Objective of Study	Population	Age (mean)	Sample Size	Length of Follow-up	Definition of CV events
Acarturk, 2004[13]	Prospective cohort	to investigate the relation between age and gender differences in plasma TG and CAD in patients with angiographically proven CAD	patients admitted for diagnostic coronary angiography due to chest pain	54.9 +/-10.26	937	NR	Coronary artery disease
Bansal, 2007 [14]	Prospective cohort	To determine the association of triglyceride levels (fasting vs nonfasting) and risk of future cardiovascular events.	healthy women	54.2 +/- 7.06	26,509	136.8 Months (median)	composite of confirmed nonfatal MI, nonfatal ischemic stroke, coronary revascularization, or death due to cardiovascular causes
Barrett-Connor, 1987 [15]	Prospective cohort	To examine the independent effect of triglyceride on the prediction of cardiovascular disease after the effects of cholesterol and other heart disease risk factors have been accounted for	healthy fasting men without known CVD	57.7	1,589	144 months	N/A
Bass, 1993 [16]	Prospective cohort	To further explore the relationships between lipid and lipoprotein levels and other conventional CVD risk factors and CVD death on women	women 30 years of age and older	58.2 +/- 5.5	1,405	Mean 168 months	N/A
Bonaventure, 2010[17]	Prospective cohort	To find the association pattern between serum TG and incident intracerebral hemorrhage as compared with coronary events and ischemic stroke	Population-based, elderly participants free from institutionalization were recruited from the electoral rolls of three French cities	74.03 years	8,393	mean of 5 years	MI, hospitalized angina pectoris, acute coronary syndrome, coronary endovascular dilatation, coronary bypass, or death due to a coronary event
Carlson, 1988 [18]	RCT	To obtain a pronounced serum lipid lowering by combined use of clofibrate and nicotinic acid in an effort to reduce the risk of IHD	Survivors of MI < 70 years of age	58.9 + -0.4 males and 62.5 + -0.9 females	Control group (n = 276)	60 months	N/A
Chan, 2005 [19]	Prospective cohort	To examine the lipid profiles in Chinese type 2 diabetic patients and their relationship with anthropometric parameters, glycemic control and cardiovascular mortality.	Chinese patients with type 2 DM	54.0 +/- 14.0	517	Mean 55.2 +/-10.8 months	N/A
Chester, 1995 [20]	Prospective cohort	To determine the standard clinical or angiographic variables or both present at initial angiography associated with the development of adverse coronary events in patients awaiting routine PTCA	Patients awaiting routine percutaneous transluminal coronary angioplasty (PTCA)	57	215	Median 8 months	fatal or non-fatal MI, unstable angina or angiographic new total coronary occlusion
Czernichow, 2007[21]	Prospective cohort	To investigated the relationship of baseline 'hypertriglyceridemic waist' (HTGW) status with CVD risk in middle-aged French men	middle-aged French men, included diabetics	51.9 +/- 4.7	3,430	90 months	new-onset angina, fatal and non-fatal MI or stroke, transient ischemic attack, sudden death or intermittent claudication

Table 1 Baseline Characteristics of Included Studies *(Continued)*

Drexel, 2005 [22]	Prospective cohort	To evaluate the atherogenicity of lipids in coronary patients with normal fasting glucose (NFG), impaired fasting glucose (IFG), and type 2 DM	Caucasian patients who were referred to coronary angiography	62.4 +/- 10.6	750	27.6 +/- 4.8 months	N/A
Eberly, 2003 [23]	Prospective cohort	To determine whether HTG is an independent risk factor for coronary heart disease (CHD), and whether fasting and nonfasting triglyceride (TG) levels are equally predictive	men at increased risk but without clinical evidence of definite CHD at baseline	46.3	2809	304.8 months	either a clinical MI or a significant serial electrocardiogram change indicative of MI
Egger, 1999 [24]	Prospective cohort	To assess the influence of differential precision in the measurement of the correlated variables total cholesterol and HDL cholesterol on estimates of risk of IHD associated with TG levels	Middle aged men living in the town of Caerphilly, South Wales, UK	52.1 +/- 4.48	2,512	5 and 10 years after baseline	death from ischemic heart disease, clinical non-fatal MI, electrocardiographic MI
Ellingsen, 2003[25]	Prospective cohort	to examine the effect of group assignment on IHD mortality in subjects with normal or high fasting TG	healthy men who had an elevated serum total cholesterol concentration or coronary risk score	46 +/-3	1232	276 months	N/A
Gaziano, 1997[26]	Case controlled study	To examine the interrelationships of the fasting TG level other lipid parameters and nonlipid risk factors with risk of MI.	Patients - coronary care and other intensive care units patients (no history of MI and angina pectoris) with whom symptoms of MI had begun 24 h of admission, control - residents of home towns.	57.7 +/- 9.65	680	NR	N/A
Goldberg, 2009[27]	Prospective/ case controlled	To ascertain coronary artery disease outcomes and predictive factors in patients with SLE and matched healthy controls prospectively	Patients with systemic lupus erythematosus (SLE) and matched healthy controls	SLE cases 44.2 +/-12.2, controls 44.5 +/- 4.4	237 controls and 241 SLE cases	86.4 months	Defined as the occurrence of MI and/or angina pectoris due to atherosclerosis.
Habib, 2006 [28]	Prospective cohort	To evaluate the association of serum TC and TG with clinical outcomes in chronic peritoneal dialysis (PD) patients.	Patients on chronic peritoneal dialysis; only in end-stage renal disease (ESRD) or patients those very ill patients who died rapidly due to unrelated conditions.	57.2 +/ 15.3	1,053	23 +/- 14 months	N/A

Table 1 Baseline Characteristics of Included Studies *(Continued)*

Haim, 1999 [29]	Prospective cohort	To investigate the association between elevated blood triglyceride levels and subsequent mortality risk in patients with established coronary heart disease (CHD)	patients with a diagnosis of CHD	59.76 +/- 6.96	11,546	61.2 months	N/A
Hoogeveen, 2001[30]	Case controlled study	To determine the effect of immigration to the USA ion plasma levels of lipoprotein a and other independent risk factors for CHD in Asian Indians	Asian Indians and Asian Indians living in the USA with and without CHD	44.2 +/- 12.79	309	NR	Coronary heart disease - incidents not specifically defined
Jonsdottir, 2002[31]	Prospective cohort	To examine the relationship between the relative risk of baseline variables and verified MI or coronary death in individuals with no prior history of MI	male and female from Reykjavik and adjusted communities	52.7 +/- 8.71	18,569	Mean 208.8 months	N/A
Lamarche, 1995[32]	Prospective cohort	To confirm the importance of both elevated plasma cholesterol and decreased high density lipoprotein cholesterol levels as risk factors for ischemic heart disease	men without ischemic heart disease	57.5	2,103	60 months	Effort angina pectoris, coronary insufficiency, nonfatal MI, and coronary death
Lloret Linares, 2008[33]	Retrospective cohort	to assess retrospectively the prevalence and the predictive factors of acute pancreatitis (AP)	Patients referred by their general practitioner or general hospital for very high TG levels.	47 +/- 10.7	129	NR	N/A
Lu, 2003[34]	Prospective cohort	To determine whether non-HDL cholesterol, a measure of total cholesterol minus HDL cholesterol, is a predictor of CVD in patients with DM	American Indians with DM	57.28 +/- 8	2,108	108 months	Coronary heart disease, MI, stroke, and other CVD
Malone, 2009 [35]	Prospective cohort	This study evaluated cardiometabolic risk factors and their relationship to prevalent diagnosis of acute MI (AMI) and stroke.	People continuously receiving health insurance benefits during study	56.8 +/- 0.03	170,648	24 months	N/A
Mazza, 2005 [36]	Prospective cohort	To evaluate whether TG level is a risk factor for CHD in elderly people from general population, and to look for interactions between TG and other risk factors.	elderly people from general population CHD in elderly people from general population	73.8 +/- 5	3,257	144 months	N/A
Mora, 2008 [37]	Prospective cohort	To evaluate levels of lipids and apolipoproteins after a typical meal and to determine whether fasting compared with non-fasting alters the association of these lipids and apolipoproteins with incident CVD.	Healthy women, aged > = 45 years, who were free of self-reported CVD or cancer at study entry and with follow-up for incident CVD.	54.7	26,330	136.8 months	Nonfatal MI, percutaneous coronary intervention, coronary artery bypass grafting, nonfatal stroke, or cardiovascular death

Table 1 Baseline Characteristics of Included Studies *(Continued)*

Noda, 2010 [38]	Case controlled study	To examine the prediction of coronary risk factors and evaluation of the predictive value for MI among Japanese middle-aged male workers.	Japanese male workers	cases 50.4 + -5.3, controls 50.4 + -5.5 years	cases 204 and controls 408	36 months	N/A
Rubins, 1999 [39]	RCT	To analyze the role of raising HDL cholesterol level and lowering triglyceride levels to reduce the rate of coronary events in patients with existing cardiovascular disease	men with coronary heart disease with absence of serious coexisting conditions	64 + -7	1267 (placebo)	61.2 months	combined incidence of nonfatal MI or death from coronary heart disease
Samuelsson, 1994[40]	Prospective cohort	To analyze the importance of DM and HTG as potential risk factors for CHD in middle-aged, treated hypertensive men	middle aged treated hypertensive men	52 +/- 2.3	686	180 months	Non-fatal MI, a fatal MI, a death certificate statement of coronary atherosclerosis as the cause of death
Schupf, 2005 [41]	Prospective cohort	To investigate the relationship between plasma lipids and risk of death from all causes in non demented elderly	Community-based sample of Medicare recipients without dementia	76.1	2,277	Mean 36 +/- 30 months	N/A
Sprecher, 2000[42]	Prospective cohort	To evaluate the predictive value of serum triglyceride levels on mortality in post coronary artery bypass graft(CABG) diabetic patients with subsequent analysis by sex	Diabetic post CABG patients at a large metropolitan hospital	63 +/- 9	1,172	84 months	N/A
Tanko, 2005 [43]	Prospective cohort	To investigate the relative utility of enlarged waist combined with elevated TG (EWET) compared with the National Cholesterol Education Program (MS-NCEP) criteria in estimating future risk of all-cause and cardiovascular mortality	Postmenopausal women	60.4 +/- 7.1	557	8.5 +/- 0.3 years	N/A
Tsai, 2008[44]	Retrospective cohort	To assess the effect of a single and a combination of "pre-disease" risk factors of metabolic syndrome on the overall and cardiac mortality.	civil servants and teachers 40 years and older	52.4 + - 8.0	35,259	median follow-up of 15 years	N/A
Upmeier, 2009[45]	Prospective cohort	To determine whether high levels of serum total cholesterol and low levels of HDL are related to increased mortality in elderly	Home dwelling older adults residents in Finland	70 years	877	144 months	N/A
Valdivielso, 2009[46]	Prospective cohort	To study the prevalence, risk factors and vascular disease associated with moderate and sever HTG in an active working population	Active working population of Spain	36 ± 10 years	594,701	NR	documented prior medical diagnosis of heart disease, cerebrovascular disease or peripheral arterial disease
Wier, 2003 [47]	Prospective cohort	To investigate the relationship between triglyceride and stroke outcome	nondiabetic patients presenting to acute stroke unit	Median 70 years	1310	mean 1195 days	N/A

UC/NR: unclear, not reported; TG: Triglycerides; HTG, hypertriglyceridemia; MI, myocardial infarction; DM, diabetes, BP, blood pressure, HTN, hypertension
Triglycerides Conversion: from mg/dL to mmol/L: multiply by (x) 0.01129; from mmol/L to mg/dL: multiply by (x) 88.6

Table 2 Quality of Included Studies

Study Label	Cohort Selection (sampling)	Outcome ascertainment*	Adjustments for variables	% lost to follow-up	Definition of hypertriglyceridemia
Acarturk, 2004[13]	not random; all patients admitted for diagnostic coronary angiography	chart review, angiography results	NR	NR	TG value in the blood was used as a continuous number (variable). OR expresses increased risk per unit of serum TG level
Bansal, 2007 [14]	derived from women health study, previously completed randomized controlled trial of aspirin and vitamin E	chart review, events adjudicated by an end point committee	adjusted for treatment assignment to ASA, vitamin E, beta carotene, age, BP, smoking status, and use of hormone therapy, levels of total cholesterol and HDL-C, history of DM, BMI, high-sensitivity C-reactive protein	0	TG value in the blood was used as a continuous number (variable). OR expresses increased risk per unit of serum TG level
Barrett-Connor, 1987 [15]	random sample	chart review, ICD or billing codes, death certificates	adjust by TG level, age, BP, BMI, smoking habit, DM, family history of heart attack	0.5%	Compared normal to "borderline HTG", defined as TG between 240-500 mg/dL (2.7-5.65 mmol/L)
Bass, 1993 [16]	subset of female participants in the Lipid Research Clinics' Follow-up Study	chart review, annual checkups	Adjusted for age, HTN, DM, smoking, history of heart disease and estrogen use	NR	Compared TG < 200 mg/dL (< 2.25 mmol/L) to elevated 200 to 399 mg/dL (2.25 to 4.49 mmol/L) and high > 400 mg/dL (> 4.50 mmol/L)
Bonaventure, 2010[17]	not random and not consecutive: recruited from electoral rolls	Death certificates and autopsy reports, ascertained the same way in cases and controls	medical history of MI, stroke, or peripheral arterial disease, as well as smoking and alcohol consumption status (never, former, current), excess weight, elevated BP, DM, apolipoprotein E (APOE) genotype, low-dose aspirin intake, and lipid-lowering treatment	NR	They compared tertiles or quintiles: TG < 83.4 mg/dL (< 0.94), 84.2-117.8 mg/L (0.95-1.33), and > 118.7 mg/dL (1.34 mmol/L)
Carlson, 1988 [18]	consecutive sample (all patients presenting with HTG)	chart review, ascertained the same way in cases and controls, done without knowledge of patients' TG level	NR	13.4%	3 groups according to TG levels. Low = TG < 132.9 mg/dL (1.5 mmol/L), intermediate = TG 132.9-177.2 mg/dL (1.5-2.0 mmol/L), high = TG > 177.2 (2.0 mmol/L).

Table 2 Quality of Included Studies *(Continued)*

Chan, 2005 [19]	not random; consecutive patients with type 2 DM, not HPTG	chart review, death registry	Adjusted for sex and age. stepwise linear regression with BMI, WC, HbA1c, FPG and HOMA as independent variables and lipid profile as dependent variable	0	Unclear
Chester, 1995 [20]	consecutive sample (all men presenting with HTG and are awaiting routine angioplasty)	chart review, done without knowledge of patients' TG level	The potential predictor variables-that is, risk factors assessed at baseline angiography, for adverse events were analyzed using the multiple logistic regression models.	2	TG value in the blood was used as a continuous number (variable). Here OR expresses increased risk per unit of serum TG level: mmol/L
Czernichow, 2007[21]	consecutive sample	self report, chart review, ICD or billing codes, ascertained differently: self report in all patients, however if a CVD event was reported – chart review and ICD billing codes were reviewed for those individuals only	Age	NR	Age-adjusted relative risk correlate to one standard deviation increase in TG levels
Drexel, 2005 [22]	consecutive sample	follow up investigation after 2.3 years, Time and causes of death were obtained from national surveys, hospital records	age, sex, and use of lipid-lowering medication	0	Unclear
Eberly, 2003 [23]	not random; likely consecutive sample: 2863 men with both nonfasting and fasting TG levels measured at screens 1 and 2	self report, chart review, ICD or billing codes, death certificates	age, lipids subfractions, glucose level, BP, cigarettes smoked per day, alcohol use, BMI and race	0	TG value in the blood was used as a continuous number (variable). Here OR expresses increased risk per unit of serum TG level: mg/dL
Egger, 1999 [24]	not random; likely consecutive sample: Participants of the Caerphilly Heart Disease Study	self report, chart review, ICD or billing codes	age, all three lipid factors, laboratory error and within person variation, blood glucose and diastolic BP, BMI, smoking and markers for pre-existent disease	12.5	TG value in the blood was used as a continuous number (variable). Here OR expresses increased risk per unit of serum TG level: mmol/L

Table 2 Quality of Included Studies *(Continued)*

Ellingsen, 2003[25]	not random; likely consecutive sample: 1232 healthy men with elevated cholesterol or coronary risk score included in the study from a pool of 16202 screened men	chart review, ICD or billing codes, ascertained the same way in cases and controls	adjusted for age, BMI, cigarette smoking, total cholesterol, triacylglycerol, glucose, BP, dietary score, alcohol intake, and activity level	0	TG value in the blood was used as a continuous number (variable). Here OR expresses increased risk per unit of serum TG level: high TG > or = 178.1 mg/dL (2.01 mmol/L)
Gaziano, 1997[26]	not random, likely consecutive sample: Men/women < 76 yrs. age with no prior history of CAD discharged from one of 6 Boston area hospitals with the diagnosis of confirmed MI	chart review, medical exam/lab analysis, ascertained differently: cases were interviewed 8 weeks after MI	Adjusted for age, sex, history of HTN, history of DM, body mass index, type A personality, family history of previous MI, alcohol consumption, physical activity, smoking, caloric intake	12	they compared quintiles, highest compared to lowest
Goldberg, 2009[27]	consecutive sample (all patients presenting with HTG)	chart review, telephone calls, ascertained the same way in cases and controls	A time-to-event regression model was performed to establish the role of baseline lipid subfractions, other metabolic risk factors, lifestyle variables, and demographic characteristics in relation to the development of CAD.	3.8	high triglyceride level > = 248.1 mg/dL (2.8 mmol/L)
Habib, 2006 [28]	Data from the United States Renal Data System database collected during the prospective Dialysis Morbidity and Mortality Study Wave 2 study	chart review	age, gender, race, weight, height, primary cause of ESRD, hemoglobin, serum albumin, serum calcium phosphate product, serum bicarbonate, residual kidney creatinine clearance, PD parameters (dialysate effluent volume, dialysis creatinine clearance, D/P creatinine ratio after a 4 h dwell), use of lipid-modifying medications and comorbidity characteristics	0	TG value in the blood was used as a continuous number (variable). Here OR expresses increased risk per unit of serum TG level: HR is using a reference of TG levels 200-300 mg/dl (2.2-3.4 mmol/L)
Haim, 1999 [29]	not random; likely consecutive sample	chart review, ICD or billing codes	age, previous MI, DM, NYHA class, HTN, LDL cholesterol, glucose, chronic obstructive pulmonary disease, peripheral vascular disease, stroke, angina pectoris, smoking, and lipids	0.37	TG value in the blood was used as a continuous number (variable). Here OR expresses increased risk per unit of serum TG level: mg/dL

Table 2 Quality of Included Studies *(Continued)*

Hoogeveen, 2001[30]	Random sample	chart review, clinical exam and investigations, ascertained the same way in cases and controls	Logistic regression applied but no specific adjustments are mentioned	12	TG value in the blood was used as a continuous number (variable). Here OR expresses increased risk per unit of serum TG level: 10 mg/dL (0.11 mmol/L)
Jonsdottir, 2002[31]	not random; likely consecutive: subjects of the Reykjavik Study	self report, chart review, ICD or billing codes	age, high-density lipoprotein cholesterol, total/low-density lipoprotein cholesterol, smoking, body mass index and BP	0.6	TG value in the blood was used as a continuous number (variable). Here OR expresses increased risk per unit of serum TG level: mmol/L
Lamarche, 1995[32]	random sample	chart review, Examination/EKG/ death certificate	Adjusted for age, systolic BP, DM, alcohol consumption, and tobacco use	27	TG value in the blood was used as a continuous number (variable). Here OR expresses increased risk per unit of serum TG level: TG > 203.8 mg/dL (2.3 mmol/L)
Lloret Linares, 2008[33]	not random and not consecutive: Patients referred by their general practitioner or general hospital for very high TG levels to Endocrinology Dept. between 2000 and 2005	self report, chart review	Adjusted for age at hospitalization	NR	TG: lowest 95.1-180 mg/dL (1.1-2.0 mmol/L) vs. highest 360-1505 gm/dL (4.1-17 mmol/L).
Lu, 2003[34]	not random; likely consecutive: cohort chosen from the strong heart study to include only DM, no baseline CVD	through death certificates and tribal and Indian Health Service hospital records and by direct contact of study personnel with the study participants and their families	Adjusted for age, BMI, smoking status, study center, systolic BP, HbA1c, fibrinogen, insulin, and ratio of albumin to creatinine	0	They compared tertiles or quintiles: TG: lower < 111; 111-175; higher > 175 mg/dL (lower < 1.2; 1.2-2.0; higher > 2.0 mmol/L)
Malone, 2009 [35]	Not random; likely consecutive: Retrospective data from 3 integrated health-care systems that systematically collect and store detailed patient-level data.	Chart review, ICD or billing codes	Adjusted for age, sex, smoking status and site	N/A	lower/normal TG - 80.0 mg/dl (0.9 mmol/L); higher TG - TG = 217.4 mg/dl (2.4 mmol/L)
Mazza, 2005 [36]	random sample	chart review, ICD or billing codes, through the Register Office, general practitioners	Gender, age, DM, obesity, lipids subfractions, serum uric acid, BP, smoking, alcohol and proteinuria	0	They compared tertiles or quintiles: TG: First (low) < 97.5 mg/dL (1.01 mmol/L); Fifth (high) > = 156.8 mg/dL (1.77 mmol/L)
Mora, 2008 [37]	Random sample enrolled in the Women's Health Study	Follow-up questionnaires every 6-12 months	Adjusted for age, randomized treatment assignment, smoking status, menopausal status, postmenopausal hormone use, BP, DM, and BMI	NR	They compared tertiles or quintiles: TG: First (low) < 89.5 mg/dL (1.01 mmol/L); Fifth (high) > = 180.7 mg/dL (2.04 mmol/L)

Table 2 Quality of Included Studies *(Continued)*

Noda, 2010 [38]	not random and not consecutive: death related to a MI defined a case, then 2 controls were selected randomly matched by age	Death registration from 1997-2000, done without knowledge of patients' TG level, ascertained the same way in cases and controls	Adjusted for age and 6 risk factors for MI	NR	TG value in the blood was used as a continuous number (variable). Here OR expresses increased risk per unit of serum TG level: High TG > = 150 mg/dL (1.7 mmoml/L)
Rubins, 1999 [39]	not random and not consecutive: to obtain population with appropriate lipid levels, a multi stage screening method that included two lipid profiles obtained one week apart	chart review, clinical and radiologic data, ascertained the same way in cases and controls	Adjustment for baseline variables in the Cox models had a trivial effect on the estimates of the hazard ratios	2.3%	Two groups: TG < 150 mg/dl (1.7 mmol/L) and TG > 150 mg/dl (1.7 mmol/L)
Samuelsson, 1994[40]	random sample	chart review	traditional risk factors, end-organ damage status	NR	TG value in the blood was used as a continuous number (variable). Here OR expresses increased risk per unit of serum TG level: RR reported for every 88.6 mg/dL (1 mmol/L) increase in TG level
Schupf, 2005 [41]	random sample	self report, chart review, interviewing relatives	Adjusted for age, sex, ethnicity, and level of education, for BMI or APOE; a history of HTN, DM, heart disease, stroke, or cancer; or current smoking	0	They compared tertiles or quintiles: Lowest - < = 98.9 mg/dl (1.1 mmol/L), highest - > 191.2 mg/dl (2.1 mmol/L); RR compared the lowest quartile to the highest quartile.
Sprecher, 2000[42]	not random; likely consecutive: diabetic patients undergoing primary isolated CABG between 1982 and 1992 at Cleveland Clinic	chart review, clinical exam, labs and CVIR (Cardiovascular Information Registry)	age, sex, left ventricular function, coronary anatomy, history of HTN, BMI, and total cholesterol		highest quartile compared to lower three quartiles (normal)
Tanko, 2005 [43]	not random and not consecutive: recruited via a questionnaire surveys	self report, chart review: Central Registry of the Danish Ministry of Health	Adjusted for age, smoking, and LDL-C), waist circumference	NR	TG value in the blood was used as a continuous number (variable). Here OR expresses increased risk per unit of serum TG level: presented as 2 cutoffs - > 128.5 mg/dL (1.45 mmol/L) - > 149.7 mg/dL (1.69 mmol/L)

Table 2 Quality of Included Studies *(Continued)*

Tsai, 2008[44]	not random; likely consecutive: civil servants and teachers who took the annual physical examination at the Taipei Outpatient Center	chart review, annual exam, national death files	Adjusted for age, gender, fasting glucose, BP, BMI, smoking	NR	They compared tertiles or quintiles: TG normal < 150 mg/dL (1.7 mmol/L, abnormal 150 mg/dL (1.7 mmol/L)-199 mg/dL (2.2 mmol/L), and high abnormal > 200 mg/dL (2.25 mmol/L)
Upmeier, 2009[45]	not random and not consecutive: mailed invitation to participate to all residents of Turku born in 1920	Self report, chart review, ICD or billing codes	Adjusted for gender, body mass index, smoking and any history of angina pectoris, stroke, DM, and HTN	NR	They compared TG level quartiles, highest to lowest
Valdivielso, 2009[46]	not random; likely consecutive	Chart review and self report	age, sex, smoking, HTN, DM, and lipids fractions	NR	Categorized as normal when TG was < 150 mg/dL (< 1.69 mmol/L); the remainder were considered to be HTG
Wier, 2003 [47]	not random; likely consecutive	chart review, done without knowledge of patients' TG level	age, time of resolution of symptoms, smoking, BP, presence of atrial fibrillation and hyperglycemia	0	They compared tertiles or quintiles: TG, mmol/l: < = 0.9; 1.0-1.3; 1.4-1.8; > = 1.9. Mg/dL: < = 79.7; 88.6-115.2; 124.0-159.5; > = 168.3

UC/NR: unclear, not reported; TG: Triglycerides; HTG, hypertriglyceridemia; MI, myocardial infarction; DM, diabetes, BP, blood pressure, HTN, hypertension

* It was unclear in most studies if enrolled patients did not have the outcomes pre-existent at baseline. In most studies, it was also unclear if patients were treated with drugs that can affect TG level (both of these elements lower the observed strength of association)

Triglycerides Conversion from mg/dL to mmol/L: multiply by (x) 0.01129; from mmol/L to mg/dL: multiply by (x) 88.6

All-cause mortality

	Odds ratio	Lower limit	Upper limit	p-Value
Barrett-Connor, 1987	1.00	0.90	1.11	1.00
Carlson, 1988	0.96	0.56	1.64	0.88
Habib, 2006	0.45	0.34	0.59	0.00
Haim, 1999 (men)	1.09	0.94	1.26	0.25
Haim, 1999 (women)	1.10	0.80	1.51	0.56
Schupf, 2005	1.01	0.79	1.29	0.94
Sprecher, 2000	1.26	1.00	1.59	0.05
Tanko, 2005	1.90	1.18	3.05	0.01
Tsai, 2008	1.01	0.85	1.20	0.88
Upmeier, 2009	1.03	0.73	1.46	0.86
Weir, 2003	2.42	1.93	3.04	0.00
	1.10	0.90	1.36	0.35

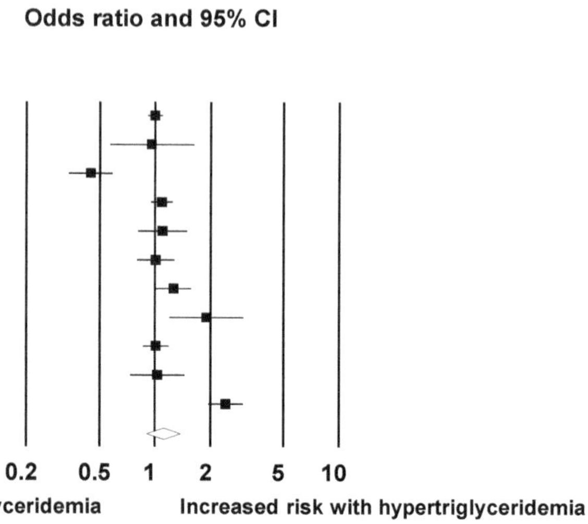

Meta Analysis

Figure 2 Random effects meta-analysis (all-cause mortality).

Cardiovascular death

	Statistics for each study			
	Odds ratio	Lower limit	Upper limit	p-Value
Barrett-Connor, 1987	1.00	0.90	1.11	1.00
Bass, 1993	6.92	3.40	14.08	0.00
Chan, 2005	2.97	1.00	8.80	0.05
Eberly, 2003	1.26	0.99	1.61	0.06
Ellingsen, 2003	1.43	0.88	2.31	0.15
Mazza, 2005	2.45	1.48	4.05	0.00
Tanko, 2005	3.10	1.40	6.86	0.01
Tsai, 2008	1.08	0.78	1.50	0.64
Weir, 2003	1.95	1.44	2.63	0.00
	1.80	1.31	2.49	0.00

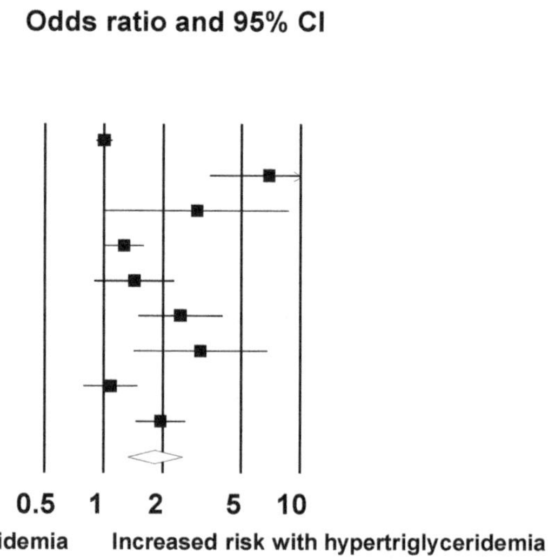

Meta Analysis

Figure 3 Random effects meta-analysis (cardiovascular death).

Cardiovascular events

	Odds ratio	Lower limit	Upper limit	p-Value
Acarturk, 2004	1.62	1.02	2.58	0.04
Bansal, 2007	1.11	0.92	1.34	0.28
Bonaventure, 2010	1.49	1.24	1.79	0.00
Chester, 1995	2.30	1.68	3.16	0.00
Czernichow, 2007	1.30	1.21	1.39	0.00
Drexel, 2005	1.17	1.00	1.37	0.05
Eberly, 2003	1.64	1.20	2.24	0.00
Egger, 1999	1.12	0.88	1.43	0.36
Goldberg, 2009	7.96	2.65	23.94	0.00
Hoogeveen, 2001	1.07	0.98	1.16	0.12
Lamarche, 1995	3.10	1.54	6.25	0.00
Lu, 2003	1.42	1.11	1.81	0.00
Mora, 2008	1.47	1.00	2.16	0.05
Rubins, 1999	1.12	0.86	1.46	0.39
Samuelsson, 1994	1.21	1.03	1.43	0.02
Valdivielso, 2009	4.41	1.59	12.22	0.00
	1.37	1.23	1.53	0.00

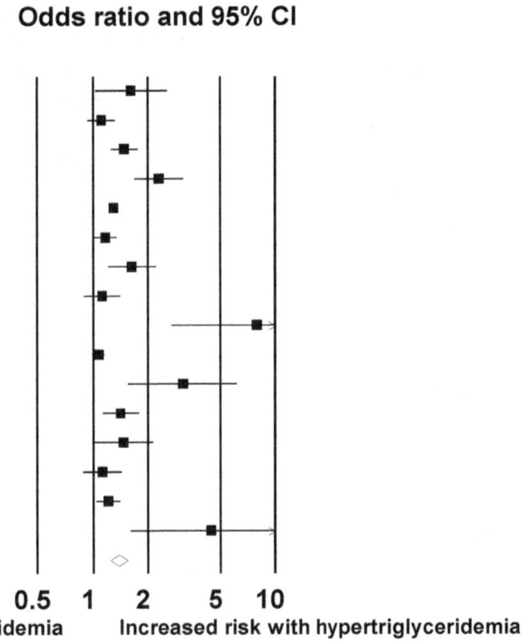

Meta Analysis

Figure 4 Random effects meta-analysis (cardiac events).

The overall confidence in the estimated magnitude of associations is low [10]considering the described methodological limitations in evaluating the association with cardiovascular events; and imprecision (small number of events) in evaluating the association with pancreatitis.

The strengths of this study stems from the comprehensive literature search that spans across multiple databases and duplicate appraisal and study selection. Our results are consistent with previous evidence synthesis reports about the association of hypertriglyceridemia with cardiovascular events. We estimated increased odds by 37% (odds ratio of 1.37). Hokanson and Austin [3] estimated adjusted relative risks of 1.14 (95% Cl 1.05-1.28) in men and 1.37 (95% Cl 1.13-1.66) in women. Sarwar et al. [2] reported odds ratio of 1.73 in prospective cohort studies published prior to 2006. A systematic review by Labreuche et al. [49] demonstrated that baseline triglyceride levels in randomized trials is associated with increased stroke risk (adjusted RR, 1.05 per 10-mg/dL (0.1 mmol/L) increase; 95% CI, 1.03-1.07). To our knowledge, this is the first systematic review that sought to identify controlled studies evaluating the association with pancreatitis.

Implications

The associations demonstrated between hypertriglyceridemia and cardiovascular risk should not necessarily translate into a recommendation for treatment. It is plausible that the benefits of lowering triglycerides do not merely depend on how much the level is lowered, but rather on how it is lowered (i.e., lifestyle interventions vs. pharmacological therapy). Therefore, randomized trials of the different approaches with patient-important outcomes [50] used as primary endpoints are needed for making policy and clinical decisions.

Several systematic reviews and meta-analyses [49,51-54] have summarized the evidence from randomized trials of fibrate therapy and demonstrated that fibrate therapy reduced the risk of vascular events (RR 0.75, 95% CI 0.65 to 0.86) in patients with high triglyceride levels or atherogenic dyslipidemia (low HDL cholesterol combined with high triglyceride level) although all-cause mortality and non cardiovascular mortality were both significantly increased in clofibrate trials. Meta-analyses [55,56] of niacin therapy demonstrate significant reduction in the risk of major coronary events (25% reduction in relative odds; 95% CI 13, 35), stroke (26%; 95% CI 8, 41) and any

Myocardial Infarction

	Odds ratio	Lower limit	Upper limit	p-Value
Gaziano, 1997	2.70	1.36	5.35	0.00
Jonsdottir, 2002 (men)	1.21	1.08	1.36	0.00
Jonsdottir, 2002 (women)	1.40	1.15	1.70	0.00
Lu, 2003	2.04	1.12	3.70	0.02
Malone, 2009	1.17	1.08	1.27	0.00
Noda, 2010	1.46	0.89	2.39	0.13
	1.31	1.15	1.49	0.00

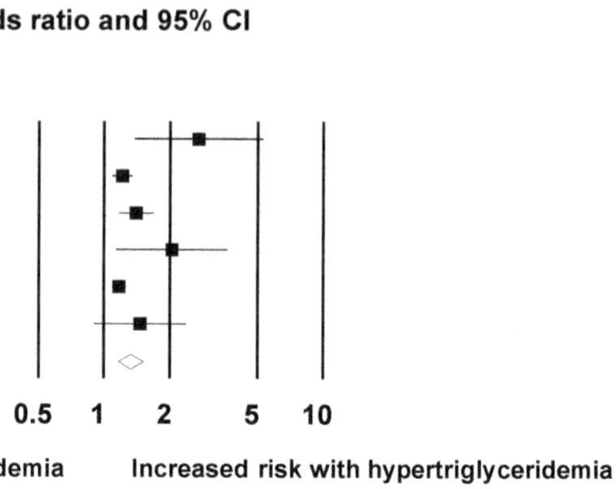

Meta Analysis

Figure 5 Random effects meta-analysis (myocardial infarction).

Table 3 Subgroup analysis

Subgroup	No. studies	OR	LL	UL	P-effect Size	P-interaction
			Mortality			
Men	3	1.03	0.95	1.12	0.49	0.04
Women	3	1.55	1.05	2.27	0.03	
adequate adjustment	9	1.09	0.83	1.43	0.55	0.54
inadequate adjustment	3	1.22	0.94	1.59	0.14	
General population	10	1.09	0.87	1.37	0.46	0.49
Diabetes	2	1.37	0.75	2.50	0.31	
			Cardiovascular death			
Men	3	1.14	0.92	1.40	0.23	0.00
Women	2	4.73	2.15	10.37	0.00	
adequate adjustment	5	1.88	1.12	3.15	0.02	0.84
inadequate adjustment	4	1.76	1.18	2.62	0.01	
General population	8	1.75	1.26	2.43	0.00	0.36
Diabetes	1	2.97	1.00	8.80	0.05	
			Cardiovascular events			
Men	6	1.29	1.13	1.47	0.00	0.67
Women	2	1.21	0.94	1.57	0.14	
adequate adjustment	12	1.39	1.23	1.58	0.00	0.91
inadequate adjustment	4	1.37	1.01	1.84	0.04	
General population	15	1.37	1.22	1.54	0.00	0.81
Diabetes	1	1.42	1.11	1.81	0.00	
			Myocardial infarction			
Men	2	1.22	1.09	1.37	0.00	0.24
Women	1	1.40	1.15	1.70	0.00	
adequate adjustment	3	1.72	0.98	3.01	0.06	0.29
inadequate adjustment	3	1.26	1.15	1.39	0.00	
General population	5	1.27	1.13	1.44	0.00	0.13
Diabetes	1	2.04	1.12	3.70	0.02	

*Only feasible analyses are shown

cardiovascular events (27%; 95% CI 15, 37). However, contemporary trials in the statin era have failed to substantiate these findings with fenofibrate among patients with diabetes [57] and with niacin in high risk patients [58]. Also, to our knowledge, there are no trials assessing the value of triglyceride lowering to reduce the risk of pancreatitis. Thus, lifestyle changes should remain the mainstay of therapy. Treatment of the underlying metabolic disorder (e.g., insulin resistance) should also be an essential and first step in the management plan of hypertriglyceridemia.

Conclusions

The current evidence suggests that hypertriglyceridemia is associated with increased risk of cardiovascular death, MI, cardiovascular events, and acute pancreatitis. The strength of inference is limited by the unexplained inconsistency of results and high risk of confounding and publication bias.

Acknowledgements

This review was funded by a contract from the Endocrine Society. The funder had no role in study design; in the collection, analysis, and interpretation of data; in the writing of the manuscript; and in the decision to submit the manuscript for publication.

Disclosure statement

MM, AH, FC, SD, SG, IB, ML, LB and VM have nothing to declare.

Financial support

This review was funded by a contract from the Endocrine Society.

Author details

[1]Knowledge and Evaluation Research Unit, Mayo Clinic, Rochester, MN, USA. [2]Division of Preventive Medicine, Mayo Clinic, Rochester, MN, USA. [3]Department of Internal Medicine, University of North Dakota, Fargo, ND, USA. [4]Davis and the VA Northern California Health Care System, University of California, Sacramento, USA. [5]Division of Endocrinology, Diabetes, Metabolism, Nutrition, Mayo Clinic, Rochester, MN, USA.

Authors' contributions

MHM, VMM, LB and PJE conceived and designed the study and acquired funding. HM, AH, FCY, SD, SG, IB, ML and TE collected data. MHM, VMM and AH conducted analysis. MHM, VMM and LB drafted the manuscript. All authors provided critical revisions to the manuscript and made substantive intellectual contributions to the study. All authors read and approved the final manuscript.

Competing interests

The authors declare that they have no competing interests.

References

1. Ford ES, Li C, Zhao G, Pearson WS, Mokdad AH: **Hypertriglyceridemia and its pharmacologic treatment among US adults.** *Arch Intern Med* 2009, **169(6)**:572-578.
2. Sarwar N, Danesh J, Eiriksdottir G, Sigurdsson G, Wareham N, Bingham S, Boekholdt SM, Khaw KT, Gudnason V: **Triglycerides and the risk of coronary heart disease: 10,158 incident cases among 262,525 participants in 29 Western prospective studies.** *Circulation* 2007, **115(4)**:450-458.
3. Hokanson JE, Austin MA: **Plasma triglyceride level is a risk factor for cardiovascular disease independent of high-density lipoprotein cholesterol level: a meta-analysis of population-based prospective studies.** *J Cardiovasc Risk* 1996, **3(2)**:213-219.
4. Patel A, Barzi F, Jamrozik K, Lam TH, Ueshima H, Whitlock G, Woodward M: **Serum triglycerides as a risk factor for cardiovascular diseases in the Asia-Pacific region.** *Circulation* 2004, **110(17)**:2678-2686.
5. Toskes PP: **Hyperlipidemic pancreatitis.** *Gastroenterol Clin North Am* 1990, **19(4)**:783-791.
6. Brunzell JD, Schrott HG: **The interaction of familial and secondary causes of hypertriglyceridemia: role in pancreatitis.** *Trans Assoc Am Physicians* 1973, **86**:245-254.
7. **Familial lipoprotein lipase deficiency, ApoC-II deficiency, and hepatic lipase deficiency.** In *The Metabolic Basis of Inherited Disease.*. 8 edition. Edited by: Scriver C, Beaudet A, Sly W, Valle D, Brunzell J, Deeb SI. New York: McGraw-Hill; 2001:2789-2816.
8. Moher D, Liberati A, Tetzlaff J, Altman DG: **Preferred reporting items for systematic reviews and meta-analyses: the PRISMA statement.** *PLoS Med* 2009, **6(7)**:e1000097.
9. Wells G, Shea B, O'Connell D, Peterson J, Welch V, Losos M, Tugwell P: **The Newcastle-Ottawa Scale (NOS) for assessing the quality of nonrandomised studies in meta-analyses.** *Ottawa Hospital Research Institute* .
10. Swiglo BA, Murad MH, Schunemann HJ, Kunz R, Vigersky RA, Guyatt GH, Montori VM: **A case for clarity, consistency, and helpfulness: state-of-the-art clinical practice guidelines in endocrinology using the grading of recommendations, assessment, development, and evaluation system.** *J Clin Endocrinol Metab* 2008, **93(3)**:666-673.
11. DerSimonian R, Laird N: **Meta-analysis in clinical trials.** *Control Clin Trials* 1986, **7(3)**:177-188.
12. Egger M, Davey Smith G, Schneider M, Minder Minder C: **Bias in meta-analysis detected by a simple, graphical test.** *BMJ* 1997, **315(7109)**:629-634.
13. Acarturk E, Cayli M, Akpinar O, Attila G, Demir M: **Relation between age and gender differences in plasma triglyceride concentrations and coronary artery disease in Southern Turkey.** *Clin Chim Acta* 2004, **339(1-2)**:123-128.
14. Bansal S, Buring JE, Rifai N, Mora S, Sacks FM, Ridker PM: **Fasting compared with nonfasting triglycerides and risk of cardiovascular events in women.** *JAMA* 2007, **298(3)**:309-316.
15. Barrett-Connor E, Khaw KT: **Borderline fasting hypertriglyceridemia: absence of excess risk of all-cause and cardiovascular disease mortality in healthy men without hypercholesterolemia.** *Prev Med* 1987, **16(1)**:1-8.
16. Bass KM, Newschaffer CJ, Klag MJ, Bush TL: **Plasma lipoprotein levels as predictors of cardiovascular death in women.** *Arch Intern Med* 1993, **153(19)**:2209-2216.
17. Bonaventure A, Kurth T, Pico F, Barberger-Gateau P, Ritchie K, Stapf C, Tzourio C: **Triglycerides and risk of hemorrhagic stroke vs. ischemic vascular events: the three-city study.** *Atherosclerosis* 2010, **210(1)**:243-248.
18. Carlson LA, Rosenhamer G: **Reduction of mortality in the Stockholm ischaemic heart disease secondary prevention study by combined treatment with clofibrate and nicotinic acid.** *Acta Med Scand* 1988, **223(5)**:405-418.
19. Chan WB, Tong PC, Chow CC, So WY, Ng MC, Ma RC, Osaki R, Cockram CS, Chan JC: **Triglyceride predicts cardiovascular mortality and its relationship with glycaemia and obesity in Chinese type 2 diabetic patients.** *Diabetes Metab Res Rev* 2005, **21(2)**:183-188.
20. Chester M, Chen L, Kaski JC: **Identification of patients at high risk for adverse coronary events while awaiting routine coronary angioplasty.** *Br Heart J* 1995, **73(3)**:216-222.
21. Czernichow S, Bruckert E, Bertrais S, Galan P, Hercberg S, Oppert JM: **Hypertriglyceridemic waist and 7.5-year prospective risk of cardiovascular disease in asymptomatic middle-aged men.** *Int J Obes (Lond)* 2007, **31(5)**:791-796.
22. Drexel H, Aczel S, Marte T, Benzer W, Langer P, Moll W, Saely CH: **Is atherosclerosis in diabetes and impaired fasting glucose driven by elevated LDL cholesterol or by decreased HDL cholesterol?** *Diabetes Care* 2005, **28(1)**:101-107.
23. Eberly LE, Stamler J, Neaton JD: **Relation of triglyceride levels, fasting and nonfasting, to fatal and nonfatal coronary heart disease.** *Arch Intern Med* 2003, **163(9)**:1077-1083.
24. Egger M, Smith GD, Pfluger D, Altpeter E, Elwood PC: **Triglyceride as a risk factor for ischaemic heart disease in British men: effect of adjusting for measurement error.** *Atherosclerosis* 1999, **143(2)**:275-284.
25. Ellingsen I, Hjermann I, Abdelnoor M, Hjerkinn EM, Tonstad S: **Dietary and antismoking advice and ischemic heart disease mortality in men with normal or high fasting triacylglycerol concentrations: a 23-y follow-up study.** *Am J Clin Nutr* 2003, **78(5)**:935-940.
26. Gaziano JM, Hennekens CH, O'Donnell CJ, Breslow JL, Buring JE: **Fasting triglycerides, high-density lipoprotein, and risk of myocardial infarction.** *Circulation* 1997, **96(8)**:2520-2525.

27. Goldberg RJ, Urowitz MB, Ibanez D, Nikpour M, Gladman DD: **Risk factors for development of coronary artery disease in women with systemic lupus erythematosus.** *J Rheumatol* 2009, **36(11)**:2454-2461.
28. Habib AN, Baird BC, Leypoldt JK, Cheung AK, Goldfarb-Rumyantzev AS: **The association of lipid levels with mortality in patients on chronic peritoneal dialysis.** *Nephrol Dial Transplant* 2006, **21(10)**:2881-2892.
29. Haim M, Benderly M, Brunner D, Behar S, Graff E, Reicher-Reiss H, Goldbourt U: **Elevated serum triglyceride levels and long-term mortality in patients with coronary heart disease: the Bezafibrate Infarction Prevention (BIP) registry.** *Circulation* 1999, **100(5)**:475-482.
30. Hoogeveen RC, Gambhir JK, Gambhir DS, Kimball KT, Ghazzaly K, Gaubatz JW, Vaduganathan M, Rao RS, Koschinsky M, Morrisett JD: **Evaluation of Lp[a] and other independent risk factors for CHD in Asian Indians and their USA counterparts.** *J Lipid Res* 2001, **42(4)**:631-638.
31. Jonsdottir LS, Sigfusson N, Guonason V, Sigvaldason H, Thorgeirsson G: **Do lipids, blood pressure, diabetes, and smoking confer equal risk of myocardial infarction in women as in men? The Reykjavik study.** *J Cardiovasc Risk* 2002, **9(2)**:67-76.
32. Lamarche B, Despres JP, Moorjani S, Cantin B, Dagenais GR, Lupien PJ: **Prevalence of dyslipidemic phenotypes in ischemic heart disease (prospective results from the Quebec Cardiovascular study).** *Am J Cardiol* 1995, **75(17)**:1189-1195.
33. Lloret Linares C, Pelletier AL, Czernichow S, Vergnaud AC, Bonnefont-Rousselot D, Levy P, Ruszniewski P, Bruckert E: **Acute pancreatitis in a cohort of 129 patients referred for severe hypertriglyceridemia.** *Pancreas* 2008, **37(1)**:12-13.
34. Lu W, Resnick HE, Jablonski KA, Jones KL, Jain AK, Howard WMJ, Robbins DC, Howard BV: **Non-HDL cholesterol as a predictor of cardiovascular disease in type 2 diabetes: The strong heart study.** *Diabetes Care* 2003, **26(1)**:16-23.
35. Malone DC, Boudreau DM, Nichols GA, Raebel MA, Fishman PA, Feldstein AC, Ben-Joseph RH, Okamoto LJ, Boscoe AN, Magid DJ: **Association of cardiometabolic risk factors and prevalent cardiovascular events.** *Metab Syndr Relat Disord* 2009, **7(6)**:585-593.
36. Mazza A, Tikhonoff V, Schiavon L, Casiglia E: **Triglycerides + high-density-lipoprotein-cholesterol dyslipidaemia, a coronary risk factor in elderly women: the CArdiovascular STudy in the ELderly.** *Intern Med J* 2005, **35(10)**:604-610.
37. Mora S, Rifai N, Buring JE, Ridker PM: **Fasting compared with nonfasting lipids and apolipoproteins for predicting incident cardiovascular events.** *Circulation* 2008, **118(10)**:993-1001.
38. Noda H, Maruyama K, Iso H, Dohi S, Terai T, Fujioka S, Goto K, Horie S, Nakano S, Hirobe K: **Prediction of myocardial infarction using coronary risk scores among Japanese male workers: 3M study.** *J Atheroscler Thromb* 2010, **17(5)**:452-459.
39. Rubins HB, Robins SJ, Collins D, Fye CL, Anderson JW, Elam MB, Faas FH, Linares E, Schaefer EJ, Schectman G, *et al*: **Gemfibrozil for the secondary prevention of coronary heart disease in men with low levels of high-density lipoprotein cholesterol. Veterans Affairs High-Density Lipoprotein Cholesterol Intervention Trial Study Group.** *N Engl J Med* 1999, **341(6)**:410-418.
40. Samuelsson O, Hedner T, Persson B, Andersson O, Berglund G, Wilhelmesen L: **The role of diabetes mellitus and hypertriglyceridaemia as coronary risk factors in treated hypertension: 15 years of follow-up of antihypertensive treatment in middle-aged men in the Primary Prevention Trial in Goteborg, Sweden.** *J Intern Med* 1994, **235(3)**:217-227.
41. Schupf N, Costa R, Luchsinger J, Tang MX, Lee JH, Mayeux R: **Relationship between plasma lipids and all-cause mortality in nondemented elderly.** *J Am Geriatr Soc* 2005, **53(2)**:219-226.
42. Sprecher DL, Pearce GL, Park EM, Pashkow FJ, Hoogwerf BJ: **Preoperative triglycerides predict post-coronary artery bypass graft survival in diabetic patients: a sex analysis.** *Diabetes Care* 2000, **23(11)**:1648-1653.
43. Tanko LB, Bagger YZ, Qin G, Alexandersen P, Larsen PJ, Christiansen C: **Enlarged waist combined with elevated triglycerides is a strong predictor of accelerated atherogenesis and related cardiovascular mortality in postmenopausal women.** *Circulation* 2005, **111(15)**:1883-1890.
44. Tsai SP, Wen CP, Chan HT, Chiang PH, Tsai MK, Cheng TY: **The effects of pre-disease risk factors within metabolic syndrome on all-cause and cardiovascular disease mortality.** *Diabetes Res Clin Pract* 2008, **82(1)**:148-156.
45. Upmeier E, Lavonius S, Lehtonen A, Viitanen M, Isoaho H, Arve S: **Serum lipids and their association with mortality in the elderly: A prospective cohort study.** *Aging Clin Exp Res* 2009, **21(6)**:424-430.
46. Valdivielso P, Sanchez-Chaparro MA, Calvo-Bonacho E, Cabrera-Sierra M, Sainz-Gutierrez JC, Fernandez-Labandera C, Fernandez-Meseguer A, Quevedo-Aguado L, Moraga MR, Galvez-Moraleda A, *et al*: **Association of moderate and severe hypertriglyceridemia with obesity, diabetes mellitus and vascular disease in the Spanish working population: results of the ICARIA study.** *Atherosclerosis* 2009, **207(2)**:573-578.
47. Weir CJ, Sattar N, Walters MR, Lees KR: **Low triglyceride, not low cholesterol concentration, independently predicts poor outcome following acute stroke.** *Cerebrovasc Dis* 2003, **16(1)**:76-82.
48. Furukawa TA, Watanabe N, Omori IM, Montori VM, Guyatt GH: **Association between unreported outcomes and effect size estimates in Cochrane meta-analyses.** *JAMA* 2007, **297(5)**:468-470.
49. Labreuche J, Deplanque D, Touboul PJ, Bruckert E, Amarenco P: **Association between change in plasma triglyceride levels and risk of stroke and carotid atherosclerosis: systematic review and meta-regression analysis.** *Atherosclerosis* 2010, **212(1)**:9-15.
50. Gandhi GY, Murad MH, Fujiyoshi A, Mullan RJ, Flynn DN, Elamin MB, Swiglo BA, Isley WL, Guyatt GH, Montori VM: **Patient-important outcomes in registered diabetes trials.** *JAMA* 2008, **299(21)**:2543-2549.
51. Bruckert E, Labreuche J, Deplanque D, Touboul PJ, Amarenco P: **Fibrates effect on cardiovascular risk is greater in patients with high triglyceride levels or atherogenic dyslipidemia profile: a systematic review and meta-analysis.** *J Cardiovasc Pharmacol* 2011, **57(2)**:267-272.
52. Loomba RS, Arora R: **Prevention of cardiovascular disease utilizing fibrates-a pooled meta-analysis.** *Am J Ther* 2010, **17(6)**:e182-e188.
53. Jun M, Foote C, Lv J, Neal B, Patel A, Nicholls SJ, Grobbee DE, Cass A, Chalmers J, Perkovic V: **Effects of fibrates on cardiovascular outcomes: a systematic review and meta-analysis.** *Lancet* 2010, **375(9729)**:1875-1884.
54. Lee M, Saver JL, Towfighi A, Chow J, Ovbiagele B: **Efficacy of fibrates for cardiovascular risk reduction in persons with atherogenic dyslipidemia: A meta-analysis.** *Atherosclerosis* 2011.
55. Bruckert E, Labreuche J, Amarenco P: **Meta-analysis of the effect of nicotinic acid alone or in combination on cardiovascular events and atherosclerosis.** *Atherosclerosis* 2010, **210(2)**:353-361.
56. Duggal JK, Singh M, Attri N, Singh PP, Ahmed N, Pahwa S, Molnar J, Singh S, Khosla S, Arora R: **Effect of niacin therapy on cardiovascular outcomes in patients with coronary artery disease.** *J Cardiovasc Pharmacol Ther* 2010, **15(2)**:158-166.
57. Chew EY, Ambrosius WT, Davis MD, Danis RP, Gangaputra S, Greven CM, Hubbard L, Esser BA, Lovato JF, Perdue LH, *et al*: **Effects of medical therapies on retinopathy progression in type 2 diabetes.** *N Engl J Med* 2010, **363(3)**:233-244.
58. AIM-HIGH Investigators: **The role of niacin in raising high-density lipoprotein cholesterol to reduce cardiovascular events in patients with atherosclerotic cardiovascular disease and optimally treated low-density lipoprotein cholesterol Rationale and study design. The Atherothrombosis Intervention in Metabolic syndrome with low HDL/ high triglycerides: Impact on Global Health outcomes (AIM-HIGH).** *Am Heart J* 2011, **161(3)**:471-477, e472.

2

Relationship between hyperglycemia, hormone disturbances, and clinical evolution in severely hyperglycemic post surgery critically ill children

Yolanda Ballestero[1], Jesús López-Herce[1,3,4*], Rafael González[1,3,4*], Maria José Solana[1,3,4], Jimena del Castillo[1,3,4], Javier Urbano[1,3,4], Marta Botran[1], Ana García[1], Nieves López[2] and Jose María Bellón[3]

Abstract

Background: To study hormonal changes associated with severe hyperglycemia in critically ill children and the relationship with prognosis and length of stay in intensive care.

Methods: Observational study in twenty-nine critically ill children with severe hyperglycemia defined as 2 blood glucose measurements greater than 180 mg/dL. Severity of illness was assessed using pediatric index of mortality (PIM2), pediatric risk of mortality (PRISM) score, and pediatric logistic organ dysfunction (PELOD) scales. Blood glucose, glycosuria, insulin, C-peptide, cortisol, corticotropin, insulinlike growth factor-1, growth hormone, thyrotropin, thyroxine, and treatment with insulin were recorded. β-cell function and insulin sensitivity and resistance were determined on the basis of the homeostatic model assessment (HOMA), using blood glucose and C-peptide levels.

Results: The initial blood glucose level was 249 mg/dL and fell gradually to 125 mg/dL at 72 hours. Initial β-cell function (49.2%) and insulin sensitivity (13.2%) were low. At the time of diagnosis of hyperglycemia, 50% of the patients presented insulin resistance and β-cell dysfunction, 46% presented isolated insulin resistance, and 4% isolated β-cell dysfunction. β-cell function improved rapidly but insulin resistance persisted. Initial glycemia did not correlate with any other factor, and there was no relationship between glycemia and mortality. Patients who died had higher cortisol and growth hormone levels at diagnosis. Length of stay was correlated by univariate analysis, but not by multivariate analysis, with C-peptide and glycemic control at 24 hours, insulin resistance, and severity of illness scores.

Conclusions: Critically ill children with severe hyperglycemia initially present decreased β-cell function and insulin sensitivity. Nonsurvivors had higher cortisol and growth hormone levels and developed hyperglycemia later than survivors.

Keywords: Hyperglycemia, Critically ill children, Length of stay, Hormone disturbances

* Correspondence: pielvi@hotmail.com; darthrafa@hotmail.com
[1]Pediatric Intensive Care Department, Hospital General Universitario Gregorio Marañón Complutense University of Madrid, Madrid, Spain
[3]Instituto de Investigación biomédica del Hospital Gregorio Marañón, Madrid, Spain
Full list of author information is available at the end of the article

Background

The incidence of hyperglycemia is very high, between 56 and 86%, and it is an independent risk factor for morbidity and mortality in critically ill patients [1-3].

Many studies have analyzed the effect of treatment of hyperglycemia on the prognosis of critically ill patients. Although initial studies found that intensive insulin treatment improved the prognosis, subsequent research has not confirmed these findings and has detected a higher incidence of hypoglycemia [1-7].

Few studies have investigated the pathophysiological mechanisms involved in hyperglycemia of the critically ill patient [8-11]. Hyperglycemia of critically ill adults and children have different characteristics. An understanding of the mechanisms that give rise to hyperglycemia in the critically ill child could help to define the most appropriate treatment.

The objectives of the present study were to investigate the pathophysiological mechanisms of severe hyperglycemia in the critically ill child, to analyze the clinical factors associated with hyperglycemia, and to evaluate the association of hyperglycemia with prognosis and length of hospital stay.

Methods

A prospective observational study was performed in patients aged between 1 month and 16 years admitted to the Pediatric Intensive Care Unit (PICU) between July 2009 and March 2010 and who developed significant hyperglycemia, defined as 2 blood glucose measurements greater than 180 mg/dL, separated by at least 2 hours, at any time during admission to the PICU. Children with type 1 diabetes mellitus were excluded from the study.

The study was approved by the Investigation and Ethics Committee of the Gregorio Marañón Hospital. Parents or legal guardians gave their parental permission for the child to participate in the study and to publish the results.

Clinical severity was assessed using the pediatric index of mortality 2 (PIM2) [12], pediatric risk of mortality (PRISM) score [13], and pediatric logistic organ dysfunction (PELOD) scale [14]. PIM score calculates the risk of mortality based in the first clinical and analytical data after admission. They include the kind of admission (programmed or no), the diagnosis classified in high and low-risk, photomotor reflex, mechanical ventilation, blood pressure, base deficit and FiO2/PaO2 [12]. PRISM score calculates the risk of mortality based on the worst values in the first 24 h of admission of several physiological values (heart rate, blood pressure, Glasgow scale and pupillary reaction) and analytical values (PaO2/FiO2, PaCO2, prothrombine time, billirubin, calcium, potassium, glycemia) [13]. PELOD score evaluates the risk of mortality analyzing the number of failure of different systems by different parameters: cardiovascular (heart rate, blood pressure), respiratory (PaO2/FiO2, PaCO2, mechanical ventilation), neurologic (Glasgow score, pupillary reactions), hematologic (leucocytes, platelets), renal (creatinine), hepatic (AST, prothrombine time). Scores was recorded at the time of diagnosis of hyperglycemia and 24 and 72 hours later. Treatment with corticosteroids, the doses of vasoactive drugs, the vasoactive score calculated by the following formula: dopamine dose (μg/kg/min) + dobutamine dose (μg/kg/min) + 100 epinephrine dose (μg/kg/min) + 10 milrinone dose (μg/kg/min) + 10.000 vasopresine dose (U/kg/min) + 100 noerpinephrine dose (μg/kg/min) [15], blood glucose, glycosuria, insulin, C-peptide, cortisol, corticotropin (ACTH), insulinlike growth factor (IGF-1), growth hormone (GH), thyrotropin (TSH), free thyroxine (T_4), and dose of insulin treatment were recorded at the time of diagnosis of hyperglycemia and 24 and 72 hours later.

Insulin, C-peptide, cortisol, and IGF-1 were measured using a solid-phase chemoluminescent enzyme immunometric assay (Immulite 2000, Siemens), ACTH and GH using an immunoradiometric assay (DiaSorin), TSH using a solid-phase paramagnetic-particle chemoluminescent enzyme immunometric assay (Access®Beckman Coulter™), and free T_4 using a 2-step, paramagnetic-particle competitive chemoluminescent enzyme immunoassay (Access®Beckman Coulter™).

β-cell function and insulin sensitivity and resistance were determined on the basis of the homeostatic model assessment (HOMA) calculated by computer software (www.OCDEM.ox.ac.uk) [16,17]. HOMA model is used to estimate insulin sensitivity (HOMA-%S) and β-cell function (HOMA-%B) using blood glucose and C-peptide levels [16]. Normal β-cell function is a HOMA-%B of 100%, normal insulin sensitivity is a HOMA-%S of 100%, and normal insulin resistance is 1 [16].

In accordance with our protocol, insulin was administered to those patients who presented blood glycemia above 200 mg/dL in 2 measurements separated by 4 hours. Treatment was started with 0.05-0.1 IU/kg/h, with hourly monitoring of the glycemia and glycosuria and adjustment of the insulin infusion to achieve glycemia between 120 and 150 mg/dL; subsequent monitoring was performed at least every 4 hours and the insulin infusion was interrupted if the glycemia fell below 120 mg/dl. The dose and duration of insulin treatment and the adverse effects attributable to treatment were recorded. Hypoglycemia was defined as glycemia less than 60 mg/dL.

The presence of infection, the need for and duration of mechanical ventilation, continuous renal replacement therapy (CRRT), and extracorporeal membrane oxygenation (ECMO), the duration of PICU admission, and mortality and its causes were also recorded.

Statistical analysis of the results was performed with the SPSS statistical package, version 18. The nonparametric

Wilcoxon, Mann–Whitney and Kruskal-Wallis tests were used to compare quantitative variables, the Pearson χ^2 test was used to compare frequencies, and the nonparametric Spearman rank correlation (ρ) was used to determine the correlation between quantitative variables. A P value less than .05 was considered significant. Multiple logistic regression analysis was made to study the association of variables with length of PICU admission and mortality.

Results

Characteristics of patients

Thirty-one hyperglycemic episodes were detected in 29 patients (2 patients presented 2 episodes separated by more than 7 days), aged between 1 and 204 months (median, 36 months) and weighing between 4 and 70 kg (median, 16.3 kg).

The reasons for admission were the following: postoperative period of cardiac surgery in 22, postoperative period of colectomy for ulcerative colitis in 1, cardiogenic shock in 4 and respiratory disease in 2.

Mechanical ventilation was required by 74% of patients, ECMO by 41%, and renal replacement therapy by 41% during admission to the PICU, and 48% developed nosocomial infection (respiratory tract in 24%, sepsis in 17%, and other sites in 6%). 96.5% of patients received vasoactive drugs (initial vasoactive score was 3.5 (IQR 3–5) and it did not change during the study. Four patients (13%) died during admission to the PICU, 3 due to multiorgan failure and 1 due to cerebral hemorrhage.

Initially all patients received intravenous glucose infusion and during the study enteral nutrition was started and increased progressively. Carbohydrate delivery is showed in Table 1. None of patients received parenteral nutrition.

Evolution of blood glucose and hormone levels

The changes in the blood glucose, hormone levels, clinical severity scores, and clinical parameters over the 72 hours of the study are shown in Table 1. The median initial blood glucose was 249 mg/dL, and this fell significantly to reach values of 125 mg/dL at 72 hours, despite a progressive increase in carbohydrate ingestion (Table 1). Intravenous insulin treatment was required in 83% of the episodes (mean dose, 0.11 ± 0.09 U/kg/h; mean duration of treatment, 45.2 ± 74.6 hours). The minimum blood glucose was 74 mg/dL. None of the patients developed hypoglycemia.

The insulin and C-peptide levels were elevated initially in 64% and 72% of patients, respectively, and did not show significant variations over the 72 hours of the study. β-cell function and insulin sensitivity were initially low but increased over the first 24 hours, although only the change in β-cell function reached statistical significance.

At the time of diagnosis of hyperglycemia, 50% of the patients presented insulin resistance and β-cell dysfunction, 46% presented isolated insulin resistance, and 4% isolated β-cell dysfunction.

Cortisol levels were initially elevated (levels above 25 μg/dL in 64% of patients), though ACTH levels were normal. During the course of the study, there was a significant fall in cortisol levels but no change in ACTH. Patients did not received steroids during the three days of the study. 15 patients received steroids previously to the diagnosed of hyperglycemia. There were no significant differences in initial cortisol levels of patients treated with steroids (47.3 μg/dL) than of the rest of patients (57.9 μg/dL).

T_4 levels were initially normal, whereas 44% of patients presented low TSH levels. Over the course of the study there was a significant fall in T_4 (36% of patients had low T_4 levels at 72 hours), though there were no significant changes in TSH levels.

The levels of GH and IGF-1 were initially low and there were no significant changes over the course of the study.

Correlation between parameters

No relationship was observed between the blood glucose at any time during the evolution and most of hormone parameters, clinical variables, and treatments. Nor were there differences in the changes in blood glucose over the course of the study according to age, sex, diagnosis, need for mechanical ventilation, ECMO or CRRT, or the presence of nosocomial infection.

Only at 24 and 72 hours there was a significant correlation between the blood glucose and insulin and C-peptide levels and between these 3 parameters and the PRIMS, PIM2, and PELOD clinical severity scores (data not showed). There was a relationship between the maximum blood glucose and the maximum dose of insulin administered (ρ = 0.596, P = .001), but not with the duration of insulin treatment.

Correlation with prognosis

There was no relationship between glucose levels over the course of the study and mortality. However, the onset of hyperglycemia occurred later in nonsurvivors than in survivors. The following factors were associated with mortality: cardiogenic shock (P = .014), nosocomial infection (P = .008), and the need for ECMO (P < .001) or CRRT (P < .001). Compared to survivors, patients who died had higher cortisol levels at the time of diagnosis of hyperglycemia and 24 hours later. GH values at the time of diagnosis of hyperglycemia were also higher in the patients who died. Compared to survivors, patients who died presented greater insulin resistance 72 hours after diagnosis (Table 2). There was no relationship between mortality and the values of the other hormones. Multiple logistic regression analysis could not be performed because only four patients died.

Table 1 Changes in hormone levels and clinical parameters

	At diagnosis of hyperglycemia		At 24 hours		At 72 hours		*P*
	Median	(IQR)	Median	(IQR)	Median	(IQR)	
Blood glucose, mg/dl	249	217-315	153	112-194	125	109-166	0.0001
Insulinemia, mUI/L	20	8.5-32.5	13	6.5-27.5	16	7-29	0.401
C-peptide, nmol/L	2	0.8-2.7	1.6	1-2.6	2	0.9-3.9	0.903
β-cell function with C-peptide %	49.2	30.8-91.3	96.3	78.4-139.8	135.9	95.2-187.8	0.001
Insulin sensitivity % with C-peptide	13.2	10.3-32.2	21.9	11.9-33.0	20.6	11.9-38.7	0.085
Insulin resistance with C-peptide	7.6	3.1 -9.6	4.5	3-8.4	4.9	2.7-8.3	0.081
Carbohydrate delivery, g/kg/day	2	1.8 -4.4	4.8	1.9-8.5	7.3	4.8-9.2	0.001
TSH, mUI/L	0.5	0.3-0.8	0.3	0.2-0.9	0.6	0.2-3.3	0.091
Free T4, ng/dL	1	0.8-1.2	0.9	0.7-1.2	0.7	0.5-1.2	0.009
ACTH, ng/L	21.5	12.8-41	21	12-33.5	20.8	11.6-34.4	0.410
Cortisol, μg/dL	43.7	12.6-77.3	16.1	7.9 -30.1	15.5	8.9-34.9	0.001
GH, μg/L	0.8	0.5-7.1	1.2	0.5-2.9	1.8	0.6-3.4	0.708
IGF1, μg/L	26	25-89.	25	25-54	25	25-48	0.132
PRIMS %	15.6	5.7-42.5	13.2	4.2-33.6	7.5	1.4-29.2	0.349
PIM2 %	2.7	1.4-11.8	3.4	2-18.9	5.4	0.5-25.2	0.397
PELOD %	6.7	1-19.5	1.5	0.1-1.7	1.3	0-2.3	0.787
HR, bpm	125	113.7-150.2	130	112.5-150	127.5	110-148.5	0.482
MAP, mmHg	62	55.5-72.2	67	54.5-73.5	63	58-79.5	0.837

Abbreviations: *ACTH* corticotrophin, *bpm* beats per minute, *GH* growth hormone, *HR* heart rate, *IGF* insulinlike growth factor, *IQR* interquartile range, *MAP* mean arterial pressure, *PELOD* pediatric logistic organ dysfunction, *PIM2* pediatric index of mortality 2, *PRIMS* pediatric risk of mortality, *T4* thyroxine, *TSH* thyrotropin.

The mean length of stay in the PICU was 16.4 ± 14.8 days. Length of stay was associated with the severity of illness scores, the blood glucose, C-peptide levels, insulinemia (Table 3), the time from admission to the onset of hyperglycemia (r = 0.532, p = 0.002), the maximum dose of insulin (r = 0.539, p = 0.004), and the duration of treatment with insulin (r = 0.602, p = 0.001). There were also statistically significant correlations between the length of PICU stay and the presence of nosocomial infection (*P* = .001) or the need for ECMO (*P* = .012), CRRT (*P* = .012), or mechanical ventilation (*P* = .001).

Table 2 Comparison between survivors and nonsurvivors

	Survivors		Nonsurvivors		*P*
	Median	(IQR)	Median	(IQR)	
Onset of hyperglycemia, h	6.5	(3.7 -27)	59	(13.5-137.5)	.028
Baseline cortisol, μg/dL	37	(12.4-66)	100	(74–138)	.024
Cortisol at 24 h, μg/dL	13	(5.6 -22.4)	39.7	(29.9-59.3)	.003
Baseline GH, μg/dL	0.7	(0.5-3.6)	15	(1.8-31)	.026
Sensitivity with C-peptide at 72 h, %	29.0	(14.3-67.8)	11.9	(10.7-12.9)	.026
IR with C-peptide at 72 h	3.4	(1.5-6.9)	8.4	(7.7 -9.3)	.026
Cardiogenic shock	7.3%		60%		.014
Nosocomial infection	30.7%		100%		.008
ECMO	0%		100%		.001
CRRT	0%		100%		.001

Abbreviations: *CCRT* continuous renal replacement therapy, *ECMO* extracorporeal membrane oxygenation, *GH* growth hormone, *IR* insulin resistance, *IQR* interquartile range.

Multiple logistic regression analysis did not identify factors associated with a length of PICU stay more than 14 days, possibly due to the low number of patients studied. The univariate and multivariate analyses of the patients in the postoperative period of cardiac surgery did not show different results than analysis of the total population (data not shown).

Discussion

Critical illness hyperglycemia (CIH) is probably due to endogenous counter-regulatory hormones and other diabetogenic factors, such as proinflammatory mediators and therapeutic interventions, including the administration of glucocorticoids and catecholamines, which interfere with insulin-receptor signaling and/or glucose transport and utilization within cells [8-11,18-21]. On the other hand insulin therapy acts to suppress counterregulatory hormones and proinflammatory transcription factors.

Our study is the first to analyze the relationship of severe hyperglycemia in the critically ill child with the values of various hormones and with the clinical course.

Table 3 Correlation between length of pediatric intensive care stay and other variables

	Time of diagnosis of hyperglycemia		24 h after the diagnosis		72 h after diagnosis	
	Correlation (r)	*P*	Correlation (r)	*P*	Correlation (r)	*P*
PRIMS			0.508	0.060	0.480	0.037
PIM2	0.568	0.004	0.626	0.001	0.548	0.015
PELOD	0.499	0.013	0.497	0.007	0.615	0.005
MAP	−0.429	0.018			−0.515	0.020
Blood glucose			0.531	0.004		
C-peptide			0.697	0.001	0.618	0.002
Insulinemia			0.542	0.030		
IGF-1	−0.500	0.011	−0.393	0.043		

Mechanisms of production of hyperglycemia and relationship with hormonal alterations

Hyperglycemia is a state of metabolic dysregulation due to an imbalance between insulin production and insulin sensitivity in the target tissues [8].

C-peptide and insulin levels

Studies in adults suggest that CIH is primarily due to insulin resistance in spite of a situation of supranormal β-cell function, because beta cell could not secrete as much insulin as that necessary to compensate insulin resistance [17,22]. However, in CIH in children, the C-peptide levels may be low or elevated [8]. Our patients presented elevated C-peptide levels, although these levels were relatively low given the blood glucose levels at that time, which would suggest the presence both of reduced β-cell function and of increased insulin resistance.

Preissig et al., found in 41 critically ill children with hyperglycemia, that low levels of insulin were associated with a rapid onset of hyperglycemia, greater clinical severity, greater insulin requirements and increased duration of mechanical ventilation and length of PICU stay [8]. We found higher C-peptide levels in more severely ill patients (higher PRISM, PIM2, and PELOD scores) and that higher C-peptide levels were associated with a longer PICU stay, probably because C-peptide levels were a marker of more severe ill. In contrast to the findings of Preissig et al., in our study the onset of hyperglycemia occurred later in the more seriously ill patients.

In a study of children with meningococcal sepsis and hyperglycemia 62% presented isolated insulin resistance, 17% β-cell dysfunction and 21% combined β-cell dysfunction and insulin resistance [17]. In our patients, there was a reduction both in β-cell function and in insulin sensitivity at the time of diagnosis of the hyperglycemia. Both improved at 24 hours and β-cell function normalized at 72 hours, though a degree of insulin resistance persisted. This would suggest that the mechanism of hyperglycemia in critically ill children with severe hyperglycemia is probably multifactorial and involve both a relative reduction in insulin production due to beta cell dysfunction whose cause of the is not well known, and peripheral resistance to insulin.

It has been reported that treatment with exogenous insulin improves insulin sensitivity [23]. In our study there was a slight improvement in insulin sensitivity at 24 hours, coinciding with insulin treatment, though sensitivity continued to be low at 72 hours.

Inotropic index

Catecholamines may directly suppress β-cell function and insulin secretion [8]. Some authors have reported that the inotropic index is inversely related to C-peptide levels and that hyperglycemic children have a higher inotropic index [18]. In contrast, other authors have found no correlation between the inotropic index and blood glucose, insulin or C-peptide levels [17], as occurred in our study.

Corticosteroids

Corticotropin-releasing hormone and ACTH control cortisol secretion in the acute phase of critical illness, whereas non-ACTH-mediated pathways (interleukin [IL] 1, IL6, and tumor necrosis factor-α) are involved during prolonged critical illness. Protracted critical illness is associated with a fall in plasma ACTH concentrations despite the persistence of a state of hypercortisolism [24].

Our results, with very high initial cortisol levels, coincide with previous reports. The absence of elevated ACTH levels suggests that other factors contributed to the hypercortisolism in the majority of our patients. We found no relationship between cortisol and blood glucose levels at any time. We cannot therefore state that corticosteroids played a fundamental role in the onset of hyperglycemia in our patients.

Growth hormone and insulinlike growth factor-1

GH secretion is induced by stress and the mean serum GH level may be elevated early in the course of trauma or surgery and fall progressively during the first week [25]. Serum IGF-1 levels are almost invariably low in critically ill patients. In acute stress situations, a low IGF-1 level in presence of enhanced GH secretion indicates GH resistance [25]. In our study, GH and IGF-1 levels were initially low and they showed no significant modifications over the course of the study. There was no relationship of the GH and IGF-1 levels with blood glucose, insulin, or C-peptide levels, suggesting that these hormones do not play a role in the onset of hyperglycemia.

Thyrotropin and thyroxine

In critically ill patients, T_3 is typically low on admission, with normal or slightly elevated TSH and T_4 levels. TSH levels subsequently normalize while T_3 levels remain low and, in serious diseases such as meningococcal sepsis, T_4 levels fall [26]. In our study, a large proportion of the children had low TSH levels at the time of diagnosis of hyperglycemia, with normal T_4 values. However, T_4 levels fell progressively, probably reflecting the severity of the illness. We are therefore unable to state that there is a clear link between thyroid hormone alterations and the onset of hyperglycemia.

Relationship of blood glucose levels and treatment with prognosis

Most studies have reported that hyperglycemia occurs early in critical illness and is independently associated with death [1,2,18,19]. However, it is unclear whether this association is indicative of the severity of the underlying illness or that hyperglycemia is itself a risk factor. Other studies in critically ill children have found no association between the blood glucose levels and mortality [27] or length PICU stay [20].

Our study showed that children with persistent severe hyperglycemia had a high mortality (13%)—the overall mortality in our PICU over the study period was 3%. This fact suggest that hyperglycemia is a marker of severity and an indicator of risk of death [28]. However, although the number of patients was low, we did not find a relationship between the absolute blood glucose, C-peptide, or insulin values and mortality. The presence of hyperglycemia would therefore appear to be a marker of severity in the critically ill patient but not itself worsen the prognosis.

On the other hand, we found that the onset of hyperglycemia occurred later in patients that died than in survivors and nonsurvivors presented greater insulin resistance at 72 hours after diagnosis. This could indicate the existence of two types of hyperglycemia in the critically ill patient. An initial, frequently transitory hyperglycemia caused by the stress of admission to the PICU and that is not associated with a poor prognosis, and another of later onset that could reflect more serious metabolic dysregulation with persistent insulin resistance and that is an indicator of mortality.

In our study, the main factors associated with mortality and the length of PICU stay were the clinical severity scores and the presence of severe multiorgan failure with the need for CRRT and ECMO.

Initial studies in critically ill patients found short-term benefits to maintaining normoglycemia [1,29]. However recent studies have found that intensive treatment with insulin does not decrease mortality [6,7,30] and may even be associated with a higher mortality and hypoglycemia [6,7,27,29]. A large proportion of our patients received insulin treatment despite our use of more restrictive indications for insulin treatment and less strict glycemic control objectives. None of our patients developed hypoglycemia, which confirms that insulin treatment with moderate objectives reduces the risk of hypoglycemia.

Corticosteroids and prognosis

The higher corticosteroids levels in the patients who died support the hypothesis that these patients had more serious illness and therefore had a more marked adrenal response. Many studies have analyzed the relationship of corticosteroid levels and the adrenal response with the prognosis of septic patients, reporting contradictory results [31,32]. The data from our study only allow us to state that critically ill children with hyperglycemia very often present elevated corticosteroid levels and that patients who die have higher levels than survivors. In critically ill children, both low and elevated corticosteroid levels may be indicators of severity and of risk of death. However, the number of patients who died in our study was small and further studies are necessary to confirm these results.

Limitations

Our study has certain limitations. The number of patients was low and most of them were in the postoperative period of cardiac surgery. The number of patients could not permit to perform a multiple logistic regression analysis and it is a small sample size to detect a difference in mortality. There was no control group without hyperglycemia to compare hormonal changes. However it is very difficult to achieve a control group with the same characteristics and severity as the study group but without hyperglycemia. To use HOMA in critically ill patients in those glucose and insulin concentrations are not in a steady state and/or are receiving exogenous insulin has limitations because this method has not been verified in these situations and for this reason the interpretation of the results has to be made with caution. The duration of the study was limited, as patients were only studied for 72 hours and we therefore do not know the changes in the hormone levels over the subsequent days, although the majority of the patients achieved adequate glycemic control at 72 hours. PRISM and PIM was measured to evaluate the severity of illness at different times although these scores only have been validated in the first 24 hours of admission. Analytical measures were made at fixed times, independently of the hour of the day and this fact could influence in some hormone values as ACTH or cortisol. Finally, we did not measure other factors that could mediate in the onset of hyperglycemia in the critically ill patient, such as catecholamines, cytokines, glucagonlike peptide-1 or nonesterified fatty acids [33].

Conclusions

We conclude that critically ill children with severe hyperglycemia initially have reduced β-cell function and insulin sensitivity. β-cell function recovers rapidly but peripheral resistance to insulin persists. There was no relationship between glycemia and the majority of the hormonal changes detected. Patients who died had higher cortisol and growth hormone levels and developed hyperglycemia later than survivors. There was no relationship between glycemia and mortality although the number of patients is too small to detect differences. Length of stay was associated with C-peptide, insulin, and blood glucose levels, insulin resistance, and severity of illness at 24 hours.

Competing interests

The authors declare that they have no competing interests.

Authors' contributions

All authors have made substantial contributions to conception and design, or acquisition of data, or analysis and interpretation of data; have been involved in drafting the manuscript or revising it critically for important intellectual content; and have given final approval of the version to be published. YB and JL-H: conceived the study and participated in the design, data collection and analysis, and drafting of the manuscript. RG, MJS, JC, JU, MB, and AGS participated in the design of the study, data collection and analysis of data, and drafting of the manuscript. NL performed hormonal laboratory analysis and drafted the manuscript. JMB participated in the design of the study and performed the statistical analysis. All authors read and approved the final manuscript.

Acknowledgements

To the nurses of the Pediatric Intensive Care Department of the Hospital Gregorio Marañón for their contribution to this study.

Author details

[1]Pediatric Intensive Care Department, Hospital General Universitario Gregorio Marañón Complutense University of Madrid, Madrid, Spain. [2]Laboratory Department, Hospital General Universitario Gregorio Marañón, Madrid, Spain. [3]Instituto de Investigación biomédica del Hospital Gregorio Marañón, Madrid, Spain. [4]Red de Salud Materno Infantil y del Desarrollo, Red SAMID II, Madrid, Spain.

References

1. Vlasselaers D, Milants I, Desmet L, Wouters PJ, Vanhorebeek I, van den Heuvel I, Mesotten D, Casaer MP, Meyfroidt G, Ingels C, Muller J, Van Cromphaut S, Schetz M, Van den Berghe G: **Intensive insulin therapy for patients in paediatric intensive care: a prospective, randomised controlled study.** *Lancet* 2009, **373:**547–556.
2. Yung M, Wilkins B, Norton L, Slater A: **Glucose control, organ failure, and mortality in pediatric intensive care.** *Pediatr Crit Care Med* 2008, **9:**147–152.
3. Hirshberg E, Larsen G, Van Duker H: **Alterations in glucose homeostasis in the pediatric intensive care unit: Hyperglycemia and glucose variability are associated with increased mortality and morbidity.** *Pediatr Crit Care Med* 2008, **9:**361–366.
4. The NICE-SUGAR Study Investigators: **Intensive versus conventional glucose control in critically ill patients.** *N Engl J Med* 2009, **360:**1283–1297.
5. Van den Berghe G, Wouters P, Weekers F, Verwaest C, Bruyninckx F, Schetz M, Vlasselaers D, Ferdinande P, Lauwers P, Bouillon R: **Intensive insulin therapy in the critically ill patients.** *N Engl J Med* 2001, **345:**1359–1367.
6. Agus MS, Steil GM, Wypij D, Costello JM, Laussen PC, Langer M, Alexander JL, Scoppettuolo LA, Pigula FA, Charpie JR, Ohye RG, Gaies MG, SPECS Study Investigators: **Tight glycemic control versus standard care after pediatric cardiac surgery.** *N Engl J Med* 2012, **367:**1208–1219.
7. Macrae D, Grieve R, Allen E, Sadique Z, Morris K, Pappachan J, Parslow R, Tasker RC, Elbourne D, CHiP Investigators: **A randomized trial of hyperglycemic control in pediatric intensive care.** *N Engl J Med* 2014, **370:**107–118.
8. Preissig CM, Rigby MR: **Hyperglycaemia results from beta-cell dysfunction in critically ill children with respiratory and cardiovascular failure: a prospective observational study.** *Crit Care* 2009, **13:**R27.
9. Vasa FR, Molitch ME: **Endocrine problems in the chronically critically ill patient.** *Clin Chest Med* 2001, **22:**193–208.
10. Delarue J, Magnan C: **Free fatty acids and insulin resistance.** *Curr Opin Clin Nutr Metab Care* 2007, **10:**142–148.
11. Mesotten D, Swinnen JV, Vanderhoydonc F, Wouters PJ, Van der Berghe G: **Contribution of circulating lipids to the improved outcome of critical illness by glycemic control with intensive insulin therapy.** *J Clin Endocrinol Metab* 2004, **89:**219–226.
12. Slater A, Shann F, Pearson G: **PIM II. A revised version of the Paediatric Index of Mortality.** *Intensive Care Med* 2003, **29:**278–285.
13. Pollack MM, Ruttimann UE, Getson PR: **The pediatric risk of mortality (PRISM) score.** *Crit Care Med* 1988, **16:**1110–1116.
14. Leteurtre S, Martinot A, Duhamel A, Proulx F, Grandbastien B, Cotting J, Gottesman R, Joffe A, Pfenninger J, Hubert P, Lacroix J, Leclerc F: **Validation of pediatric logistic organ dysfunction (PELOD) score. Prospective, observational, multicenter study.** *Lancet* 2003, **362:**192–197.
15. Haterill M, Tibby SM, Hillirad T, Turner C, Murdoch IA: **Adrenal insufficiency in septic shock.** *Arch Dis Child* 1999, **80:**51–55.
16. Matthews DR, Hosker JP, Rudenski AS, Naylor BA, Treacher DF, Turner RC: **Homeostasis model assessment: insulin resistance and β-cell function from fasting plasma glucose and insulin concentrations in man.** *Diabetologia* 1985, **28:**412–419.
17. Verhoeven JJ, den Brinker M, Hokken-Koelega AC, Hazelzet JA, Joosten KF: **Pathophysiological aspects of hyperglycemia in children with meningococcal sepsis and septic shock: a prospective, observational cohort study.** *Crit Care* 2011, **15:**R44.
18. Preissig CM, Rigby MR, Maher KO: **Glycemic control for postoperative pediatric cardiac patients.** *Pediatr Cardiol* 2009, **30:**1098–1104.
19. Faustino EV, Bogue CW: **Relationship between hypoglycemia and mortality in critically ill children.** *Pediatr Crit Care Med* 2010, **11:**690–698.
20. Branco RG, Tasker RC: **Glycemic level in mechanically ventilated children with bronchiolitis.** *Pediatr Crit Care Med* 2007, **8:**546–550.
21. Allen HF, Rake A, Roy M, Brenner D, McKiernan CA: **Prospective detection of hyperglycemia in critically ill children using continuous glucose monitoring.** *Pediatr Crit Care Med* 2008, **9:**153–158.
22. Soop M: **Stress induced insulin resistance: recent developments.** *Curr Opin Clin Nutr Metab Care* 2007, **10:**181–186.
23. Fram RY, Cree MG, Wolfe RR, Mlcak RP, Qian T, Chinkes DL, Herndon DN: **Intensive insulin therapy improves insulin sensitivity and mitochondrial function in severely burned children.** *Crit Care Med* 2010, **38:**1475–1483.
24. Arafah BM: **Review: Hypothalamic pituitary adrenal function during critical illness: limitations of current assessments methods.** *J Clin Endocrinol Metab* 2006, **91:**3725–3745.
25. Baxter RC: **Changes in the IGF-IGFBP axis in critical illness.** *Best Pract Res Clin Endocrinol Metab* 2001, **15:**421–434.
26. Mebis L, van den Berghe G: **The hypothalamus-pituitary-thyroid axis in critical illness.** *Neth J Med* 2009, **67:**332–340.
27. Garcia Branco R, Xabier L, Celiny P, Piva JP, Fiori HH, Baldisserotto M, Fiori RM, Tasker RC: **Prospective operationalization and feasibility of a glycemic control protocol in critically ill children.** *Pediatr Crit Care Med* 2011, **12:**265–270.
28. Bhutia TD, Lodha R, Kabra SK: **Abnormalities in glucose homeostasis in critically Ill children.** *Pediatr Crit Care Med* 2012. Epub ahead of print.
29. Rake AJ, Srinivasan V, Nadkarni V, Kaptan R, Newth CJ: **Glucose variability and survival in critically ill children: allostasis or harm?** *Pediatr Crit Care Med* 2010, **11:**707–712.

30. Treggiari MM, Karir V, Yanez ND, Weiss NS, Daniel S, Deem SA: **Intensive insulin therapy and mortality in critically ill patients.** *Crit Care* 2008, **12:**R29.
31. Hebbar KB, Stockwell JA, Leong T, Fortenberry JD: **Incidence of adrenal insufficiency and impact of corticosteroid supplementation in critically ill children with systemic inflammatory syndrome and vasopressor-dependent shock.** *Crit Care Med* 2011, **39:**1145–1150.
32. COIITSS Study Investigators, Annane D, Cariou A, Maxime V, Azoulay E, D'honneur G, Timsit JF, Cohen Y, Wolf M, Fartoukh M, Adrie C, Santré C, Bollaert PE, Mathonet A, Amathieu R, Tabah A, Clec'h C, Mayaux J, Lejeune J, Chevret S: **Corticosteroid treatment and intensive insulin therapy for septic shock in adults: a randomized controlled trial.** *JAMA* 2010, **303:**341–348.
33. Mechanick JI: **Metabolic mechanisms of stress hyperglycemia.** *J Parenter Enteral Nutr* 2006, **30:**157–163.

3

A case report of syndrome of inappropriate antidiuretic hormone secretion with Castleman's disease and lymphoma

Chong-Gui Zhu[1], Qiu-Zi Zhang[1], Mei Zhu[1*], Qiong-Li Zhai[2], Xiao-Yu Liang[3], Zong-Hong Shao[4], Emily C Ver Hoeve[5] and Hui-Qi Qu[5]

Abstract

Background: Syndrome of inappropriate antidiuretic hormone secretion (SIADH) is a common cause of hyponatremia in hospitalized patients and is often described in patients with small-cell carcinoma of the lung. In this report, we described both Castleman's disease and lymphoma coexisting in one patient with SIADH.

Case presentation: A 70-year-old Chinese woman with a history of diabetes mellitus and insulin therapy had severe hyponatremia and gastrointestinal symptoms. Through a series of examinations, common causes such as pulmonary carcinoma were excluded. An abdominal mass was detected by computed tomography. Although the peripheral lymph node biopsy showed the pathological result as Castleman's disease, the pathology of the abdominal lymph node revealed diffuse large B-cell lymphoma. After chemotherapy, the hyponatremia was treated during a period of follow-up.

Conclusion: This patient presented with the rare clinical condition of inappropriate antidiuretic hormone secretion alongside Castleman's disease and lymphoma. Asymptomatic hyponatremia may persist for some time suggesting that clinical physicians should pay attention to the mild cases of hyponatremia. We also hypothesized that Castleman's disease is a condition of pre-lymphoma with both having the ability to cause SIADH. The possibility of lymphoma as well as Castleman's disease triggering the development of SIADH should also be taken into consideration for conducting recurrent biopsies.

Keywords: Castleman's disease, Hyponatremia, Lymphoma, Syndrome of inappropriate antidiuretic hormone secretion (SIADH)

Background

The syndrome of inappropriate antidiuretic hormone secretion (SIADH) is caused by the excessive release of antidiuretic hormone (ADH, also known as vasopressin) from the posterior pituitary gland [1,2] and can cause hyponatremia in hospitalized patients with an incidence as high as 30% [3]. SIADH is generally seen in patients diagnosed with small-cell lung cancer (SCLC) which was first described by Schwartz et al. in two patients with lung cancer [4].

* Correspondence: meichuqin@yahoo.com.cn
[1]Department of Endocrinology, Tianjin Medical University General Hospital, No 154 Anshan Road, Heping District, Tianjin 300052, China
Full list of author information is available at the end of the article

SIADH is not difficult to diagnose in clinic. It can be secondary to a variety of disorders, such as medications, malignancies, surgery, and HIV infection or be idiopathic [1,2]. While SCLC is the primary malignancy causing SIADH, lymphoma can also induce this condition [5,6]. In this report, the diagnosis of Castleman's disease was established before we suspected SIADH was caused by a malignancy. After extensive examinations, we made the final diagnosis of diffuse large B-cell lymphoma. Chemotherapy treatment was recommended for the patient and significantly ameliorated the SIADH symptoms.

Case presentation

In October 2011, a 70-year-old Han Chinese woman with Type 2 diabetes (T2D) was admitted to Department of Endocrinology at the Tianjin Medical University General Hospital for uncontrolled hyperglycemia. The patient had a history of T2D for 21 years and received continuous long-term insulin treatment with a dosage of about fifty units per day. On the seventh day after admission, the patient developed symptoms of nausea and vomiting accompanied by left leg radiating pain without diarrhea and fever. She did not present with headache, dizziness, disturbance of consciousness, melana or hematemesis. The medications used in the hospital are listed in Table 1. The patient had no recent history of using diuretic agents. Serum sodium levels decreased to 112 mmol/l and chloride levels to 81 mmol/l with an effective osmolality at 267 mOsm/kg.H_2O (normal range: 280–310 mOsm/kg. H_2O). Urinary sodium increased to 85 mmol/l and chloride to 86 mmol/l with an osmolality of 257 mOsm/kg. H_2O indicating hypotonicity during normal dietary salt intake. She was clinically normovolemic with no signs of fluid retention. Her hepatic and renal functions were normal with a serum creatinine of 68 (normal range: 44–115) umol/L. Fractional sodium excretion was calculated as 1.56%. Thyroid and adrenal function were measured with ACTH = 59.8 pg/mL(normal range: 0–46), cortisol = 25.6 ug/dL(normal range: 5–25), 24-hour cortisol in urine = 64.4 ug(normal range: 30–110), FT3 = 3.04 pmol/L(normal range: 3.5–6.5), FT4 = 19.76 pmol/L (normal range: 11.5–23.5), TSH = 3.657 uIU/mL(normal range: 0.3–5.0) and rT3 = 1.76 nmol/l (normal range: 0.43–1.15). The magnetic resonance imaging (MRI) of her pituitary gland showed herniation of the suprasellar cistern. Based on the MRI result, our first diagnosis was hypopituitarism, which was treated with intravenous hydrocortisone at 50 mg/day. Both the serum sodium and serum chloride increased from 112 to 116 mmol/l and from 81 to 84 mmol/l, respectively, on the following day.

After further inquiry, the patient informed us of a past history of Mucosal-associated lymphoid tissue lymphoma (MALT) which had not received further treatment. We also discovered that she was last hospitalized on March 2011 for uncontrolled hyperglycemia without symptoms of nausea and vomiting. Nevertheless, hyponatremia had been noticed with serum sodium of 131 mmol/L and serum chloride of 95 mmol/l. Urinary investigation showed increased levels of sodium (90 mmol/l) and chloride (83 mmol/l) without corresponding osmolality data. Her renal function was normal with a serum creatinine of 63 umol/L. This information led us to believe that SIADH caused the patient's hyponatremia. Three days after restricting fluid intake to 1000 ml/day, the serum sodium rose to 128 mmol/L from 116 mmol/L. Ten days later, the patient's serum sodium levels increased to 142 mmol/l, and the symptoms of nausea and vomiting disappeared.

Table 1 Medications used in the current hospitalization

Medicine	Dose	Times
Voglibose	0.3 mg	3
Glimepiride	4 mg	Once in the morning
Glimepiride	2 mg	Once in the evening
Insulin Aspart 30	28 IU	2
Irbesartan	150 mg	1

Since the patient had a past history of MALT, we performed a gastric endoscopy, which indicated the absence of lymphoma. Additionally, the serology result was negative for purified protein derivative (PPD), and the serum and urine protein electrophoresis were also negative for monoclonal gammopathy. Additional laboratory findings were listed in Table 2. A negative chest computed tomography (CT) scan excluded the possibility of SCLC as the cause of SIADH in this patient. However, we noticed that the patient had obvious pain in the left leg, abdominal distension, and skin itching on a clinical exam and further discovered that her abdomen circumference had increased significantly in the last six months. An abdominal CT scan showed that a mass measuring approximately 49 mm*70 mm*90 mm was located on front lumbar vertebra 1–4 and the surrounding abdominal aorta. A subsequent abdominal enhancement CT revealed that the mass might be lymphoma (Figure 1). As the pathological result was critical for her diagnosis, we conducted a left inguinal lymph node puncture showing no abnormal lymphocytes. Consequently, a whole left inguinal (2 × 1 × 0.5 cm) lymph node was resected. The pathological morphology revealed that the lymph node structure was replaced with substantial amounts of lymphoid tissue and fibrosis. Thus, the diagnosis of Castleman's disease was established according to the pathological exam (Figure 2A, B, C).

Although hyponatremia was corrected, her hemoglobulin levels decreased from 109 g/L to 96 g/L. With her consent, we conducted a biopsy of the enlarged abdominal lymph node by using a celioscope. The pathological exam disclosed diffuse large B-cell lymphoma with an anaplastic subtype (Figure 3A, B).

After the diagnosis of lymphoma was established, the patient was transferred to the Department of Hematology for further treatment. For the etiology treatment of B-cell lymphoma, the chemotherapy of cyclophosphamide, hydroxydaunorubicin, oncovin and prednisone (CHOP) with rituximab (a monoclonal antibody against the protein CD20) was administered. The patient's serum sodium level stabilized without fluid restriction.

Discussion

In this case, the hyponatremia had existed for a long time and failed to gain proper attention until serious

Table 2 Laboratory findings in the current hospitalization

Exam	Value	Reference range	Unit
HbA1c	10.50%	4-6%	
FBG	12.5	3.9-6.1	mmol/L
24-h proteinuria	124.2	0-150	mg
Blood urea nitrogen	4	1.7-8.3	mmo/L
Serum uric acid	144	140-414	μmol/L
Serum creatinine	68	44-115	μmol/L
Ccr	86.8	80-120	ml/min
ACTH	59.8	0-46	pg/mL
Cortisol	25.6	5-25	μg/dL
24-hour cortisol in urine	64.4	30-110	ug
FT3	3.04	3.5-6.5	pmol/L
FT4	19.76	11.5-23.5	pmol/L
TSH	3.657	0.3-5.0	μIU/mL
rT3	1.76	0.43-1.15	nmol/l
ESR	21	0-20	mm/h
Lactic acid dehydrogenase	186	94-250	U/L
ß2-microglobulin	2.04	0.8-2.0	mg/L
Antinuclear antibody	Negative		
Immunoglobulin G	811	751-1560	mg/dl
Immunoglobulin A	64.8	82-453	mg/dl
Immunoglobulin M	48.1	46-304	mg/dl
C3	88.9	79-152	mg/dl
C4	17.10.	16-38	mg/dl
C-reactive protein	1.07	<0.80	mg/dl
Circulating immunologic complex	4.2	<13	U/ml
Immunoglobulin E	<5.00	<165	IU/ml
Alpha Fetoprotein	4.42	0-20	ng/ml
Ferritin	272.87	4.6-204	ng/ml
Carcinoembryonic antigen	1.42	0-5	ng/ml
Carbohydrate antigen19-9	<0.60	0-37	U/ml
Carbohydrate antigen 242	0.05	0-20	U/ml
Carbohydrate antigen 153	16.3	0-30	U/ml
HIV	Negative		

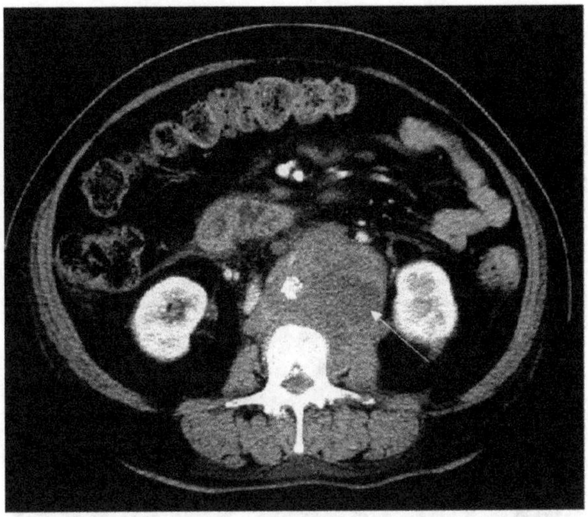

Figure 1 CT scan of abdomen showing a mass. Axial contrast-enhanced CT image shows a large lobulated irregular mass with inhomogenous enhancement that is encasing and anteriorly displacing the abdominal aorta.

clinical manifestations developed. Her past history of MALT as well as the success of fluid restriction and failure of hydrocortisone infusion suggested the possibility of hyponatremia caused by SIADH. One limitation of our investigation was the failure to measure urine uric acid and urea levels. Fractional uric acid excretion (FE-UA) has been demonstrated as a useful criterion in the diagnosis of SIADH particularly when attempting to differentiate between SIADH and hypovolaemic hyponatremia [7].

The main therapeutic issue in SIADH is fluid excess, and hyponatremia is dilutional in essence. Fluid restriction is the primary treatment option for SIADH. The vasopressin V2 receptor antagonist is effective for assisting the SIADH treatment [8]. Urea administration could be used in patients with chronic SIADH but also in acute SIADH like in critically ill patients [9].

Once a diagnosis of SIADH is established, determining its cause is most important. Castleman's disease is characterized by non-cancerous growths that may develop in the lymph node tissue throughout the body [10]. Lesions often occur in the chest, abdomen, or neck, where the abnormal enlargement of lymph nodes could usually be found. Although SIADH is reported to be associated with Castleman's disease [11], the possibility of general lymphoma in this case could not be excluded. Several major points supported this conclusion including: (1) past history of MALT; (2) occurrence of itching (characteristic symptom of lymphoma); (3) CT scan findings suggested lymphoma; and (4) the manifestation of progressive anemia. Moreover, the patient had a long history of T2D treated with insulin. Recent studies suggest that insulin treatment may be associated with an higher risk of the developing certain types cancers including lymphoma [12].

Although Castleman's disease is inherently a non-neoplastic process, an association with concurrent or subsequent lymphoma has been well described [13]. The hyaline-vascular type of Castleman's disease which contains numerous lymphoid follicles should be differentiated from Hodgkin lymphoma and low-grade B-cell lymphomas [14]. Several B-cell lymphomas with prominent atrophic germinal centers and hyaline vascular penetration including follicular lymphoma, mantle cell lymphoma, and

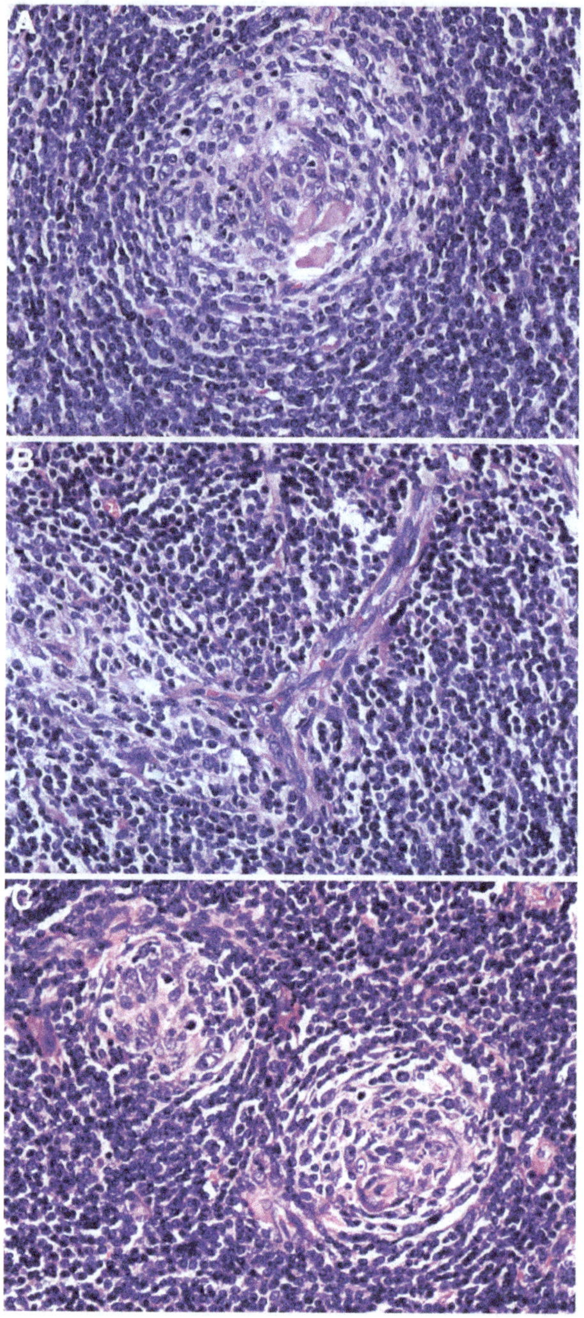

Figure 2 The pathological exam suggests Castleman's disease. The gross examination of the inguenal lymph node biopsy specimen shows a fairly well-encapsulated, soft tan lesion with a largest dimension of 1.2 cm. Microscopy reveals areas of hyaline-vascular Castleman's disease-like pattern. The majority of the lymphoid follicles had atrophic or regressive germinal centers, and some of them are penetrated by capillaries. There was concentric layering of lymphocytes in an onion-skin appearance and one or more penetrating blood vessels. The interfollicular stroma was also prominent with numerous hyperplastic vessels of the post-capillary venule type and plump endothelial lining. (**A**) concentric layering of lymphocytes in an onion-skin appearance; (**B**) a "lollipop" appearance; (**C**) two atrophic germinal centers within a single mantle zone.

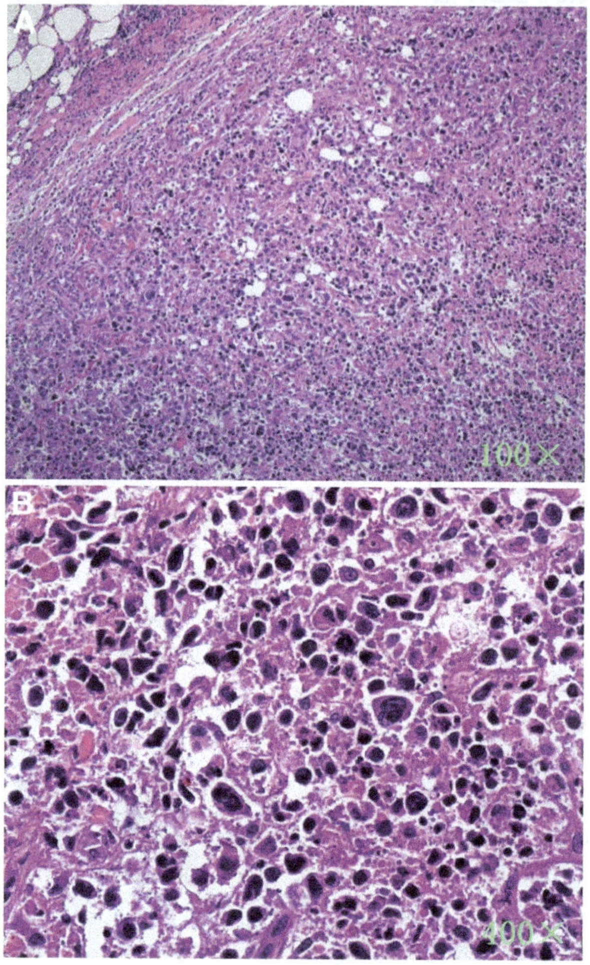

Figure 3 An abdominal lymph node biopsy suggests the diagnosis of diffuse large-B cell lymphoma, anaplastic subtype. (**A**) At low magnification, the normal nodal architecture was totally effaced and the node was diffusely infiltrated by a population of large atypical lymphocytes with a highly characteristic morphology. Extensive infiltration of the perinodal adipose tissue was observed as well. (Haematoxylin and eosin). (**B**) High magnification show that nuclei were round to oval with fine chromatin; Extensive areas of coagulative necrosis and karyorrhectic nuclei were present. Reed-Sternberg–like forms and giant cells are also prominent and conspicuous nucleoli are seen in these cells. Eosinophilic region was seen near the nucleus, probably representing a prominent Golgi apparatus.

nodal marginal zone lymphoma tend to be misdiagnosed as Castleman's disease due to the similar clinicopathologic features [15]. Furthermore, multicentric Castleman's disease could show similar FDG PET/CT appearance mimicking lymphoma, which reveals that Castleman's disease and lymphoma exhibit similar functions [16]. After consulting the literaure and examining the presentation of SIADH caused by both diseases, we hypothesized that Castleman's disease can develop into lymphoma, and a variety of pathological lymphomas may result in the development of SIADH [6,17]. One possible mechanism is the effect of hypercytokinemia. Some cytokines, such as interleukin (IL)-2, IL-6, IL-1β, and tumor necrosis factor (TNF)-α, have been reported to stimulate parvicellular and magnocellular neurons to secrete more ADH thus causing SIADH [18,19].

In our case, three separate biopsies showed differing results suggesting that this procedure is so imperative for certain conditions that several biopsies may be needed for a final diagnosis.

Conclusion

This report describes a rare case, in which an older woman had both Castleman's disease and lymphoma coexisting with SIADH. We wish to highlight the following key points: First, lymphoma as well as Castleman's disease, though uncommon, is an important cause of SIADH, and mild hyponatemia should get proper attention by clinical endocrinologists. Second, repeated lymph node biopsy may be crucial for the etiological diagnosis of SIADH.

Consent

Written informed consent was obtained from the patient for publication of this case report and the accompanying images. A copy of the written consent is available upon request for review by the Journal Editor.

Abbreviations

SIADH: Syndrome of inappropriate antidiuretic hormone secretion; ADH: Antidiuretic hormone; ACTH: Adreno-corticotrophic hormone; IL: Interleukin.

Competing interests

The authors declare that they have no competing interests.

Authors' contributions

MZ and CGZ led the conception and design, acquisition of data, review of literature, and drafted the manuscript. ZHS reviewed the manuscript. HQQ contributed the concept of research paper and critically reviewed the manuscript. QLZ expatiated the pathology and provided the pictures. All authors read and approved the manuscript.

Authors' information

MZ is the director of the Department of Endocrinology, Tianjin Medical University General Hospital. CGZ is the resident of Department of Endocrinology. HQQ is an Assistant Professor, Division of Epidemiology, Human Genetics and Environmental Sciences at School of Public Health, University of Texas Health Science Center at Houston.

Author details

[1]Department of Endocrinology, Tianjin Medical University General Hospital, No 154 Anshan Road, Heping District, Tianjin 300052, China. [2]Department of Pathology, Tianjin Medical University Cancer Hospital, Huan-Hu-Xi Road, Tiyuanbei, Hexin District, Tianjin 300060, China. [3]Department of Surgery, Tianjin Medical University General Hospital, No 154 Anshan Road, Heping District, Tianjin 300052, China. [4]Department of Hematology, Tianjin Medical University General Hospital, No 154 Anshan Road, Heping District, Tianjin 300052, China. [5]Division of Epidemiology, Human Genetics and Environmental Sciences, University of Texas School of Public Health, 1200 Herman Pressler, Houston, Texas 77030, USA.

References

1. Pillai BP, Unnikrishnan AG, Pavithran PV: **Syndrome of inappropriate antidiuretic hormone secretion: Revisiting a classical endocrine disorder.** *Indian J Endocrinol Metab* 2011, **15**(Suppl 3):S208–S215.
2. Esposito P, Piotti G, Bianzina S, Malul Y, Dal Canton A: **The syndrome of inappropriate antidiuresis: pathophysiology, clinical management and new therapeutic options.** *Nephron Clin Pract* 2011, **119**(1):c62–c73. discussion c73.
3. Upadhyay A, Jaber BL, Madias NE: **Incidence and prevalence of hyponatremia.** *Am J Med* 2006, **119**(7 Suppl 1):S30–S35.
4. Schwartz WB, Bennett W, Curelop S, Bartter FC: **A syndrome of renal sodium loss and hyponatremia probably resulting from inappropriate secretion of antidiuretic hormone.** *J Am Soc Nephrol* 1957, **12**(12):2860–2870.
5. Morimoto K, Ogihara T, Shiomi T, Awaya N: **Intravascular large B-cell lymphoma with preceding syndrome of inappropriate secretion of antidiuretic hormone.** *Intern Med* 2007, **46**(18):1569–1572.
6. Kobayashi K, Yokote T, Akioka T, Takubo T, Tsuji M, Hanafusa T: **Inappropriate antidiuretic hormone production in diffuse large B-cell lymphoma.** *Br J Haematol* 2008, **143**(1):2.
7. Fenske W, Stork S, Koschker AC, Blechschmidt A, Lorenz D, Wortmann S, Allolio B: **Value of fractional uric acid excretion in differential diagnosis of hyponatremic patients on diuretics.** *J Clin Endocrinol Metab* 2008, **93**(8):2991–2997.
8. Schrier RW, Gross P, Gheorghiade M, Berl T, Verbalis JG, Czerwiec FS, Orlandi C: **Tolvaptan, a selective oral vasopressin V2-receptor antagonist, for hyponatremia.** *N Engl J Med* 2006, **355**(20):2099–2112.
9. Coussement J, Danguy C, Zouaoui-Boudjeltia K, Defrance P, Bankir L, Biston P, Piagnerelli M: **Treatment of the syndrome of inappropriate secretion of antidiuretic hormone with urea in critically ill patients.** *Am J Nephrol* 2012, **35**(3):265–270.
10. Roca B: **Castleman's disease: a condition with protean manifestations.** *Onkologie* 2011, **34**(8–9):412–414.
11. Galmarini O, Garrido CM, Felgueres M, Saccoliti M, Duran M, Sanchez B: **Giant lymph node hyperplasia (Castleman's disease) with peripheral nerve diseases and syndrome of inappropriate secretion of antidiuretic hormone.** *Medicina (B Aires)* 1987, **47**(1):75–79.
12. Janghorbani M, Dehghani M, Salehi-Marzijarani M: **Systematic Review and Meta-analysis of Insulin Therapy and Risk of Cancer.** *Horm Cancer* 2012, **3**(4):137–146.
13. Larroche C, Cacoub P, Soulier J, Oksenhendler E, Clauvel JP, Piette JC, Raphael M: **Castleman's disease and lymphoma: report of eight cases in HIV-negative patients and literature review.** *Am J Hematol* 2002, **69**(2):119–126.
14. Kojima M, Shimizu K, Ikota H, Ohno Y, Motoori T, Itoh H, Masawa N, Nakamura S: **"Follicular variant" of hyaline-vascular type of Castleman's disease: histopathological and immunohistochemical study of 11 cases.** *J Clin Exp Hematop* 2008, **48**(2):39–45.
15. Siddiqi IN, Brynes RK, Wang E: **B-cell lymphoma with hyaline vascular Castleman disease-like features: a clinicopathologic study.** *Am J Clin Pathol* 2011, **135**(6):901–914.
16. Elboga U, Narin Y, Urhan M, Sahin E: **FDG PET/CT appearance of multicentric Castleman's disease mimicking lymphoma.** *Rev Esp Med Nucl Imagen Mol* 2012, **31**(3):142–144.
17. Onishi C, Ikejiri F, Kawakami K, Miyake T, Kumanomido S, Inoue M, Takahashi T, Tanaka J, Yamamoto M, Sugimoto T, *et al*: **Asian variant of intravascular large B cell lymphoma causes patients to frequently develop the syndrome of inappropriate antidiuretic hormone secretion.** *Ann Hematol* 2011, **90**(11):1293–1297.
18. Lim GW, Lee M, Kim HS, Hong YM, Sohn S: **Hyponatremia and syndrome of inappropriate antidiuretic hormone secretion in kawasaki disease.** *Korean Circ J* 2010, **40**(10):507–513.
19. Mastorakos G, Weber JS, Magiakou MA, Gunn H, Chrousos GP: **Hypothalamic-pituitary-adrenal axis activation and stimulation of systemic vasopressin secretion by recombinant interleukin-6 in humans: potential implications for the syndrome of inappropriate vasopressin secretion.** *J Clin Endocrinol Metab* 1994, **79**(4):934–939.

4

Differences and associations of metabolic and vitamin D status among patients with and without sub-clinical hypothyroid dysfunction

Naji J Aljohani[1,3], Nasser M Al-Daghri[2,3*], Omar S Al-Attas[2,3,4], Majed S Alokail[2,3], Khalid M Alkhrafy[2,3,5], Abdulaziz Al-Othman[2,6], Sobhy Yakout[2,3], Abdulaziz F Alkabba[1], Ahmed S Al-Ghamdi[1], Mussa Almalki[1], Badurudeen Mahmood Buhary[1] and Shaun Sabico[2,3]

Abstract

Background: Sub-clinical hypothyroid dysfunction, a relatively understudied disorder in the Kingdom of Saudi Arabia (KSA), has significant clinical implications if not properly monitored. Also from KSA, more than 50% of the population suffer from hypovitaminosis D (<50 nmol/l). In this cross-sectional case-control study, we described the differences and associations in the metabolic patterns of adult Saudis with and without hypothyroid dysfunction in relation to their vitamin D status, PTH, calcium and lipid profile.

Methods: A total of 94 consenting adult Saudis [52 controls (without subclinical hypothyroidism), 42 cases (previously diagnosed subjects)] were included in this cross-sectional study. Anthropometrics were obtained and fasting blood samples were taken for ascertaining lipid and thyroid profile, as well as measuring PTH, 25(OH) vitamin D and calcium.

Results: Cases had a significantly higher body mass index than the controls ($p < 0.001$). Circulating triglycerides was also significantly higher in cases than the controls ($p = 0.001$). A significant positive association between HDL-cholesterol and PTH (R = 0.56; $p = 0.001$), as well as a negative and modestly significant negative association between LDL-cholesterol and PTH (R = - 20.0; $p = 0.04$) were observed. FT3 was inversely associated with circulating 25 (OH) vitamin D (R = -0.25; $p = 0.01$).

Conclusions: Patients with hypothyroid dysfunction possess several cardiometabolic risk factors that include obesity and dyslipidemia. The association between PTH and cholesterol levels as well as the inverse association between vitamin D status and FT3 needs to be reassessed prospectively on a larger scale to confirm these findings.

Keywords: Thyroid dysfunction, Obesity, Dyslipidemia, Saudi

Background

Thyroid diseases are one of the more commonly encountered endocrine disorders in the Kingdom of Saudi Arabia (KSA), next to diabetes mellitus (DM) [1]. While current demographics point to less alarming prevalence of thyroid dysfunction, certain populations such as children with Down syndrome appear to manifest conditions related to thyroid dysfunction [2]. In the Middle East in general, thyroid dysfunction, specifically subclinical hypothyroid dysfunction, is a relatively understudied field as compared to other metabolic disorders such as obesity and insulin resistance. In a recent study, Bahammam and colleagues observed that subclinical hypothyroid dysfunction was prevalent among Saudi patients suffering from obstructive sleep apnea (OSA), with an estimated 1 out of 10 OSA patients harboring the condition [3]. Granted that hypothyroid dysfunction is not as endemic as the previously mentioned disorders, it nevertheless deserves attention as it can lead to serious repercussions if left ignored. Several studies point to an association between thyroid diseases, particularly Grave's disease and vitamin D status

* Correspondence: aldaghri2011@gmail.com
[2]Biochemistry Department, Biomarkers Research Program, College of Science, King Saud University, Riyadh, Saudi Arabia
[3]Prince Mutaib Chair for Biomarkers of Osteoporosis, King Saud University, Riyadh, Saudi Arabia
Full list of author information is available at the end of the article

in several ethnic groups, but none if not limited in the Middle East [4-6]. In this cross-sectional case-control study, we describe the differences and associations in the metabolic patterns of adult Saudis with and without subclinical hypothyroid dysfunction in relation to lipid and calcium metabolism in an attempt to stimulate further clinical investigations with respect to this under-studied disorder.

Methods

Subjects

A total of 94 consenting adult Saudis [52 control (6 males; 46 females), 42 cases (3 males, 39 females)] were included in this cross-sectional study. All subjects were recruited at the Endocrinology Unit of King Fahad Medical City, Riyadh Saudi Arabia. Adult Saudis aged 20-50, who are known cases of subclinical hypothyroid dysfunction based on previous clinical assessment (elevated TSH with normal FT4 levels), medications taken and laboratory tests with no complications were included. Control subjects were those who tested negative for subclinical hypothyroid dysfunction with no history of thyroid medications. Non-Saudis and pregnant women as well as children were excluded. Written and informed consent were secured prior to inclusion. Ethical approval was obtained from the Institutional Review Board of King Fahad Medical City, Riyadh, KSA.

Anthropometrics

Anthropometric parameters were obtained while the subject was standing erect and barefoot. Height and weight were determined using standardized conventional methods. Body mass index (BMI) was calculated using the formula: weight in kilograms (kg) divided by height in squared meters (m^2).

Blood measurements

Blood (≈ 10cc) was withdrawn after an overnight fast (> 10 hours). Serum calcium was measured using standard analytical techniques (Konelab, Finland). Fasting blood lipids which included triglycerides, total, HDL- and LDL-cholesterol as well as calcium were measured routinely using a chemical analyzer (Konelab, Finland). Serum TSH, FT3, and FT4 were estimated using commercially available kits by Roche Elecsys Modular Analytics Cobas e411 utilizing electrochemiluminescence immunoassay (Roche Diagnostics, Mannheim, Germany). TSH upper normal limit for males is 3.69 μIU/ml and 3.94 μIU/ml for females. Intact PTH and 25(OH)D were measured by specific ELISAs in accordance with the instructions provided by the manufacturer (IDS, Tyne & Wear, UK). 25(OH) vitamin D has been the preferred metabolite for the measurement of vitamin D status instead of 1, 25(OH)D, and remains the basis for the diagnosis of vitamin D deficiency [7]. The inter- and intra-assay variabilities were 5.8% and 3.4% respectively for the intact PTH ELISA, 5.3% and 4.6% respectively for the 25(OH)D ELISA. Anti-thyroid peroxidase (TPO) antibodies (Ab) were also measured using commercially available ELISA kits (Bio-Line S.A, Brussels, Belgium) with a sensitivity of 1.4 U/ml (intra-assay variability 6.9%; inter-assay variability 13.4%).

Data analysis

Data was analyzed using the Statistical Package for the Social Sciences (SPSS) version 16.5 (Chicago, IL, USA). Frequencies were presented as N and continuous variables if normal were presented as mean ± standard deviation and median (inter-quartile range) for variables with non-normal distribution. For group comparisons (controls versus cases), independent T-test if normally distributed continuous variables, and Mann-Whitney U-test for variables with non-Gaussian distribution were utilized. Significance set at $p < 0.05$.

Results

Table 1 shows the general characteristics of both cases and controls. There was no significant difference in the mean age of both groups. Subjects with thyroid dysfunction had a significantly higher body mass index than controls ($p < 0.001$). Circulating triglycerides were also

Table 1 Differences in metabolic characteristics of controls versus cases

	Controls	Cases	P value
N	52	42	
Age (years)	36.1 ± 8.1	35.5 ± 10.1	0.75
Gender (M/F)	6/46	3/39	
Body Mass Index (kg/m^2)	27.8 ± 3.9	32.3 ± 6.8	<0.001
Triglycerides (mmol/l)	1.2 ± 0.26	1.9 ± 0.46	0.001
Total Cholesterol (mmol/l)	5.1 ± 0.80	5.2 ± 1.0	0.56
LDL-Cholesterol (mmol/l)	3.9 ± 0.88	3.9 ± 0.87	0.99
HDL-Cholesterol (mmol/l)	0.90 ± 0.37	0.88 ± 0.30	0.78
Iodine (μg/l)	119.5 ± 35.9	97.6 ± 38.5	0.009
TSH (mIU/l)#	2.4 (1.6, 3.3)	3.7 (1.5, 7.6)	0.04
FT3 (pmol/l)	6.0 ± 1.3	4.8 ± 1.2	<0.001
FT4 (pmol/l)	17.2 ± 1.3	17.5 ± 1.2	0.80
TPOAb (U/ml) #	17.7 (14.1, 25.0)	164.9 (15.8, 582.9)	0.001
PTH (pg/ml)	5.3 ± 1.5	8.0 ± 1.2	0.15
Albumin (g/l)	33.8 ± 5.4	36.5 ± 6.8	0.03
Corrected Ca (mmol/l)	2.4 ± 0.23	2.1 ± 0.18	< 0.001
Ca (mmol/l)	2.5 ± 0.19	2.1 ± 0.45	0.002
25 (OH) Vitamin D (nmol/l)	18.3 ± 1.5	37.3 ± 1.9	< 0.001

Note: # denotes non-Gaussian distribution and presented as median (interquartile range); *p*-value significant at < 0.05.

Table 2 Correlation coefficients (R) of Lipids to thyroid function tests, PTH and vitamin D adjusted for age and BMI

	TSH	FT3	FT4	PTH	Iodine	TPO Ab	Vitamin D
Total Cholesterol (mmol/l)	-0.05	-0.02	-0.06	-0.04	0.05	0.03	-0.02
HDL-Cholesterol (mmol/l)	-0.12	-0.13	-0.13	**0.56****	-0.04	0.08	-0.04
Triglycerides (mmol/l)	0.12	0.04	-0.10	-0.16	-0.09	0.01	-0.19
LDL-Cholesterol (mmol/l)	-0.04	0.02	0.003	**-0.20***	0.08	0.001	0.04

Note: * denotes significance at < 0.05; ** denotes significance at < 0.01; *p*-value significant at < 0.05.

significantly higher among the cases than the controls ($p = 0.001$). The rest of the lipid parameters (Total, LDL- and HDL-cholesterol) were not significant. Among the thyroid tests, median TSH and median TPO Ab were significantly higher in the cases (consistent with Hashimoto's Thyroiditis) who also had a significantly lower mean FT3 and iodine than the controls (p values 0.03, 0.001, 0.009 and < 0.001, respectively). Only 2 subjects had TPOAb levels below 1.7 U/ml (cases). Mean FT4 was similar in both cases and controls. Lastly, mean serum calcium as well as corrected calcium were significantly lower in cases than controls ($p = 0.002$ and $p \leq 0.001$, respectively). Cases also had a significantly higher 25 (OH) vitamin D levels than the controls ($p < 0.001$), although both groups fall below sufficiency levels. Intact PTH was not significantly different between groups. Table 2 shows the regression coefficients of the lipid parameters versus the different thyroid tests, as well as 25(OH) vitamin D and PTH. A significant positive association between HDL-cholesterol and PTH ($R = 0.56$; $p = 0.001$) as well as a negative and modestly significant association between LDL-cholesterol and PTH were detected ($R = -20.0$; $p = 0.04$). The rest of the associations were not significant. Finally, Figure 1 shows the inverse and significant association between FT3 and circulating 25 (OH) vitamin D ($R = -0.25$; $p = 0.01$). TSH was not significantly associated with 25(OH) vitamin D.

Discussion

The main finding of this study is that aside from the conventional and expected differences in the expression of thyroid tests, including iodine and TPOab, patients with hypothyroid dysfunction also exhibited obesity and elevated levels of triglycerides as compared to controls. How subclinical hypothyroid dysfunction influences weight gain can be explained via the peripheral effects of thyroid hormones and their local regulation of central nervous system (CNS) in the physiologic regulation of appetite that is independent of their conventional role in basal energy expenditure as well as regulation of resting energy expenditure [8,9]. With respect to obesity per se, it has been found out that visceral adipose tissue has a direct effect in TSH levels among obese, and this is independent of insulin resistance [10]. Regarding triglycerides, our results were in accordance with the study of Wanjia and colleagues, who also observed elevated TSH levels among patients with hypertriglyceridemia [11]. The exact mechanisms accountable for the effects of thyroid function with respect to lipid profile are unclear. Nevertheless it is almost established that TSH receptors are present in tissues other than the thyroid gland which include kidneys, bone marrow and adipose tissue, and that variations ion TSH levels among euthyroid patients are partially explained by lipid components and hypercholesterolemia which are independent of thyroid hormones [12,13]. Furthermore, there are several factors not accounted for in this study that may influence thyroid function and lipid profile, including smoking and insulin resistance [14], as well as obesity and abnormalities in glucose tolerance.

One striking and unexpected finding in this study is the significantly higher mean 25(OH) vitamin D levels among patients with subclinical hypothyroid dysfunction

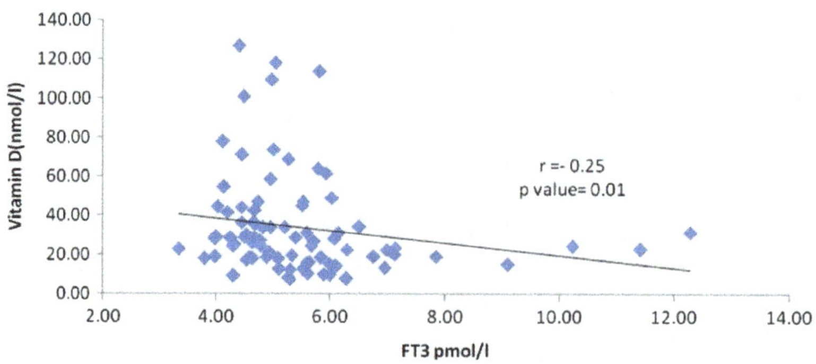

Figure 1 Inverse association between FT3 and 25(OH) Vitamin D.

than controls despite the presence of established risk factors for vitamin D deficiency including obesity and hypetriglyceridemia [15-17]. Calcium levels while also significantly different, still fall within normal range, although the possibility of other causes such as malabsorption or decreased dietary calcium intake in some subjects cannot be ruled out. Furthermore, PTH levels were higher, although not significant in the case group than controls. These differences this can be attributed to several confounders unaccounted for in the study which include differences in dietary calcium and vitamin D intake, undocumented comorbidities such as malabsorption and existing renal disorders which were not evident at the time of selection, as well as sun exposure, and needs further investigation. Nevertheless, while the vitamin D status of cases was significantly higher as compared to controls, both mean levels were still far below sufficiency levels and the corresponding PTH levels were not significantly different from one another, and as such the interpretation is comparable. Furthermore we recently observed that PTH levels do not correlate with 25(OH) vitamin D levels in Saudis despite severely low levels [18].

The association of PTH with lipid concentrations, specifically the cholesterol levels was demonstrated earlier and we suggest that this is mainly due to the positive association of PTH to body composition and adiposity, rather than the cholesterol itself [19,20]. Also, the inverse association of FT3 to circulating levels of 25(OH) D should be interpreted with caution. It was previously reported that higher vitamin D status was associated with low TSH only among younger individuals and not in adults [21]. Furthermore, while vitamin D deficiency has been implicated in several autoimmune thyroid diseases, no association was elicited between the antibodies measured in the present study and vitamin D, confirming a recent study among Dutch natives about the lack of correlation of low vitamin D levels and the early stages of thyroid auto-immunity [22]. Similarly, polymorphisms of vitamin D alpha-hydroxylase (CYP)1alpha, a key enzyme for regulating both systemic and tissue levels of 1, 25-dihydroxyvitamin D3 [23], did not correlate with known auto-immune disorders such as type 1 diabetes mellitus, Grave's disease and Hashimoto's thyroidits among Caucasian pedigrees [24]. In this context, it should be taken into account that TSH may have direct and independent effects on bone metabolism regardless of thyroid hormones [25,26].

The authors acknowledge several limitations. The cross-sectional nature of the study and the small sample size limits the findings of the study to at best, suggestive. Several major confounders were also not included including season which has a counterintuitive effect in the vitamin D status of citizens residing in the Gulf region [27]. Gender difference could not be elicited due to the big discrepancy in the numbers between male and female subjects. Nevertheless, the study has its own strength as being the first to document several metabolic differences among Saudi patients with and without hypothyroid dysfunction and the first to associate vitamin D status in relation to thyroid function profile.

Conclusions

In summary, adult Saudi patients with subclinical hypothyroid dysfunction harbor several cardiometabolic abnormalities, including obesity and dyslipidemia, the latter being associated positively with PTH levels. Higher vitamin D levels were associated with lower FT3 in the patents. Further prospective studies are needed to determine whether the associations elicited are causal to one another.

Competing interests

The authors declare that they have no competing interest.

Authors' contributions

NJA and NMA conceived the study. OSA, MSA, KMA and AA carried out data acquisition and interpretation. SY, AFA, ASA, MA and BMB analyzed the data and prepared the manuscript. NJA and SS drafted the revised and final version of the manuscript. All authors provided intellectual contributions to the manuscript and has read and approved the final version.

Acknowledgments

The author would like to thank the nursing staff of KFMC for the recruitment, data and sample collection of patients. The authors also thank Mr. Benjamin Vinodson for the statistical analysis of the data.

Author details

[1]Faculty of Medicine, King Saud bin Abdulaziz University for Health Sciences, King Fahad Medical City, Riyadh, Saudi Arabia. [2]Biochemistry Department, Biomarkers Research Program, College of Science, King Saud University, Riyadh, Saudi Arabia. [3]Prince Mutaib Chair for Biomarkers of Osteoporosis, King Saud University, Riyadh, Saudi Arabia. [4]Center of Excellence in Biotechnology Research Center, King Saud University, Riyadh, Saudi Arabia. [5]Clinical Pharmacy Department, College of Pharmacy, King Saud University, Riyadh, Saudi Arabia. [6]College of Applied Medical Sciences, King Saud University, Riyadh, KSA, Saudi Arabia.

References

1. Akbar DH, Ahmed MM, Al-Mughales J: **Thyroid dysfunction and thyroid autoimmunity in Saudi type 2 diabetics.** *Acta Diabetol* 2006, **43:**14–18.
2. Abdullah MA, Salman H, Al-Habib S, Ghareeb A, Abanamy A: **Antithyroid antibodies and thyroid dysfunction in Saudi children with Down syndrome.** *Ann Saudi Med* 1994, **14:**283–285.
3. Bahammam SA, Sharif MM, Jammah AA, Bahammam AS: **Prevalence of thyroid disease in patients with obstructive sleep apnea.** *Respir Med* 2011, **105:**1755–1760.
4. Yasuda T, Okamoto Y, Hamada N, Miyashita K, Takahara M, Sakamoto F, Miyatsuka T, Kitamura T, Katakami N, Kawamori D, Otuski M, Matsuoka TA, Kaneto H, Shinomura I: **Serum vitamin D levels are decreased and associated with thyroid volume in female patients with newly onset Grave's disease.** *Endocrine* 2012, **42:**739–741.
5. Yasuda T, Okamoto Y, Hamada N, Miyashita K, Takahara M, Sakamoto F, Miyatsuka T, Kitamura T, Katakami N, Kawamori D, Otsuki M, Matsuoka TA, Kaneto TH, Shimomura I: **Serum vitamin D levels are decreased in patients without remission of Grave's disease.** *Endocrine* 2013, **43:**230–232.

6. Rotondi M, Chiovato L: **Vitamin D deficiency in patients with Grave's disease: probably something more than a casual association.** *Endocrine* 2013, **43**:3–5.
7. Rizzoli R, Boonen S, Brandi ML, Bruyere O, Cooper C, Kanis JA, Kaufman JM, Ringe JD, Weryha G, Reginster JY: **Vitamin D supplementation in elderly or postmenopausal women: a 2013 update of the 2008 recommendations from the European Society for Clinical and Economic Aspects of Osteoporosis and Osteoarthritis (ESCEO).** *Curr Med Res Opin* 2013, **29**:305–313.
8. Amin A, Dhillo WS, Murphy KG: **The central effects of thyroid hormones on appetite.** *J Thyroid Res* 2011, **2011**:306510.
9. Al-Adsani H, Hoffer LJ, Silva JE: **Resting energy expenditure is sensitive to small dose changes in patients on chronic thyroid hormone replacement.** *J Clin Endocrinol Metab* 1997, **82**:1118–1125.
10. Muscogiuri G, Sorice GP, Mezza T: **High normal TSH values in obesity: is it insulin resistance or adipose tissue's guilt?** *Obesity (Silver Spring)* 2013, **21**:101–106.
11. Wanjia X, Chenggang W, Aihong W, Xiaomei Y, Jiajun Z, Chunxiao Y, Jin X, Yinglong H, Ling G: **A high normal TSH levels is associated with an atherogenic lipid profile in euthyroid non-smokers with newly diagnosed asymptomatic coronary heart disease.** *Lipids Health Dis* 2012, **11**:44.
12. Williams GR: **Extrathyroidal expression of TSH receptor.** *Ann Endocrinol (Paris)* 2011, **72**:68–73.
13. Wang F, Tan Y, Wang C, Zhang X, Zhao Y, Song X, Zhang B, Guan Q, Xu J, Zhang J, Zhang D, Lin H, Yu C, Zhao J: **Thyroid-stimulating hormone levels within the reference range are associated with serum lipid profiles independent of thyroid hormones.** *J Clin Endocrinol Metab* 2012, **97**:2724–2731.
14. Palmieri EA, Fazio S, Lombardi G, Biondi B: **Subclinical hypothyroidism and cardiovascular risk: a reason to treat?** *Treat Endocrinol* 2004, **3**:233–244.
15. Al-Daghri NM, Al-Attas OS, Al-Okail MS, Alkharfy KM, Al-Yousef MA, Nadhrah HM, Sabico SB, Chrousos GP: **Severe hypovitaminosis D is widespread in Saudi adults and is more common in non-diabetics than diabetics.** *Saudi Med J* 2010, **31**:775–780.
16. Al-Daghri NM, Al-Attas OS, Alokail MS, Alkharfy KMK, Yousef M, Nadhrah HM, Al-Othman A, Al-Saleh Y, Sabico S, Chrousos GP: **Hypovitaminosis D and cardiometabolic risk factors among non-obese youth.** *Cent Eur J Med* 2010, **5**:752–757.
17. Tamer G, Mesci B, Tamer I, Kilic D, Arik S: **Is vitamin D deficiency an independent risk factor for obesity and abdominal obesity in women?** *Endokrynol Pol* 2012, **63**:196–201.
18. Al-Saleh Y, Al-Daghri NM, Alkharfy KM, Al-Attas OS, Alokail MS, Al-Othman A, Sabico S, Chrousos GP: **Normal circulating PTH in Saudi healthy individuals with hypovitaminosis D.** *Horm Metab Res* 2013, **45**:43–46.
19. Williams DM, Fraser A, Lawlor DA: **Association of vitamin D, parathyroid hormone and calcium with cardiovascular risk factors in US adolescents.** *Heart* 2011, **97**:315–320.
20. Kayaniyil S, Vieth R, Harris SB, Retnakaran R, Knight JA, Gerstein HC, Perkins BA, Zinman B, Hanley AJ: **Association of 25(OH)D and PTH with metabolic syndrome and its traditional and nontraditional components.** *J Clin Endocrinol Metab* 2011, **96**:168–175.
21. Chailurkit LO, Aekplakorn W, Ongphiphadhanakul B: **High vitamin D status in younger individuals is associated with low circulating thyrotropin.** *Thyroid* 2013, **23**:25–30.
22. Effraimidis G, Badenhoop K, Tijssen JG, Wiersinga WM: **Vitamin D deficiency is not associated with early stages of thyroid autoimmunity.** *Eur J Endocrinol* 2012, **167**:43–48.
23. Kozai M, Yamamoto H, Ishiguro M, Harada N, Masuda M, Kagawa T, Takei Y, Otani A, Nakahashi O, Ikeda S, Taketani Y, Takeyama K, Kato S, Takeda E: **Thyroid hormones decrease plasma 1α,25-dihydroxyvitamin D levels through transcriptional repression of the renal 25-hydroxyvitamin D3 1α-hydroxylase gene (CYP27B1).** *Endocrinology* 2013, **154**:609–622.
24. Pani MA, Regulla K, Segni M, Krause M, Hofmann S, Hufner M, Herwig J, Pasquino AM, Usadel KH, Badenhoop K: **Vitamin D1alpha-hydroxylase (CYP1alpha) polymorphism in Grave's disease, Hashimoto's thyroidits and type 1 diabetes mellitus.** *Eur J Endocrinol* 2002, **146**:777–781.
25. Mazziotti G, Porcelli T, Patelli I, Vescovi PP, Giustina A: **Serum TSH values and risk of vertebral fractures in euthyroid post-menopausal women with low bone mineral density.** *Bone* 2010, **46**:747–751.
26. Maziotti G, Sorvillo F, Piscopo M, Cioffi M, Pilla P, Biondi B, Iorio S, Giustina A, Amato G, Carella C: **Recombinant human TSH modulates in vivo C-telopeptides of type-1 collagen and bone alakaline phosphatase, but not osteoprotegerin production in postmenopausal women monitored for differentiated thyroid carcinoma.** *J Bone Miner Res* 2005, **20**:480–486.
27. Al-Daghri NM, Al-Attas OS, Alokail MS, Alkharfy KM, El-Kholie E, Yousef M, Al-Othman A, Al-Saleh Y, Sabico S, Kumar S, Chrousos GP: **Increased vitamin D supplementation recommended during summer season in the gulf region: a counterintuitive seasonal effect in vitamin D levels in adult, overweight and obese Middle Eastern residents.** *Clin Endcrinol (Oxf)* 2012, **76**:346–350.

5

A case of Aromatase deficiency due to a novel *CYP19A1* mutation

Lucia Gagliardi[1,2,3*], Hamish S Scott[2,3,4,5,6], Jinghua Feng[4,5] and David J Torpy[1,3]

Abstract

Background: Aromatase deficiency is a rare, autosomal recessive disorder of which there are approximately twenty four case reports. The aromatase enzyme is crucial in the biosynthesis of oestrogens from androgens. The phenotype of aromatase deficiency therefore is the result of androgen excess and oestrogen deficiency in the absence of normal aromatase activity. We report the first case of aromatase deficiency diagnosed in a female adult, at the age of 32 years, due to a novel duplication in the aromatase gene.

Case presentation: A 32 year old Indian woman presented with a history of gender assignment difficulties at birth, lack of pubertal development, osteopaenia with fracture and tall stature. She had central obesity, impaired fasting glucose and borderline hypertension. Past examinations had revealed partial fusion of urethra and vagina, hypoplastic uterus and streak ovaries. The ovaries had been excised due to malignant risk after an initial clinical diagnosis of Turner's syndrome with Y mosaicism. Oestrogen replacement commenced shortly after her fracture, in adulthood. After reassessment, aromatase deficiency was diagnosed. Sequencing of the coding exons of the aromatase (*CYP19A1*; OMIM 109710) gene revealed a novel 27-base duplication in exon 8 (p.Ala306_Ser314*dup*). This duplication, occurring within the aromatase α-helix, would be likely to disrupt substrate (androgen) and cofactor (protoporphyrin IX) binding, resulting in a lack of oestrogen synthesis.

Conclusions: We report a female with a phenotype compatible with aromatase deficiency which was unrecognised until adulthood and found she had a novel duplication in *CYP19A1*. Previous case reports have described polycystic ovarian morphology, especially in childhood and adolescence, but never streak ovaries. This may reflect the few adult cases reported, that aromatase deficiency in females is generally diagnosed at birth and oestrogen treatment commences decades earlier than occurred in our patient. Streak ovaries are consistent with the phenotype of the aromatase knockout mouse followed through adulthood. The observed clinical features of obesity, dysglycaemia and hypertension, are compatible with the observation that lack of a counterbalancing effect of oestrogen on tissue androgens until adulthood may lead to a metabolic syndrome phenotype. This report broadens the spectra of phenotype and genetic mutations underlying this rare disorder.

Keywords: Aromatase deficiency, Pubertal development, Streak ovaries, Androgens

Background

Human aromatase is a 58KDa protein which was first isolated from the placenta in the 1980s [1]. Tissues expressing aromatase include the granulosa cells and lutea corpora of the ovary, Leydig and Sertoli cells of the testis, breast, syncytiotrophoblast of the placenta, neurons, brain (including hypothalamus), liver, pre-adipocytes and fibroblasts, vascular smooth muscle cells, chondrocytes and osteoblasts [2]. Aromatase is a cytochrome P450 critical in the biosynthesis of oestrogen since it converts androgenic substrates, primarily testosterone and androstenedione, to oestradiol and oestrone, respectively [2]. In pregnancy, placental aromatisation of 16-hydroxy-dehydroepiandrosterone sulphate, arising from foetal liver hydroxylation of dehydroepiandrosterone sulphate produced by the foetal adrenal, is the major source of circulating oestrogens; the activity of placental aromatase protects the foetus against the virilising action of foetal androgens [3]. Placental aromatisation of foetal androgens also prevents high levels from reaching the maternal circulation, where they would result in maternal virilisation during pregnancy, subsiding post-partum.

* Correspondence: lucia.gagliardi@health.sa.gov.au
[1]Endocrine and Metabolic Unit, Royal Adelaide Hospital, North Terrace, Adelaide, SA 5000, Australia
[2]Department of Genetics and Molecular Pathology, Centre for Cancer Biology, SA Pathology, Frome Road, Adelaide, SA 5000, Australia
Full list of author information is available at the end of the article

The single gene encoding human aromatase (*CYP19A1;* OMIM 109710) is a 120Kb gene on chromosome 15q21.1, comprising nine coding exons (2-10) spanning approximately 35Kb; there are multiple first exons that are involved in tissue-specific expression [4-6]. These exons generate alternative splicing such that the coding region, and hence protein sequence, is conserved in every tissue. Within the aromatase protein, the most highly conserved region (the core region), consists of a four-helix bundle, two β sheets and the haem-binding region [7].

Aromatase deficiency is an autosomal recessive disorder due to mutations of the *CYP19A1* gene which result in reduced aromatase activity. There have been approximately twenty four cases of aromatase deficiency reported, including the original case reported by Shozu and colleagues in 1991 [8-12].

Clinical features of CYP19A1 deficiency include maternal virilization during pregnancy due to non-aromatization of foetal-derived androgens which resolves gradually postpartum, foetal virilisation of external genitalia and symptoms of haemorrhagic ovarian cysts in childhood [13-18]. Adrenarche is reportedly normal; however there is primary amenorrhoea and lack of breast development [15]. Elevated gonadotropins and hyperandrogenism are often present [16]. Virilization may progress with age – factors determining the presence and rate of progression are not established [15,19]. Delayed epiphyseal fusion and decreased bone density are reported [15,16]. Variation in phenotypic expression including some breast and uterine development may be due to partial aromatase activity. The natural history of CYP19A1 deficiency in females is largely unknown because early diagnosis leads to timely treatment. Males are usually diagnosed later in life, are tall due to delayed epiphyseal closure and have osteoporosis due to impaired bone mineralisation; these clinical features are comparable to those seen in patients with oestrogen receptor mutations; altered testis size and spermatogenesis may also be due to aromatase deficiency [15,20]. A metabolic syndrome-like picture of abdominal obesity, hepatic steatosis and insulin resistance has been well described in males; in females metabolic syndrome has been noted to be more prominent in cases where oestrogen treatment was delayed until adulthood [12,21-24].

Here, we report for the first time a female patient diagnosed with aromatase deficiency during adulthood. We found this patient to have a novel mutation in exon 8 of *CYP19A1,* which broadens the spectrum of mutations underlying aromatase deficiency.

Case presentation

The patient was referred for endocrine review for a past diagnosis of "Turner's syndrome". She was born to consanguineous parents and reportedly had abnormal genitalia at birth. Growth and development were unremarkable until the teenage years when spontaneous puberty did not occur. At age 25, she came to medical attention after fracturing her right radius following a fall onto her outstretched hand. Bone densitometry revealed osteoporosis (T-score spine -2.5, total hip -1.7). Oestradiol 1 mg per day, Alendronate and Calcium carbonate with Vitamin D2 were commenced. Abnormal genitalia were again noted. She was referred to a surgical centre in India, where an examination under anaesthesia and laparoscopy revealed clitoromegaly, partial fusion of urethra and vagina (Prader classification 3), hypoplastic uterus and bilateral streak ovaries which were excised (Figure 1) [25]. Histological examination of the

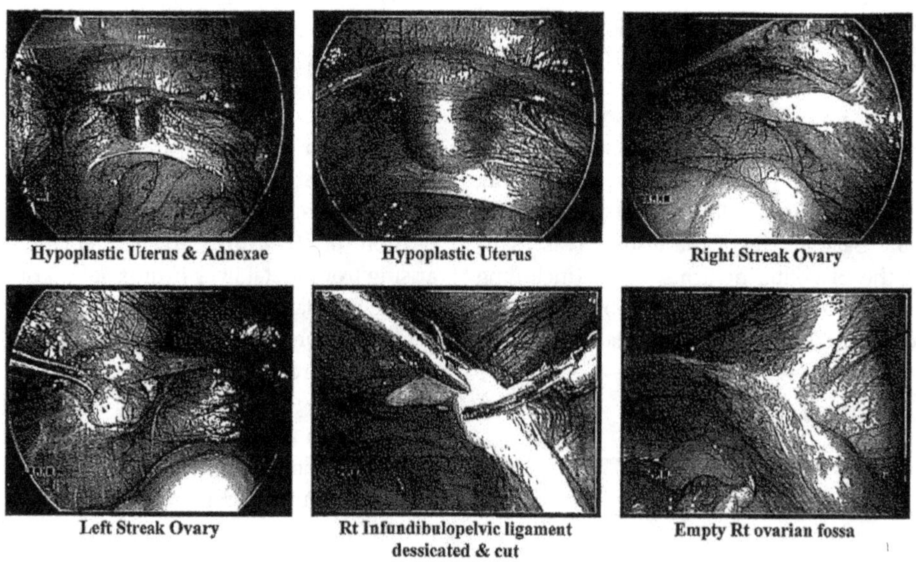

Figure 1 Clinical photographs taken at the patient's laparoscopy. The hypoplastic uterus and adnexae, including bilateral streak ovaries are shown.

streak ovaries revealed atretic and primordial follicles, but no evidence of ovulation.

On referral to us after migration to Australia, the patient, aged 32, reported good health other than recurrent perineal infections which had been treated with antibiotics and drainage via abscess incision on several occasions. Surgical reconstruction of the urogenital sinus is planned. Her height was 180 cm, she had predominant abdominal obesity (waist circumference 131 cm, hip circumference 115 cm) and eunuchoidal proportions (arm span 191 cm, lower segment 103 cm). Her height was well above her mid-parental predicted height of 161 cm (father 170 cm, mother 165 cm). Her only sibling, a younger brother, has a height of 193 cm at age 30, but was unavailable for detailed examination. She did not have a webbed neck, goitre or high arched palate. Her blood pressure was in the upper normal - borderline hypertensive range at 130–145/80–100 mmHg. She was not hirsute; breasts, pubic and axillary hair were normal (Tanner stage 5). Appearance of the external genitalia has been described. Her general examination was otherwise within normal limits. The results of hormonal evaluation (on oestrogen) are shown in Table 1. Biochemical testing revealed impaired fasting glucose, dyslipidaemia and insulin resistance (Table 1). Repeat densitometry revealed osteopenia (T-score spine -2.1, T-score total hip -1.0). Moderate hepatic steatosis was evident on abdominal ultrasound.

The karyotype obtained on both peripheral blood lymphocytes and cultured fibroblasts ($n = 134$) was 46, XX. Based on the clinical history, we suspected aromatase deficiency and Sanger sequenced the nine coding exons of *CYP19A1*. We also sequenced the coding exons of P450-oxidoreductase (POR), the electron donor for cytochrome P450 enzymes (including *CYP19A1*), which has been associated with a phenotype of ambiguous genitalia and, via consequent dysfunction of *CYP19A1*, could result in maternal virilisation in pregnancy [26]. Prior written, informed consent was obtained from the patient. Primers and sequencing methods are presented in Additional file 1 (Methods).

Sequencing of *POR* revealed two synonymous single nucleotide polymorphisms (rs1057870 and rs2228104), unrelated to the patient's phenotype. The patient had a novel 27-base pair duplication in exon 8 of *CYP19A1* (p.Ala306_Ser314*dup*) (Figure 2a, 2b; full genomic reference presented in Additional file 1 (Results)). Whilst she is most likely to be homozygous for the observed mutation, her parents were unavailable for testing and hence we are unable to exclude hemizygosity. The *CYP19A1* mutation would be expected to result in a duplication of nine amino acids (p.Ala306_Ser314*dup*) in the protein. This duplication occurs within the aromatase α-helix, a region crucial for binding of the cofactor protoporphyrin IX and the substrate androstenedione [7,27]. The insertion of this long sequence (approximately one third of the α-helix; Figure 2c, 2d and Additional file 2) would induce a major disruption of the α-helix conformation. Prediction tools of protein secondary structure consistently suggest a break of the α-helix around the middle, turning a continuous helix into the structure of helix-coil-helix [28-30]. This would be likely to disrupt substrate and cofactor binding resulting in a lack of oestrogen synthesis (Figure 2c).

Table 1 Biochemical evaluation of the patient

Test	Patient	Reference range
Follicle stimulating hormone	32	<12 mIU/L**
Luteinizing hormone	17	<12 mIU/L**
Testosterone	0.89	<2 nmol/L
Progesterone	<2	<6 nmol/L*
Sex-hormone binding globulin	45	25-90 nmol/L
Dehydroepiandrosterone sulphate	5.2	1-8.5 μmol/L
17-hydroxyprogesterone	2.4	0.2-11.3 nmol/L
Anti-mullerian hormone	<3 pmol/L	(below 25th percentile for age)
Thyroid-stimulating hormone	2.2	0.5-4 mIU/L
Free thyroxine	15	10-25 pmol/L
Oral glucose tolerance test - fasting glucose	6.1	<5.2 mmol/L
Oral glucose tolerance test – 2 hour glucose	7.5	<7.8 mmol/L
Glycosylated haemoglobin	6.7, 7.1	<5.5%
Fasting insulin	57	<12 mU/L
Total cholesterol	5.9	<5.5 mmol/L
HDL-cholesterol	1.4	1.0-2.2 mmol/L
LDL-cholesterol	3.6	<3.7 mmol/L
Triglycerides	2	0.3-2 mmol/L
Bilirubin	8	2-24 μmol/L
Gamma-glutamyl transpeptidase (GGT)	21	<60 U/L
Alkaline phosphatase (ALP)	134	30-100 U/L
Alanine aminotransferase (ALT)	41	<55 U/L
Aspartate aminotransferase (AST)	38	<45 U/L

*Hormone measurements were made whilst the patient was on oestrogen replacement.
**Reference range quoted is for the follicular phase of the menstrual cycle.

Most individuals reported with *CYP19A1* deficiency have been homozygous for loss-of-function mutations and born to consanguineous parents [8-13]. Up until recently, all reported mutations have been in coding exons, mostly in exons 9 and 10, which encode the substrate (androgen) binding site and haem-binding domains, respectively [9]. Recently, a patient with aromatase deficiency was found to be heterozygous for a novel mutation (p.Asn411Ser) in exon 9 [10]. *In vitro* studies

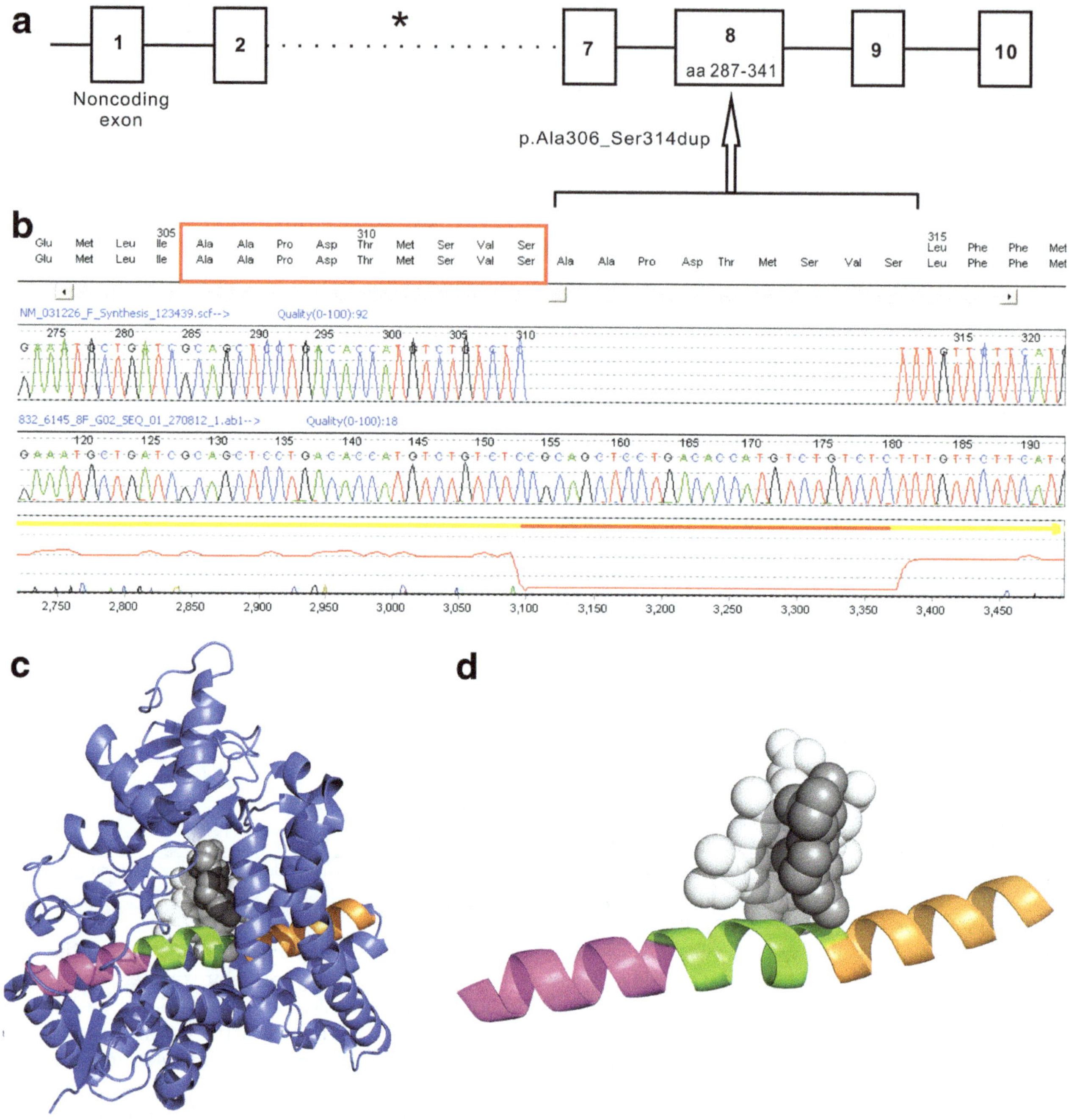

Figure 2 A novel duplication of 27 base pairs in the *CYP19A1* gene, was identified in the patient reported here. This duplication is predicted to disrupt a critical α-helix of the aromatase enzyme. **a.** A schematic diagram of the aromatase gene, comprised of nine coding exons (exons 2-9). The location of the novel duplication identified in our patient in exon 8 is shown. **b.** Results of Sanger sequencing showing a 27 base pair duplication in exon 8 of the *CYP19A1* gene from the patient (chr15 (hg19): g.51507347_51507373dup, NM_031226.2: c.915_941dup; NP_112503.1: p.Ala306_Ser314*dup*) (visualised in Mutation Surveyor® software (Version 2.51, SoftGenetics LLC, Philadelphia, USA)). **c.** Crystallographic structure of human wild-type aromatase in complex with the cofactor protoporphyrin IX and the substrate androstenedione. The segment of an α-helix in green shows where the duplication occurs. N- and C-terminuses of the α-helix are in orange and magenta, respectively. The rest of aromatase is shown in blue. Protoporphyrin IX, white, and androstenedione, grey. The crystallographic structure is from reference 1 and visualised in PyMOL (Version 1.5.0.3, Schrödinger, LLC). A three-dimensional image of this is provided in the accompanying Additional file 2. **d.** A close-up showing the α-helix providing binding sites of protoporphyrin IX (white) and androstenedione (grey).

confirmed this was a loss-of-function mutation; when co-expressed with the wildtype, the enzyme activity of the mutant was approximately 65% of wildtype; compatible with a recessive disease and thus the mutation alone did not explain the phenotype. There was a heterozygous, paternally inherited C > T variant -41 base pairs upstream of exon 1, in placental promoter I.1, a previously observed polymorphism (rs6493497) [10,31]. *In vitro* studies revealed a 50% reduction in transactivation ability of the placental promoter harbouring the mutation, compared with wildtype [10].

Our patient had several clinical features in common with the first female patient recently described with oestrogen resistance due to a novel homozygous missense mutation in a highly conserved region of exon 5 of the oestrogen receptor α (*ESR1*) [32]. Both lacked spontaneous breast development, and had primary amenorrhoea and osteopaenia. The patient with oestrogen resistance had delayed bone age and unfused epiphyses; in our patient whilst x-rays were not available we surmise from her eunuchoidal proportions that epiphyseal fusion of long bones was delayed [32]. The phenotype of tall stature, continuing linear growth into adulthood, delayed bone age, osteoporosis and eunuchoidal skeletal proportions is also well described in adult aromatase deficient males [33]. That it corrects with oestrogen treatment in both genders, reflects the common role across genders of oestrogen in bone development [34].

Our patient had a phenotype of metabolic syndrome not present in the patient with oestrogen resistance [32]. The absence of the metabolic phenotype in the latter case is in contrast with the only previously reported patient with an *ESR1* mutation [35,36]. In aromatase deficient females, the relationship between insulin resistance and oestrogen deficiency is unclear. A 14 year old female had normalisation of mild dyslipidaemia with oestrogen treatment [13]. However, a nine year old female had severe insulin resistance despite treatment with oestrogen and metformin [23]. It was postulated that *in utero* exposure to high levels of androgens or lack of oestrogens altered foetal programming of insulin sensitivity. Aromatase deficient adult men have a variable phenotype of metabolic syndrome, which improves with oestrogen treatment [14,34,37-39]. The development of central obesity post-menopausally is also considered a result of oestrogen deficiency.

The phenotype of the *CYP19A1* knockout (ArKO) mouse suggests an association between aromatase deficiency and metabolic perturbations [40,41]. Aging ArKO mice had progressively greater accumulation of visceral adiposity than wild-type, which regressed after administration of oestrogen [42]. Elevated cholesterol, insulin levels and glucose intolerance and hepatic steatosis have also been noted [42,43]. Oestrogen treatment improved glucose tolerance and reversed hepatic steatosis in male ArKO mice [43,44]. Thus, the majority of the available data infer that prolonged oestrogen deficiency is associated with a metabolic syndrome. However, there may be a gender difference in the mechanisms. High androgen levels have been associated with peripheral insulin resistance in women, but not in men [45,46]. This may be due to differences in the androgen-oestrogen ratio and its effects on cellular metabolism.

The patient we report exhibited evidence of *in utero* androgenisation of genitalia [47]. Subsequent failure of pubertal development, untreated during the adolescent years, ensued and she eventually came to medical attention with a minimal trauma fracture at age 25, prompting oestrogen replacement. She did not have features of progressive virilisation. This may reflect relatively early loss of ovarian function as a source of androgens. She had eunuchoidal proportions, a result of continued linear growth in adulthood due to unfused epiphyses in the absence of oestrogen. Genetic analyses revealed a novel 27 base duplication in exon 8 of *CYP19A1*, likely to result in a complete loss of function of the aromatase enzyme, the key enzyme regulating the oestradiol:testosterone ratios in tissues. A limitation of this work is that we have not performed functional studies to verify the effect of the duplication on protein function; however the clinical presentation and the correlation with cases already reported and with the ArKO mouse model is compelling for this being a loss of function mutation.

Unexpectedly, our patient had had streak ovaries excised. We caution that the histological slides were unavailable for verification and streak ovaries have not been described in association with aromatase deficiency. Polycystic ovaries and regression of ovarian cysts have been described previously in cases of aromatase deficiency [14-18,48]. Other cases had normal ovarian morphology, even in the absence of prior oestrogen treatment [10,11]. Thus, there is no consistent ovarian phenotype in aromatase deficiency and, furthermore, the phenotype may be modulated by treatment. In our patient, the ovarian morphology may be a result of oestrogen treatment.

Alternatively, extrapolating from observations in the ArKO mouse, we speculate that the streak ovaries may be an inherent manifestation of *CYP19A1* deficiency [40,41]. Follicular development in ArKO is abnormal in an age dependent manner, with an early block in follicular development at the antral stage with absent corpora lutea, then haemorrhagic cysts and later, absent secondary and antral follicles and atresia of primary follicles with increased collagen deposition [40,41]. The longer life span of the human may permit more complete follicular atresia and collagen deposition mimicking the classical streak ovaries seen in Turner's syndrome. Streak ovaries may not have been previously described in

CYP19A1 deficiency because of infrequent laparoscopic visualization of the ovaries and some of the cases may have been too young to develop this manifestation. In addition, some of the cases may have had *CYP19A1* mutations that allowed some residual aromatase function with a less severe ovarian atretic phenotype.

Another possibility is that our patient may have another cause of the streak ovaries such as XO mosaicism localised to the ovaries, although the normal XX karyotype makes this less likely. Streak ovaries are not clearly associated with any other disorder but Turner's syndrome. In view of the small numbers of CYP19A1 deficiency cases reported, this manifestation should be noted particularly since this finding may be relevant to ovarian developmental biology.

Conclusions

We report a case of the very rare condition, aromatase deficiency, due to a novel aromatase mutation and corresponding enzyme region distinct from previous reports. Our case is unique because it is the first reported case of aromatase deficiency in a female not treated until adulthood, and it depicts, for the first time, the natural history of aromatase deficiency in females. This comprises a phenotype of osteopaenia, tall stature and metabolic syndrome, as occurs in aromatase deficient males in whom, similarly to our patient, diagnosis and treatment are delayed. Streak ovaries may represent an extension of the clinical spectrum of this disorder and appears to correlate with findings in the aromatase knockout mouse model.

Abbreviation

CYP19A1: Aromatase gene.

Competing interests

The authors declare that they have no competing interests.

Authors' contributions

LG carried out the sequencing of the aromatase gene and drafted and revised the manuscript. HSS participated in the study design and drafted the manuscript. JF performed the protein prediction work, generated the figures of the protein structure presented in the manuscript and drafted the manuscript. DJT performed the clinical work. All authors read and approved the final manuscript.

Acknowledgements

We thank the patient for providing the clinical photographs presented in Figure 1. This work was supported by the "Gum Bequest" administered by the Endocrine and Metabolic Unit, Royal Adelaide Hospital (LG) and an NHMRC fellowship APP1023059 (HSS).

Author details

[1]Endocrine and Metabolic Unit, Royal Adelaide Hospital, North Terrace, Adelaide, SA 5000, Australia. [2]Department of Genetics and Molecular Pathology, Centre for Cancer Biology, SA Pathology, Frome Road, Adelaide, SA 5000, Australia. [3]School of Medicine, University of Adelaide, Adelaide, SA 5000, Australia. [4]Cancer Genomics Facility, Centre for Cancer Biology, SA Pathology, Adelaide, SA 5000, Australia. [5]School of Molecular and Biomedical Science, University of Adelaide, Adelaide, SA 5000, Australia. [6]Division of Health Sciences, School of Pharmacy and Medical Sciences, University of South Australia, Adelaide, SA 5000, Australia.

References

1. Corbin CJ, Graham-Lorence S, McPhaul M, Mason JI, Mendelson CR, Simpson ER: **Isolation of a full-length cDNA insert encoding human aromatase system cytochrome P-450 and its expression in non-steroidogenic cells.** *Proc Natl Acad Sci USA* 1988, **85:**8948–8952.
2. Simpson ER, Mahendroo MS, Means GD, Kilgore MW, Hinshelwood MM, Graham-Lorence S, Amarneh B, Ito Y, Fisher R, Michael MD, Mendelson CR, Bulun SE: **Aromatase cytochrome P450, the enzyme responsible for oestrogen biosynthesis.** *Endocr Rev* 1994, **15:**342–355.
3. Belgorosky A, Rivarola MA: **Physiology and pathophysiology of oestrogens: lessons from paediatric patients with complete aromatase deficiency.** *Endocrinologist* 2004, **14:**1–8.
4. Means GD, Mahendroo MS, Corbin CJ, Mathis JM, Powell FE, Mendelson CR, Simpson ER: **Structural analysis of the gene encoding human aromatase cytochrome P-450, the enzyme responsible for estrogen biosynthesis.** *J Biol Chem* 1989, **264:**19385–19391.
5. Harada N, Yamada K, Saito K, Kibe N, Dohmaet S, Takagi Y: **Structural characterization of the human estrogen synthesis (aromatase) gene.** *Biochem Biophys Res Commun* 1990, **166:**365–372.
6. Mahendroo MS, Means GD, Mendelson CR, Simpson ER: **Tissue-specific expression of human P-450AROM. The promoter responsible for expression in adipose tissue is different from that utilised in placenta.** *J Biol Chem* 1991, **266:**11276–11281.
7. Graham-Lorence S, Amarneh B, White RE, Peterson JA, Simpson ER: **A three-dimensional model of aromatase cytochrome 450.** *Protein Sci* 1995, **4:**1065–1080.
8. Shozu M, Akasofu K, Harada T, Kubota Y: **A new cause of female pseudohermaphroditism: placental aromatase deficiency.** *J Clin Endocrinol Metab* 1991, **72:**560–566.
9. Belgorosky A, Guercio G, Pepe C, Saraco N, Rivarola MA: **Genetic and clinical spectrum of aromatase deficiency in infancy, childhood and adolescence.** *Horm Res* 2009, **72:**321–330.
10. Hauri-Hohl A, Meyer-Böni M, Lang-Muritano M, Hauri-Hohl M, Schoenle EJ, Biason-Lauber A: **Aromatase deficiency owing to a functional variant in the placenta promoter and a novel missense mutation in the *CYP19A1* gene.** *Clin Endocrinol (Oxf)* 2011, **75:**39–43.
11. Ludwikowski B, Heger S, Datz N, Richter-Unruh A, González R: **Aromatase deficiency: rare cause of virilization.** *Eur J Pediatr Surg* 2013, **23:**418-422.
12. Verma N, Jain V, Birla S, Jain R, Sharma A: **Growth and hormonal profile from birth to adolescence of a girl with aromatase deficiency.** *J Pediatr Endocrinol Metab* 2012, **25:**1185–1190.
13. Lin L, Ercan O, Raza J, Burren CP, Creighton SM, Auchus RJ, Dattani MT, Achermann JC: **Variable phenotypes associated with aromatase (CYP19) insufficiency in humans.** *J Clin Endocrinol Metab* 2007, **92:**982–990.
14. Ito Y, Fisher CR, Conte FA, Grumbach MM, Simpson ER: **Molecular basis of aromatase deficiency in an adult female with sexual infantilism and polycystic ovaries.** *Proc Natl Acad Sci USA* 1993, **90:**11673–11677.
15. Morishima A, Grumbach MM, Simpson ER, Fisher C, Qin K: **Aromatase deficiency in male and female siblings caused by a novel mutation and the physiological role of oestrogens.** *J Clin Endocrinol Metab* 1995, **80:**3689–3698.
16. Mullis PE, Yoshimura N, Kuhlmann B, Lippuner K, Jaeger P, Harada H: **Aromatase deficiency in a female who is compound heterozygote for two new point mutations in the P450arom gene: impact of oestrogens on hypergonadotropic hypogonadism, multicystic ovaries, and bone densitometry in childhood.** *J Clin Endocrinol Metab* 1997, **82:**1739–1745.
17. Belgorosky A, Pepe C, Marino R, Guercio G, Saraco N, Vaiani E, Rivarola MA: **Hypothalamic-pituitary-ovarian axis during infancy, early and late prepuberty in an aromatase-deficient girl who is a compound heterozygote for two new point mutations of the CYP19 gene.** *J Clin Endocrinol Metab* 2003, **88:**5127–5131.
18. Janner M, Flück CE, Mullis PE: **Impact of oestrogen replacement throughout childhood on growth, pituitary-gonadal axis and bone in a 46, XX patient with CYP19A1 deficiency.** *Horm Res Paediatr* 2012, **78:**261–268.

19. Lubahn DB, Moyer JS, Golding TS, Couse JF, Korach KS, Smithies O: **Alteration of reproductive function but not prenatal sexual development after insertional disruption of the mouse oestrogen receptor gene.** *Proc Natl Acad Sci USA* 1993, **90**:11162–11166.
20. Lanfranco F, Zirilli L, Baldi M, Pignatti E, Corneli G, Ghigo E, Aimaretti G, Carani C, Rochira V: **A novel mutation in the human aromatase gene: insights on the relationship among serum oestradiol, longitudinal growth and bone mineral density in an adult man under oestrogen replacement treatment.** *Bone* 2008, **43**:628–635.
21. Maffei L, Rochira V, Zirilli L, Antunez P, Aranda C, Fabre B, Simone ML, Pignatti E, Simpson ER, Houssami S, Clyne CD, Carani C: **A novel compound heterozygous mutation of the aromatase gene in an adult man: reinforced evidence on the relationship between congenital oestrogen deficiency, adiposity and the metabolic syndrome.** *Clin Endocrinol (Oxf)* 2007, **67**:218–224.
22. Rochira V, Madeo B, Zirilli L, Caffagni G, Maffei L, Carani C: **Oestradiol replacement treatment and glucose homeostasis in two men with congenital aromatase deficiency: evidence for a role of oestradiol and sex steroids imbalance on insulin sensitivity in men.** *Diabet Med* 2007, **24**:1491–1495.
23. Guercio G, Di Palma MI, Pepe C, Saraco NI, Prieto M, Saure C, Mazza C, Rivarola MA, Belgorosky A: **Metformin, estrogen replacement therapy and gonadotropin inhibition fail to improve insulin sensitivity in a girl with aromatase deficiency.** *Horm Res* 2009, **72**:370–376.
24. Czajka-Oraniec IK, Chik C, Mitchell R, Yuen AHL, Brown KA, Clyne C, Simpson ER: **Long-term effects of estrogen deprivation in an aromatase deficient woman.** In *Program of the 90th Annual Meeting of The Endocrine Society, San Francisco, CA.* 2008:1–610.
25. Von Prader A: **Der genitalbefund beim pseudohermaphroditismus femininus des kongenitalen adrenogenitalen syndromes.** *Helv Pediatr Acta* 1954, **9**:231–248.
26. Flück CE, Miller WL: **P450 oxidoreductase deficiency: a new form of congenital adrenal hyperplasia.** *Curr Opin Pediatr* 2006, **18**:435–441.
27. Ghosh D, Griswold J, Erman M, Pangborn W: **Structural basis for androgen specificity and oestrogen synthesis in human aromatase.** *Nature* 2009, **457**:219–223.
28. Rost B, Yachdav G, Liu J: **The predict-protein server.** *Nucleic Acids Res* 2004, **32**:W321–W326.
29. Adamczak K, Porollo A, Meller J: **Accurate prediction of solvent accessibility using neural networks-based regression.** *Proteins* 2004, **56**:753–767.
30. Pollastri G, McLysaght A: **Porter: a new, accurate server for protein secondary structure prediction.** *Bioinformatics* 2005, **21**:1719–1720.
31. Ma CX, Adjei AA, Salavaggione OE, Coronel J, Pelleymounter L, Wang L, Eckloff BW, Schaid D, Wieben ED, Adjei AA: **Human aromatase: gene resequencing and functional genomics.** *Cancer Res* 2005, **65**:11071–11082.
32. Quaynor SD, Stradtman EW Jr, Kim HG, Shen Y, Chorich LP, Schreihofer DE, Layman LC: **Delayed puberty and estrogen resistance in a woman with estrogen receptor α variant.** *New Engl J Med* 2013, **369**:164–171.
33. Rochira V, Carani C: **Aromatase deficiency in men: a clinical perspective.** *Nat Rev Endocrinol* 2009, **5**:559–568.
34. Carani C, Qin K, Simoni M, Faustini-Fustini M, Serpenter S, Boyd J, Korach KS, Simpson ER: **Effect of testosterone and estradiol in a man with aromatase deficiency.** *New Engl J Med* 1997, **337**:91–95.
35. Smith EP, Boyd J, Frank GR, Takahashi H, Cohen RM, Specker B, Williams TC, Lubahn DB, Korach KS: **Oestrogen resistance caused by a mutation in the oestrogen-receptor gene in a man.** *New Engl J Med* 1994, **331**:1056–1061.
36. Heine PA, Taylor JA, Iwamoto GA, Lubahn DB, Cooke PS: **Increased adipose tissue in male and female oestrogen receptor-α knockout mice.** *Proc Natl Acad Sci* 2000, **97**:12729–12734.
37. Herrmann BL, Saller B, Janssen OE, Gocke P, Bockisch A, Sperling H, Mann K, Broecker M: **Impact of estrogen replacement therapy in a male with congenital aromatase deficiency caused by a novel mutation in the CYP19 gene.** *J Clin Endocrinol Metab* 2002, **87**:5476–5484.
38. Maffei L, Murata Y, Rochira V, Tubert G, Aranda C, Vazquez M, Clyne CD, Davis S, Simpson ER, Carani C: **Dysmetabolic syndrome in a man with a novel mutation of the aromatase gene: effects of testosterone, alendronate, and oestradiol treatment.** *J Clin Endocrinol Metab* 2004, **89**:61–70.
39. Herrmann BL, Janssen OE, Hahn S, Brocker-Preuss M, Mann K: **Effect of estrogen replacement therapy on bone and glucose metabolism in a male with congenital aromatase deficiency.** *Horm Metab Res* 2005, **37**:178–183.
40. Britt KL, Drummond AE, Cox VA, Dyson M, Wreford NG, Jones MEE, Simpson ER, Findlay JK: **An age-related ovarian phenotype in mice with targeted disruption of the *Cyp19* (Aromatase) gene.** *Endocrinology* 2000, **141**:2614–2623.
41. Britt KL, Drummond AE, Dyson M, Wreford NG, Jones ME, Simpson ER, Findlay JK: **The ovarian phenotype of the aromatase knockout (ArKO) mouse.** *J Steroid Biochem Mol Biol* 2001, **79**:181–185.
42. Jones MEE, Thorburn AW, Britt KL, Hewitt KN, Wreford NG, Proietto J, Oz OK, Lewy BJ, Robertson KM, Yoo S, Simpson ER: **Aromatase-deficient (ArKO) mice have a phenotype of increased adiposity.** *Proc Natl Acad Sci USA* 2000, **97**:12735–12740.
43. Takeda K, Toda K, Saibara T, Nagakawa M, Saika K, Onishi T, Sugiura T, Shizuta Y: **Progressive development of insulin resistance phenotype in male mice with complete aromatase (CYP19) deficiency.** *J Endocrinol* 2003, **176**:237–246.
44. Hewitt KN, Pratis K, Jones MEE, Simpson ER: **Estrogen replacement reverses the hepatic steatosis in the male aromatase knockout mouse.** *Endocrinology* 2004, **145**:1842–1848.
45. Peiris AN, Aiman EJ, Drucker WD, Kissebah AH: **The relative contribution of hepatic and peripheral tissues to insulin resistance in hyperandrogenic women.** *J Clin Endocrinol Metab* 1989, **68**:715–720.
46. Friedl KE, Jones RE, Hannan CJ Jr, Plymate SR: **The administration of pharmacological doses of testosterone or 19-nortestosterone to normal men is not associated with increased insulin secretion or impaired glucose tolerance.** *J Clin Endocrinol Metab* 1989, **68**:971–975.
47. Wilson PD, Barker G, Barnard RJ, Siddle NC: **Steroid receptors in the lower female urinary tract.** *Urol Int* 1984, **39**:39–58.
48. Conte FA, Grumbach MM, Ito Y, Fisher CR, Simpson ER: **A syndrome of female pseudohermaphrodism, hypergonadotropic hypogonadism, and multicystic ovaries associated with missense mutations in the gene encoding aromatase.** *J Clin Endocrinol Metab* 1994, **78**:1287–1292.

6

Current practice of glucocorticoid replacement therapy and patient-perceived health outcomes in adrenal insufficiency

M Forss[1*], G Batcheller[1], S Skrtic[2] and G Johannsson[3]

Abstract

Background: The aim was to survey current practice in glucocorticoid replacement therapy and self-perceived health outcomes in patients with adrenal insufficiency.

Methods: Participants were recruited via patient organizations to respond anonymously to a web-based survey developed by clinical experts. Unique entries were set up for each patient organization enabling geographical localization of the entries.

Results: 1245 participants responded (primary adrenal insufficiency: 84%; secondary adrenal insufficiency: 11%; unsure: 5%). Therapies included hydrocortisone (75%), prednisone/prednisolone (11%), cortisone acetate (6%) and dexamethasone (4%). Dosing regimens were once daily (10%), twice daily (42%), thrice daily (32%) or other (17%). Compromised subjective health necessitating changes to physical activity or social-, work- or family life was reported by 64% of the participants. 40% of the participants reported absence from work/school in the last 3 months. Irrespective of diagnosis, 76% were concerned about long-term side-effects of therapy, mainly osteoporosis (78%), obesity (64%) and cardiovascular morbidity (46%). 38% of the participants had been hospitalized in the last year.

Conclusions: Glucocorticoid replacement therapy among the respondents consisted primarily of hydrocortisone administered twice or thrice daily. A majority reported impact of their disease or treatment on subjective health requiring alterations in e.g. physical activity or family life. Three quarters reported concerns about long-term side-effects of the treatment. These data demonstrate - from the patients' perspective - a need for improvement in the management of adrenal insufficiency.

Background

Recent data indicate that replacement therapy with glucocorticoids in adrenal insufficiency (AI) is associated with poor long-term outcome. In the two largest registry-based studies on mortality in patients with Addison's disease, the relative risk of death was more than 2-fold compared to the background population despite treatment [1,2]. Patients with hypopituitarism and secondary AI also have increased relative risk of death [3]. Based on the increase in cardiovascular risk factors [4,5] and reduced bone mineral density (mainly in female AI patients) [6-10], overly high glucocorticoid exposure is likely to occur at least during parts of the day/night. This is supported by data showing an inverse relationship between dose exposure and bone mineral density [7]. Due to the short half-life of hydrocortisone, each oral dose is followed by a rapid increase and often an overly high peak in serum cortisol concentration followed by a rapid decline. Multiple doses of immediate-release hydrocortisone tablets are needed in order to cover the active part of the day but result in a peak after each dose and a trough between doses. It has been estimated that AI patients are on average over-substituted by 6-7 mg hydrocortisone/day based on an

* Correspondence: maria.forss@duocort.com
[1]DuoCort Pharma, Medicinaregatan 8A, 413 46, Gothenburg, Sweden
Full list of author information is available at the end of the article

ideal body mass area-dose ratio of 11 mg/m^2 [11]. Besides symptoms indicating over-exposure to glucocorticoids, e.g. a tendency to gain weight, symptoms indicating underexposure, e.g. salt craving, were also commonly reported in a previous survey [12].

The subjective health-related quality of life (QoL) of AI patients is impaired on a group level [13-16] with health scores inferior to those of the background population. General health and vitality have been found to be consistently impaired [13], with fatigue being the most characteristic subjective health feature of AI [12,13]. Working ability is reduced to various degrees in different countries [11-14]. Attempts to re-establish the normal cortisol exposure-time profile have in an open study demonstrated improvement in well-being [17], and improved QoL was observed in another study when changing from a twice daily (BID) to a thrice daily (TID) regimen [18]. These data suggest that the peaks and troughs between doses may to some extent explain the poor self-perceived well-being reported by patients.

The aim of this patient survey was to investigate current practice in glucocorticoid replacement therapy (therapy and dosage regimen) in patients with primary or secondary AI in different countries and the participants' self-perceived health status and outcomes by type of disease and therapy.

Methods

This was an open cross-sectional survey. Participants were recruited via patient organizations (e-mail contact lists and newsletters) to respond anonymously to the web-based survey. The following patient organizations actively approached their members to participate in the survey and had links to the survey on their home page: National Adrenal Diseases Foundation (NADF) in the US, Australian Addison's Disease Foundation, Addison's Disease Self Help Group (ADSHG) in the UK and Cushing's Support and Research Foundation (CSRF) in the US. Some additional patient organizations also had information about and/or links to the survey on their respective websites: CARES foundation in the US, Association Surrénales in France, two Swedish associations (The Swedish Addison Association and Hypofysis), two Danish associations (Addisonforeningen in Denmark and Danish Morbus Addison Site), the Dutch Addison & Cushing Society (NVACP) and Associazioni Italiana Pazienti Addison in Italy. A link was also set up on the sponsor's website for other patients wanting to complete the survey.

The questionnaire covered a range of questions (39 questions in total), including patient demographics (country, type of disease, etc.), medication and satisfaction with the current medication. It also covered impact of the disease on self-perceived subjective health, the prevalence and impact of fatigue, views on long-term side effects related to treatment, hospitalizations and absenteeism from work or school. The questionnaire consisted of a mix of single select, multiple select and open questions. A pilot survey was conducted with four members from different patient organizations to ensure the validity of the questions in the questionnaire. Revisions were then made to the questionnaire before the survey was conducted. In order to ensure the privacy of the participants' contact details, it was agreed that each patient organization should send out alerts via e-mail and newsletters to inform its members about the survey and its objectives. Although no research ethics committee approval is needed for the conduct of this kind of patient survey [19], a research application had to be completed for the UK patient organization ADSHG, in order to be able to recruit volunteers from their membership registry. No remuneration was given to the participants. No data on age and gender were collected in order to further protect the individual identity of the participants.

Unique links for each patient organization were set up in the web survey tool Easyresearch (by QuestBack, Oslo, Norway), the technical platform used for administration and analysis of the survey. The unique entries enabled geographical localization of the entries. The intention was to have the survey open for approximately 6 weeks, but the survey opening time was extended as a result of the high degree of interest from individual patients and additional patient organizations. The survey was open from September 12th to December 19th 2008.

The data were analyzed descriptively (frequency analysis) by disease type (primary or secondary AI), treatment and dosing regimen. The country-specific analyses included only countries with more than 20 participants. The denominator for the calculation of frequency varied between the questions since not all participants answered all questions. The asking of some of the questions, such as on subjective general health, was dependent on previous answers (e.g. degree of impact on QoL was only asked if the participant had answered that the disease affected their QoL). No statistical tests were performed.

Results

A total of 1281 persons visited the webpage of the survey whereof 1245 responded to at least the first question ("In which country do you live?"). The respondents were from (by number of participants): US (801), Australia (90), France (81), UK (80), Canada (37), Sweden (35), Denmark (19), the Netherlands (8), Germany (7), Belgium (6), New Zealand (5), Mexico (4), Ecuador (3), Ireland (3), Spain (3), Chile (2), Dominican Republic (2), India (2), Norway (2), Philippines (2), Poland (2), South Africa (2), Switzerland (2), Argentina (1), Dubai (1),

Greece (1), Hungary (1), Israel (1), Italy (1), Jamaica (1), Martinique (1), Portugal (1), Serbia (1) and Uruguay (1).

When asked "What type of cortisol deficiency are you suffering from?", 939 participants (84%) defined their AI as primary (Addison's disease, congenital adrenal hyperplasia, adrenal disease causing dysfunction of adrenal glands or removed glands) and 125 (11%) as secondary (pituitary or hypothalamic disease) while 51 (5%) were unsure.

Glucocorticoid treatment regimen

Overall, hydrocortisone was used by 75% of the participants, prednisone/prednisolone by 11%, cortisone acetate by 6% and dexamethasone by 4% of the participants, Table 1. A high proportion of participants (40%) in Australia reported using cortisone acetate. Among the countries with at least 20 respondents, the use of prednisone/prednisolone was most common in Canada (27%), the US (14%) and Australia (11%) and dexamethasone was most commonly used in Australia (5%) and the US (4%). The distribution of therapies was similar between patients with primary and secondary AI. The majority of the patients were on BID (42%), or TID (32%), while 10% were on an OD regimen, Table 1. Of the patients on a BID regimen, 58% took their medication in the morning and afternoon and 42% in the morning and evening. Patients with secondary AI took their BID dosing in the morning and afternoon (39%) rather than in the morning and evening (9%). 53% of the patients on prednisone/prednisolone were on BID and 5% on TID. For treatment regimen by therapy, please see Table 2.

One quarter (23%) of the participants were dissatisfied or very dissatisfied with their current treatment, 18%

Table 1 Therapy and dosing regimen, by type of adrenal insufficiency, reported in an international patient survey

		Primary AI	Secondary AI	All
		n (%)	n (%)	n (%)
Therapy	Hydrocortisone	697 (75%)	98 (80%)	833 (75%)
	Prednisone, prednisolone	100 (11%)	12 (10%)	124 (11%)
	Cortisone acetate	57 (6%)	4 (3%)	63 (6%)
	Dexamethasone	35 (4%)	4 (3%)	39 (4%)
	Other	38 (4%)	4 (3%)	50 (5%)
	N	N = 927	N = 122	N = 1109
Dosing regimen	Once daily	80 (9%)	14 (12%)	104 (10%)
	Twice daily	360 (42%)	58 (48%)	437 (42%)
	Thrice daily	291 (34%)	25 (21%)	328 (32%)
	Other	135 (16%)	23 (19%)	173 (17%)
	N	N = 866	N = 120	N = 1042

Note: The number of patients responding to the question about therapy was not the same as the number of patients reporting dosing regimen (different questions).

Table 2 Dosing regimen, by therapy, reported in an international patient survey

	Hydrocortisone	Prednisone/ prednisolone	Cortisone acetate	All
	n (%)	n (%)	n (%)	n (%)
	(N = 772)	(N = 116)	(N = 60)	(N = 1042)
Once daily	47 (6%)	35 (30%)	4 (7%)	104 (10%)
Twice daily	304 (39%)	61 (53%)	44 (73%)	437 (42%)
Thrice daily	301 (39%)	6 (5%)	8 (13%)	328 (32%)
Other	120 (16%)	14 (12%)	4 (7%)	173 (17%)

Note: The number of patients recording dosing regimen was not the same as the number of patients reporting therapy (Table 1).

were indifferent and 59% were satisfied or very satisfied. Patients with secondary AI reported less satisfaction with their current therapy than patients with primary AI. The ratings of satisfaction were similar among the different therapies.

Multiple daily dosing was reported as a problem by 38% of the participants whereof 15% were on OD, 35% on BID, 32% on TID and 17% on another regimen. Of those who did not find multiple daily dosing to be a problem 7% were on OD, 45% on BID, 32% on TID and 16% on another regimen. Among respondents answering that multiple daily dosing was a problem 94% reported one or more of the following: difficulties to remember/forgetting doses (particularly the midday and afternoon doses), difficulties in taking the medication at a specific time every day and/or difficulties to remember to bring the medication. Many reported that their days are planned according to their dose intake and for those who lead a busy life and are working, this was found to be challenging as some also reported that they do not want to be seen by their colleagues when taking their medication. Several reported that multiple daily dosing becomes very restrictive to an active life and that multiple daily dosing is a reminder several times per day that they have this disease. Many also reported health issues such as being fatigue and exhausted in the day, evening and the following day(s) if missing a dose. In addition, many reported that taking a missed dose too late disrupts their sleep and causes issues with insomnia. Some reported instability of physical and mental well-being with mood swings and ups and downs in energy levels. The patients who reported multiple daily dosing to be a problem also reported higher frequencies of impacted QoL, more fatigue and more activities altered due to their disease (data not shown).

Enduring efficacy over 24 hours was considered the most important feature of an optimal replacement medication (29%) followed by few side effects (25%) and low risk of adrenal crisis (22%). Similar responses were obtained from patients with primary and secondary AI.

Health-related questions and hospitalizations

A majority of the patients (648 of 1026 [64%]) reported impacted quality of life (QoL) due to their illness, 87% (99 of 114) of patients with secondary AI and 60% (515 of 857) of the patients with primary AI. Approximately three quarters (73 of 99 [74%]) of the patients with secondary AI graded the impact on QoL as "quite a lot" or "very much", Table 3. The proportion of patients who reported impaired QoL varied with dosing regimen (OD > BID > TID). However, the level of impairment did not differ between the dosing regimens. A lower proportion of patients treated with hydrocortisone reported impaired QoL compared with patients receiving cortisone acetate or prednisone/prednisolone but the level of impairment did not differ between the therapies (data not country-adjusted).

All patients were asked "What activities do you need to alter due to your AI?", regardless of whether they had answered that their QoL was impaired or not. A large percentage of the participants reported that they had had to alter their physical activity (56%), social life (40%), work life (39%) or family life (31%) due to their illness (the participants were allowed to choose more than one alternative). A higher proportion of patients with secondary AI (90%) than with primary AI (68%) reported that they had had to alter work life, social life, physical activity or family life, Figure 1.

A majority of the participants reported fatigue in the morning (57%) and during the day (65%) to be a problem. Fatigue was more pronounced in patients with secondary AI than in patients with primary AI, Table 4. Of those reporting morning fatigue to be a problem, 75% also reported fatigue during the day to be a problem. Similarly, of those reporting fatigue during the day to be a problem, 85% also reported morning fatigue to be a problem.

In this survey, 61% of the respondents considered themselves fit to work while 17% did not. Additionally 5% of the respondents both considered themselves unfit to work and were on sick leave, 10% were retired and 7% were unemployed. Of those considering themselves fit to work, 72% considered themselves fit to work full-time, while 18% could work 75%, 9% could work 50% and 1% could work <50%. Overall, 40% of the participants had been absent from work in the last 3 months and, again, this was more common among patients suffering from secondary AI (50%) than for patients with primary AI (38%). Almost one third (28%) of those being away from work or school reported more than 3 weeks' absence in the 3 months preceding their participation in the survey, Table 5. A higher percentage of patients treated with prednisone/prednisolone reported absenteeism compared with patients on hydrocortisone and they also reported more lengthy absenteeism (data not shown).

A majority of the participants were worried about long-term side effects. The participants were most worried about osteoporosis (79%), followed by obesity (64%), fatigue (52%) and cardiovascular problems (46%) (more than one alternative could be chosen), Table 6. A higher proportion of those treated with prednisone/prednisolone were worried about long-term side effects than those treated with hydrocortisone (data not shown).

Overall, 32% of the participants reported that they increased their dose due to physical activity at least once per week (primary AI patients: 30%; secondary AI patients: 49%) and 66% increased their dose due to illness at least once per month (primary AI patients: 65%; secondary AI patients: 76%).

Overall, 38% of the participants responding to the question about hospitalizations (N = 977) answered that they had been hospitalized at least once during the last 12 months (37% of patients with primary AI and 43% of patients with secondary AI). One third of the patients (32%) had been hospitalized more than once during the last 12 months. The reported reason for hospitalization was adrenal crisis, vomiting or an acute infection for 17% of the patients who had been hospitalized.

Table 3 Impact of adrenal insufficiency on quality of life (QoL) captured in an international survey

		Primary AI	Secondary AI	All
		n (%)	n (%)	n (%)
Impact on QoL	Yes	515 (60%)	99 (87%)	658 (64%)
	N	N = 857	N = 114	N = 1026
Degree of impacton QoL	A little	73 (14%)	10 (10%)	86 (13%)
	Intermediate	170 (33%)	16 (16%)	195 (30%)
	Quite a lot or very much	267 (52%)	73 (74%)	372 (57%)
	N	N = 510	N = 99	N = 653

Discussion

The conduct of this survey was similar to previous cross-sectional surveys with participants recruited via patient organizations [5,11,12]. The current survey of 1245 respondents is to our knowledge the largest patient survey to date in patients with AI. Previous studies have shown that outcomes in patients with AI are compromised [12-14]. The responses from this survey provide more information on the impact of the disease and its treatment on patient-perceived outcomes, and support previous data showing a large impact of the disease and its treatment on the daily life of these patients.

Therapy traditions differ to some extent between countries but hydrocortisone was the most commonly used therapy in this survey (75%), irrespectively of country, which is also in line with previous studies from Europe [4,20]. The distribution of therapies, i.e. type of

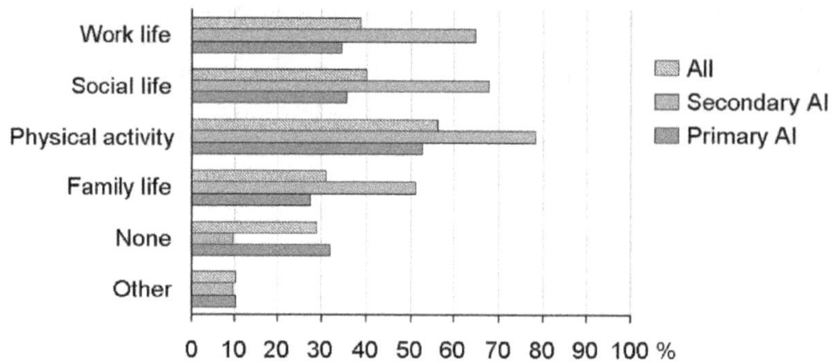

Figure 1 Change in activities due to adrenal insufficiency. Responses to the question "What activities do you need to alter due to your adrenal insufficiency"? in an international patient survey. A total of 1001 subjects responded to this question.

glucocorticoid, was similar between patients with primary and secondary AI. Three quarters of the patients were on a BID or TID regimen. One unexpected observation in this survey was the high percentage (58%) of patients on prednisone/prednisolone who were on a BID or TID regimen.

That multiple daily dosing is a problem from a compliance point of view is well known from other therapies [21]. The free-text answers to the open questions of this survey confirmed that multiple daily dosing is not optimal in AI and has an impact on patients' social life and work life. More specifically, 4 of 10 patients in this survey found multiple daily dosing to be a problem. The impact on leading a normal life was attributed both to multiple dosing and to fluctuations in mental/physical energy over the day as multiple daily dosing with hydrocortisone/cortisone acetate causes peaks and low trough values in-between dosing occasions. When asked about the most important features of an optimal replacement medication, the patients ranked efficacy over 24 hours first and few side effects second. More patients on TID were satisfied with their treatment compared to those on BID or OD treatment. This might be attributable to the better cortisol coverage of TID during the active part of the day [22,23] over the convenience of fewer dosing times.

The results from this survey are in line with a recently published clinical study [24] which showed that a majority of the patients preferred the four-daily dosing regimen to twice daily when comparing equal doses of hydrocortisone given either twice daily or four times daily. The reasons reported were less fatigue, more alertness during the day, less headache and a feeling that the treatment effect was less varying during the day. The patients had complaints after the study that a four-dose regimen may be difficult to manage in the long run [24]. Another study has shown that a thrice-daily administration with weight-adjusted doses provides a better PK profile within the constraints of immediate-release hydrocortisone formulations [25]. 85% of the patients opted to remain on the TID regimen given in that study. These data suggest that patients experience benefits of having increased cortisol coverage during the active part of the day. One caveat of the above studies is that the total exposure of cortisol is higher when the same daily dose of hydrocortisone is administered divided into three or four daily doses than at BID administration. This is due to the fact that increasing the dose of hydrocortisone at one dose occasion does not result in a proportional increase in total exposure of cortisol due to the non-linear bioavailability of orally administered hydrocortisone [26]. Thus, there might be a short-term

Table 4 Fatigue in the morning and during the day reported by patients with adrenal insufficiency in an international patient survey

		Primary AI	Secondary AI	All
		n (%)	n (%)	n (%)
Fatigue experienced as a problem in the morning	Yes	438 (53%)	91 (81%)	571 (57%)
	N	N = 832	N = 113	N = 998
Fatigue experienced as a problem during the day	Yes	508 (61%)	99 (87%)	644 (65%)
	N	N = 830	N = 114	N = 995

Table 5 Absenteeism from work or school due to adrenal insufficiency in the last 3 months reported in an international patient survey

		Primary AI	Secondary AI	All
		n (%)	n (%)	n (%)
Any abseenteism	Yes	299 (38%)	54 (50%)	379 (40%)
	N	N = 796	N = 108	N = 951
No. of days of abseenteism	1-5	174 (59%)	17 (33%)	198 (53%)
	6-10	37 (13%)	6 (12%)	46 (12%)
	11-15	16 (5%)	5 (10%)	23 (6%)
	>16	70 (24%)	24 (46%)	107 (29%)
	N	N = 297	N = 52	N = 374

Table 6 Worries about long-term effects reported by patients with adrenal insufficiency in an international patient survey

		Primary AI	Secondary AI	Respondents
		n (%)	n (%)	n (%)
Any worry	Yes	612 (75%)	93 (82%)	740 (76%)
	N	N = 819	N = 113	N = 977
Pre-specified long-term effects	Osteoporosis	477 (79%)	76 (82%)	578 (79%)
	Obesity	374 (62%)	72 (77%)	464 (64%)
	Fatigue	301 (50%)	63 (68%)	381 (52%)
	Cardiovascular	258 (43%)	58 (62%)	334 (46%)
	Infectious disease	230 (38%)	52 (56%)	300 (41%)
	Other	117 (20%)	15 (16%)	138 (19%)
	N	N = 601	N = 93	N = 728

perceived benefit of the increased cortisol exposure whereas the long-term risk may increase.

It is difficult to mimic physiological cortisol profiles with immediate release hydrocortisone replacement therapies [22,25]. Therefore, attempts to better mimic the normal cortisol profiles have been made by developing new treatment regimens using the concept of chronotherapy, i.e. considering circadian rhythms in determining the timing and amount of the medication to optimize the desired effects and minimize the undesired ones [17,27]. A once-daily treatment with dual action, combining immediate release and extended release hydrocortisone has shown benefit over immediate release hydrocortisone with the same daily dosing administered thrice daily in patients with adrenal insufficiency [28].

Two thirds of the participants reported impacted QoL from their illness. In line with this being a patient survey (capturing the patient's general perception of their subjective health at only one time point) and not a clinical trial, the questionnaire used in this survey did not include validated QoL questions from specific QoL questionnaires. Instead, the included questions were focused on the patients' general perception of how and to what degree their disease and/or treatment affected their QoL. This survey showed that patients with secondary AI perceived their QoL as more impaired than patients with primary AI, which is in agreement with a previous study using validated QoL questionnaires showing that patients with AI have compromised QoL and that the impairment of QoL is worse in patients with secondary AI [14]. The current survey did not collect data on comorbidities. Patients with secondary adrenal insufficiency may have other hormone deficiencies which could impact on QoL. However, data from previous studies are inconsistent and while some impact was observed in a Norwegian study of patients with Addison's disease [13], another study [14] showed that the impairment in health-related subjective health status in AI patients is largely independent of concomitant diseases.

More than half of the AI patients needed to alter their physical activity and many needed to change their social life, work life or family life due to their illness. The level of impact on social life is in line with data from another international survey, conducted in 2003, in which one-third reported that their condition impacted on their ability to participate in social activities [29]. A Dutch patient survey reports similar impact on lifestyle [5]. Detailed questions on fatigue were included in the current survey as fatigue is the most commonly reported subjective health-related problem in AI [5,11-13,29,30]. This survey showed that 57% of the participants experienced fatigue in the morning as a problem and 65% reported fatigue during the day to be a problem. This response is in some contrast to the general perception that morning fatigue is a much larger clinical problem than fatigue during the day in patients with AI who have low or undetectable serum morning cortisol levels when using hydrocortisone BID or TID. Fatigue was more common in secondary AI than in primary AI and often necessitated changes in daily activities or changes in dose or the timing of dosing.

The current survey demonstrated a high absenteeism from work or school. More specifically, 4 of 10 patients reported absenteeism from work or school due to AI in the last 3 months and one third of those reported more than 3 weeks' absence. Furthermore, 17% of the participants did not consider themselves to be fit to work. Among those who considered themselves fit to work, 28% worked part-time instead of full-time. These data are similar to those of a survey conducted across the UK, Canada, Australia and New Zealand (n = 850) [29], in which over 10% of the respondents reported that they were unable to work compared with 1% in the matched control group. Moreover, in the study by Hahner et al. [14], 18% of the AI patients (primary and secondary) did not work vs. 4% in the general population. In a Norwegian study, working disability amounted to 26% among patients with primary AI vs. 10% in the general population [13].

Patients with AI are educated to increase their glucocorticoid dose in stressful situations and in association with other illnesses. This survey showed that 60-75% of the patients increased their replacement dose due to illness every month. The high rate of hospitalizations in this survey (38% of the patients had been hospitalized at least once in the last year) is in line with the Dutch survey in which 3 of 10 patients had been hospitalized [5]. The reported reason for hospitalization was adrenal crisis, vomiting or an acute infection in 17% of the patients. As a comparison, the incidence rate of adrenal crises was 6.3 per 100 patient years in a study by Hahner et al.

[31]. The reason for this discrepancy is most likely the differences in methods of collecting data and that the definition of adrenal crisis is not the same, e.g. only cases of hospitalization necessitating i.v. glucocorticoid administration were counted as adrenal crises in the study by Hahner.

Because of the relatively small disease population, age and gender were not included in the questionnaire in order to protect personal integrity and anonymity. Internet use and behaviours linked to it are hypothetical confounding factors in the interpretation of the survey results. Patients who seek information about their disease usually tend to be more active than other patients, which can also affect the results. Despite the fact that congenital adrenal hyperplasia (CAH) constitutes one form of primary AI, it would have been interesting to analyse data on this patient group separately as recent data published by Arlt et al. (2010) showed significantly impaired health status and adverse metabolic and skeletal health in adult CAH patients [32], however, data were not separately collected for patients with CAH in this survey.

Conclusions

This international survey showed that the glucocorticoid replacement regimens in AI differ to some degree between countries. Three quarters of the AI patients participating in the survey received hydrocortisone administered two or three times daily. A large majority of the participants reported that their disease and the current treatment have an impact on QoL leading to alterations in physical activity, social life, work life and family life. Furthermore, 76% of the participants reported concerns of long-term side-effects of their treatment. These data demonstrate - from the AI patients' perspective – an obvious need for improvement in the management of AI including the regimen of glucocorticoid replacement therapy.

Competing interests
This survey was funded by DuoCort Pharma. MF works for DuoCort Pharma AB. *GB, SS and GJ* have equity interests in DuoCort AB.

Acknowledgements
We thank the participants in the survey and the patient organizations supporting their members to participate and share their experience. We also thank Karin Gewert, Writewise, who provided medical writing services on behalf of DuoCort Pharma.

Author details
[1]DuoCort Pharma, Medicinaregatan 8A, 413 46, Gothenburg, Sweden. [2]Department of Clinical Pharmacology, Sahlgrenska Academy, University of Gothenburg, Gothenburg, Sweden. [3]Department of Endocrinology, Sahlgrenska Academy, University of Gothenburg, Gothenburg, Sweden.

Authors' contributions
All authors contributed to the design of the survey and writing/review of the manuscript. All authors read and approved the final manuscript.

References

1. Bergthorsdottir R, Leonsson-Zachrisson M, Odén A, Johannsson G: **Premature mortality in patients with Addison's disease: a population-based study.** *J Clin Endocrinol Metab* 2006, **91**:4849–4853.
2. Bensing S, Brandt L, Tabaro F, Sjöberg O, Nilsson B, Ekbom A, Blomqvist P, Kämpe O: **Increased death risk and altered cancer incidence pattern in patients with isolated or combined autoimmune primary adrenocortical insufficiency.** *Clin Endocrinol (Oxf)* 2008, **69**:697–704.
3. Mills JL, Schonberger LB, Wysowski DK, Brown P, Durako SJ, Cox C, Kong F, Fradkin JE: **Long-term mortality in the United States cohort of pituitary-derived growth hormone recipients.** *J Pediat* 2004, **144**:430–436.
4. Filipsson H, Monson JP, Koltowska-Häggström M, Mattsson A, Johannsson G: **The impact of glucocorticoid replacement regimens on metabolic outcome and comorbidity in hypopituitary patients.** *Clin Endocrinol Metab* 2006, **91**:3954–3961.
5. Holleman J: **Illness, healthcare, and the quality of life.** In *A survey among patients with Addison's disease, Cushing's syndrome or congenital adrenal Hyperplasia (CAH)*. the Netherlands: Dutch Addison and Cushing Society: NVACP; 2006 (English version: November 2007). ISBN 90-78441-02-X.
6. Zelissen PM, Croughs RJ, van Rijk PP, Raymakers JA: **Effect of glucocorticoid replacement therapy on bone mineral density in patients with Addison disease.** *Ann Intern Med* 1994, **120**:207–210.
7. Løvås K, Gjesdal CG, Christensen M, Wolff AB, Almås B, Svartberg J, Fougner K, Syversen U, Bollerslev J, Falch JA, Hunt PJ, Chatterjee VKK, Husebye ES: **Glucocorticoid replacement therapy and pharmacogenetics in Addison's disease: effects on bone.** *Eur J Endocrinol* 2009, **160**:993–1002.
8. Devogelaer JP, Crabbé J, Nagant de Deuxchaisnes C: **Bone mineral density in Addison's disease: evidence for an effect of adrenal androgens on bone mass.** *Br Med J (Clin Res Ed)* 1987, **294**:798–800.
9. Florkowski CM, Holmes SJ, Elliot JR, Donald RA, Espiner EA: **Bone mineral density is reduced in female but not male subjects with Addison's disease.** *N Z Med J* 1994, **107**:52–53.
10. Ragnarsson O, Nyström HF, Johannsson G: **Glucocorticoid replacement therapy is independently associated with reduced bone mineral density in women with hypopituitarism.** *Clin Endocrinol (Oxf)* 2012, **76**:246–252.
11. Wass J, White K, Elliott A, Baker S, Arlt W, Chatterjee K, Croxson M, Gurnell E, Hunt P, Howlett T: **Medication management and quality of life in patients with primary adrenal insufficiency.** In *International Addison's survey 2003*. 2005. Poster presentation in Harrogate 2005. http://www.addisons.org.uk/comms/meetings/harrogateposter2005.pdf.
12. Margulies PL, Mullen J, National Adrenal Diseases Foundation: *North American survey of individuals with Addison's disease*. 1997. http://www.nadf.us/news/survey1997_text.pdf.
13. Løvås K, Loge JH, Husebye ES: **Subjective health status in Norwegian patients with Addison's disease.** *Clin Endocrinol (Oxf)* 2002, **56**:581–588.
14. Hahner S, Loeffler M, Fassnacht M, Weismann D, Koschker AC, Quinkler M, Decker O, Arlt W, Allolio B: **Impaired subjective health status in 256 patients with adrenal insufficiency on standard therapy based on cross-sectional analysis.** *J Clin Endocrinol Metab* 2007, **92**:3912–3922.
15. Gurnell EM, Hunt PJ, Curran SE, Conway CL, Pullenayegum EM, Huppert FA, Compston JE, Herbert J, Chatterjee VKK: **Long-term DHEA replacement in primary adrenal insufficiency: a randomized, controlled trial.** *J Clin Endocrinol Metab* 2008, **93**:400–409.
16. Erichsen MM, Løvås K, Skinningsrud B, Wolff AB, Undlien DE, Svartberg J, Fougner KJ, Berg TJ, Bollerslev J, Mella B, Carlson JA, Erlich H, Husebye ES: **Clinical, immunological, and genetic features of autoimmune primary adrenal insufficiency: observations from a Norwegian registry.** *J Clin Endocrinol Metab* 2009, **94**:4882–4890.
17. Løvås K, Husebye ES: **Continuous subcutaneous hydrocortisone infusion in Addison's disease.** *Eur J Endocrinol* 2007, **157**:109–112.
18. Groves RW, Toms GC, Houghton BJ, Monson JP: **Corticosteroid replacement therapy: twice or thrice daily?** *J R Soc Med* 1988, **81**:514–516.
19. British Healthcare Business Intelligence Association (BHBIA): *Legal and ethical guidelines for healthcare market research*. October 2011th edition. http://www.bhbia.org.uk/guidelines/legalandethicalguidelines.aspx.
20. Reynolds RM, Stewart PM, Seckl JR, Padfield PL: **Assessing the HPA axis in patients with pituitary disease: a UK survey.** *Clin Endocrinol (Oxf)* 2006, **64**:82–85.
21. World Health Organization: *Adherence to long-term therapies: evidence for action*. Geneva, Switzerland: 2003. http://www.who.int/chp/knowledge/publications/adherence_full_report.pdf.

22. Simon N, Castinetti F, Ouliac F, Lesavre N, Brue T, Oliver C: **Pharmacokinetic evidence for suboptimal treatment of adrenal insufficiency with currently available hydrocortisone tablets.** *Clin Pharmacokinet* 2010, **49:**455–463.
23. Blomgren J, Ekman B, Andersson PO, Arnqvist HJ: **Non-physiological levels of circulating cortisol in growth hormone-treated hypopituitary adults after conventional cortisone substitution.** *Scand J Clin Lab Invest* 2004, **64:**132–139.
24. Ekman B, Bachrach-Lindström M, Lindström T, Wahlberg J, Blomgren J, Arnqvist HJ: **A randomized double blind crossover study comparing two and four dose hydrocortisone regimen with regard to quality of life, cortisol and ACTH profiles in patients with primary adrenal insufficiency.** *Clin Endocrinol (Oxf)* 2012, **77:**18–25.
25. Mah PM, Jenkins RC, Rostami-Hodjegan A, Newell-Price J, Doane A, Ibbotson V, Tucker GT, Ross RJ: **Weight-related dosing, timing and monitoring hydrocortisone replacement therapy in patients with adrenal insufficiency.** *Clin Endocrinol (Oxf)* 2004, **61:**367–375.
26. Toothaker RD, Craig WA, Welling PG: **Effect of dose size on the pharmacokinetics of oral hydrocortisone suspension.** *J Pharm Sci* 1982, **71:**1182–1185.
27. Debono M, Ghobadi C, Rostami-Hodjegan A, Huatan H, Campbell MJ, Newell-Price J, Darzy K, Merke DP, Arlt W, Ross RJ: **Modified-release hydrocortisone to provide circadian cortisol profiles.** *J Clin Endocrinol Metab* 2009, **94:**1548–1554.
28. Johannsson G, Nilsson AG, Bergthorsdottir R, Burman P, Dahlqvist P, Ekman B, Engström BE, Olsson T, Ragnarsson O, Ryberg M, Wahlberg J, Biller BM, Monson JP, Stewart PM, Lennernäs H, Skrtic S: **Improved cortisol exposure-time profile and outcome in patients with adrenal insufficiency: a prospective randomized trial of a novel hydrocortisone dual-release formulation.** *J Clin Endocrinol Metab* 2012, **97:**473–481.
29. White KG, Wass JAHW, Elliott AE, Baker SJK: **Medication management and quality of life in patients with primary adrenal insufficiency. British Endocrine Societies Joint Meeting.** In *Endocrine Abstracts 9 P142.* 2005. http://www.endocrine-abstracts.org/ea/0009/ea0009p142.htm.
30. Løvås K, Curran S, Oksnes M, Husebye ES, Huppert FA, Chatterjee VK: **Development of a disease-specific quality of life questionnaire in Addison's disease.** *J Clin Endocrinol Metab* 2010, **95:**545–551.
31. Hahner S, Loeffler M, Bleicken B, Drechsler C, Milovanovic D, Fassnacht M, Ventz M, Quinkler M, Allolio B: **Epidemiology of adrenal crisis in chronic adrenal insufficiency: the need for new prevention strategies.** *Eur J Endocrinol* 2010, **162:**597–602.
32. Arlt W, Willis DS, Wild SH, Krone N, Doherty EJ, Hahner S, Han TS, Carroll PV, Conway GS, Rees DA, Stimson RH, Walker BR, Connell JM, Ross RJ: **United Kingdom Congenital Adrenal Hyperplasia Adult Study Executive (CaHASE): Health status of adults with congenital adrenal hyperplasia: a cohort study of 203 patients.** *J Clin Endocrinol Metab* 2010, **95:**5110–5121.

The clinical significance of aldosterone synthase deficiency: report of a novel mutation in the *CYP11B2* gene

Elaine Hui[1], Matthew CW Yeung[2], Pik To Cheung[3], Elaine Kwan[3], Louis Low[3], Kathryn CB Tan[1], Karen SL Lam[1] and Angel OK Chan[2*]

Abstract

Background: Aldosterone synthase (*CYP11B2*) deficiency is a rare autosomal recessive disorder, usually presenting with severe salt-wasting in infancy or stress-induced hyperkalaemia and postural hypotension in adulthood. Neonatal screening for congenital adrenal hyperplasia, another cause of salt wasting, using 17-hydroxyprogesterone measurement would fail to detect aldosterone synthase deficiency, a diagnosis which may be missed until the patient presents with salt-wasting crisis. Due to this potential life-threatening risk, comprehensive hormonal investigation followed by genetic confirmation for suspected patients would facilitate clinical management of the patient and assessment of the genetic implication in their offspring.

Case presentation: We describe a 33-year old Chinese man who presented in infancy with life-threatening hyponatraemia and failure to thrive, but remained asymptomatic on fludrocortisone since. Chromosomal analysis confirmed a normal male karyotype of 46, XY. Plasma steroid profile showed high plasma renin activity, low aldosterone level, and elevated 18-hydroxycorticosterone, compatible with type 2 aldosterone synthase deficiency. The patient was heterozygous for a novel *CYP11B2* mutation: c.977C > A (p.Thr326Lys) in exon 3. He also carried a heterozygous mutation c.523_525delAAG (p.Lys175del) in exon 6, a known pathogenic mutation causing aldosterone synthase deficiency. Sequencing of *CYP11B2* in his parents demonstrated that the mother was heterozygous for c.977C > A, and the father was heterozygous for c.523_525delAAG.

Conclusion: Although a rare cause of hyperreninaemic hypoaldosteronism, aldosterone synthase deficiency should be suspected and the diagnosis sought in patients who present with life-threatening salt-wasting in infancy, as it has a good long-term prognosis when adequate fludrocortisone replacement is instituted. To our knowledge, this is the first Chinese patient in which the molecular basis of aldosterone synthase deficiency has been identified.

Keywords: Aldosterone synthase deficiency, Salt-wasting, Hypoaldosteronism

Background

Aldosterone is the main mineralocorticoid hormone in humans that regulates sodium excretion and intravascular volume. It acts via distal renal tubules and cortical collecting ducts by increasing sodium reabsorption from and potassium excretion into the urine. It is synthesized by aldosterone synthase (*CYP11B2*), an enzyme encoded by *CYP11B2*, expression of which is almost entirely confined to the adrenal cortex and exclusively in the zona glomerulosa layer. Aldosterone synthase is a cytochrome P450 enzyme that catalyses the final 3 steps of aldosterone biosynthesis: first by the hydroxylation of deoxycorticosterone (DOC) at position 11β to form corticosterone (B), then the hydroxylation at position 18 to form 18-hydroxycorticosterone (18OHB), and lastly the oxidation at position 18 to aldosterone [1]. Isolated deficiencies of aldosterone biosynthesis are caused by inactivating mutations in the *CYP11B2* gene [2,3]. Aldosterone deficiency leads to excessive sodium excretion and potassium retention, resulting in hyponatraemia, hyperkalaemia, and

* Correspondence: cok436@ha.org.hk
[2]Department of Pathology, The University of Hong Kong, Queen Mary Hospital, Pokfulam Road, Pokfulam, Hong Kong
Full list of author information is available at the end of the article

metabolic acidosis. Cases of aldosterone synthase deficiency (ASD) have been identified in Iranian Jews, Europeans and North Americans [4]. In Asians, it has been reported in Thai, Japanese and Indian individuals [5,6]. To our knowledge, there has been no report of Chinese cases with confirmed genetic analysis. Here, we describe a case of aldosterone synthase deficiency in a Chinese man and results of *CYP11B2* analysis in the patient and his family.

Case presentation

Case report

The index patient, at the time of this report aged 33 years old, was delivered normally at term with a birth weight of 3.1 kg. He had repeated vomiting with poor feeding and failure to thrive at 5 weeks of age. He was found to have hyponatraemia and was started on cortisone acetate 2.5 mg three times daily and fludrocortisone 50 µg daily on the presumptive diagnosis of congenital adrenal hyperplasia. He had normal male phenotype and chromosomal analysis confirmed a normal male karyotype of 46, XY. He was evaluated with supervised treatment withdrawal by 6 months old. 24-hour urinary ketosteroid was normal but plasma renin activity was high and aldosterone was low, suggestive of hypoaldosteronism. Cortisone acetate was subsequently stopped. Plasma steroid profiling, which was performed after withholding therapy for a week at the age of 14.5 years old, gave characteristic findings of type 2 ASD (Table 1). Developmental milestones, electrolytes and blood pressure were normal while on fludrocortisone 100 µg daily. Both his unrelated parents and his older brother were phenotypically normal.

Genetic analysis

During family planning, genetic analysis was performed to ascertain the diagnosis at the age of 33 years. Blood samples were obtained and genomic DNA extracted from the patient, his brother and both non-consanguineous parents with informed consent. The nine coding exons and flanking intronic regions (15 bp) of the *CYP11B2* gene were amplified by polymerase chain reaction on the patient's genomic DNA, followed by direct DNA sequencing using primers and conditions as previously described [5]. Targeted mutational analysis was also performed on both parents and his brother's genomic DNA. The patient and family members' DNA sequences were compared to NCBI Reference Sequences, NG_008374.1, NM_000498.3 and NP_000489.3. The affected patient carried a novel heterozygous missense mutation: c.977C > A (p.Thr326Lys) in exon 3 (Figure 1), which has not previously been reported. He also carried a heterozygous mutation c.523_525delAAG (p.Lys175del) in exon 6, a known pathogenic frameshift mutation causing ASD [7]. Sequencing of *CYP11B2* in the parents demonstrated that the mother was heterozygous for c.977C > A (p.Thr326Lys) and the father was heterozygous for c.523_525delAAG (p.Lys175del). Neither mutation was detected in the patient's brother.

Table 1 Plasma steroid profile of the patient

	Basal (nmol/L)	Post-ACTH stimulation (nmol/L)
Aldosterone	0.166 (0.39-2.44)	0.19 (0.01 – 0.55)
18-OH-Corticosterone (18-OHB)	7.06 (0.56 – 1.46)	12.1 (0.83 – 5.5)
Corticosterone	44.4 (0.14 – 14.23)	151.8 (34.0 - 208.4)
18-OH-deoxycorticosterone	1.64 (0.13-0.72)	5.28 (0.58 – 6.1)
Deoxycorticosterone	0.57 (0.09 – 0.57)	2.36 (0.27 – 1.35)
Progesterone	1.94 (0.095 – 3.15)	2.96 (0.52 – 2.55)
17-hydroxyprogesterone	3.09 (0.24 – 4.93)	15.2 (1.88 – 10.96)
11-Deoxycortisol	2.22 (0.15-2.58)	14.5 (1.36 - 9.44)
Cortisol	274.3 (59.9 - 480)	721.5 (317.3 – 979.3)
Cortisone	161.2 (6.37-123.6)	59.9 (34.8 – 79.7)
Ratio		
B/18-OHB	6	12
18-OHB/ aldo	43	63

Plasma steroid profile showed low aldosterone level, elevated 18-hydroxycorticosterone (18-OHB), low corticosterone/18-OHB and high 18-OHB/aldosterone ratios, compatible with type 2 aldosterone synthase deficiency.

Discussion

We describe a Chinese man who presented with severe salt-wasting in infancy and hyperreninaemic hypoaldosteronism, and in whom genetic analysis confirmed aldosterone synthase deficiency. He remained clinically well in adulthood with normal electrolytes and blood pressure whilst on fludrocortisone.

Inadequate aldosterone production results in decreased renal sodium reabsorption and potassium excretion in ASD. Clinical severity varies, with the most severe forms presenting in infancy. Affected infants usually develop vomiting, dehydration, hypovolaemia, and failure to thrive at a few days to weeks following delivery [8]. However, salt-losing crisis in isolated ASD is usually indistinguishable clinically from other forms of defective steroid biosynthesis, such as 21-hydroxylase deficiency in congenital adrenal hyperplasia. Therefore, life-threatening salt-wasting in affected infants is usually treated initially with both hydrocortisone and fludrocortisone pending steroid hormone analysis [9]. Phenotypically, infants with ASD have normal external genitalia [5]. Hydrocortisone can be withdrawn once characteristic steroid profile or genetic mutations of *CYP11B2* gene are confirmed. A typical biochemical profile of this disorder includes hyponatraemia, hyperkalaemia, raised plasma

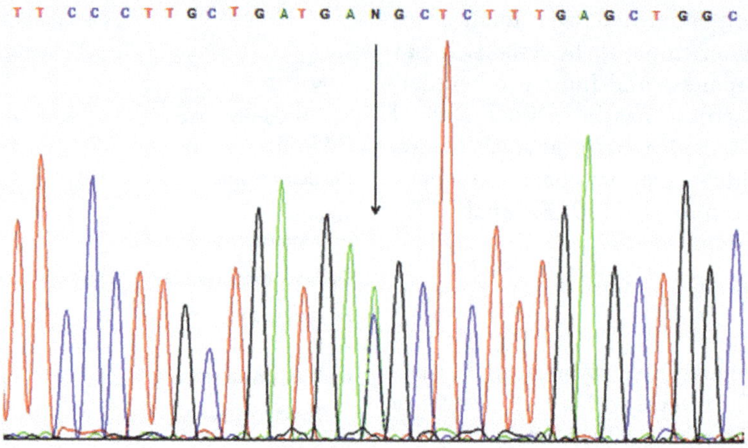

Figure 1 Electropherogram of segment of *CYP11B2* showing the heterozygous c.977C > A mutation. The mutation site is denoted by the letter N and is indicated by an arrow.

renin activity, undetectable or low aldosterone level, and normal or elevated cortisol levels.

Aldosterone synthase deficiency has been classified based on biochemical phenotypes: in type 1 ASD, the enzymatic *CYP11B2* activity is completely abolished. Affected individuals have low to normal levels of 18OHB, and undetectable to low levels of plasma aldosterone or its urinary metabolite, tetrahydroaldosterone [10]. In type 2 deficiency, the mutations in the *CYP11B2* gene only decrease 18-hydroxylase and 18-oxidase activities, but not 11β-hydroxylase activity. It differs from type 1 in that 18-OHB levels are markedly elevated, whilst plasma aldosterone levels and urinary tetrahydroaldosterone are low [7]. However, it is now recognised that these biochemical phenotypes have clinical, hormonal and genotypic overlapping features [11] and that type 1 and type 2 ASD would be better considered a continuous spectrum of the same disease [5].

As clinical severity gradually improves with age, affected adults are usually asymptomatic despite no mineralocorticoid therapy [5,12]. However, termination of mineralocorticoid may lead to postural hypotension and hyperkalaemia when triggered by stress due to dehydration or reduced salt intake in some affected adults [12]. Generalised weakness with marked hyperkalaemia and dehydration has been reported as the first presentation in a middle-aged man after concurrent institution of indapamide for hypertension and bowel preparation for barium enema. Interestingly, further questioning revealed a past history of vomiting and failure to thrive in early infancy that resolved without any mineralocorticoid replacement [13]. Therefore, detailed childhood history would be a helpful clue in suspected ASD case presenting in adulthood. Possible mechanisms for reduced clinical severity of ASD with advancing age include increasing sensitivity to mineralocorticoid action and sodium intake with age. It has been shown that mineralocorticoid receptor expression in human kidneys begins with low levels in late gestation and rises progressively after birth [14]. Another potential mechanism is age-dependent impaired 11β-hydroxysteroid dehydrogenase type 2 activity, leading to greater cortisol availability for the mineralocorticoid receptor with age [15].

Neonatal screening for CAH using 17-hydroxyprogesterone measurement would fail to detect ASD, as infants with ASD usually have normal [12] or slightly elevated basal and stimulated 17-hydroxyprogesterone [9]. The diagnosis of ASD may therefore be missed until the patient presents with salt-wasting crisis. Therefore, comprehensive hormonal investigation followed by genetic confirmation for suspected adults and their respective partners would be useful to assess the genetic implication in their offspring and to minimize the potential life-threatening risk.

Compound heterozygosity has been reported when phenotypically unaffected parents contribute to each allele with a heterozygous mutation, rendering phenotypes of ASD type 1 in the affected offspring [6,10]. Our current case inherited one of the heterozygous mutations c.977C > A (p.Thr326Lys) maternally, and the other c.523_525delAAG (p.Lys175del) paternally. The unaffected parents are heterozygous for their respective mutations, in accordance with an autosomal recessive inheritance. *In silico* protein function prediction using PolyPhen-2 and Align GVGD both predict the novel missense variant c.977C > A (p.Thr326Lys) to be damaging. Multiple sequence alignment of the *CYP11B2* gene also showed that the threonine residue is highly conserved across multiple mammal species (Table 2). The threonine residue in codon 326 is located in the I-helix of *CYP11B2* protein (Figure 2). A previous study mapping the amino acid difference between *CYP11B2*

Table 2 Multiple sequence alignment of a segment of the *CYP11B2* gene

Homo sapiens	GSVDTTAFPLLM**T**LFELARNPDV
Canis lupus	GSVDTTAYPLWM**T**LFELARNPDV
Mus musculus	GSVDTTAIPLVM**T**LFELARNPDV
Macaca mulatta	GSVDTTAFPLLM**T**LFELARNPDV
Rattus norvegicus	GSVDTTAIPLVM**T**LFELARNPDV

Codon 326 of the *CYP11B2* gene in *homo sapiens* and the corresponding codon in other species are in bold phase. The threonine residue at codon 326 (in bold) is highly conserved across different mammal species.

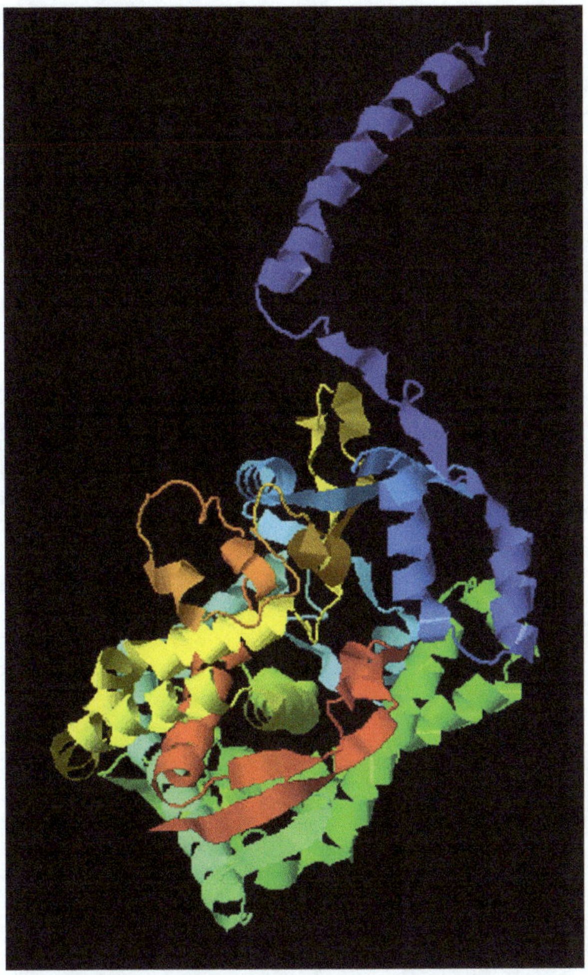

Figure 2 3-D model of the *CYP11B2* mutant with the novel missense c.977C > A mutation. The threonine residue in codon 326 is located in the I-helix of *CYP11B2* protein, which is implicated in 18-hydroxylation/oxidation due to the clusters of *CYP11B2* isoform-specific residues in that region. In particular, the alanine residue in position 320 is required for methyloxidase reaction and the p.Thr318Met in the I-helix is a known deleterious mutation causing aldosterone synthase deficiency. This structural information and functional correlation suggest that the I-helix region, where the novel variant c.977C > A (p.Thr326Lys) is located, is important for the enzyme activity of *CYP11B2*.

and *CYP11B1* showed that *CYP11B2* isoform-specific residues are clustered around the H-helix and in the I-helix and are essential for 18-hydroxylation/oxidation [16]. In particular, the alanine residue in position 320 in *CYP11B2* is required for methyloxidase reaction. Also, p.Thr318Met in the I-helix is a known deleterious mutation causing aldosterone synthase deficiency [11]. This structural information and functional correlation suggest that the I-helix region, where the novel variant c.977C > A (p.Thr326Lys) is located, is important for enzyme activity of CYP11B2. Taking all the aforementioned factors into consideration, the variant c.977C > A (p.Thr326Lys) is likely to be pathogenic, in keeping with our case.

Homozygous p.Lys175del (previously described as homozygous deletion of codon 173 before the use of the latest HGVS nomenclature) has been reported in a girl presenting with salt-wasting during infancy [7]. *CYP11B2* is polymorphic at this position, encoding arginine or lysine. Amino acid residue 173 is positioned in α-helix D, and the secondary structure of aldosterone synthase was presumed to be altered by the single amino acid deletion. Indeed, using fission yeast system, Tin *et al.* demonstrated that the deletion mutation at codon 173 displayed markedly reduced 11-β-hydroxylation activity (16.3%), and no 18-hydroxylation and 18-oxidation activities [17].

Conclusion

Aldosterone synthase deficiency is a rare cause of hyperreninaemic hypoaldosteronism and its genetic and molecular basis is more heterogeneous than previously described. It should be suspected in infants without virilisation presenting with salt-wasting or in adults presenting with stress-induced hyperkalaemia and a history of failure to thrive in childhood. Our case illustrates the clinical significance to recognize this condition as it has a good long-term prognosis when adequate fludrocortisone replacement is instituted.

Competing interests

The authors declare that they have no competing interests.

Authors' contributions

EH and MY drafted the manuscript. PTC, EK, LL, MY and AC performed the biochemical and genetic analysis. KT, KL and AC revised the manuscript critically. All authors read and approved the final manuscript.

Acknowledgement

We thank the patient and his family for their support.

Author details

[1]Department of Medicine, The University of Hong Kong, Queen Mary Hospital, Pokfulam Road, Pokfulam, Hong Kong. [2]Department of Pathology,

The University of Hong Kong, Queen Mary Hospital, Pokfulam Road, Pokfulam, Hong Kong. [3]Department of Pediatrics and Adolescent Medicine, The University of Hong Kong, Queen Mary Hospital, Pokfulam Road, Pokfulam, Hong Kong.

Reference

1. Lisurek M, Bernhardt R: **Modulation of aldosterone and cortisol synthesis on the molecular level.** *Mol Cell Endocrinol* 2004, **215**:149–159.
2. Pascoe L, Curnow KM, Slutsker L, Rosler A, White PC: **Mutations in the human CYP11B2 (aldosterone synthase) gene causing corticosterone methyloxidase II deficiency.** *Proc Natl Acad Sci U S A* 1992, **89**:4996–5000.
3. Portrat-Doyen S, Tourniaire J, Richard O, Mulatero P, Aupetit-Faisant B, Curnow KM, Pascoe L, Morel Y: **Isolated aldosterone synthase deficiency caused by simultaneous E198D and V386A mutations in the CYP11B2 gene.** *J Clin Endocrinol Metab* 1998, **83**:4156–4161.
4. White PC: **Aldosterone synthase deficiency and related disorders.** *Mol Cell Endocrinol* 2004, **217**:81–87.
5. Klomchan T, Supornsilchai V, Wacharasindhu S, Shotelersuk V, Sahakitrungruang T: **Novel CYP11B2 mutation causing aldosterone synthase (P450c11AS) deficiency.** *Eur J Pediatr* 2012, **171**:1559–1562.
6. Kondo E, Nakamura A, Homma K, Hasegawa T, Yamaguchi T, Narugami M, Hattori T, Aoyagi H, Ishizu K, Tajima T: **Two novel mutations of the CYP11B2 gene in a Japanese patient with aldosterone deficiency type 1.** *Endocr J* 2013, **60**:51–55.
7. Peter M, Dubuis JM, Sippell WG: **Disorders of the aldosterone synthase and steroid 11beta-hydroxylase deficiencies.** *Horm Res* 1999, **51**:211–222.
8. Ulick S, Wang JZ, Morton DH: **The biochemical phenotypes of two inborn errors in the biosynthesis of aldosterone.** *J Clin Endocrinol Metab* 1992, **74**:1415–1420.
9. Wasniewska M, De LF, Valenzise M, Lombardo F, De LF: **Aldosterone synthase deficiency type I with no documented homozygous mutations in the CYP11B2 gene.** *Eur J Endocrinol* 2001, **144**:59–62.
10. Nguyen HH, Hannemann F, Hartmann MF, Malunowicz EM, Wudy SA, Bernhardt R: **Five novel mutations in CYP11B2 gene detected in patients with aldosterone synthase deficiency type I: functional characterization and structural analyses.** *Mol Genet Metab* 2010, **100**:357–364.
11. Zhang G, Rodriguez H, Fardella CE, Harris DA, Miller WL: **Mutation T318M in the CYP11B2 gene encoding P450c11AS (aldosterone synthase) causes corticosterone methyl oxidase II deficiency.** *Am J Hum Genet* 1995, **57**:1037–1043.
12. Lovas K, McFarlane I, Nguyen HH, Curran S, Schwabe J, Halsall D, Bernhardt R, Wallace AM, Chatterjee VK: **A novel CYP11B2 gene mutation in an Asian family with aldosterone synthase deficiency.** *J Clin Endocrinol Metab* 2009, **94**:914–919.
13. Kayes-Wandover KM, Schindler RE, Taylor HC, White PC: **Type 1 aldosterone synthase deficiency presenting in a middle-aged man.** *J Clin Endocrinol Metab* 2001, **86**:1008–1012.
14. Martinerie L, Viengchareun S, Delezoide AL, Jaubert F, Sinico M, Prevot S, Boileau P, Meduri G, Lombes M: **Low renal mineralocorticoid receptor expression at birth contributes to partial aldosterone resistance in neonates.** *Endocrinology* 2009, **150**:4414–4424.
15. Henschkowski J, Stuck AE, Frey BM, Gillmann G, Dick B, Frey FJ, Mohaupt MG: **Age-dependent decrease in 11beta-hydroxysteroid dehydrogenase type 2 (11beta-HSD2) activity in hypertensive patients.** *Am J Hypertens* 2008, **21**:644–649.
16. Strushkevich N, Gilep AA, Shen L, Arrowsmith CH, Edwards AM, Usanov SA, Park HW: **Structural insights into aldosterone synthase substrate specificity and targeted inhibition.** *Mol Endocrinol* 2013, **27**:315–324.
17. Tin MK, Hakki T, Bernhardt R: **Fission yeast Schizosaccharomyces pombe as a new system for the investigation of corticosterone methyloxidase deficiency-causing mutations.** *J Steroid Biochem Mol Biol* 2011, **124**:31–37.

8

Evaluating hormonal mechanisms of vitamin D receptor agonist therapy in diabetic kidney disease: the VALIDATE-D study

Jenifer M Brown, Kristina Secinaro, Jonathan S Williams and Anand Vaidya*

Abstract

Background: Insufficient vitamin D status and increased renin-angiotensin system (RAS) activity have been associated with renal-vascular disease and nephropathy in diabetes. Accumulating evidence indicates that vitamin D receptor (VDR) activation lowers unfavorable RAS activity; however, more human intervention studies evaluating whether this mechanism could influence diabetic kidney disease are needed. We previously reported that both vitamin D levels and genetic variation at the VDR predict human RAS activity, and that vitamin D therapy can lower RAS activity in non-diabetics. The VALIDATE-D study is a randomized, placebo-controlled, intervention study designed to extend these findings by evaluating whether direct VDR activation in diabetes lowers circulating and local renal-vascular tissue RAS activity (Aims 1 and 2) in a manner similar to the action of ACE inhibitors (Aim 3).

Methods/Design: Forty subjects with type 2 diabetes, microalbuminuria, and without chronic kidney disease will be recruited to undergo detailed assessment of the RAS before and after randomization to calcitriol 0.75 mcg/day or placebo. Primary analyses will evaluate whether calcitriol therapy reduces circulating and renal-vascular tissue-RAS activity in comparison to placebo. All subjects will thereafter be treated with lisinopril and followed for 3.5 months to evaluate whether combination therapy (calcitriol + lisinopril vs. placebo + lisinopril) additively or synergistically improves renal-vascular function, and lowers proteinuria.

Discussion: The VALIDATE-D study is the first human intervention study to evaluate whether direct VDR activation can lower the human RAS in diabetes, compared to the effect of an ACE inhibitor, and whether this mechanism can translate to clinically relevant endpoints for diabetic kidney disease. The outcomes of VALIDATE-D will have major implications for the recommendation of vitamin D supplementation for the primary prevention of kidney complications in diabetes.

Keywords: Vitamin D, Calcitriol, Renin, Angiotensin, Diabetes, Kidney

Background

The link between vitamin D and kidney disease, particularly in the setting of human diabetes, has received much attention [1,2]. Observational and limited interventional studies have supported a renoprotective benefit to higher vitamin D levels and vitamin D supplementation [3-7]; however, there is a need for more dedicated human intervention studies to confirm these findings. One of the main proposed mechanisms linking vitamin D with renal-vascular and kidney disease is regulation of the renin-angiotensin system (RAS) [8,9]. Since both of these hormonal systems have complex genetic and environmental regulatory steps (Figure 1), carefully controlled interventional studies that evaluate both *mechanisms of action and clinical outcomes* are needed to distinguish the hormonal interplay that is likely involved for vitamin D therapy to influence kidney disease.

Both excess activity of the renin-angiotensin system (RAS) and insufficient vitamin D status have been implicated in the development of renal-vascular disease that

* Correspondence: avaidya1@partners.org
Division of Endocrinology, Diabetes, and Hypertension, Brigham and Women's Hospital and Harvard Medical School, 221 Longwood Ave, RFB, Boston, MA 02115, USA

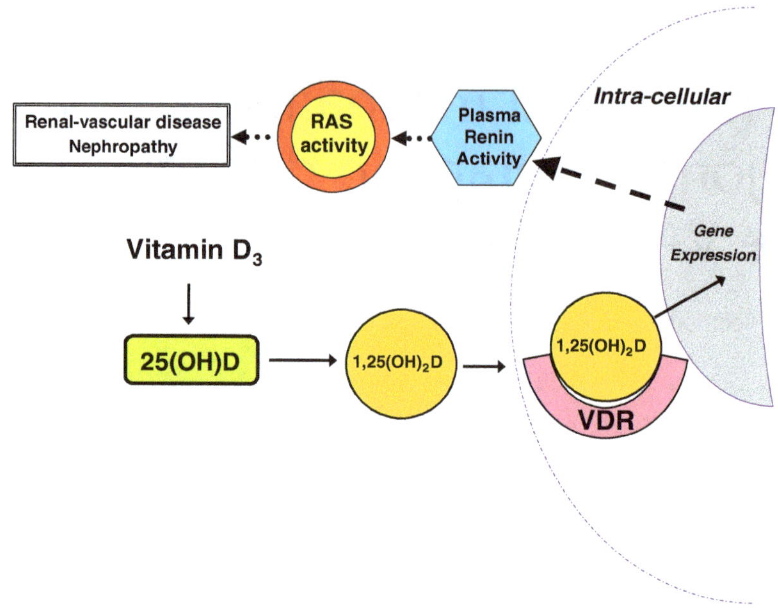

Figure 1 The proposed interaction between vitamin D and RAS metabolism. Renin catalyzes the conversion of angiotensinogen to angiotensin I, which is further converted to the vasoactive peptide angiotensin II. Angiotensin II is a direct vasoconstricter, and can also ilicit aldosterone secretion from the adrenal cortex. Under physiologic situations, activation of the RAS in response to renal-vascular hypo-perfusion serves to increase blood pressure and renal salt retention. However, in pathologic states (such as in diabetes and obesity), inappropriately high RAS activity contributes to vascular and kidney diseases. Vitamin D_3 is largely produced in the skin with exposure to ultraviolet radiation, but may also be ingested orally. This precursor is hydroxylated to 25-hydroxyvitamin D (25[OH]D) and 25(OH)D serves as the stable barometer of clinical "vitamin D status." Under the control of parathyroid hormone and calcium status, 25(OH)D can be hydroxylated to form the active vitamin D receptor (VDR) agonist 1,25-dihydroxyvitamin D ($1,25[OH]_2D$). Activation of the VDR by $1,25(OH)_2D$ is known to influence the regulation and expression of a myriad of genes, including renin.

results in diabetic nephropathy [1,2,10]. The RAS can mediate renal-vascular disease via its circulating components, and additionally the locally expressed renal-vascular tissue-RAS also contributes to the development of kidney disease [11,12]. Excess renal-vascular tissue-RAS activity has been implicated in the development of diabetic nephropathy; RAS inhibitors [13-15], as well as favorable vitamin D status [5,16,17], may mitigate this effect.

Animal studies have shown that the activation of the vitamin D receptor (VDR) by 1,25-dihydroxyvitamin D ($1,25[OH]_2D$) negatively regulates renin expression and thereby lowers RAS activity [9,18] (Figure 1). In mouse models of diabetes, both VDR-agonists and RAS-inhibitors blunted the development of diabetic nephropathy when given alone, but the combination (VDR-agonist + RAS-inhibitor) *synergistically* prevented the development of diabetic nephropathy via down-regulation of the renal-vascular tissue-RAS [19-21]. We, and others, have reported findings that translate these animal experiments to humans: the combination of vitamin D levels and genetic variation at the human VDR predicts RAS activity [22-24]. Large observational studies have shown that the prevalence of chronic kidney disease and proteinuria (a marker of kidney disease progression) are associated with lower 25(OH)D levels [3,25,26]. Due to their cross-sectional design, these aforementioned studies could not reveal causality or confirm the mechanism linking vitamin D-VDR interactions and renal outcomes. A few human interventions have demonstrated that VDR agonists may reduce proteinuria [2,7], but these studies were confined to populations with established chronic kidney disease (CKD), and evaluation of the RAS was not undertaken. We recently completed a pilot human intervention study in non-diabetics without CKD that demonstrated that high-dose vitamin D_3 therapy improved renal-vascular hemodynamics by lowering renal-vascular tissue-RAS activity [5]. This latter effect was similar to that induced by an angiotensin converting enzyme (ACE) inhibitor, thereby further supporting a renoprotective effect of vitamin D therapy [5].

In light of these novel human results translated from animal experiments, we hypothesize that activation of the VDR represents a method to lower renal-vascular tissue-RAS activity in human diabetes, and could therefore play an important role in the *primary prevention* of diabetic nephropathy. We therefore designed the VALIDATE-D study: an ongoing randomized, double-blinded, placebo-controlled study to assess whether direct VDR activation: Aim 1) lowers circulating RAS activity in human diabetes; Aim 2) lowers renal-vascular tissue-RAS activity in human diabetes; and Aim 3) in combination with ACE inhibition, exerts an additive or synergistic effect on the renal-vascular tissue-RAS and proteinuria.

Methods/Design

Study population and recruitment

The VALIDATE-D study will enroll 40 adults, aged 18–70 years, with Type 2 diabetes (T2DM), microalbuminuria, and without known CKD (estimated glomerular filtration rate > 60 mL/min). Subjects will be recruited from the local community and from the outpatient clinics of the Division of Endocrinology, Diabetes, and Hypertension within the Department of Medicine at Brigham and Women's Hospital, Boston, USA. Eligibility will be assessed at an in-person screening visit involving detailed history, physical examination, and laboratory assessment.

Inclusion criteria include T2DM that is controlled with diet, oral hypoglycemic agents, incretin analogues, or a single basal insulin injection; microalbuminuria; normal blood pressure or stage 1 hypertension treated with 0–1 antihypertensive agents; and normal blood cell counts, liver function, and electrocardiogram.

Exclusion criteria include CKD (glomerular filtration rate < 60 mL/min); poorly controlled T2DM (defined as HbA1c > 8.5% or the use of >1 daily insulin injection or a history or retinopathy); stage 2–3 hypertension or the use of more than one antihypertensive agent; kidney stones, parathyroid or granulomatous disorders, liver or heart failure, or coronary artery disease or congestive heart failure or cerebrovascular accidents. All subjects provide informed consent, and all study procedures have been approved by the Brigham & Women's Hospital institutional and ethics board as well as the Brigham and Women's Hospital Center for Clinical Investigation. Recruitment was initiated in September 2012 and is expected to be completed by September 2016.

Study protocol overview

A detailed study schema is shown in Figure 2. All study visits will occur in the Clinical Research Center (CRC) at Brigham and Women's Hospital. Studies will be performed in the CRC in order to control posture, time of day, dietary intake, and medication administration, since all of these factors are known to influence RAS activity. In brief, detailed profiling of the RAS will be performed at baseline before any intervention (Visits 2 & 3), again after double-blinded randomization to calcitriol or placebo (Visits 5 & 6) to assess whether calcitriol lowers RAS activity, and again after the addition of lisinopril to the blinded study drug to assess for an additive or synergistic relationship between VDR-agonist and ACE inhibitor therapy on the RAS and proteinuria (Visits 8 & 13).

Washout

It is well known that many medications interfere with physiologic RAS responses or with the assays that measure the RAS. To optimize the reliability and accuracy of RAS measurements, medications that interfere with RAS assessments will be withdrawn. Subjects using RAS inhibitors (such as angiotensin converting enzyme [ACE] inhibitors, angiotensin receptor blockers, or mineralocorticoid receptor antagonists) will stop their medications for 2 months prior to study. Subjects using beta-blockers or diuretics will stop their medications for 1 month prior to study, whereas those on calcium channel blockers will stop for 2 weeks prior to study. Medication washout will

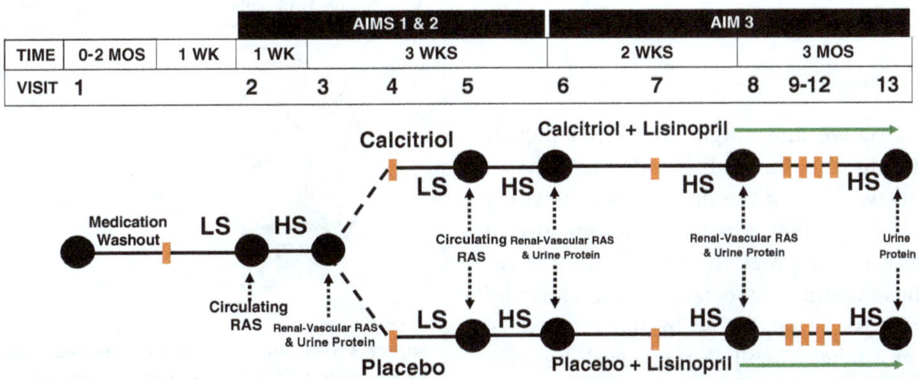

Figure 2 *VALIDATE-D study schema*: subjects will be screened and then may undergo a medication washout to withdraw interfering anti-hypertensive medications (when applicable). Aim 1: The *circulating* RAS will be assessed on LS diet before and after randomization to calcitriol/placebo (visits 2 & 5). Aim 2: The *renal-vascular tissue-RAS* will be assessed on HS diet before and after calcitriol/placebo (visits 3 & 6). Aim 3: All subjects will then receive lisinopril 5 mg/d in addition to calcitriol/placebo to assess the impact of combination therapy (calcitriol + lisinopril vs. placebo + lisinopril) on the renal-vascular tissue-RAS (visits 6 & 8) and proteinuria (visits 6, 8, 13). Serum calcium and phosphate will be monitored weekly throughout the study for safety, at each visit and at designated safety checks (visits 4, 7, 9–12).

be supervised by a study staff based on previously described safety protocols [5] after providing and instructing each subject on how to use a home sphygmomanometer. As previously described, in cases where hypertension (159/99 mmHg) results following withdrawal of an antihypertensive medication, amlodipine will be used to lower blood pressure as it has a neutral effects on RAS activity.

Study diets

All study procedures will be conducted using one of two specifically designed study diets.

Low-salt diet

The low salt (LS) diet includes 10 mEq of sodium, 100 mEq of potassium, and <600 mg of calcium per day. The purpose of this diet is to induce *maximal stimulation* of RAS components to allow for adequate measurements of the *circulating RAS*. Subjects will consume the LS diet for 1 week prior to study visits where the circulating RAS will be measured (Visits 2 and 5). All daily meals and food intake during the LS dietary phase will be prepared and provided to study participants by the CRC dietary kitchen staff.

High-salt diet

The high sat (HS) diet includes 200 mEq of sodium, 50 mEq of potassium, and <600 mg of calcium per day. The purpose of this diet is to induce *maximal suppression* of the circulating RAS components in order to most effectively measure the *renal-vascular tissue-RAS*, as previously described [5,17]. Subjects will consume the HS diet for 1 week prior to study visits where the renal-vascular tissue-RAS will be evaluated (Visits 3, 6, and 8). The HS diet involves consumption of an ad lib diet, with supplements provided to achieve the sodium and potassium contents.

Low calcium diet

Subjects will be instructed and taught to restrict dietary calcium intake during the LS and HS dietary phases (<600 mg/day), and also during the duration of the study in between study visits (<1000 mg/day). The purpose of calcium restriction is to minimize the risk of hypercalcemia and hyperphosphatemia associated with calcitriol administration; this risk is negligible in the context of low dietary calcium intake [27-29]. A registered dietician will coach subjects throughout the study on restricting calcium intake and will provide materials to guide dietary intake at home (Dietary Calcium Intake Recommendations Additional file 1). Compliance with study diets will be confirmed by 24-hour urine collections obtained at every study visit.

Baseline assessments of the circulating and renal-vascular tissue-RAS (Visits 2 & 3)

After a screening visit (Visit 1) and a potential antihypertensive washout phase, all subjects will undergo baseline assessments to characterize the circulating and renal-vascular tissue-RAS.

Circulating RAS on LS diet (Visit 2)

Study visit 2 is designed to measure the baseline circulating RAS under conditions designed to induce maximal stimulation of the circulating RAS: restricted dietary sodium intake and upright posture. After one week of LS diet consumption, subjects are studied at 8 AM in the morning (Figure 2). Subjects will maintain an upright standing posture for at least 1 hour. Blood samples are obtained at the end of the postural phase to measure circulating RAS components (plasma renin activity, angiotensn II, aldosterone).

Renal-vascular tissue-RAS on HS diet (Visit 3)

Study visit 3 is designed to assess baseline renal-vascular tissue-RAS activity by measuring changes in renal plasma flow (RPF) in response to an infusion of exogenous angiotensin II. Angiotensin II is a vasopressor that specifically interacts with angiotensin receptors to induce renal-vascular vasoconstriction resulting in a decrease in RPF. *The magnitude of the decline in RPF to angiotensin II is inversely related to renal-vascular tissue-RAS activity* (Figure 3); greater renal-vascular responses to angiotensin II signify lower local tissue-RAS activity [5,30,31]. Using this physiologic methodology,

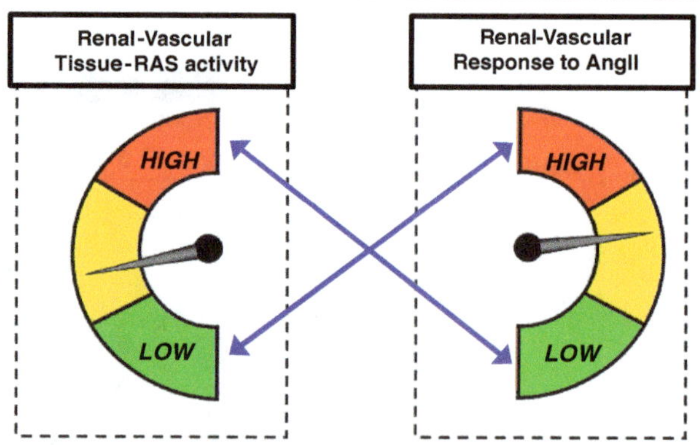

Figure 3 Reciprocal relationship between renal-vascular tissue-RAS activity and the renal-vascular response to angiotensin II. A blunted response to angiotensin II reflects a high level of local, endogenous, renal-vascular tissue-RAS activity (the smaller the decline in renal plasma flow in response to an infusion of angiotensin II, the greater the activity of the local renal-vascular tissue-RAS). Conversely, a robust response to angiotensin II is observed when tissue-RAS activity is low.

measurement of RPF responses to angiotensin II provide an indirect method to assess the human renal-vascular tissue-RAS.

To adequately measure the renal-vascular tissue-RAS, subjects are studied on a HS diet and in overnight supine posture to suppress endogenous circulating RAS components, thereby amplifying measurable RPF responses to angiotensin II [32]. After completing one week of HS diet, subjects will be admitted to the CRC and maintained supine overnight and throughout the study procedures on the following morning. In the morning, two intravenous lines will be placed to facilitate infusion of study drugs and frequent blood sampling. Weight-based *para*-aminohippurate (PAH) will then be infused and its clearance used to measure RPF throughout the duration of the study visit [5]. After allowing PAH concentrations to reach a steady state over 60 minutes, blood will be sampled to establish the baseline RPF. Angiotensin II will then be infused at 0.3 ng/kg/min for 45 minutes and escalated to 1 ng/kg/min for an additional 45 minutes to assess dose–response characteristics. PAH will be measured during and after each angiotensin II infusion to measure RPF dynamics. Blood pressure will be monitored closely throughout the infusions based on standardized safety protocols [5] that we have extensive experience performing in our CRC. The study visit will end upon completion of the angiotensin II infusions, and subjects will be discharged to undergo randomization to the study drug.

Randomization to study drug

Following study visit 3, subjects will be randomized to either calcitriol 0.75 mcg/day or placebo arm using a 2 block randomization. Double-blinded randomization will be performed by the investigational drug pharmacy at our institution, and neither the subjects nor the investigators will know the identity of the randomized study drug.

The influence of calcitriol on the RAS (Visits 5 & 6)

Circulating RAS on LS diet (Visit 5)

After 2 weeks of daily calcitriol or placebo, subjects will return on LS diet and complete visit 5, which is identical to visit 2. Aim 1 of this study (to assess whether direct VDR activation lowers circulating RAS activity in human diabetes) is executed in study visits 2 and 5. *Anticipated Results:* It is anticipated that calcitriol therapy will lower circulating RAS components (plasma renin activity and angiotensin II) when compared to placebo, demonstrating for the first time that VDR agonism can inhibit the circulating RAS in human diabetes.

Renal-vascular tissue-RAS on HS diet (Visit 6)

After a third week on the study drug, subjects will return on HS diet for an overnight CRC study visit 6, that is identical to Visit 3. This visit will permit assessment of study Aim 2 (to assess whether direct VDR activation lowers renal-vascular tissue-RAS activity in human diabetes) by comparing the renal-vascular tissue-RAS activity before and after calcitriol/placebo. *Anticipated Results:* It is anticipated that calcitriol therapy will raise basal RPF and increase the RPF sensitivity to angiotensin II, thereby demonstrating that VDR activation improves renal-vascular hemodynamics by lowering local renal-vascular RAS activity in human diabetics without CKD.

The influence of combination VDR-agonist and ACE inhibitor therapy on the renal-vascular tissue RAS (Visit 8)

Upon completing study visit 6, all subjects will receive lisinopril (initially 2.5 mg daily, which will be increased to 5 mg daily after one week, unless blood pressures are below 90/50 mmHg or subjects experience orthostatic symptoms) in addition to their randomized study drug (Figure 2). After 2 weeks of daily combined therapy (calictirol + lisinopril or placebo + lisinopril), subjects will return on the HS diet for a final inpatient CRC visit that is identical to study visits 3 & 6. Comparing the outcomes of study visits 6 and 8 will permit evaluation of Aim 3 of this study (to assess whether direct VDR activation in combination with ACE inhibition exerts an additive or synergistic effect on the renal-vascular tissue-RAS and proteinuria). *Anticipated Results:* Combination therapy (calcitriol + lisinopril) will additively or synergistically raise RPF and increase the RPF sensitivity to angioensin II infusion, reflecting decreased renal-vascular tissue-RAS activity when compared to placebo + lisinopril.

The influence of chronic combination therapy on proteinuria (Visit 13)

Following completion of study visit 8, subjects will be discharged home to continue both the study drug and lisinopril for three months of long-term therapy (Figure 2). For the final visit of the study, subjects will return after one week of HS diet with a completed 24-hour urine collection, which will be analyzed for protein. The 24-hour urine protein measured at this visit will be compared using repeated measures analyses to the urine protein levels obtained from 24-hour urine collections completed at each inpatient visit on HS dietary balance (visits 3, 6, 8). *Anticipated Results:* Combination therapy (calcitriol + lisinopril) will additively or synergistically lower proteinuria when compared to placebo + lisinopril, thereby paralleling prior animal studies that showed that the combination of VDR agonist + conventional RAS inhibitor therapy induced synergistic renoprotective benefits in mouse models of diabetes [19-21].

Safety & monitoring

Calcium/Phosphate

To minimize the risk of hypercalcemia due to calcitriol, all subjects will undergo laboratory evaluation of serum calcium and phosphate at 1–3 week intervals throughout the study duration, including at the aforementioned study visits and additionally at designated safety visits (visits 4, 7, 9–12). If calcium or phosphate rises above the upper limit of normal, the test will be repeated in 3 days and subjects will be counseled by our dedicated study dietician on adherence to a low calcium diet (Dietary Calcium Intake Recommendations Additional file 1). If calcium or phosphate levels remain elevated, or the calcium-phosphate product exceeds 50, the dose of study drug will be reduced by one third. Based on several prior studies that have employed chronic VDR-agonist therapy in combination with lowered dietary calcium intake, our dosing and study duration are unlikely to invoke hypercalcemia or hyperphosphatemia [27-29].

Blood pressure

During PAH and angiotensin II infusion, blood pressure (BP) will be monitored every 2 minutes using an automated sphyngomanometer. An increase in BP is an expected effect of angiotensin II infusion, and the following protocol has been used safely in over 1500 subjects [5]. The 0.3 ng/kg/min dose was selected because it does not induce a pressor effect but still influences renal-vascular hemodynamics [30], and the 1 ng/kg/min dose was selected because it has previously been shown to induce minimal BP elevations well within a safety range [5,30]. A study physician will supervise all angiotensin II infusions as previously described [5].

All subjects will monitor their BP daily with a home sphygmomanometer while on the washout phase (when applicable) and while on lisinopril and will communicate their readings to study staff twice weekly. Study staff will monitor for unsafe high BP during the washout period (>159/99 mmHg) or unsafe hypotension during lisinopril treatment (<90/50 mmHg). Subjects who develop high BPs during the washout period may be treated with amlodipine which has a neutral effect on RAS components. Subjects who develop low BPs on lisinopril may have their dose reduced 50%, however, if a 2.5 mg daily dose is not tolerated, subjects will be removed from the study.

Blood glucose

Subjects will be asked to check their home blood glucose daily, and study staff will monitor their glycemic control throughout the study. If fasting morning blood glucose is consistently >150 mg/dL, medications will be adjusted by a study physician. Such adjustments include increasing the dose of a home medication or adding a second oral hypoglycemic agent.

Lipids

Any subject who has a screening LDL cholesterol greater than 100 mg/dL, will either be prescribed simvastatin 20-40 mg daily, or if already taking a statin medication, have their pre-existing statin dose increased, to remain consistent with clinical standards of care for diabetes.

Laboratory measurements

25(OH)D (Diasorin, Inc., Stillwater, MN), $1,25(OH)_2D$ (Diasorin), parathyroid hormone (Beckman Coulter, Fullerton, CA), and serum and urine electrolytes (including calcium and phosphate) will be measured at baseline at all visits. Components of the circulating RAS, including plasma renin activity (Diasorin) and aldosterone (Siemens, Los Angeles, CA), will be measured from samples drawn in upright and supine posture (Visits 2, 5, 13) and before and during angiotensin II infusion (Visits 3, 6, 8) [5]. For assessment of RPF, *para*-aminohippurate will be measured in triplicate at steady-state and during angiotensin II infusion and will then be adjusted by body surface area in all RPF calculations (Visits 3, 6, 8).

Statistical analyses

Sample size calculations

Sample size calculations were made using our prior data evaluating the impact of vitamin D on the systemic [23] and renal-vascular tissue-RAS [5] by paired analyses with an alpha-error of 0.05. For Aim 1, prior data suggest that therapy with a VDR agonist could reduce plasma renin activity, a measure of the circulating RAS, by 1 ng/mL/hr (SD = 0.54). A minimum of 5 subjects would be required in each study arm for a paired comparison to detect this difference with a power of 0.9. In our pilot intervention study, we demonstrated an effect of vitamin D therapy on the renal-vascular tissue-RAS (Aims 2 & 3) in a sample of 14 subjects. To account for underestimation of sample-size, variability in measurements, and to permit non-paired comparisons, we intend to study 20 subjects in each intervention group.

Outcomes

Paired and repeated measures analyses will be used to evaluate intra-individual changes in the circulating RAS, RPF responses to angiotensin II infusion (i.e. renal-vascular tissue-RAS), and urine protein levels. Non-paired comparisons will be used to evaluate changes in these parameters between the calcitriol and placebo groups. A two-tailed P-value < 0.05 will be considered statistically significant.

Discussion

The VALIDATE-D study is a unique randomized and double-blinded human intervention study that is designed to elucidate the *mechanism* by which vitamin D therapy may impart renoprotective benefits in diabetes. Vitamin D metabolism and regulation of the RAS are complex processes that involve multiple genes, gene-products, and environmental inputs (Figure 1); the genetic variation, dietary intake, and other environmental exposures for each individual have been shown to alter the balance of each of these hormonal systems [33-35]. In this regard, using supplementation with vitamin D_3 in an intervention study to induce a clinical outcome that is mediated by the interaction between $1,25(OH)_2D$ and the VDR (such as RAS inhibition to influence renal-vascular function) is analogous to administering a pre- or pro-drug that is dependent on multiple subsequent enzymatic steps, each regulated and modified by genetics and environment. The strengths of the VALIDATE-D study are that it focuses on overcoming this individual variability by investigating the influence of *direct* VDR-agonist therapy in modulating RAS activity and renal-vascular function, and employs a meticulous design to evaluate the underlying mechanism of potential findings (regulation of RAS activity).

Increasing evidence highlights a relationship between vitamin D and the RAS, with relevant implications for renal-vascular and kidney disease [1,36]. Lowering unfavorable RAS activity has known vascular benefits in diabetes [37], and the use of RAS inhibitors is common practice to prevent or delay the progression of diabetic nephropathy. Animal studies have elegantly shown that activating the VDR results in lowering of the renal-vascular tissue-RAS, and that this interaction translates to reduced kidney injury, particularly in the setting of animal models of diabetes [19-21]. While human studies often focus on influencing clinical outcomes by supplementing with vitamin D_3 [5,38], research studies that employ direct VDR-agonists may be most effective at invoking VDR-mediated effects such as RAS modulation [2,39]. The advantage of using direct VDR-agonists in intervention studies is that they likely maximize any effect mediated by the VDR, eliminate inter-individual variations in vitamin D metabolism, and may influence clinical outcomes in a shorter duration of time than would take with vitamin D_3 supplementation. The disadvantage of using VDR-agonists is that they are not commonly used in individuals without CKD and therefore direct clinical translation of study findings is limited; however, positive findings would support any therapy (vitamin D_3 or VDR-agonist) that raises $1,25(OH)_2D$ levels or activates the VDR as an equal surrogate.

The results of the VALIDATE-D study will shed light on: 1) the mechanism by which VDR activation influences renal-vascular function in human diabetes (via modulation of the RAS), and 2) whether VDR activation modulates renal hemodynamics and proteinuria in human diabetes. These findings would not only carry major implications for the recommendation of vitamin D supplementation in the primary prevention of diabetic nephropathy, but they could help interpret the findings of many other studies that evaluated clinical outcomes of vitamin D therapy without accounting for the mechanisms involved. In this regard, the VALIDATE-D study may explain the reasons prior negative studies failed to see outcomes and why positive studies may have succeeded.

At least three unique findings will emerge from the VALIDATE-D study. First, this intervention study will conclusively evaluate whether vitamin D therapy lowers the *circulating* human RAS. By using direct VDR agonists and a meticulous study design to account for confounders of the RAS (diet, posture, medications, time of day), this study will investigate whether calcitriol therapy lowers the maximally stimulated RAS on a LS diet in comparison to placebo. Second, this study will evaluate whether direct VDR activation improves renal-vascular hemodynamics by increasing renal blood flow and the renal-vascular sensitivity to angiotensin II; both of these observations are consistent with reductions in the renal-vascular tissue-RAS as would be induced by an ACE inhibitor. The study design includes a comparison of renal-vascular hemodynamics (while the circulating RAS is suppressed on a HS diet) during treatment with calcitriol vs. placebo, and then again during treatment with calcitriol + lisinopril vs. placebo + lisinopril (Figure 2). In this regard, the study design is optimized to decipher the individual role of VDR activation, and the effect of combining VDR activation with conventional RAS inhibition, since this combination therapy has been shown to provide synergistic renoprotection in animal models of diabetes [19-21]. The assessment of the renal-vascular tissue-RAS in humans is a unique and defining aspect of this study protocol. The renal vasculature is specifically sensitive to the effects of angiotensin II, and the magnitude of renal-vascular responses to angiotensin II is inversely proportional to the degree of local tissue-RAS activity [5,11,16]. High endogenous tissue-RAS activity results in a blunted local sensitivity to the effect of angiotensin II, while inhibiting the local renal-vascular tissue-RAS (for example with an ACE inhibitor) improves the renal-vascular sensitivity to angiotensin II [30] (Figure 3). Therefore, our ability to measure renal hemodynamics via *para*-aminohippurate clearance permits us to objectively ascertain the state of the renal-vascular tissue-RAS in response to drug intervention (calcitriol, lisinopril, placebo) and in response to provocation by angiotensin II. Lowering renal-vascular tissue-RAS activity in pathologic states such as diabetes and obesity with conventional pharmacotherapy (ACE inhibitor or angiotensin receptor blocker) has shown efficacy for the primary prevention of diabetic nephropathy [15,40,41]. Thirdly, the impact of adding chronic VDR-agonist therapy to ACE inhibitor therapy on proteinuria will be assessed. Since the study population is strategically selected to have diabetes without CKD, together these study findings will have implications for recommending vitamin D supplementation to lower unfavorable RAS activity for the *primary prevention* of diabetic nephropathy.

We have previously shown in a pilot study that high-dose vitamin D_3 therapy to markedly raise $1,25(OH)_2D$ concentrations can lower renal-vascular tissue-RAS activity in non-diabetics with normal renal function [5]. Like an ACE inhibitor, this intervention induced a favorable state of low tissue-RAS resulting in increased renal-vascular sensitivity to angiotensin II [5]. The VALIDATE-D study will extend these findings by employing a double-blinded randomization, employing direct VDR agonist therapy, and focusing on patients with diabetes without CKD. In prior clinical studies of secondary prevention in diabetes with pre-existing CKD, direct VDR agonists (calcitriol and paracalcitol) reduced proteinuria [7,42-45]; whether this effect was mediated by the RAS, or could be extrapolated for the *primary* prevention of diabetic nephropathy, are questions that the VALIDATE-D study will clarify.

VALIDATE-D is the first human study to investigate whether vitamin D therapy to activate the VDR can lower circulating and renal-vascular tissue-RAS activity in diabetics without CKD. This study is designed to specifically focus on whether modulating the RAS represents a key mechanism by which vitamin D intervention impacts renal-vascular hemodynamics and kidney function. In this regard, VALIDATE-D will provide evidence that may influence clinical recommendations for maintaining vitamin D status for the *primary prevention* of diabetic nephropathy. In addition, VALIDATE-D will examine whether the action of potent VDR agonist therapy complements the known beneficial effects of ACE inhibition, as has been observed in animal models [19]. If so, the results of VALIDATE-D could influence pharmacologic practices by favoring vitamin D_3 supplementation instead of, or in addition to, ACE inhibitor therapy for patients with diabetes.

Competing interests
The authors affirm they have no competing interests.

Authors' contributions
AV developed the study design and concept and is involved in the conduct and supervision of the study as the principal investigator. JMB and JSW contributed to the study design and study conduct. KS is involved in recruiting subjects and providing study coordination and dietary input. All authors contributed to the writing and editing of this manuscript.

Authors' information
The authors have unique experiences in conducting human physiology studies such as the one described here. AV and JSW have nearly ten years of experience designing and performing human research focused on the renin-angiotensin sytem and calcium-regulatory hormones. This includes research protocols with detailed dietary control and modulation of hormones using Clinical Research Center Resources. AV, JSW, and JMB have published on interactions between the renin-angiotensin system and calcium-regulatory hormones, and their reputation in this field has resulted in invitations to give regional and national talks on this topic.

Acknowledgements
We are grateful to the CRC staff and our study participants.

Funding sources
Research reported in this publication was supported by a Harvard Catalyst Clinical Research Center Resources and Services Grant, and the National Heart, Lung, And Blood Institute of the National Institutes of Health under Award Number K23HL111771. The content is solely the responsibility of the authors and does not necessarily represent the official views of the National Institutes of Health.

References
1. Vaidya A, Williams JS: **The relationship between vitamin D and the renin-angiotensin system in the pathophysiology of hypertension, kidney disease, and diabetes.** *Metabolism* 2012, **61**:450–458.
2. Vaidya A, Forman JP: **Vitamin D and vascular disease: the current and future status of vitamin D therapy in hypertension and kidney disease.** *Curr Hypertens Rep* 2012, **14**:111–119.
3. de Boer IH, Ioannou GN, Kestenbaum B, Brunzell JD, Weiss NS: **25-Hydroxyvitamin D levels and albuminuria in the third national health and nutrition examination survey (NHANES III).** *Am J Kidney Dis* 2007, **50**:69–77.
4. de Boer IH, Sachs MC, Cleary PA, Hoofnagle AN, Lachin JM, Molitch ME, Steffes MW, Sun W, Zinman B, Brunzell JD, *et al*: **Circulating vitamin D metabolites and kidney disease in type 1 diabetes.** *J Clin Endocrinol Metab* 2012, **97**(12):4780–4788.
5. Vaidya A, Sun B, Larson C, Forman JP, Williams JS: **Vitamin D3 therapy corrects the tissue sensitivity to angiotensin ii akin to the action of a converting enzyme inhibitor in obese hypertensives: an interventional study.** *J Clin Endocrinol Metab* 2012, **97**:2456–2465.
6. Huang Y, Yu H, Lu J, Guo K, Zhang L, Bao Y, Chen H, Jia W: **Oral supplementation with cholecalciferol 800 IU ameliorates albuminuria in Chinese type 2 diabetic patients with nephropathy.** *PLoS One* 2012, **7**:e50510.
7. de Zeeuw D, Agarwal R, Amdahl M, Audhya P, Coyne D, Garimella T, Parving HH, Pritchett Y, Remuzzi G, Ritz E, *et al*: **Selective vitamin D receptor activation with paricalcitol for reduction of albuminuria in patients with type 2 diabetes (VITAL study): a randomised controlled trial.** *Lancet* 2010, **376**(9752):1543–1551.
8. Vaidya A, Forman JP: **Vitamin D and hypertension: current evidence and future directions.** *Hypertension* 2010, **56**:774–779.
9. Li YC, Kong J, Wei M, Chen ZF, Liu SQ, Cao LP: **1,25-Dihydroxyvitamin D(3) is a negative endocrine regulator of the renin-angiotensin system.** *J Clin Invest* 2002, **110**:229–238.
10. Damasiewicz MJ, Magliano DJ, Daly RM, Gagnon C, Lu ZX, Sikaris KA, Ebeling PR, Chadban SJ, Atkins RC, Kerr PG, *et al*: **Serum 25-hydroxyvitamin D deficiency and the 5-year incidence of CKD.** *Am J Kidney Dis* 2013, **62**(1):58–66.
11. Bader M: **Tissue renin-angiotensin-aldosterone systems: targets for pharmacological therapy.** *Annu Rev Pharmacol Toxicol* 2010, **50**:439–465.
12. Hayden MR, Sowers KM, Pulakat L, Joginpally T, Krueger B, Whaley-Connell A, Sowers JR: **Possible mechanisms of local tissue Renin-Angiotensin system activation in the cardiorenal metabolic syndrome and type 2 diabetes mellitus.** *Cardiorenal Med* 2011, **1**(3):193–210.
13. Mallamaci F, Ruggenenti P, Perna A, Leonardis D, Tripepi R, Tripepi G, Remuzzi G, Zoccali C, Group RS: **ACE inhibition is renoprotective among obese patients with proteinuria.** *J Am Soc Nephrol* 2011, **22**:1122–1128.

14. Vejakama P, Thakkinstian A, Lertrattananon D, Ingsathit A, Ngarmukos C, Attia J: **Reno-protective effects of renin-angiotensin system blockade in type 2 diabetic patients: a systematic review and network meta-analysis.** *Diabetologia* 2012, **55:**566–578.
15. Ruggenenti P, Fassi A, Ilieva AP, Bruno S, Iliev IP, Brusegan V, Rubis N, Gherardi G, Arnoldi F, Ganeva M, *et al*: **Preventing microalbuminuria in type 2 diabetes.** *N Engl J Med* 2004, **351:**1941–1951.
16. Vaidya A, Forman JP, Williams JS: **Vitamin D and the vascular sensitivity to angiotensin II in obese Caucasians with hypertension.** *J Hum Hypertens* 2011, **25:**672–678.
17. Forman JP, Williams JS, Fisher ND: **Plasma 25-hydroxyvitamin D and regulation of the renin-angiotensin system in humans.** *Hypertension* 2010, **55:**1283–1288.
18. Zhou C, Lu F, Cao K, Xu D, Goltzman D, Miao D: **Calcium-independent and 1,25(OH)2D3-dependent regulation of the renin-angiotensin system in 1alpha-hydroxylase knockout mice.** *Kidney Int* 2008, **74:**170–179.
19. Deb DK, Sun T, Wong KE, Zhang Z, Ning G, Zhang Y, Kong J, Shi H, Chang A, Li YC: **Combined vitamin D analog and AT1 receptor antagonist synergistically block the development of kidney disease in a model of type 2 diabetes.** *Kidney Int* 2010, **77:**1000–1009.
20. Zhang Z, Zhang Y, Ning G, Deb DK, Kong J, Li YC: **Combination therapy with AT1 blocker and vitamin D analog markedly ameliorates diabetic nephropathy: blockade of compensatory renin increase.** *Proc Natl Acad Sci USA* 2008, **105:**15896–15901.
21. Ohara I, Tanimoto M, Gohda T, Yamazaki T, Hagiwara S, Murakoshi M, Aoki T, Toyoda H, Ishikawa Y, Funabiki K, *et al*: **Effect of combination therapy with angiotensin receptor blocker and 1,25-dihydroxyvitamin D(3) in type 2 diabetic nephropathy in KK-A(y)/Ta mice.** *Nephron Exp Nephrol* 2011, **117:**e124–e132.
22. Vaidya A, Sun B, Forman JP, Hopkins PN, Brown NJ, Kolatkar NS, Williams GH, Williams JS: **The Fok1 vitamin D receptor gene polymorphism is associated with plasma renin activity in Caucasians.** *Clin Endocrinol (Oxf)* 2011, **74:**783–790.
23. Vaidya A, Forman JP, Hopkins PN, Seely EW, Williams JS: **25-Hydroxyvitamin D is associated with plasma renin activity and the pressor response to dietary sodium intake in Caucasians.** *J Renin Angiotensin Aldosterone Syst* 2011, **12:**311–319.
24. Wang L, Ma J, Manson JE, Buring JE, Gaziano JM, Sesso HD: **A prospective study of plasma vitamin D metabolites, vitamin D receptor gene polymorphisms, and risk of hypertension in men.** *Eur J Nutr* 2012. epub ahead of print (Dec 21st 2012).
25. Barreto DV, Barreto FC, Liabeuf S, Temmar M, Boitte F, Choukroun G, Fournier A, Massy ZA: **Vitamin D affects survival independently of vascular calcification in chronic kidney disease.** *Clin J Am Soc Nephrol* 2009, **4:**1128–1135.
26. González EA, Sachdeva A, Oliver DA, Martin KJ: **Vitamin D insufficiency and deficiency in chronic kidney disease. a single center observational study.** *Am J Nephrol* 2004, **24:**503–510.
27. Chen JT, Shiraki M, Hasumi K, Tanaka N, Katase K, Kato T, Hirai Y, Nakamura T, Ogata E: **1-alpha-Hydroxyvitamin D3 treatment decreases bone turnover and modulates calcium-regulating hormones in early postmenopausal women.** *Bone* 1997, **20:**557–562.
28. Gallagher JC, Goldgar D: **Treatment of postmenopausal osteoporosis with high doses of synthetic calcitriol. a randomized controlled study.** *Ann Intern Med* 1990, **113:**649–655.
29. Sairanen S, Kärkkäinen M, Tähtelä R, Laitinen K, Mäkelä P, Lamberg-Allardt C, Välimäki MJ: **Bone mass and markers of bone and calcium metabolism in postmenopausal women treated with 1,25-dihydroxyvitamin D (Calcitriol) for four years.** *Calcif Tissue Int* 2000, **67:**122–127.
30. Redgrave J, Rabinowe S, Hollenberg NK, Williams GH: **Correction of abnormal renal blood flow response to angiotensin II by converting enzyme inhibition in essential hypertensives.** *J Clin Invest* 1985, **75:**1285–1290.
31. Shoback DM, Williams GH, Moore TJ, Dluhy RG, Podolsky S, Hollenberg NK: **Defect in the sodium-modulated tissue responsiveness to angiotensin II in essential hypertension.** *J Clin Invest* 1983, **72:**2115–2124.
32. Hollenberg NK, Chenitz WR, Adams DF, Williams GH: **Reciprocal influence of salt intake on adrenal glomerulosa and renal vascular responses to angiotensin II in normal man.** *J Clin Invest* 1974, **54:**34–42.
33. Wang TJ, Zhang F, Richards JB, Kestenbaum B, van Meurs JB, Berry D, Kiel DP, Streeten EA, Ohlsson C, Koller DL, *et al*: **Common genetic determinants of vitamin D insufficiency: a genome-wide association study.** *Lancet* 2010, **376:**180–188.
34. Vaidya A, Pojoga L, Underwood PC, Forman JP, Hopkins PN, Williams GH, Williams JS: **The association of plasma resistin with dietary sodium manipulation, the renin-angiotensin-aldosterone system, and 25-hydroxyvitamin D3 in human hypertension.** *Clin Endocrinol (Oxf)* 2011, **74:**294–299.
35. Levin GP, Robinson-Cohen C, de Boer IH, Houston DK, Lohman K, Liu Y, Kritchevsky SB, Cauley JA, Tanaka T, Ferrucci L, *et al*: **Genetic variants and associations of 25-hydroxyvitamin D concentrations with major clinical outcomes.** *JAMA* 2012, **308:**1898–1905.
36. Agarwal R: **Are vitamin D receptor agonists like angiotensin-converting enzyme inhibitors without side effects?** *Kidney Int* 2010, **77:**943–945.
37. Yusuf S, Sleight P, Pogue J, Bosch J, Davies R, Dagenais G: **Effects of an angiotensin-converting-enzyme inhibitor, ramipril, on cardiovascular events in high-risk patients. the heart outcomes prevention evaluation study investigators.** *N Engl J Med* 2000, **342:**145–153.
38. Forman JP, Scott JB, Ng K, Drake BF, Suarez EG, Hayden DL, Bennett GG, Chandler PD, Hollis BW, Emmons KM, *et al*: **Effect of vitamin D supplementation on blood pressure in blacks.** *Hypertension* 2013, **61:**779–785.
39. de Boer IH, Sachs M, Hoofnagle AN, Utzschneider KM, Kahn SE, Kestenbaum B, Himmelfarb J: **Paricalcitol does not improve glucose metabolism in patients with stage 3–4 chronic kidney disease.** *Kidney Int* 2013, **83:**323–330.
40. Ravid M, Brosh D, Levi Z, Bar-Dayan Y, Ravid D, Rachmani R: **Use of enalapril to attenuate decline in renal function in normotensive, normoalbuminuric patients with type 2 diabetes mellitus. A randomized, controlled trial.** *Ann Intern Med* 1998, **128:**982–988.
41. Patel A, MacMahon S, Chalmers J, Neal B, Woodward M, Billot L, Harrap S, Poulter N, Marre M, Cooper M, *et al*: **Effects of a fixed combination of perindopril and indapamide on macrovascular and microvascular outcomes in patients with type 2 diabetes mellitus (the ADVANCE trial): a randomised controlled trial.** *Lancet* 2007, **370:**829–840.
42. Agarwal R, Acharya M, Tian J, Hippensteel RL, Melnick JZ, Qiu P, Williams L, Batlle D: **Antiproteinuric effect of oral paricalcitol in chronic kidney disease.** *Kidney Int* 2005, **68**(6):2823–2828.
43. Alborzi P, Patel NA, Peterson C, Bills JE, Bekele DM, Bunaye Z, Light RP, Agarwal R: **Paricalcitol reduces albuminuria and inflammation in chronic kidney disease: a randomized double-blind pilot trial.** *Hypertension* 2008, **52**(2):249–255.
44. Szeto CC, Chow KM, Kwan BC, Chung KY, Leung CB, Li PK: **Oral calcitriol for the treatment of persistent proteinuria in immunoglobulin A nephropathy: an uncontrolled trial.** *Am J Kidney Dis* 2008, **51**(5):724–731.
45. Fishbane S, Chittineni H, Packman M, Dutka P, Ali N, Durie N: **Oral paricalcitol in the treatment of patients with CKD and proteinuria: a randomized trial.** *Am J Kidney Dis* 2009, **54**(4):647–652.

1,25-dihydroxyvitamin D and PTHrP mediated malignant hypercalcemia in a seminoma

René Rodríguez-Gutiérrez[1,2*], Maria Azucena Zapata-Rivera[1,2], Dania Lizeth Quintanilla-Flores[2,3], Carlos Rodrigo Camara-Lemarroy[2,3], Fernando Javier Lavalle-Gonzalez[1,2], José Gerardo González-González[1,2] and Jesús Zacarías Villarreal-Pérez[1,2]

Abstract

Background: Seminomas have been rarely associated with malignant hypercalcemia. The responsible mechanism of hypercalcemia in this setting has been described to be secondary to 1,25-dihydroxyvitamin D secretion. The relationship with PTHrP has not been determined or studied.
The aim of this study is to describe and discuss the case and the pathophysiological mechanisms involved in a malignant hypercalcemia mediated by 1,25-dihydroxyvitamin D and PTHrP cosecretion in a patient with seminoma.

Case presentation: A 35-year-old man was consulted for assessment and management of severe hypercalcemia related to an abdominal mass. Nausea, polyuria, polydipsia, lethargy and confusion led him to the emergency department. An abdominal and pelvic enhanced CT confirmed a calcified pelvic mass, along with multiple retroperitoneal lymphadenopathy. Chest x-ray revealed "cannon ball" pulmonary metastases. The histopathology result was consistent with a seminoma. Serum calcium was 14.7 mg/dl, PTH was undetectable, 25-dihydroxyvitamin D was within normal values and PTHrP and 1,25-dihydroxyvitamin were elevated (35.0 pg/ml, and 212 pg/ml, respectively). After the first cycle of chemotherapy with bleomycin, etoposide and cisplatin, normocalcemia was restored. Both PTHrP and 1,25-dihydroxyvitamin D, dropped dramatically to 9.0 pg/ml and 8.0 pg/ml, respectively.

Conclusion: The association of seminoma and malignant hypercalcemia is extremely rare. We describe a case of a patient with a seminoma and malignant hypercalcemia related to paraneoplastic cosecretion of 1,25-dihydroxyvitamin D and PTHrP. After successful chemotherapy, calcium, PTHrP and 1,25-Dihydroxyvitamin D returned to normal values.

Keywords: 1,25-dihydroxyvitamin D, Calcitriol, PTHrP, Malignant hypercalcemia, Seminoma

Background

Malignant hypercalcemia is the most common paraneoplastic syndrome occurring in 20-30% of patients with cancer [1]. It usually has an ominous prognosis, with a mortality of 50% within the next 30 days [2]. Both solid and hematologic malignancies have been associated with this syndrome; the most frequent etiologies being multiple myeloma, lung and breast cancer [3]. Four mechanisms of hypercalcemia in malignancy have been described: local osteolysis, parathyroid hormone related-protein (PTHrP) mediated, 1,25-dihydroxyvitamin D (1,25 $(OH)_2D_3$, calcitriol) secretion, and ectopic parathyroid hormone (PTH) [4,5].

Seminomas have seldomly been related with hypercalcemia. Less than ten cases have documented this exceptional association. Besides two cases related to bone metastasis, the mechanism of hypercalcemia in seminomas has been discussed in two previous reported cases to be secondary to $1,25(OH)_2D_3$ secretion. The underlying mechanism in the rest of the cases was not established. In the previous reports PTHrP was not measured nor related to hypercalcemia. In all of the previous documented cases, independent of the hypercalcemia related mechanism, normocalcemia was achieved soon after definitive treatment was initiated [6-9].

* Correspondence: renerodriguez@investigacion-meduanl.com
[1]Endocrinology Division, Internal Medicine Department, University Hospital "Dr. José E. González", Ave. Madero y Ave. Gonzalitos s/n, Colonia Mitras Centro, Monterrey, Nuevo León 64460, Mexico
[2]Medical School of the Universidad Autónoma de Nuevo León, Ave. Madero y Ave. Gonzalitos s/n, Colonia Mitras Centro, Monterrey, Nuevo León 64460, Mexico
Full list of author information is available at the end of the article

Herein, we present a case of a patient with a seminoma and malignant hypercalcemia mediated by 1,25 $(OH)_2D_3$ and PTHrP paraneoplastic cosecretion.

Case presentation

A 35-year-old man was referred to the Endocrinology Division for assessment and management of severe hypercalcemia related to an abdominal mass. Otherwise, he had an unremarkable medical history. One year before admission he noticed a painless hypogastric abdominal mass. The tumor progressively grew and two months before admission he developed asthenia, anorexia, general weakness, constipation, and an unintentional 10 kg weight loss. A month before admission the appearance of a left inguinal mass finally made him seek medical attention.

An abdominal ultrasound revealed a 10 × 9 × 7 cm heterogeneous (hypoechogenic with hyperechogenic areas) retroperitoneal mass along with bilateral severe hydronephrosis. Serum creatinine was 2.8 mg/dl with a modification of diet in renal disease (MDRD) calculated glomerular filtration rate (GFR) of 35 ml/min. This consequently led to an uncomplicated unilateral left nephrostomy. An abdominal and pelvic enhanced computed tomography (CT) confirmed a calcified pelvic mass, along with multiple retroperitoneal lymphadenopathy (>5 cm each) (Figure 1). A biopsy was performed and the histopathology result was consistent with a seminoma. Chest x-ray revealed "cannon ball" pulmonary metastases. Lactate dehydrogenase (LDH) was 648 UI/L and human chorionic gonadotropin was slightly elevated (35.0 µUI/ml). Alpha-fetoprotein was within its normal reference value (Table 1). A stage IIIB seminoma was

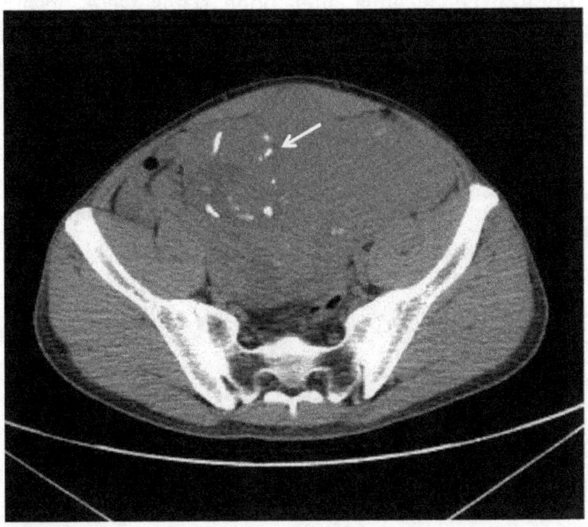

Figure 1 Pelvic enhanced computed tomography that shows a 10×9×7 cm mass with heterogeneous density and calcifications (Arrow).

Table 1 Laboratory measures

Value	Basal	Post-chemotherapy	Range
Glucose (mg/dl)	93	87	(70-100)
Creatinine (mg/dl)	3.7	2.8	(0.6-1.2)
Urea nitrogen (mg/dl)	11	13	(8-23)
MDRD GFR (ml/min)	24.0	37.1	(≥60)
Albumin (g/dl)	3.9		(3.5-5.0)
Calcium (mg/dl)	14.7	9.8	(8.2-10.2)
Phosphorus (pg/ml)	4.1	4.3	(2.3-4.7)
Magnesium (mg/dl)	1.8	2.1	(1.5-2.3)
Potassium (mmol/l)	3.8	4.1	(3.5-5.0)
Urinary calcium (mg/kg/d)	3.2	2.4	(2-4)
Alkaline phosphatase (UI/l)	146		(50-120)
LDH (UI/l)	648	110	(100-200)
AFP (ng/ml)	4.33	3.11	(≤6.0)
β-hCG (uUI/ml)	35.0		(≤3.0)
PTH (pg/ml)	<3.0	13.2	(1.5-37)
PTHrP (pg/ml)	35.0	9.0	(14-27)
$25(OH)D_3$ (ng/ml)	22.0	21.0	(>20)
$1,25(OH)_2D_3$ (pg/ml)	212.0	8.0	(18-38)

MDRD GFR, modification of diet in renal disease glomerular filtration rate; LDH, lactate dehydrogenase; APF, alpha-fetoprotein; β -hCG, human chorionic gonadotropin; PTH, parathyroid hormone; PTHrP, parathyroid hormone related protein; $25(OH)D_3$, 25, Hydroxyvitamin D; $1,25(OH)_2D_3$, 1,25-Dihydroxyvitamin D.

diagnosed and the patient was referred to oncology for chemotherapy.

Two days before admission he presented nausea, polyuria, polydipsia, lethargy, and confusion that led him to the emergency room. On physical examination he was hemodynamically stable with a heart rate of 82 per minute, blood pressure of 130/85 mmHg, a respiratory rate of 16 per minute, a temperature of 36.3°C and a room-air oxygen saturation of 97%. An irregular 10 cm abdominal mass was palpated along with bilateral inguinal adenopathy. The left testicle was not palpable. Serum calcium was 14.7 mg/dl, albumin 3.9 g/dl, alkaline phosphatase 146 UI/l, creatinine 3.7 mg/dl with a MDRD GFR of 24 ml/min. He also had a mild elevated anion-gap metabolic acidosis and a urinary calcium of 3.2 mg/kg/d (240 mg/24 h). Phosphorous, magnesium, potassium, sodium, chlorine, and glucose were normal. PTH was undetectable, 25-dihydroxyvitamin D was normal, PTHrP was 35.0 pg/ml, and calcitriol 212 pg/ml (Quest Diagnostics Nichols, Chantilly, VA) (Table 1). An electrocardiogram showed a shortened QT interval and a bone scan was negative for metastasis. Calcitonin and hydration with intravenous saline solution at 250 ml/h was started. Despite therapy, calcium lowered only to 13.5 mg/dl, but nevertheless his mental status improved. The patient received four cycles of bleomycin, etoposide and carboplatin. After the first cycle of chemotherapy, calcium, LDH and alkaline phosphatase returned to normal values. Both PTHrP and 1,25(OH)$_2$D$_3$ dropped dramatically to 9.0 pg/ml and to 8.0 pg/ml, respectively (Table 1). At 8 months follow-up, the patient was asymptomatic. CT scans showed no residual disease and calcium levels have been consistently normal without medication.

Discussion

This case illustrates, to our knowledge, the first reported case of malignant hypercalcemia in a patient with seminoma related to paraneoplastic cosecretion of PTHrP and 1,25(OH)$_2$D$_3$. Pure seminomas (no non-seminomatous elements present) account for up to 60% of all testicular germ cell tumors. They usually affect males between the second and fourth decade of life, representing 1% of all cancers in men. Undescended testes (cryptorchidism), as in our patient, is a risk factor and they are usually associated with a good prognosis with an overall five-year survival of 95% and even 80% in intermediate and high-risk patients [10,11]. Hyercalcemia associated with malignancy has been well described in both solid and hematologic malignancies (usually lymphomas) and represent the most common cause of elevated serum calcium in hospitalized patients [1]. The four mechanisms by which malignant hypercalcemia can occur are: 1) direct osteolytic metastases (20% of cases), usually related to multiple myeloma and breast cancer with release of cytokines such as interleukin (IL)-1, IL-6, IL-8 and activation of nuclear factor kappa beta; 2) PTH-rP or humoral hypercalcemia (80% of cases) usually described in nonmetastatic solid tumors (bladder, breast and squamous cell) and some non-Hodgkin lymphomas; 3) ectopic PTH secretion with only a few cases reported, and 4) 1,25(OH)$_2$D$_3$ secretion that accounts for less than 1% of cases [4,5,12,13].

Usually associated to granulomatous diseases such as sarcoidosis, tuberculosis, and systemic fungal infections, among others, calcitriol mediated hypercalcemia has been infrequently related to neoplasms [14]. Lymphomas have been the most common type of malignancy described, and other kind of tumors, such as disgerminomas, have rarely been reported [15]. Seminomas have been associated with malignant hypercalcemia almost anecdotally, with less than ten cases reported in the literature (Table 2). King et al. and Metcalfe et al. described the first two cases in the 70s. In their report, they both associated a seminoma with a pseudohyperparathyroidism and were not able to measure neither PTHrP nor vitamin D metabolites. In both cases, hypercalcemia resolved after definitive treatment with orchiectomy or corticosteroid-radiotherapy [6,7]. In 1987, Grote and Hainsworth reported the first case of a seminoma with a calcitriol mediated malignant hypercalcemia. Baseline calcitriol level was 125 pg/ml, with a normal PTH, 25-Hydroxyvitamine D and high 24 h urine calcium. PTHrP was not measured. After the first chemotherapy cycle, calcitriol concentration fell to 29 pg/mL and normocalcemia was achieved [8]. In 1992, da Silva et al. reported seven cases (four new and three previously described cases) of seminoma associated with malignant hypercalcemia. With regard to the four new cases, PTH was normal in three and was not measured in one. PTHrP and 25-hydroxyvitamin D were not measured in any case and 1,25(OH)$_2$D$_3$ was measured only in one case with an initial concentration of 79 pg/mL that decreased to 5 pg/mL after two cycles of chemotherapy and was associated afterwards with normocalcemia [9].

On the other hand, PTHrP has never been described in a patient with a pure seminoma. There are two reported cases of hypercalcemia associated with non-seminomatous germ cell tumors (NSGCTs). MacDiarmid et al. in 1995 reported a malignant hypercalcemia associated to an extragonadal NSGCT that was suspected to be probably due to a humoral hypercalcemia after bone scans were negative. PTHrP and vitamin D metabolites were not measured [16]. Later on, Sorscher described a patient with severe hypercalcemia and a NSGCT with a high PTHrP and a normal

Table 2 Reported malignant hypercalcemia in seminomas

Author (*)	Ca+	PTH	PTHrP	25D	1,25D	Tx	Ca + after Tx.	Outcome
King [6]	15.4	NS	NS	NS	NS	Orchiectomy	NL	NED 10 mo.
Metcalfe [7]	15.8	NS	NS	NS	NS	GC + RT	NL	NED 8 mo.
Grote [8]	15.4	10.0	NS	24.0	112	BEP	NL	NED 2 yr.
Da Silva [9]	12.7	NL	NS	NS	NS	NSCT	NL	Adenophaty
Da Silva [9]	18.5	NS	NS	NS	NS	BEP	NL	NED 2 mo.
Da Silva [9]	20.1	NS	NS	NS	NS	NSCT	NL	NED 4 mo.
Da Silva [9]	16.4	0.3	NS	NS	79	BEP	NL	Improved after CT
This report	14.7	≤3.0	35.0	22.0	212	BEP	NL	NED 8 mo.

(*) Reference.

Ca+, Calcium (mg/dl); PTH, parathyroid hormone; PTHrP, parathyroid hormone related protein; 25D, 25, Hydroxyvitamin D; 1,25D, 1,25-Dihydroxyvitamin D; Tx, treatment; NS, not stated; NL, normal; NED, not evidence of disease; BEP, bleomycin, etoposide and cisplatinum; NSCT, not specified chemotherapy; CT, chemotherapy.

PTH that returned to normal values after chemotherapy. No measurements of 25-hydroxyvitamin D and $1,25(OH)_2 D_3$ levels were made [17]. In our case, a diagnosis of pure seminoma was well documented. Baseline serum calcium was elevated, urinary calcium, phosphorous and 25-hydroxyvitamin D were normal, PTH was undetectable and calcitriol and PTHrP were elevated. After one cycle of chemotherapy, normocalcemia was restored and both, calcitriol and PTHrP dropped to normal levels.

The exact mechanism by which calcitriol is produced in malignancy remains open to debate. Normally, in the kidney, 1α-hydroxylase converts 25-hydroxyvitamin D into the biologically active $1,25(OH)_2D_3$, which is essential for bone and calcium metabolism/homeostasis. Nevertheless, 1α-hydroxylase has also been described in normal human tissues such as placenta, skin, gastrointestinal tract, testes, central nervous system and osteoblasts [18]. More than twenty granulomatous conditions are known to have enhanced 1α-hydroxylation of vitamin D in macrophages and increased production of active calcitriol causing hypercalcemia and/or hypercalciuria [19]. In lymphomas, Hewison et al., using inmunolocalization, showed stained sections of spleen that were negative for 1α-hydroxylase in lymphoma cells, but that were positive in surrounding macrophages [20]. Nonetheless, Evans et al. showed by reverse transcription polymerase chain reaction that mRNA for 1α-hydroxylase was increased 222-fold in disgerminoma cells compared to the surrounding non-ovarian tissue [21]. The exact mechanism in seminomas has not been explored. On the other hand, PTHrP is well recognized to be secreted by a variety of malignancies, in which there is an uncoupling of bone resorption and formation and a reduced ability of the kidney to clear calcium with the resultant hypercalcemia [22]. This last effect on the kidney could be the cause of the normal 24-h urinary calcium reported in our case, when it has been usually reported to be high in other calcitriol mediated pathologies [6-9,23]. As well, PTHrP is usually associated with hypophosphatemia due to an increase in urinary phosphorous; in this case, the concomitant renal failure could have diminished this last effect [24]. Interestingly, normocalcemia has consistently been achieved and sustained, in our case and in all previous cases, soon after definitive treatment with chemotherapy, surgery or glucocorticoids [5-8]. In this way, it is probable that bisphosphonates, denosumab, gallium nitrate, cinacalet and other medications directed to lower serum calcium could be withheld until definitive treatment is initiated.

Conclusion

Seminomas have seldom been associated with hypercalcemia. We have described the case of a patient with a seminoma and malignant hypercalcemia related to cosecretion of $1,25(OH)_2D_3$ and PTHrP. After successful treatment, calcium, PTHrP and $1,25(OH)_2D_3$ returned to normal values. The exact mechanism by which seminomas secrete $1,25(OH)_2D_3$ still remains to be elucidated.

Abbreviations

PTHrP: Parathyroid hormone related-protein; $1,25(OH)_2D_3$: 1,25-dihydroxyvitamin D, calcitriol; PTH: Parathyroid hormone; MDRD GFR: Modification of diet in renal disease calculated glomerular filtration rate; LDH: Lactate dehydrogenase; IL: Interleukin; CT: Computed tomography; NSGCTs: Non-seminomatous germ cell tumors.

Competing interests

The authors declare that they have no competing interests.

Authors' contributions

RRG and JGGG served as the principal investigators and led the conception, design, acquisition of data, review of literature, and drafted the manuscript. MAZR, DLQF, CRCL contributed in the acquisition of data, review of literature and reviewed the manuscript. FJLG and JZVP contributed the concept of research paper and critically reviewed the manuscript. All authors read and approved the manuscript.

Authors' information

RRG and MAZR are endocrinology fellows at the Endocrinology Division. DLQF and CRCL are internal medicine residents. FJLG is professor and chief of the diabetes clinic of the Endocrinology Division. JGGG is the vice-dean of research of the Medical School of the Universidad Autonoma de Nuevo Leon and professor of the Endocrinology Division. JZVP is the chief and director of the Endocrinology Division.

Acknowledgments

We wish to thank Sergio Lozano-Rodriguez for his critical reading of the manuscript.

Author details

[1]Endocrinology Division, Internal Medicine Department, University Hospital "Dr. José E. González", Ave. Madero y Ave. Gonzalitos s/n, Colonia Mitras Centro, Monterrey, Nuevo León 64460, Mexico. [2]Medical School of the Universidad Autónoma de Nuevo León, Ave. Madero y Ave. Gonzalitos s/n, Colonia Mitras Centro, Monterrey, Nuevo León 64460, Mexico. [3]Internal Medicine Department, University Hospital "Dr. José E. González", Monterrey, Nuevo León 64460, Mexico.

References

1. Stewart AF, Broadus AE: **Malignancy associated hypercalcemia.** In *Endocrinology.* 5th edition. Edited by DeGroot L, Jameson LJ. Philadelphia: Saunders. in press.
2. Stewart AF: **Clinical practice. Hypercalcemia associated with cancer.** *N Engl J Med* 2005, **352**(4):373–379.
3. Ralston SH, Gallagher SJ, Patel U, Campbell J, Boyle IT: **Cancer-associated hypercalcemia: morbidity and mortality: clinical experience in 126 treated patients.** *Ann Intern Med* 1990, **112**:499–504.
4. Horwitz MJ, Stewart AF: **Humoral Hypercalcemia Of Malignancy.** In *Primer On The Metabolic Bone Diseases And Disorders Of Mineral Metabolism.* 5th edition. Edited by Favus MF. Washington D.C: American Society for Bone and Mineral Research; 2003:246–250.
5. Roodman GD: **Mechanisms of bone metastasis.** *N Engl J Med* 2004, **350**:1655–1664.
6. King WW, Cox CE, Boyce WH: **Pseudohyperparathyroidism and seminoma.** *J Urol* 1972, **107**:809–811.

7. Metcalfe JB, Carey TC, Barry JM: **Genitourinary malignancy and pseudohyperparathyroidism.** *J Urol* 1978, **119:**702–704.
8. Grote TH, Hainsworth JD: **Hypercalcemia and elevated serum calcitriol in a patient with seminoma.** *Arch Int Med* 1987, **147:**2212–2213.
9. da Silva MA, Edmondson JW, Eby C, Loeher PJ: **Humoral hypercalcemia in seminomas.** *Med Pediatr Oncol* 1992, **20:**38–41.
10. Siegel R, Ward E, Brawley O, Jemal A: **Cancer statistics, 2011: the impact of eliminating socioeconomic and racial disparities on premature cancer deaths.** *CA Cancer J Clin* 2011, **61**(4):212.
11. Bosl GJ, Motzer RJ: **Testicular germ-cell cancer.** *N Engl J Med* 1997, **337**(4):242.
12. Doyle MA, Malcolm JC: **An unusual case of malignancy- related hypercalcemia.** *Int J Gen Med* 2014, **7:**21–27.
13. Kandil E, Noureldine S, Khalek MA, Daroca P, Friedlander P: **Ectopic secretion of parathyroid hormone in a neuroendocrine tumor: a case report and review of the literature.** *Int J Clin Exp Med* 2011, **4**(3):234–240.
14. Jacobs TP, Bilezikian JP: **Clinical review: rare causes of hypercalcemia.** *J Clin Endocrinol Metab* 2005, **90**(11):6316.
15. Seymour JF, Gagel RF: **Calcitriol: the major humoral mediator of hypercalcemia in Hodgkin's disease and non-Hodgkin's lymphomas.** *Blood* 1993, **82**(5):1383.
16. MacDiarmid SA, Norman RW: **Extragonadal nonseminomatous germ cell tumour with hypercalcemia, masquerading as renal cell carcinoma: a case report.** *Can J Surg* 1995, **38:**80–82.
17. Sorscher S: **Elevated parathyroid hormone-related peptide in a patient with an extragonadal germ-cell tumour and hypercalcemia.** *Can J Surg* 2004, **47**(2):144. No abstract available.
18. Bikle DD: **Extra renal synthesis of 1,25-dihydroxyvitamin D and its health implications.** *Clinic Rev Bone Miner Metab* 2009, **7:**114.
19. Hewison M, Burke F, Evans KN, Lammas DA, Sansom DM, Liu P, Modlin RL, Adams JS: **Extra-renal 25-hydroxyvitamin D3-1 alpha-hydroxylase in human health and disease.** *J Steroid Biochem Mol Biol* 2007, **103**(3–5):316–321.
20. Hewison M, Kantorovich V, Liker HR, Van Herle AJ, Cohan P, Zehnder D, Adams JS: **Vitamin D-mediated hypercalcemia in lymphoma: evidence for hormone production by tumor-adjacent macrophages.** *J Bone Miner Res* 2003, **18**(3):579–582.
21. Evans KN, Taylor H, Zehnder D, Kilby MD, Bulmer JN, Shah F, Adams JS, Hewison M: **Increased expression of 25-hydroxyvitamin D-1alpha-hydroxylase in dysgerminomas: a novel form of humoral hypercalcemia of malignancy.** *Am J Pathol* 2004, **165**(3):807–813.
22. Syed MA, Horwitz MJ, Tedesco MB, Garcia-Ocaña A, Wisniewski SR, Stewart AF: **Parathyroid hormone-related protein-(1–36) stimulates renal tubular calcium reabsorption in normal human volunteers: implications for the pathogenesis of humoral hypercalcemia of malignancy.** *J Clin Endocrinol Metab* 2001, **86**(4):1525–1531.
23. Giannini S, Nobile M, Castrignano R, Pati T, Tasca A, Villi G, Pellegrini F, D'Angelo A: **Possible link between vitamin D and hyperoxaluria in patients with renal stone disease.** *Clin Sci* 1993, **84:**51–54.
24. Fraher LJ, Hodsman AB, Jonas K, Saunders D, Rose CI, Henderson JE, Hendy GN, Goltzman D: **A comparison of the in vivo biochemical responses to exogenous parathyroid hormone-(1-34) [PTH-(1-34)] and PTH-related peptide-(1-34) in man.** *J Clin Endocrinol Metab* 1992, **75**(2):417.

10

Decreased levels of physical activity in adolescents with down syndrome are related with low bone mineral density

Ángel Matute-Llorente[1,2], Alejandro González-Agüero[1,3], Alba Gómez-Cabello[1,4], Germán Vicente-Rodríguez[1,2] and José Antonio Casajús[1,2*]

Abstract

Background: Down syndrome (DS) has been described as one of the main contributors for low bone mineral density (BMD). Physical activity (PA) is a key factor in skeletal health and thus, PA levels might be associated to the risk of developing osteoporosis. Therefore, the aims were (1) to describe PA patterns in adolescents with DS compared to their counterparts and (2) to determine the relationships between PA and the risk of having low bone mass in adolescents with DS.

Methods: Nineteen adolescents (10 girls) with DS and 14 without disabilities (7 girls) participated in the study. Minutes in different PA intensities were objectively assessed with accelerometers (ActiTrainer). Moreover adolescents with DS were classified into PA tertiles taking into account the amount of total minutes of PA at any intensity, resulting in those performing low, medium or high of PA (lowPA, medPA and highPA). BMD was measured at the whole body, hip and lumbar spine with dual-energy X-ray absorptiometry and the BMD Z-score was calculated for each region taking into account age- and sex-matched reference data. Student's unpaired t-tests and analysis of covariance were used to compare variables between different conditions (DS vs. control) and PA levels (low, medium and high).

Results: None of the adolescents with DS achieved the minimum of 60 min of daily moderate to vigorous PA (VPA) intensity recommended by PA guidelines; adolescents with DS group spent less time in sedentary and in VPA and more time in light PA than those without DS ($p < 0.05$). Adolescents with DS showed lower BMD Z-score values than those without ($p < 0.05$). Those adolescents with DS allocated in the lowPA tertile showed significant lower BMD Z-score at the hip and a general tendency towards lower BMD Z-score was found at whole body and lumbar spine compared to those in highPA tertile and ($p < 0.05$).

Conclusions: Adolescents with DS in the highPA tertile showed lower risk of developing future osteoporosis by having higher BMD Z-score at the hip. This data provides an idea regarding the importance of accumulated minutes of PA, and not only moderate or vigorous in the bone health in adolescents with DS.

Keywords: Osteoporosis, Osteopenia, Accelerometer, Dual energy x-ray, Actitrainer, Body composition

* Correspondence: joseant@unizar.es
[1]GENUD (Growth, Exercise, Nutrition and Development) Research Group, University of Zaragoza, Ed. Cervantes Corona de Aragón St 42, 2nd floor, Zaragoza 50009, Spain
[2]Faculty of Health and Sport Science, Department of Physiatry and Nursing, University of Zaragoza, Ronda Misericordia 5, Huesca 22001, Spain
Full list of author information is available at the end of the article

Background

Persons with Down syndrome (DS) have shown diminished levels of bone mass compared with those without DS [1-4]; therefore, DS population might be considered as a population at higher risk of suffering bone fractures and osteoporosis. The latter is a systemic skeletal diseases characterized by low bone mass and micro-architectural deterioration, resulting in an increased susceptibility to fracture [5]. Osteoporosis-related fractures constitute a major public health concern in the nowadays society [6]. Among the factors involved in fracture risk Lips et al. [7] highlighted bone mineral density (BMD), bone geometry and bone strength. Furthermore, as life expectancy in DS population has been increased over the last 70 years and this trend is expected to continue [8] the incidence of osteopenia and osteoporosis is likely to be augmented in this population within the coming years. In addition, and reinforcing this hypothesis, DS has been demonstrated as one of the main contributors for low BMD in persons with intellectual disability [9,10]. It is widely known that a increased bone mass acquisition during childhood and adolescence is determinant for a good skeletal health in adulthood [11]. Although genetic factors highly determine bone mass acquisition [12], environmental and lifestyle factors, such as physical activity (PA) have an important role in bone mass acquisition due to their osteogenic effects [13]. PA is a key factor in disease prevention and provides several benefits in overall health [14] and specifically in skeletal health [15]. Exercise has important osteogenic effect, mainly when high-impact and weight-bearing PA occur [16] in concordance with the Wolff's law [17] which postulates that bones adapt to mechanical loads. At the same time, the mechanostat theory [18,19] suggests that both systematic exercise and PA could drive to a direct osteogenic effect on bone mass and an indirect osteogenic effect by increasing muscle size and strength and hence the tensions generated on bones [16]. Persons with DS experience several barriers to participate in daily PA like transportation restrictions, low motivation and lack of integrated program options [20]. Consequently, low levels of PA [21] and physical fitness [22] have been described in this population. In addition, most of the literature regarding PA levels in children with intellectual disabilities was based on self or proxy-reported questioners, or pedometers [23] with the consequent methodological weaknesses [24]. Even with that, there was some evidence indicating that children with intellectual disabilities are less active than those without disabilities [23]. Accelerometry is an accurate, non-invasive, and relatively low-cost method that can be used with minimal interference in free-living conditions [25]; and this has been demonstrated as more reliable than pedometers [26]. Some studies using accelerometers have been performed in order to evaluate PA levels in children with DS [21,27-29]. A general tendency towards decreased levels of PA with increasing age has been shown in different studies, and also a non-achievement of the currently recommendations of PA was found in this population. As observed, information concerning bone mass in young populations with DS is scarce [30] and should therefore be given greater attention; on the other hand PA levels might have a relationship with the risk of developing osteopenia or osteoporosis.

Therefore the aims of this study were (1) to describe PA patterns in adolescents with DS compared to their counterparts and (2) to determine relationships between PA and risk of having low bone mass in adolescents with DS.

Methods

Institutions were contacted prior to the study to organize reunions in order to connect with parents and offer to participate in the study. Once the informed consents were obtained, 40 adolescents were selected taking into account their age, sex and the lack of contraindications (Figure 1). The contraindications for taking a DXA scan were: being pregnant or having had any procedure using substances such as Iodine, Barium, and Nuclear medicine isotope.

The present study was conducted on two groups: the first group was comprised by 20 adolescents with DS (10 girls, 10 boys; aged 14.7 ± 2.2 years) living at home, who were recruited from different special schools and institutions within the region of Aragon in Spain. Adolescents with DS were examined by an experienced cardiologist and all of them were healthy and given permission to participate in the study.

The second group was formed by 20 adolescents without DS (10 girls, 10 boys; aged 13.2 ± 2.8 years) and was also recruited from regular schools in the same region. All the adolescents without DS were healthy and without known illness, and all subjects had been medication-free for at least 3 months before the test. A full clinical history, including illnesses or surgical interventions and stays in a hospital, was collected for each individual. Both parents and children were informed about the aims and procedures of the study, as well as the possible risks and benefits, and then, a letter of written informed consent was obtained from all the included subjects and their parents or guardians. The study was performed in accordance with the Helsinki Declaration 1961 (revised in Edinburgh, 2000) and was approved by the Research Ethics Committee of the Government of Aragon (CEICA, Spain).

Anthropometric measures

All subjects were measured with a stadiometer without shoes and the minimum clothes to the nearest 0.1 cm

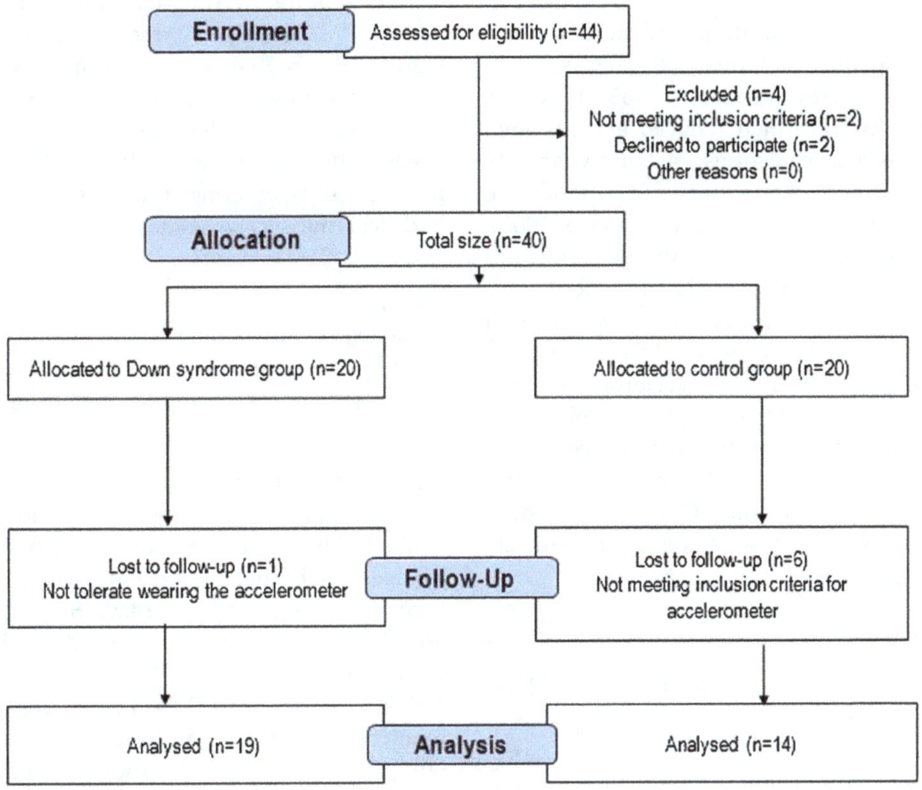

Figure 1 Consort flow diagram.

(SECA 225, SECA, Hamburg, Germany), and weighted to the nearest 0.1 kg (SECA 861, SECA, Hamburg, Germany) following the procedures by International Society for the Advancement in Kinanthropometry (ISAK) [31]. Body mass index (BMI) was calculated as weight (in kilograms) divided by height (square meters). Height, weight and BMI Z-scores were calculated using a Microsoft Excel add-in to access growth references based on the LMS method [32] using a reference European population [33].

Pubertal status assessment

Pubertal development was determined by a sport medicine physician with direct observation according to the five stages proposed by Tanner and Whitehouse [34].

Assessment of PA

Free-living PA was objectively assessed using the ActiTrainer uniaxial accelerometer (Actigraph, LLC, Pensacola, FL, USA). Actitrainer uniaxial accelerometer has been validated for assessing PA and energy expenditure [35]. ActiTrainer is a small and light device (8.6 × 3.3 × 1.5 cm, 51 g), which uses a sensor with a 0.25 to 2.5 g range capable of detecting movements in the vertical plane and a sampling frequency of 30 Hz. For this study, a 15s epoch was selected on the basis of literature recommendations [36]. The accelerometer was worn for seven consecutive days during school-term time and was mounted on the right hip of each adolescent by means of an elastic waistband. Instructions were given to the participants and caregivers both verbally and in writing on how to wear the accelerometer during all waking hours except while bathing, showering, swimming, and playing contact sports. A time sheet was used to register when the accelerometer was placed on or removed each day. In DS group, it was completed by parents or caregivers whilst in control group it was completed by themselves. A 7-day data collection period has been found to provide sufficient time to obtain a reliable estimation of normal activity in children and adolescents aged 6–17 years, as it allows for differences in PA levels across the day and between weekdays and weekends [37]. Afterwards, the previous published cut-off points proposed by Evenson et al. [38] and recommended by Trost et al. [39] were used to estimate time spent in sedentary, light-, moderate-, and VPA intensity in children and adolescents.

Data reduction

For inclusion in this study, the accelerometer had to be worn for a minimum of 10 hours per day, for at least 4 days out of the 7-day monitoring period, including one weekend day, as recommended in a previous study [21]. Data analyses involved the data processed in the R [40] program. The methodological process of this program has been described in a previous research [35]. Based on a 15 s epoch, the data were then reduced and assigned to one of the following categories: sedentary activity (counts ≤ 25), light PA (574 > counts > 25), moderate PA (1003 > counts of ≥ 574), or VPA(counts ≥ 1003). Subjects were considered compliant to the PA guidelines if their moderate to VPA, averaged over the valid days of monitoring, was ≥ 60 min a day [41]. In our study, total minutes of daily PA is equivalent to valid time being the average daily time spent wearing the accelerometer once the data reduction was done according to Ojiambo et al. [42]. A 20-min period of zero counts is produced when the accelerometer device records 20 minutes of inactivity, that is, 20 minutes of 0 counts. During data reduction 20-min period of zero counts were automatically deleted with the R program.

Bone mass

Bone mass of the participants was measured with dual-energy X-ray absorptiometry (DXA) using a pediatric version of the software QDR-Explorer (Hologic Corp. Software version 12.4, Waltham, MA). DXA equipment was calibrated daily with a lumbar spine phantom and step densities phantom following the Hologic guidelines as recommended the manufacturer. Subjects were scanned in supine position, and the scans were performed in high resolution. BMD (in grams/cm^2) was obtained from the whole body scan, lumbar spine (L_1-L_4) and proximal region of the femur (hip). BMD Z-score values were calculated for purposes of comparison. The BMD Z-score is a measurement which compares the actual BMD of a person with age- and gender-matched reference values obtaining a score of SD from the reference M. This is a more appropriate measurement for bone health in children and adolescents than t-score is [43].

Statistical analysis

All data analyses were performed using SPSS 15.0 software for Windows (SPSS Inc. Chicago, IL), and significance was set at $p \leq 0.05$. Mean (M) and Standard Deviation (SD) or Standard Error (SE) are given as descriptive statistics; otherwise they are stated. All variables included in this study showed a normal distribution, assessed by Kolmogorov-Smirnov test. Differences between DS and control groups for age, and height, weight, BMI, BMD Z-scores were established using the Student's unpaired *t*-tests. Analyses of covariance (ANCOVA) were performed to evaluate differences between DS and control groups in daily minutes in different PA intensities, with age and valid time as covariates.

Tertiles of total PA, based on the total minutes of daily PA: lowPA (min ≤ 713), medPA (795 ≥min > 713), and highPA (min > 795), were also calculated within the group of adolescents with DS. ANCOVA was also performed in order to evaluate differences in BMD Z-score values between different tertiles of PA (with further Bonferroni post-hoc test) entering Tanner stage, height and whole body lean mass as covariates.

Results

Participants

Final reduction of accelerometry data resulted in 7 participants lost for different reasons (see Figure 1).

Physical characteristics

Age and physical characteristics are summarized in Table 1. No differences between groups were observed for age, weight, height and BMI. On average, participants with DS were older (M = 14.78, SE = 0.51), lighter (M = 46.76, SE = 2.65) and smaller (M = 146.30, SE = 2.84) than those without DS (M = 13.28, SE = 0.75), (M = 50.23, SE = 4.20) and (M = 155.57, SE = 3.99). These differences were not significant $t(31)$ = −1.69, 0.73, 1.94, (all p > 0.05) (Table 1); these values did represent a medium-sized and small-sized effect r = .32, .13 and .33 respectively. When weight, height and BMI Z-scores were taken into account, adolescents with DS showed significantly differences in Height (M = −2.30, SE = 0.25), and Weight (M = −0.83, SE = 0.27) Z-scores compared with those adolescents without DS (M = 0.00, and 0.35, SE = 0.25, and 0.34 respectively) $t(31)$ 6.4 and 2.7, (all p < 0.05) (Table 1); and they represent a high and medium-sized effects r = .75, .44. However, there was no difference in BMI Z-score values between DS group (M = 0.62, SE = 0.20) and Control group (M = 0.46, SE = 0.33) $t(31)$ -0.41, (p > 0.05) (Table 1).

Table 1 Descriptive statistics for participants (M ± SD)

	Down syndrome (n = 19)	Control (n = 14)
Age (yr)	14.7 ± 2.2	13.2 ± 2.8
Weight (kg)	46.7 ± 11.5	50.2 ± 15.7
Height (cm)	146.3 ± 12.3	155.5 ± 14.9
Body mass index	21.4 ± 3.2	20.3 ± 3.7
Weight Z-score	−0.8 ± 1.2*	0.4 ± 1.3
Height Z-score	−2.3 ± 1.1*	0.0 ± 0.9
BMI Z-score	0.6 ± 0.9	0.5 ± 1.3
Lumbar spine BMD Z-score	−0.8 ± 0.9*	0.1 ± 1.1
Hip BMD Z-score	−1.1 ± 0.9*	0.1 ± 1.2
Whole body BMD Z-score	−1.7 ± 1.1*	0.5 ± 1.6

* $p \leq 0.05$ between groups. *BMD* bone mineral density.

Physical activity

Total minutes in each PA intensity adjusting by age and valid time are presented in Figure 2. There was a significant effect of the age and the valid time on sedentary PA, $F(1, 29) = 21.80$, ($p < 0.05$) and $F(1, 29) = 7.31$, $p < 0.05$. Bonferroni *post hoc* test revealed that the sedentary PA was significantly lower in DS group (M = 470.7, SD = 61.3) than in control group (M = 540.2, SD = 62.3); ($p < 0.05$). In light PA, age $F(1, 29) = 43.45$, ($p < 0.05$) and valid time $F(1, 29) = 7.38$, ($p < 0.05$) had a significant effect on it. However, in this case DS group (M = 243.5, SD = 39.5) spent more time light PA than control group (M = 181.1, SD = 39.8); ($p < 0.05$). In moderate PA, only age $F(1, 29) = 29.8$, ($p < 0.05$) had a significant effect on it; but valid time $F(1, 29) = 0.1$, ($p > 0.05$) do not and Bonferroni *post hoc* test did not reveal any different. However, adolescents with DS (M = 7.4, SD = 8.2) engaged less time in VPA than those without (M = 15.8, SD = 8.4) but neither age $F(1, 29) = 0.02$ nor valid time $F(1, 29) = 0.65$ had a significant effect on VPA (all $p > 0.05$) (See Figure 2).

None of the adolescents with DS achieved the minimum of 60 min of daily moderate to VPA recommended by guidelines; while only 3 of the control adolescents achieved that amount, which represents 21.4% of the sample (data not shown).

Bone mass

Adolescents with DS showed lower BMD Z-score values at the whole body (M = −1.75, SE = 0.24), lumbar spine (M = −0.83, SE = 0.20), and hip (M = −1.08, SE = 0.20) than the control group (M = 0.53, SE= 0.44), (M = 0.09, SE = 0.30) and (M = 0.08, SE = 0.33). All differences were significant $t(31) = 2.64$, $t(30) = 3.18$ and $t(31) = 4.48$, (all $p < 0.05$) (Table 1); and they represent a medium-sized and large-sized effects r = .43, .50 and .63.

In DS group, there was a non-significant effect of height $F(1, 13) = 0.12$, and whole body lean mass $F(1, 13) = 1.25$ on BMD Z-score at hip region but tanner stage was $F(1, 13) = 4.56$, ($p < 0.05$). Once the sample of adolescents with DS was classified within PA tertiles, Bonferroni *post hoc* test revealed that those allocated in the lowPA tertile (M = −1.79, SD = 1.3) showed lower BMD Z-score at the hip region than those in highPA tertile (M = −0.45, SD = 1.5); ($p \leq 0.05$) (Figure 3). Despite no significant differences between tertiles, a tendency towards higher BMD Z-score in medPA and highPA compared to lowPA was observed in lumbar spine and whole body BMD Z-score values (Figure 3).

Discussion

The main finding of the present study is that adolescents with DS who engage daily in more minutes of total PA present higher BMD Z-score values, mainly at the hip region. Although some previous studies described PA patterns in children and adolescents with DS [21,27-29], to our knowledge, this is the first study including objectively assessed PA and bone measurements in adolescents with and without DS. Previous studies have found lower bone mass among individuals with DS compared with others without using different equipments such as DXA [2,3,44,45] or peripheral quantitative computed tomography [4]. Our study indicates, by means of lower BMD Z-score in all studied regions, higher risk of having low bone mass of the adolescents with DS, and, as the life expectancy of persons with DS has increased [8], this is an important issue to be taken into account. Literature indicates a consistent long-term protective effect from

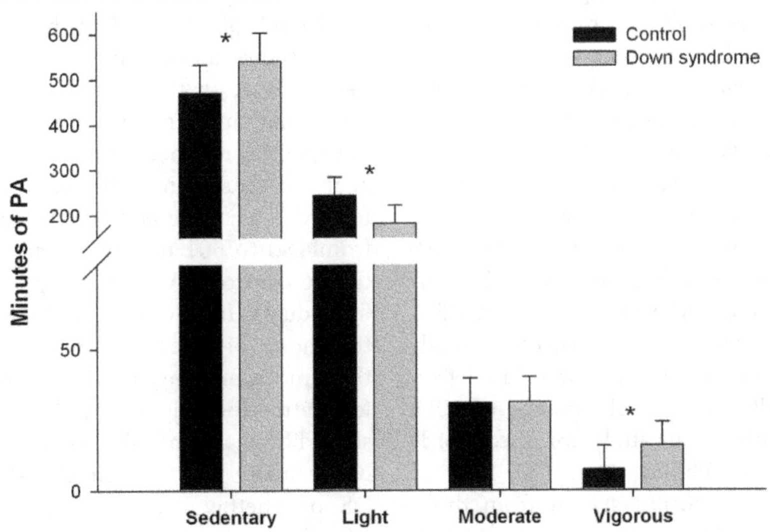

Figure 2 Daily time spent in different PA intensities adjusting by age and valid time. * $p \leq 0.05$ between groups.

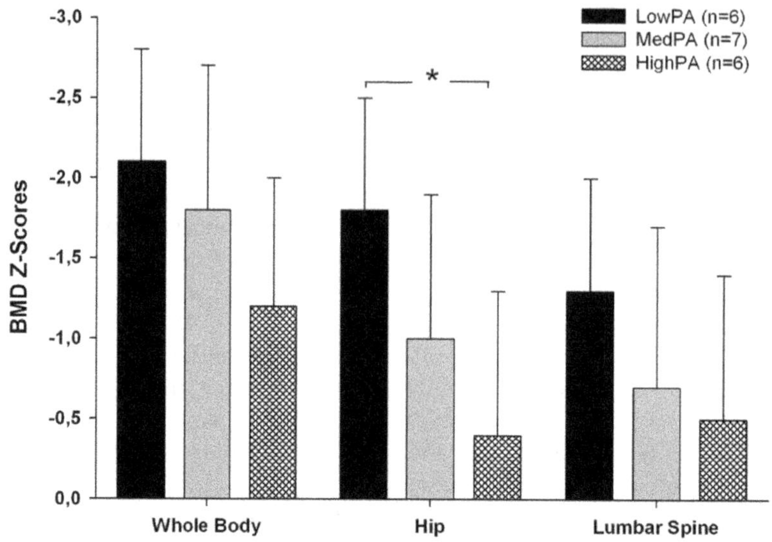

Figure 3 Bone data for PA tertiles in the DS group. Analysis adjusted for height, tanner stage and whole body lean mass. *$p \leq 0.05$ between lowPA and highPA tertiles.

PA during adolescence on bone health [46] and also that sedentary behavior during childhood is associated with poor adult health outcomes [47]. In concordance, the results of our study showed that those adolescents with DS performing more minutes of daily PA had higher BMD Z-score values, especially at hip, than those engaging less minutes of daily PA. This relationship makes us believe that total minutes of PA could be a protective factor against poor bone-health. In addition to this, a recent published study has showed that the pelvis may be the first site to show significant differences in bone mineral content and BMD between preadolescent boys with and without DS [48]. This study has reinforced the importance of this body region in relation to bone health y DS population. Therefore, PA should be promoted in adolescents with DS, not necessarily at a high intensity, in order to decrease their risk of present and future low bone mass. Adolescents with DS in the current study engaged in less minutes of sedentary PA than those without; and in addition, the average values of the adolescents with DS in our study are lower than those observed by Esposito et al. [21]. At the same time, adolescents with DS engaged in more min of light PA than those without. However, adolescents with DS engaged in less minutes of high-intensity PA such as VPA, than those without DS. A paternal overprotection in adolescents with DS might be influencing and could partially explain these results [49]. Total minutes of VPA observed in DS adolescents in our study are in concordance with those showed by Phillips et al. [27] in their sample of adolescents with DS, but are far from those achieved by children with DS in other studies [28,29]. This fact might be also explained in part due to the general trend of decreasing PA with age in individuals with DS [21,27,29]. None of the adolescents with DS in the current study met PA recommendations of at least 60 min of daily MVPA, which is in agreement with some previous research [21,27], but in contrast with others [28,29]. Our results suggest that many children with DS may not perform enough PA to maintain an overall, and specifically bone good health. In fact, a recent study [13] reported that more than 78 minute of moderate to VPA per day are needed to increase bone mass in non-DS adolescents, which is farer from the actual MVPA of young DS population. This finding emphasizes the need of adolescents with DS to increase the amount of daily MVPA, as they are predisposed to diseases associated with inactivity such as osteoporosis, artery disease or obesity in adulthood [50]. The effect that the cut-off points choice has in the results obtained is something crucial [42]. Evidence suggests that the choice of epoch and cut-off points may interact and influence PA classification in an unexpected manner. Furthermore, Reilly et al. [51] reanalyzed data using different epochs and cut-off points for sedentary time and MVPA and found values ranging from 180 to 501 min of sedentary time per day and 28 to 266 min of MVPA per day for the same periods and individuals. In addition, Ojiambo et al. [42] found that the choice of different epochs had a significant effect on the time spent engaged in sedentary or MVPA. Therefore, attention might be put on this regard, and efforts should be made in order to evaluate which cut-off points better adapt to the characteristics of adolescents with DS, or whether it could be good to develop others specifically designed for this specific population. This study is not exempt of limitations which may affect the application of these findings. PA may have been underestimated as the use of a single, waist mounted, uni-axial accelerometer will not measure PA during upper-body and non-weight bearing activities (e.g., load carrying, swimming, cycling) and during activities such as bathing, showering, swimming, or playing contact sports. To complete the information regarding total daily physical activity, in future studies would be recommended to record the time in which participants were involved in swimming/ contact sports, slept, and showered/ bathed. In addition, the use of cut-off points established for children without disabilities may not be representative in individuals with DS as pointed out by Mendoca et al. [52]. Moreover, because the results are cross-sectional, a cause-and-effect relationship between PA and bone can only be suggested. The power to detect differences between groups may be affected by the small sample size.

Conclusions

The current research provides evidence that adolescents with DS who perform more minutes of PA have lower risk of having low BMD at the hip and might be at lower risk of suffering osteoporotic fractures in the future by having a higher BMD Z-score in this region. Adolescents with DS did not achieve PA recommendations, and they engaged less minutes of VPA than those without DS. To develop specific cut-off points and/or PA recommendations for individuals with DS is an important topic to be taken into account in further research. These data remark the importance of total minutes of PA, and not only, those minutes in moderate or VPA, accumulated during the day in the population of adolescents with DS. Therefore, efforts to increase the PA levels in this population might be counteracting their intrinsic diseases of low bone mass, and preserving their future bone health.

Abbreviations

DS: Down syndrome; BMD: Bone mineral density; PA: Physical activity; VPA: Vigorous physical activity; BMI: Body mass index; DXA: Dual-energy X-ray absorptiometry; M: Mean; SD: Standard deviation; SE: Standard error; ANCOVA: Analyses of covariance.

Competing interest

The authors declare that they have no competing interest.

Authors' contributions

AML collected the accelerometers data, performed DXA scans and drafted the manuscript. AGA collected the accelerometers data, performed DXA scans, made the statistical analysis and drafted the manuscript. AGC performed DXA scans and drafted the manuscript. GVR and JAC designed and coordinated the study, and drafted the manuscript. All authors read and approved the final manuscript.

Authors' information

AML has a MSc and a predoctoral grant.
AGC has a PhD and a post doc position at Hospital Virgen del Valle, Toledo.
AGA has a PhD and is a Lecturer at Aberystwyth University.
GVR has a PhD and is a Reader at the University of Zaragoza.
JAC is MD with a PhD and is a Professor at the University of Zaragoza.

Acknowledgments

We gratefully acknowledge the help of all of the adolescents and their parents who participated in the study for their understanding and dedication to the project. Specials thanks are given to Fundación Down Zaragoza and Special Olympics Aragón for their support. This work was supported by 'Ministerio de Ciencia e Innovación' 'Plan Nacional I+D+i 2009–2011 (Project DEP 2009–09183)'. This project has been co financed by "Fondo Europeo de Desarrollo Regional" (MICINN-FEDER). AML received a Grant FPU12/02854 from the 'Ministerio de Educación Cultura y Deportes'. These authors declare that they have no conflicts of interest that may affect the contents of this work.

Author details

[1]GENUD (Growth, Exercise, Nutrition and Development) Research Group, University of Zaragoza, Ed. Cervantes Corona de Aragón St 42, 2nd floor, Zaragoza 50009, Spain. [2]Faculty of Health and Sport Science, Department of Physiatry and Nursing, University of Zaragoza, Ronda Misericordia 5, Huesca 22001, Spain. [3]Department of Sport and Exercise Science, Aberystwyth University, Ceredigion, United Kingdom. [4]Hospital Virgen del Valle, Complejo Hospitalario de Toledo, Toledo, Spain.

References

1. Angelopoulou N, Souftas V, Sakadamis A, Mandroukas K: **Bone mineral density in adults with down's syndrome.** *Eur Radiol* 1999, **9**(4):648–651.
2. Guijarro M, Valero C, Paule B, González-Macias J, Riancho JA: **Bone mass in young adults with down syndrome.** *J Intellect Disabil Res* 2008, **52**(Pt 3):182–189.
3. González-Agüero A, Vicente-Rodriguez G, Moreno LA, Casajus JA: **Bone mass in male and female children and adolescents with down syndrome.** *Osteoporos Int* 2011, **22**(7):2151–2157.
4. González-Agüero A, Vicente-Rodriguez G, Gómez-Cabello A, Casajus JA: **Cortical and trabecular bone at the radius and tibia in male and female adolescents with down syndrome: a peripheral quantitative computed tomography.** *Osteoporos Int* 2013, **24**(3):1035–1044.
5. **Consensus development conference: diagnosis, prophylaxis, and treatment of osteoporosis.** *Am J Med* 1993, **94**(6):646–650.
6. Cummings SR, Melton LJ: **Epidemiology and outcomes of osteoporotic fractures.** *Lancet* 2002, **359**(9319):1761–1767.
7. Lips P: **Epidemiology and predictors of fractures associated with osteoporosis.** *Am J Med* 1997, **103**(2A):3S–8S. discussion 8S-11S.
8. Bittles AH, Glasson EJ: **Clinical, social, and ethical implications of changing life expectancy in down syndrome.** *Dev Med Child Neurol* 2004, **46**(4):282–286.
9. Srikanth R, Cassidy G, Joiner C, Teeluckdharry S: **Osteoporosis in people with intellectual disabilities: a review and a brief study of risk factors for osteoporosis in a community sample of people with intellectual disabilities.** *J Intellect Disabil Res* 2011, **55**(1):53–62.
10. Jaffe JS, Timell AM, Elolia R, Thatcher SS: **Risk factors for low bone mineral density in individuals residing in a facility for the people with intellectual disability.** *J Intellect Disabil Res* 2005, **49**(Pt 6):457–462.
11. Rizzoli R, Bianchi ML, Garabedian M, McKay HA, Moreno LA: **Maximizing bone mineral mass gain during growth for the prevention of fractures in the adolescents and the elderly.** *Bone* 2010, **46**(2):294–305.
12. Zofkova I: **Role of genetics in prediction of osteoporosis risk.** *Vnitr Lek* 2011, **57**(1):78–84.
13. Gracia-Marco L, Moreno LA, Ortega FB, Leon F, Sioen I, Kafatos A, Martinez-Gomez D, Widhalm K, Castillo MJ, Vicente-Rodriguez G: **Levels of physical activity that predict optimal bone mass in adolescents: the HELENA study.** *Am J Prev Med* 2011, **40**(6):599–607.
14. Bauman AE: **Updating the evidence that physical activity is good for health: an epidemiological review 2000–2003.** *J Sci Med Sport* 2004, **7**(1 Suppl):6–19.
15. Bradney M, Pearce G, Naughton G, Sullivan C, Bass S, Beck T, Carlson J, Seeman E: **Moderate exercise during growth in prepubertal boys: changes in bone mass, size, volumetric density, and bone strength: a controlled prospective study.** *J Bone Miner Res* 1998, **13**(12):1814–1821.
16. Vicente-Rodriguez G: **How does exercise affect bone development during growth?** *Sports Med* 2006, **36**(7):561–569.

17. Wolff J: *The law of bone formation.* Berlin: Hirschwald; 1892.
18. Rauch F, Bailey DA, Baxter-Jones A, Mirwald R, Faulkner R: **The 'muscle-bone unit' during the pubertal growth spurt.** *Bone* 2004, **34**(5):771–775.
19. Schoenau E, Frost HM: **The "muscle-bone unit" in children and adolescents.** *Calcif Tissue Int* 2002, **70**(5):405–407.
20. Sayers Menear K: **Parents' perceptions of health and physical activity needs of children with down syndrome.** *Downs Syndr Res Pract* 2007, **12**(1):60–68.
21. Esposito PE, Macdonald M, Hornyak JE, Ulrich DA: **Physical activity patterns of youth with down syndrome.** *Intellect Dev Disabil* 2012, **50**(2):109–119.
22. Fernhall B, Pitetti KH: **Limitations to physical work capacity in individuals with mental retardation.** *Clin Exer Physiol* 2001, **3**:176–185.
23. Hinckson EA, Curtis A: **Measuring physical activity in children and youth living with intellectual disabilities: a systematic review.** *Res Dev Disabil* 2012, **34**(1):72–86.
24. Shephard RJ: **Limits to the measurement of habitual physical activity by questionnaires.** *Br J Sports Med* 2003, **37**(3):197–206. discussion 206.
25. Toschke JA, von Kries R, Rosenfeld E, Toschke AM: **Reliability of physical activity measures from accelerometry among preschoolers in free-living conditions.** *Clin Nutr* 2007, **26**(4):416–420.
26. Eston RG, Rowlands AV, Ingledew DK: **Validity of heart rate, pedometry, and accelerometry for predicting the energy cost of children's activities.** *J Appl Physiol* 1998, **84**(1):362–371.
27. Phillips AC, Holland AJ: **Assessment of objectively measured physical activity levels in individuals with intellectual disabilities with and without down's syndrome.** *PLoS One* 2011, **6**(12):e28618.
28. Whitt-Glover MC, O'Neill KL, Stettler N: **Physical activity patterns in children with and without down syndrome.** *Pediatr Rehabil* 2006, **9**(2):158–164.
29. Shields N, Dodd KJ, Abblitt C: **Do children with down syndrome perform sufficient physical activity to maintain good health? A pilot study.** *Adapt Phys Activ Q* 2009, **26**(4):307–320.
30. González-Agüero A, Vicente-Rodriguez G, Moreno LA, Guerra-Balic M, Ara I, Casajus JA: **Health-related physical fitness in children and adolescents with Down syndrome and response to training.** *Scand J Med Sci Sports* 2010, **20**(5):716–724.
31. Marfell-Jones M: *International standars for anthropometric assessment.* Potchefstroom, South Africa: International Society for the Advancement of Kinanthropometry; 2006.
32. Pan H, Cole TJ: **ImsGrowth, a Microsoft Excel add-in to access growth references based on the LMS method. Version 2.77.** www.healthforallchildren.co.uk.
33. Cole TJ, Freeman JV, Preece MA: **British 1990 growth reference centiles for weight, height, body mass index and head circumference fitted by maximum penalized likelihood.** *Stat Med* 1998, **17**(4):407–429.
34. Tanner JM, Whitehouse RH: **Clinical longitudinal standards for height, weight, height velocity, weight velocity, and stages of puberty.** *Arch Dis Child* 1976, **51**(3):170–179.
35. Ojiambo R, Konstabel K, Veidebaum T, Reilly J, Verbestel V, Huybrechts I, Sioen I, Casajus JA, Moreno LA, Vicente-Rodriguez G, *et al*: **Validity of hip-mounted uniaxial accelerometry with heart-rate monitoring vs. triaxial accelerometry in the assessment of free-living energy expenditure in young children: the IDEFICS Validation Study.** *J Appl Physiol* 2012, **113**(10):1530–1536.
36. Pfeiffer KA, McIver KL, Dowda M, Almeida MJ, Pate RR: **Validation and calibration of the Actical accelerometer in preschool children.** *Med Sci Sports Exerc* 2006, **38**(1):152–157.
37. Trost SG, Pate RR, Freedson PS, Sallis JF, Taylor WC: **Using objective physical activity measures with youth: how many days of monitoring are needed?** *Med Sci Sports Exerc* 2000, **32**(2):426–431.
38. Evenson KR, Catellier DJ, Gill K, Ondrak KS, McMurray RG: **Calibration of two objective measures of physical activity for children.** *J Sports Sci* 2008, **26**(14):1557–1565.
39. Trost SG, Loprinzi PD, Moore R, Pfeiffer KA: **Comparison of accelerometer cut points for predicting activity intensity in youth.** *Med Sci Sports Exerc* 2011, **43**(7):1360–1368.
40. R Development Core Team: *R: a Language and Environment for Statistical Computing R Foundation for Statistical Computing (Online).* Vienna, Austria: R Development Core Team; 2011. http://www.R-project.org/.
41. U.S. Department of Health and Human Services: *2008 Physical Activity Guidelines for Americans.* Washington (DC); 2008.
42. Ojiambo R, Cuthill R, Budd H, Konstabel K, Casajus JA, González-Agüero A, Anjila E, Reilly JJ, Easton C, Pitsiladis YP: **Impact of methodological decisions on accelerometer outcome variables in young children.** *Int J Obes (Lond)* 2011, **35**(Suppl 1):S98–S103.
43. Leonard MB: **Assessment of bone health in children and adolescents with cancer: promises and pitfalls of current techniques.** *Med Pediatr Oncol* 2003, **41**(3):198–207.
44. Angelopoulou N, Matziari C, Tsimaras V, Sakadamis A, Souftas V, Mandroukas K: **Bone mineral density and muscle strength in young men with mental retardation (with and without down syndrome).** *Calcif Tissue Int* 2000, **66**(3):176–180.
45. Baptista F, Varela A, Sardinha LB: **Bone mineral mass in males and females with and without down syndrome.** *Osteoporos Int* 2005, **16**(4):380–388.
46. Khan K, McKay HA, Haapasalo H, Bennell KL, Forwood MR, Kannus P, Wark JD: **Does childhood and adolescence provide a unique opportunity for exercise to strengthen the skeleton?** *J Sci Med Sport* 2000, **3**(2):150–164.
47. Hallal PC, Victora CG, Azevedo MR, Wells JC: **Adolescent physical activity and health: a systematic review.** *Sports Med* 2006, **36**(12):1019–1030.
48. Wu J: **Bone mass and density in preadolescent boys with and without Down syndrome.** *Osteoporos Int* 2013. May 17 [Epub ahead of print] PMID: 23681086.
49. Sharav T, Bowman T: **Dietary practices, physical activity, and body-mass index in a selected population of Down syndrome children and their siblings.** *Clin Pediatr (Phila)* 1992, **31**(6):341–344.
50. Pate RR, Pratt M, Blair SN, Haskell WL, Macera CA, Bouchard C, Buchner D, Ettinger W, Heath GW, King AC, *et al*: **Physical activity and public health. A recommendation from the Centers for Disease Control and Prevention and the American College of Sports Medicine.** *Jama* 1995, **273**(5):402–407.
51. Reilly JJ, Penpraze V, Hislop J, Davies G, Grant S, Paton JY: **Objective measurement of physical activity and sedentary behaviour: review with new data.** *Arch Dis Child* 2008, **93**(7):614–619.
52. Mendonca GV, Pereira FD, Fernhall B: **Walking economy in male adults with Down syndrome.** *Eur J Appl Physiol* 2009, **105**(1):153–157.

11

Changes in the vitamin D endocrine system and bone turnover after oral vitamin D3 supplementation in healthy adults

Kristin Holvik[1,2,4*], Ahmed A Madar[2], Haakon E Meyer[1,2], Cathrine M Lofthus[3] and Lars C Stene[1]

Abstract

Background: There is uncertainty as to which intake of vitamin D is needed to suppress PTH and maintain normal bone metabolism throughout winter at northern latitudes. We aimed to investigate whether four weeks' daily supplementation with 10 µg vitamin D3 from fish oil produced a greater change in serum vitamin D metabolites, parathyroid hormone, and bone turnover in healthy adults compared with solid multivitamin tablets. Furthermore, it was studied whether age, gender, ethnic background, body mass index, or serum concentrations at baseline predicted the magnitude of change in these parameters.

Methods: Healthy adults aged 19–48 years living in Oslo, Norway (59°N) were randomised to receive a daily dose of 10 µg vitamin D3 given as fish oil capsules or multivitamin tablets during four weeks in late winter. Serum samples from baseline and after 28 days were analysed for 25-hydroxyvitamin D (s-25(OH)D), 1,25-dihydroxyvitamin D (s-1,25(OH)$_2$D), intact parathyroid hormone (s-iPTH), and osteoclast-specific tartrate-resistant acid phosphatase 5b (s-TRACP). Fifty-five eligible participants completed the intervention (74% of those randomised).

Results: S-25(OH)D increased by mean 34.1 (SD 13.1) nmol/l, $p < 0.001$; s-iPTH decreased by mean 1.2 (SD 2.5) pmol/l, $p = 0.001$; s-1,25(OH)$_2$D increased by mean 13 (SD 48) pmol/l, $p = 0.057$; and s-TRACP increased by mean 0.38 (SD 0.33) U/l, $p < 0.001$. For all these parameters, there was no difference between fish oil and multivitamin formulation. Baseline concentrations were the only independent predictors of changes in biochemical parameters.

Conclusions: Four weeks of daily supplementation with 10 µg vitamin D3 decreased mean s-iPTH and increased s-TRACP concentration, and this did not differ by mode of administration. Our results suggest an increased bone resorption following vitamin D supplementation in young individuals, despite a decrease in parathyroid hormone levels.

Keywords: Supplementation, Randomised trial, Vitamin D3, Cholecalciferol, 25-hydroxyvitamin D, 1,25-dihydroxyvitamin D, Parathyroid hormone, Tartrate-resistant acid phosphatase, Bone turnover

* Correspondence: kristin.holvik@fhi.no
[1]Division of Epidemiology, Norwegian Institute of Public Health, Oslo, Norway
[2]Institute of Health and Society, University of Oslo, Oslo, Norway
Full list of author information is available at the end of the article

Background

Low vitamin D status is commonly observed at northern latitudes such as in Scandinavia during wintertime, with a drop in serum concentrations of 25-hydroxyvitamin D (s-25(OH)D) and a corresponding increase in serum parathyroid hormone levels (PTH) and bone turnover [1,2]. In addition to latitude and season, individual sun exposure and vitamin D supplementation are strong predictors of vitamin D status [1]. Maintaining s-25(OH)D and suppressing PTH through winter is expected to be beneficial in order to prevent bone resorption. Possible direct means of increasing wintertime vitamin D status at northern latitudes may be increased fortification of foods [3], or increased supplementation. Current recommended dietary intake of vitamin D for adults in European countries and the US varies between 0–15 µg/day (20 µg/day for elderly in the US) [4,5]. Daily supplementation with 10 µg (400 IU) vitamin D is recommended to elderly individuals with low sun exposure in the Nordic countries [6]. However, there is uncertainty as to which supplemental dose is needed in order to maintain 25(OH)D levels associated with PTH suppression and normal bone metabolism. In an experimental study performed in Omaha (41°N) it was estimated that daily oral supplementation with 12.5 µg (500 IU) may be required in order to maintain autumn s-25(OH)D levels of 70 nmol/l through winter [7]. Daily oral supplementation with 10 µg (400 IU) or 20 µg (800 IU) vitamin D3 prevented increase in PTH and bone turnover during winter in healthy men in Helsinki, Finland (60°N) (n = 48) [8]. There seems to be large variation in s-25(OH)D in response to oral supplementation. According to a summary of various studies published up to 1999 [9], a daily dose of 10 µg (400 IU) vitamin D led to an average increase in s-25(OH)D of 31 nmol/l, although with large variation between studies, suggesting that additional factors may influence the degree of increase. A systematic review concluded that the degree of PTH suppression achieved by vitamin D supplementation depends not only on baseline PTH and increase in s-25(OH)D, but also on the subjects' age and mobility [10]. Healthy young students in Coleraine, Northern Ireland (55°N) who received a daily oral supplement of 15 µg (600 IU) vitamin D3 for 8 weeks in late winter, increased their mean s-25(OH)D from 47.9 to 86.5 nmol/l, but the supplementation did not influence PTH levels or bone turnover significantly [11]. In a recent 2-center double-blind placebo-controlled study from the same group, 215 persons aged 20–40 received 0, 5, 10, or 15 µg vitamin D3 daily during 22 weeks in late winter, but supplementation did not affect PTH levels or bone turnover [12]. Elderly osteoporotic women in sunshine abundant São Paulo, Brazil (23°S) who received 10 µg (400 IU) vitamin D3 daily for three months increased their mean s-25(OH)D from 46.7 to 59.5 nmol/l, whereas PTH levels or bone turnover were not significantly affected [13].

In our experimental study performed in Oslo (59°N) during late winter, we found a similar effect of fish oil capsules and multivitamin D tablets on increase in s-25(OH)D [14]. We here present results for the predefined secondary objectives of the study: (a) to compare changes in s-1,25(OH)$_2$D, s-iPTH and s-TRACP in the fish oil capsule vs. multivitamin tablet groups, and (b) in the supplement groups combined, to investigate whether the magnitude of change in s-25(OH)D and the above mentioned metabolites was predicted by ethnic background, body mass index, age, gender, or serum concentrations at baseline.

Methods

Study subjects

Subjects with Norwegian (in the following quoted as Norwegians) and other ethnic background were recruited primarily among medical students and nurse students in Oslo. In addition, subjects with Sri Lankan Tamil background (in the following quoted as Tamils) were recruited through an organisation for Tamils in Oslo (Tamil Resource and Counselling Centre). The participants recruited through medical or nursing school attended pre-test baseline examination within the period 14–17 February, and the participants recruited through the Tamil Resource and Counselling Centre attended within the period 11–14 March. The four-week intervention was thus completed in mid-April by the latest, i.e. prior to Easter holidays when sunlight exposure would be expected to increase. Those who already took a vitamin D supplement regularly, defined as once a week or more, or had been travelling to sunny areas or used a tanning bed during the previous three months, were defined as ineligible to participate. A total of 74 subjects of the 143 subjects who had agreed to participate (51.7%), were randomised to receive multivitamin tablets or fish oil capsules [14].

Intervention

The participants each received a daily supplement of 10 µg (400 IU) vitamin D3 from one multivitamin tablet of type Vitaplex ABCD (Cederroth AS, Revetal, Norway), or one fish oil capsule, specially manufactured for this study by Peter Möller (now Möller's, Oslo, Norway). Vitamin D3 content of the supplements was determined by an independent laboratory (AS Vitas, Oslo, Norway). Mean content was 9.79 µg per multivitamin tablet (SD 1.51), and 9.99 µg per fish oil capsule (SD 0.23), respectively. In addition to vitamin D3, the multivitamin tablets were declared by the manufacturer to contain 750 µg vitamin A, 1.5 mg vitamin B1, 1.7 mg vitamin B2, 1.5 mg vitamin B6, 20 mg niacin, 5 mg pantothenic acid, and 30 mg vitamin C. The fish oil capsules contained 660 μg vitamin A, 3.7 mg vitamin E, and 0.5 g n-3 polyunsaturated fatty acids, as analysed by the manufacturer. Retinol concentration in the fish oil capsules was standardised to be similar to the multivitamin tablets. Supplements were handed out to each participant at baseline, along with a self-administered compliance form. Participants were encouraged to maintain their usual diet during the study period. The tablets or capsules were ingested daily for 4 weeks, which is considered to be a sufficient duration in order to reach equilibrium (plateau concentration) in s-25(OH)D [9].

Data collection

A venous serum sample was drawn on day 1, prior to the intervention, and on day 29, the day subsequent to ingesting the final tablet or capsule. The participants completed a self-administered three-page questionnaire at baseline. During completion of the questionnaire, they had the possibility to ask for assistance (i.e. clarification of questions, or language issues) from one of the project leaders. The questionnaire included questions about usual intake of vitamin D-containing foods, supplement use, clothing and sun exposure habits, self-reported height and weight, date of birth, education, and ethnic background. At follow-up, all participants' height and weight were measured with an electronic height- and weight-measuring device.

Serum sample handling and analyses

Blood samples were centrifuged (10 min, 2000 g at 10 °C) within 30 minutes after blood collection and sera were immediately frozen and kept at −70 °C until analyzed. Pre- and post-intervention serum from all participants were analysed blinded, in one batch at the Hormone Laboratory (Department of Endocrinology, Oslo University Hospital Aker, Oslo, Norway).

S-25(OH)D was measured by radioimmunoassay (RIA) (DiaSorin, Stillwater, MN, USA). This assay measures both 25(OH)D_3 and 25(OH)D_2. The intra- and interassay coefficients of variation (CV) were 6% and 14-15%, respectively. The detection limit was 6 nmol/l.

Intact PTH (iPTH) were measured by chemiluminoimmunometric assay (DPC, Los Angeles, CA, USA). The intra- and interassay CVs for iPTH were 4% and 10%, respectively.

S-1,25$(OH)_2$D was measured by competitive RIA (DiaSorin, Stillwater, MN, USA). Prior to the 1,25$(OH)_2$D determination, serum lipids and interfering vitamin D metabolites were removed by chromatography on a C18OH column. Cross reaction with 25(OH)D after chromatography is noted to be 0.002%. The intra- and interassay CVs for the s-1,25$(OH)_2$D assay were 7 and 14%, respectively. The limit of detection was 12 pmol/l.

S-TRACP was measured by enzyme activity assessment after immune extraction (Suomen Bioanalytiikka Oy, Oulu, Finland). This assay measures the active isoform 5b derived from osteoclasts. The intra- and interassay CVs for s-TRACP were 5–12 and 8–14% respectively.

Statistical analysis

The data were analysed in SPSS and Stata. According to normality plots, the dependent variables: Δ25(OH)D, Δ PTH, Δ1,25$(OH)_2$D and ΔTRACP did not deviate substantially from a normal distribution, and non-parametric tests yielded similar results. Therefore, means and distributions are presented for continuous variables, and percentages are presented for categorical variables. Pre- and post-intervention concentration of biochemical parameters were compared by paired samples t tests. Crude differences between the two intervention groups were tested using *t* test. Potential predictors of change in biochemical parameters were analysed using linear regression.

Results

Participants

Of the 74 subjects included in the study, 10 violated the eligibility criteria according to the questionnaire at baseline, three reported an intake of less than 26 tablets or capsules during the 28-day intervention period, three were lost to follow-up, two had their second blood sample taken three days before schedule, and one withdrew. The number of participants excluded was similar in the two intervention groups (nine and ten, respectively). Thus, 55 eligible participants completed the study. Of these, 36 had ethnic Norwegian background, 12 had Tamil background, and seven had various other ethnic backgrounds. Characteristics of the study participants are presented in Table 1.

Effect of supplementation on vitamin D status

Mean (SD) s-25(OH)D in the sample increased from 44.3 (23.6) nmol/l to 78.4 (24.5) nmol/l, with a mean (SD) increase (Δ25(OH)D) of 34.1 (13.1) nmol/l (Table 2). Individual Δ25(OH)D ranged from −12 nmol/l to 58 nmol/l. Δ25(OH)D did not differ by type of supplement, as previously published [14]. At baseline, one person had s-25(OH)D <12.5 nmol/l and 13 persons (24%) had s-25(OH)D <25 nmol/l. Four persons (7%) had s-25(OH)D >75 nmol/l. At follow-up, none had s-25(OH)D <25 nmol/l. Five participants (9%) had s-25(OH)D <50 nmol/l. Twenty-nine participants (53%) had s-25(OH)D >75 nmol/l at follow-up.

Effect of supplementation on PTH and TRACP

S-iPTH decreased by mean 1.2 pmol/l, from 5.9 pmol/l to 4.7 pmol/l (Table 2), and the decrease did

Table 1 Background characteristics of participants (n = 55)

Age, years, mean (range)	28 (19–48)
Gender, n (%) women	35 (63.6)
Body mass index, kg/m^2, mean (SD)	23.7 (3.8)
Daily use of vitamin D-containing butter or margarine on bread or in cooking, n (%)	25 (45.5)
Regular consumption of vitamin D enriched milk, n (%)	14 (25.5)
Intake of fatty fish at least twice a week, n (%)	32 (58.2)
Habitual use of dietary supplements other than vitamin D, n (%)	7 (12.7)
Common use of sunscreen on sunny days, n (%)	18 (32.7)
Exposes skin to direct sunlight > 10 minutes on sunny days, n (%)	49 (89.1)
Spends on average more than 2 hours outdoors during a sunny week, n (%)	36 (65.5)

not differ significantly by type of supplement. The decrease was significant in the multivitamin group where s-iPTH at baseline was accidentally higher. There was an overall borderline statistically significant increase in s-1,25(OH)$_2$D. Individual Δs-1,25(OH)$_2$D showed a large variation, from −135 to 120 pmol/l. S-TRACP increased significantly from mean 2.65 to mean 3.03 U/L during supplementation.

Potential predictors of effect of supplementation

Results of linear regression analysis are shown in Table 3. Baseline s-25(OH)D was predicted only by ethnic background, Norwegians having unadjusted mean 33 (95% CI 20, 46) nmol/l higher baseline s-25(OH)D than Tamils. However, ethnic background did not affect increase in vitamin D status. Mean (SD) increase in s-25(OH)D was 33.8 (14.1) in Norwegians and 36.2 (10.0) in

Table 2 Mean (SD) unadjusted serum levels of markers of the vitamin D endocrine system and bone turnover at baseline and follow-up according to type of supplement

Variable	*n*	*Mean (SD) serum level at baseline*	*Mean (SD) serum level at follow-up*	*Mean (SD) change during intervention*	*p value* [(2)]
s-25(OH)D (nmol/l)					
Overall	55	44.3 (23.6)	78.4 (24.5)	34.1 (13.1)	<0.001
Fish oil capsules	27	48.5 (24.8)	80.4 (25.0)	31.9 (15.3)	<0.001
Multivitamin tablets	28	40.3 (22.0)	76.5 (24.3)	36.2 (10.4)	<0.001
p value [(1)]		0.20	0.56	0.22	
s-iPTH (pmol/l)					
Overall	55	5.9 (2.6)	4.7 (2.1)	−1.2 (2.5)	0.001
Fish oil capsules	27	5.7 (2.6)	4.9 (2.5)	−0.9 (2.8)	0.13
Multivitamin tablets	28	6.0 (2.7)	4.5 (1.6)	−1.4 (2.2)	0.002
p value [(1)]		0.77	0.52	0.40	
s-1,25(OH)$_2$D (pmol/l)					
Overall	53	121 (41)	134 (38)	13 (48)	0.057
Fish oil capsules	27	128 (38)	136 (34)	8 (45)	0.37
Multivitamin tablets	26	113 (43)	131 (42)	18 (50)	0.09
p value [(1)]		0.20	0.64	0.46	
s-TRACP (U/l)					
Overall	54	2.65 (0.70)	3.03 (0.69)	0.38 (0.33)	<0.001
Fish oil capsules	27	2.59 (0.80)	3.01 (0.77)	0.43 (0.31)	<0.001
Multivitamin tablets	27	2.71 (0.61)	3.04 (0.60)	0.34 (0.36)	<0.001
p value [(1)]		0.53	0.87	0.32	

[(1)] Differences between types of supplement are tested using *t* test.

[(2)] Paired-samples *t* test for comparison of individual pre- and post-intervention concentration.

Table 3 Predictors of change in biochemical parameters during four weeks of vitamin D3 supplementation (n = 55)

Dependent variable	Δs-25(OH)D (nmol/l)		Δs-iPTH (pmol/l)		Δs-1,25(OH)$_2$D (pmol/l)		Δs-TRACP (U/L)	
	B (95% CI)	*p value*	B (95% CI)	*p value*	B (95% CI)	*p value*	B (95% CI)	*p value*
Type of supplement (solid multivitamin tablet vs. gelatine fish oil capsule with n-3 fatty acids) [(1)]	3.5 [(2)] (−3.6, 10.6)	0.33	−0.4 (−1.5, 0.6)	0.39	−1 (−22, 19)	0.89	−0.08 (−0.25, 0.10)	0.40
Age, per 10 years	1.4 (−3.2, 6.0)	0.54	−0.5 (−1.3, 0.4)	0.31	−10 (−27, 7)	0.24	0.07 (−0.05, 0.19)	0.25
Gender, men vs. women	1.0 (−6.4, 8.5)	0.78	−1.3 (−2.5, 0.3)	0.11	18 (−8, 46)	0.17	0.04 (−0.16, 0.23)	0.71
Body mass index, per 5 kg/m2	−1.0 (−5.7, 3.7)	0.68	−0.3 (−1.2, 0.6)	0.48	−9 (−26, 8)	0.30	0.05 (−0.07, 0.17)	0.41
Ethnic background, Tamil vs. Norwegian	2.7 (−6.0, 11.3)	0.54	−0.5 (−2.2, 1.2)	0.54	−18 (−51, −14)	0.26	0.27 (0.05, 0.49)	0.016
Baseline s-25(OH)D, per 10 nmol/l	−1.1 (−2.6, 0.4)	0.13	0.2 (−0.1, 0.5)	0.10	−3 (−8, 3)	0.31	−0.03 (−0.07, 0.01)	0.10
Baseline s-iPTH, per 5 pmol/l	4.4 (−2.3, 11.2)	0.20	−3.2 (−4.2, −2.3)	< 0.001	−13 (−38, 12)	0.30	−0.04 (−0.22, 0.14)	0.66
Baseline s-1,25(OH)$_2$D, per 10 pmol/l	−0.3 (−1.2, 0.6)	0.51	0.0 (−0.2, 0.1)	0.71	−8 (−10, −5)	< 0.001	< −0.01 (−0.03, 0.02)	0.81
Baseline s-TRACP, per U/l	−4.7 (−9.8, 0.3)	0.07	0.1 (−0.9, 1.1)	0.86	9 (−10, 28)	0.34	−0.13 (−0.26, -0.01)	0.039

[1] Groups are randomised with regard to type of supplement. The analysis of type of supplement is adjusted for baseline serum concentration of the respective dependent variables, while the other analyses in the table are unadjusted.

[2] Result previously published in: Holvik K *et al.*, Br J Nutr 2007; 98: 620–5.

Tamils, p = 0.60. No background characteristics were significantly associated with increase in s-25(OH)D during supplementation (Table 3). The changes in the biochemical parameters (except 25(OH)D) were inversely associated with their baseline concentrations. Decrease in s-iPTH during supplementation tended to be larger when baseline s-25(OH)D was lower (Figure 1).

There was a significant association between ethnic background and ΔTRACP, Tamils having higher increase in s-TRACP than Norwegians (Table 3). This was not significant when adjusting for the lower baseline s-TRACP in Tamils (p = 0.07).

There was no effect of type of supplement (fish oil capsule or multivitamin tablet) on change in any biochemical parameter.

Discussion

We found that supplementation with 10 μg vitamin D3/day administered for four weeks in late winter led to vitamin D sufficiency (s-25(OH)D > 50 nmol/l) in healthy adults of ethnic Norwegian background, but not completely so in Tamils living in Oslo (59°N). This was due to a very low baseline vitamin D status in Tamils, which we have also observed previously [15]. In spite of the strict exclusion criteria, vitamin D status at baseline was not very low in ethnic Norwegian participants. A large proportion of the study sample were medical and nursing students, probably more health-conscious than the general population, and may have had a relatively high intake of vitamin D intake during winter. However, the supplementation was equally efficient regardless of ethnic background, and led to an overall mean increase in s-25(OH)D of 34.1 nmol/l in the course of four weeks. We found no effect of type of vitamin D supplement (solid multivitamin tablet or fish oil capsule containing n-3 fatty acids) on either increase in vitamin D status [14] or in the change in parathyroid hormone, the active vitamin D hormone, or osteoclast activity. As far as we are aware, this is the first randomised trial to compare the effect of two different modes of administration of vitamin D3 on markers of the vitamin D endocrine system and bone turnover.

S-25(OH)D above 50 nmol/l has been associated with optimal musculoskeletal function in elderly [16], and this level is commonly used as cut-off for vitamin D sufficiency in European populations [17-19]. However, some advocate a target s-25(OH)D in the adult European and US population of at least 75 nmol/l for optimal fall and fracture prevention, and this requires daily supplementation of at least 18–25 μg (700–1000 IU) [20]. However, few intervention studies have focused on supplementation in young adult individuals and its influence on markers of bone health.

Unlike other intervention studies with a similar dose of vitamin D [8,11-13], we observed a significant suppression of PTH as well as increased bone turnover in our study.

Vitamin D supplementation is expected to prevent bone loss mainly by slowing bone resorption. Due to the short follow-up time, we expected any effect on bone turnover likely to be observed in resorption rather than formation. The TRACP isoform 5b is released by osteoclasts early in their differentiation, and this enzyme is specifically a marker of number of osteoclasts rather than of their resorptive activity. In healthy individuals, however, the osteoclast number and their resorptive activity is expected to be highly correlated [21]. TRACP 5b was also studied in the recent Finnish supplementation study in healthy men aged 21–49 years (n = 48) [8]. The

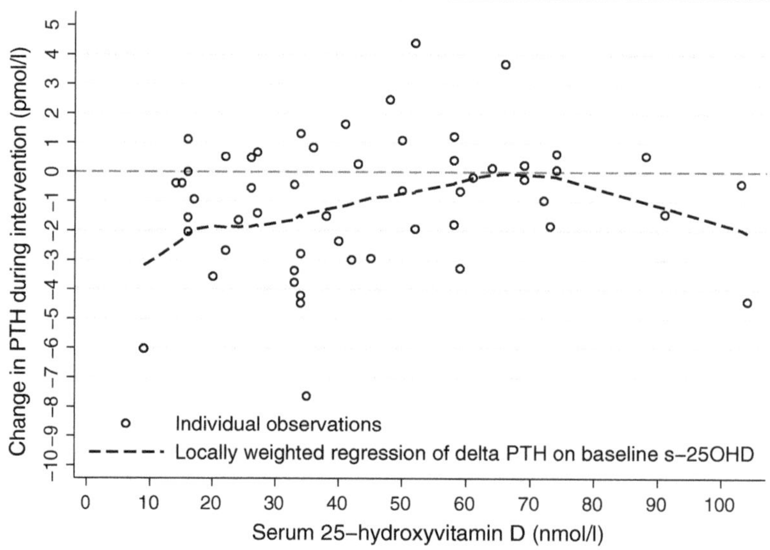

Figure 1 Relationship between vitamin D status at baseline and change in PTH (n = 55).

investigators observed a decrease in this marker throughout winter (6 months) regardless of whether the participants received placebo, 10, or 20 μg vitamin D. The bone formation marker (bone alkaline phosphatase) decreased in the groups receiving vitamin D supplementation but was unaltered in the placebo group.

The suggested increase in osteoclast activity in our data in spite of the improvement in vitamin D status and corresponding PTH suppression is surprising, but may represent a transient high turnover state with increased bone turnover as a result of increased bone formation. The participants were relatively young, and 40% were below 25 years of age. Peak bone mass may not have been acquired in all participants [22]. An increased bone turnover may thus suggest an improved rate of bone growth in young adults. As bone formation and resorption are coupled processes, increased formation will follow the increase in resorption. A decrease in PTH would be expected to suppress bone resorption, but bone resorption is also stimulated by $1,25(OH)_2D$. Local production of $1,25(OH)_2D$ in the tissues may have increased, while we have only measured circulating $1,25(OH)_2D$. There is evidence that 25(OH)D affects osteoclastogenesis and bone turnover (and thereby TRACP production) by local activation in bone cells [23]. In a recent review, it was considered that due to this local activation, circulating levels of 25(OH)D, and not $1,25(OH)_2D$, may represent the better correlate to parameters of bone health [24].

There is ongoing research concerning the role of n-3 fatty acids in bone health, as bone loss due to increased osteoclast activity may be mediated by inflammatory cytokines, and some studies suggest a protective effect of n-3 fatty acids on bone resorption [25,26]. In bone marrow from ovarioectomized mice, addition of eicosapentaenoic acid and docosahexaenoic acid led to significantly reduced TRACP activity and osteoclastogenesis [27]. A protective effect of n-3 fatty acids (0.5 g/day) in fish oil on bone resorption was not supported in our data in young adults, as subjects' s-TRACP increased regardless of being randomised to ingest fish oil capsules containing omega-3 fatty acids, or solid tablets. The increase in s-TRACP was even slightly higher in the group ingesting fish oil capsules (not shown/not significant).

It cannot be excluded that an independent effect of the supplementation on bone turnover regardless of the observed decrease in PTH could be brought about by factors other than vitamin D. Both intervention supplements contained vitamin A (retinol). Although the evidence of an effect of vitamin A on bone health is inconsistent, some in vitro studies have shown that retinoic acid directly stimulate osteoclastic bone resorption, and high intakes and serum levels of retinol have been associated with reduced bone mineral density or increased fracture risk in some population-based studies [28].

Our study was a parallel-group intervention and we did not include a placebo group. Due to the late wintertime intervention period we did not expect any notable background increase in vitamin D status. Moreover, any background change in vitamin D status would be the consequence of any unexpected behaviour in relation to diet or sun exposure in both parallel-groups regardless of supplement. Our study sample was restricted to not take a regular supplement other than the intervention supplement, use a tanning bed, or travel to sunny areas. Any extraordinary dietary intake (e.g. large fatty fish dinner) would be noted on the participants' individual compliance form, and no such behaviour was reported. Also, only those who were compliant defined as consuming at least 26 of the 28 tablets were included in the analyses. Thus, there is reason to expect that any observed change in the vitamin D endocrine system is an effect of the supplementation.

A limitation of the ethnic comparison was the different age distributions between participants with ethnic Norwegian and Sri Lankan Tamil background. Mean age in the two groups differed by 14 years. While more than half of the subjects with ethnic Norwegian background were below 30 years of age, none of those with Sri Lankan Tamil background were below that age. Age is an important predictor of serum PTH [10], but limited overlap in age between the ethnic groups in our study makes it difficult to rule out the influence of age and ethnic background, respectively.

Conclusions

We conclude that four weeks of daily supplementation with 10 μg (400 IU) vitamin D3 to healthy adults during wintertime led to a decrease in s-iPTH and an increase in circulating TRACP. These effects did not differ by mode of administration. In spite of different serum levels at baseline in Norwegians and Tamils, the effect was similar in the two ethnic groups.

Competing interests

One of the intervention supplements used was provided freely for this research project by the manufacturer (Möller's). We declare that the Authors have no employment or personal financial interest in relation to the work described.

Acknowledgements

Specially manufactured fish oil capsules were provided by Möller's. The blood sample analyses were funded by Aktieselskabet Freia Chocolade Fabriks Medisinske fond. KH's doctoral grant was financed with the aid of EXTRA funds from the Norwegian Foundation for Health and Rehabilitation. We are grateful to those who participated in the study, and to bioengineer Eva Kristensen at the Institute of Health and Society who drew the blood samples.

Author details

[1]Division of Epidemiology, Norwegian Institute of Public Health, Oslo, Norway. [2]Institute of Health and Society, University of Oslo, Oslo, Norway. [3]Department of Endocrinology, Oslo University Hospital, Oslo, Norway. [4]Norwegian Institute of Public Health, P.O. Box 4404 Nydalen 0403 Oslo, Norway.

Authors' contribution

KH and AAM planned and carried out the data collection under guidance of HEM and LCS. AAM prepared the data file. KH analysed the data and wrote the manuscript. HEM and LCS initiated the study and contributed to the methods and the design of the paper. CML was responsible for the serum sample analyses. All co-authors have critically revised and approved the manuscript.

References

1. Brot C, Vestergaard P, Kolthoff N, Gram J, Hermann AP, Sørensen OH: **Vitamin D status and its adequacy in healthy Danish perimenopausal women: relationships to dietary intake, sun exposure and serum parathyroid hormone.** *Br J Nutr* 2001, **86**(Suppl 1):S97–S103.
2. Holick MF, Chen TC: **Vitamin D deficiency: a worldwide problem with health consequences.** *Am J Clin Nutr* 2008, **87:**1080S–1086S.
3. Pedersen JI: **Vitamin D requirement and setting recommendation levels - current Nordic view.** *Nutr Rev* 2008, **66:**S165–S169.
4. Doets EL, de Wit LS, Dhonukshe-Rutten RA, Cavelaars AE, Raats MM, Timotijevic L, Brzozowska A, Wijnhoven TM, Pavlovic M, Totland TH, Andersen LF, Ruprich J, Pijls LT, Ashwell M, Lambert JP, Veer P, de Groot LC: **Current micronutrient recommendations in Europe: towards understanding their differences and similarities.** *Eur J Nutr* 2008, **47**(Suppl 1):17–40.
5. Committee to Review Dietary Reference Intakes for Vitamin D and Calcium: *Food and Nutrition Board: Dietary Reference Intakes for Calcium and Vitamin D.* Washington D.C: National Academies Press; 2011.
6. Nordic Council of Ministers: *Nordic Nutrition Recommendations.* Copenhagen:; 2004.
7. Heaney RP, Davies KM, Chen TC, Holick MF, Barger-Lux M: **Human serum 25-hydroxycholecalciferol response to extended oral dosing with cholecalciferol.** *Am J Clin Nutr* 2003, **77:**204–210.
8. Viljakainen HT, Väisänen M, Kemi V, Rikkonen T, Kröger H, Laitinen EK, Rita H, Lamberg-Allardt C: **Wintertime vitamin D supplementation inhibits seasonal variation of calcitropic hormones and maintains bone turnover in healthy men.** *J Bone Miner Res* 2009, **24:**346–352.
9. Vieth R: **Vitamin D supplementation, 25-hydroxyvitamin D concentrations, and safety.** *Am J Clin Nutr* 1999, **69:**842–856.
10. Björkman M, Sorva A, Tilvis R: **Responses of parathyroid hormone to vitamin D supplementation: a systematic review of clinical trials.** *Arch Gerontol Geriatr* 2009, **48:**160–166.
11. Barnes MS, Robson PJ, Bonham MP, Strain JJ, Wallace JM: **Effect of vitamin D supplementation on vitamin D status and bone turnover markers in young adults.** *Eur J Clin Nutr* 2006, **60:**727–733.
12. Seamans KM, Hill TR, Wallace JM, Horigan G, Lucey AJ, Barnes MS, Taylor N, Bonham MP, Muldowney S, Duffy EM, Strain JJ, Kiely M, Cashman KD: **Cholecalciferol supplementation throughout winter does not affect markers of bone turnover in healthy young and elderly adults.** *J Nutr* 2010, **140:**454–460.
13. Pignotti GA, Genaro PS, Pinheiro MM, Szejnfeld VL, Martini LA: **Is a lower dose of vitamin D supplementation enough to increase 25(OH)D status in a sunny country?** *Eur J Nutr* 2010, **49:**277–283.
14. Holvik K, Madar AA, Meyer HE, Lofthus CM, Stene LC: **A randomised comparison of increase in serum 25-hydroxyvitamin D concentration after 4 weeks of daily oral intake of 10 μg cholecalciferol from multivitamin tablets or fish oil capsules in healthy young adults.** *Br J Nutr* 2007, **98:**620–625.
15. Meyer HE, Holvik K, Lofthus CM, Tennakoon SU: **Vitamin D status in Sri Lankans living in Sri Lanka and Norway.** *Br J Nutr* 2008, **99:**941–944.
16. Wicherts IS, van Schoor NM, Boeke AJ, Visser M, Deeg DJ, Smit J, Knol DL, Lips P: **Vitamin D status predicts physical performance and its decline in older persons.** *J Clin Endocrinol Metab* 2007, **92:**2058–2065.
17. Lips P: **Vitamin D deficiency and secondary hyperparathyroidism in the elderly: consequences for bone loss and fractures and therapeutic implications.** *Endocr Rev* 2001, **22:**477–501.
18. Mejborn H, Brot C, Hansen HB, Koch B, Hyldstrup L, Mortensen L, Mosekilde L, Mølgård C, Petersen T, Rasmussen SE, Rasmussen LB: *D-vitaminstatus i den danske befolkning bør forbedres (Vitamin D status in the Danish population should be improved).* Copenhagen: Danish Ministry of Food, Agriculture and Fisheries; 2004.
19. Meyer HE, Brunvand L, Brustad M, Holvik K, Johansson L, Paulsen JE: *Tiltak for å sikre en god vitamin D-status i befolkningen (Measures to ensure a good vitamin D status in the population).* Oslo: Norwegian National Nutrition Council; 2006.
20. Bischoff-Ferrari H: **Vitamin D: What is an adequate vitamin D level and how much supplementation is necessary?** *Best Pract Res Clin Rheumatol* 2009, **23:**789–795.
21. Henriksen K, Tanko LB, Qvist P, Delmas PD, Christiansen C, Karsdal MA: **Assessment of osteoclast number and function: application in the development of new and improved treatment modalities for bone diseases.** *Osteoporos Int* 2007, **18:**681–685.
22. Matkovic V, Jelic T, Wardlaw GM, Ilich JZ, Goel PK, Wright JK, Andon MB, Smith KT, Heaney RP: **Timing of peak bone mass in Caucasian females and its implication for the prevention of osteoporosis. Inference from a cross-sectional model.** *J Clin Invest* 1994, **93:**799–808.
23. Kogawa M, Anderson PH, Findlay DM, Morris HA, Atkins GJ: **The metabolism of 25-(OH)vitamin D3 by osteoclasts and their precursors regulates the differentiation of osteoclasts.** *J Steroid Biochem Mol Biol* 2010, **121:**277–280.
24. Anderson PH, Atkins GJ: **The skeleton as an intracrine organ for vitamin D metabolism.** *Mol Aspects Med* 2008, **29:**397–406.
25. Poulsen RC, Moughan PJ, Kruger MC: **Long-chain polyunsaturated fatty acids and the regulation of bone metabolism.** *Exp Biol Med* 2007, **232:**1275–1288.
26. Salari P, Rezaie A, Larijani B, Abdollahi M: **A systematic review of the impact of n-3 fatty acids in bone health and osteoporosis.** *Med Sci Monit* 2008, **14:**RA37–RA44.
27. Sun D, Krishnan A, Zaman K, Lawrence R, Bhattacharya A, Fernandes G: **Dietary n-3 fatty acids decrease osteoclastogenesis and loss of bone mass in ovariectomized mice.** *J Bone Miner Res* 2003, **18:**1206–1216.
28. Ahmadieh H, Arabi A: **Vitamins and bone health: beyond calcium and vitamin D.** *Nutr Rev* 2011, **69:**584–598.

12

A case of osmotic demyelination syndrome occurred after the correction of severe hyponatraemia in hyperemesis gravidarum

Giovanni Corona[1], Luigi Simonetti[2], Corinna Giuliani[3], Alessandra Sforza[1] and Alessandro Peri[3*]

Abstract

Background: Osmotic demyelination syndrome (ODS) may be observed as a result of a rapid change in serum osmolarity, such as that induced by an overly rapid correction of serum sodium levels in hyponatraemic patients.

Case presentation: We describe the case of a 21-year-old woman who was hospitalized at week 10 of gestation because of severe hyperemesis. At admission the patient appeared restless and confused and severe hyponatraemia (serum sodium 107 mmol/L) and hypokalemia (serum potassium 1.1 mmol/L) were detected. Active and simultaneous correction of these imbalances led to an overly rapid increase of serum sodium levels (17 mmol/L in the first 24 hours). Isotonic saline solution was stopped and replaced by 5% dextrose solution infusion. However, the neurological alterations worsened and the radiological features were consistent with the diagnosis of extra-pontine ODS. Steroids were administered intravenously with progressive improvement of biochemical and clinical abnormalities. At the time of discharge, 20 days later, the patient was able to walk and eat autonomously with only minimal external support.

Conclusions: This report illustrates an unusual case of ODS, occurred after an excessive rate of correction of hyponatraemia obtained with isotonic saline infusion. Hypokaliemia and its active correction very likely played a crucial role in facilitating the onset of ODS. This interesting aspect will be explained in detail in the article. A more cautious and thoughtful correction of electrolyte alterations, would have probably prevented the onset of ODS in this patient. Physicians should be aware of the possibly fatal consequences that an exceedingly rapid change of serum osmolarity may have and should strictly follow the known safety measures in order to prevent it to occur.

Keywords: Osmotic demyelination syndrome, Hyponatraemia, Pregnancy

Background

Osmotic demyelination syndrome (ODS) is an uncommon disorder, characterized by non-inflammatory demyelination involving the pons and other areas of the central nervous system, which may occur for instance as a consequence of an overly rapid correction of hyponatraemia [1]. Here we report a case of ODS occurred after correction of hyponatraemia with isotonic saline solution in a pregnant woman with hyperemesis gravidarum and concomitant other electrolyte disorders, which are additional risk factors for the development of this syndrome. Some criticisms in the management of the patient, which undoubtedly eased the occurrence of ODS, will be highlighted.

Case presentation

Hyperemesis gravidarum is a condition characterized by severe vomiting resulting in dehydration, fluid electrolyte imbalance and weight loss [2]. We report the case of a 21-year-old woman who was hospitalized at week 10 of gestation due to severe hyperemesis. The condition appeared at week 4 of pregnancy and caused her weight to drop from 51 kg to 46 kg. The day of admission to the hospital she became restless and confused. Clinical examination performed in the emergency room revealed the presence of mild dehydration (dry mouth and skin) with normal blood pressure, increased heart rate and slightly reduced breath frequency (Table 1). Biochemical assessment performed at

* Correspondence: alessandro.peri@unifi.it
[3]Department of Experimental and Clinical Biomedical Sciences, Endocrine Unit, University of Florence, Florence, Italy
Full list of author information is available at the end of the article

Table 1 Clinical and biochemical features of the patient

Clinical data		
Weight (kg)	46	
Height (cm)	160	
BMI (Kg/m^2)	17.9	
SBP (mmHg)	120	
DBP (mmHg)	60	
HR (bpm)	120	
RF (bpm)	10	
Laboratory parameters		
Serum data	**Value**	**Normal range**
Glycaemia (mmol/L)	4.17	(3.3-6.5)
Na^+ (mmol/L)	107	(135-146)
K^+ (mmol/L)	1.1	(3.5-5.0)
Ca^{++} (mmol/L)	2.5	(2.18-2.58)
Mg^{++} (mmol/L)	0.90	(1.02-1.84)
Phosphate (mmol/L)	0.41	(0.48-1.45)
Creatinine (μmol/L)	36.24	(50-90)
Urea (mmol/L)	1.83	(2.5-8)
Total protein (g/L)	52	(60-80)
Albumin (g/L)	30	(35-50)
Prealbumin (mg/L)	127	(200-400)
Osmolarity (mmol/kg)	254	(275-295)
Retinol binding protein (mg/dl)	1.33	(1.55-4.59)
TSH (mIU/L)	0.01	(0.4-5.0)
fT3 (pmol/L)	7.06	(3.5-6.5)
fT4 (pmol/L)	28.31	(9-21.80)
ACTH (pmol/L)	2.26	(1.3-16.7)
Cortisol (nmol/L)	606.98	(110-607)
Urinary data		
Na^+ (mmol/L)	3	
K^+ (mmol/L)	2	
Osmolarity (mmol/kg)	418	(500-1500)
Hemogasanalysis data		
pH	7.65	
pO_2 mmHg	69	
pCO_2 mmHg	58	
BE mmol/L	37.4	
HCO_3^- mmol/L	63.9	
AG mmol/L	-10	

BMI = body mass index, *SBP* = systolic blood pressure, *DBR* = diastolic blood pressure, *HR* = heart rate, *RF* = respiratory frequence, *bpm* = beats per minute, *BE* = base excess, *AG* = anion gap.

admission revealed severe hyponatraemia (107 mmol/L) and hypokalemia (1.1 mmol/L) (Table 1 and Figure 1) with secondary metabolic alkalosis and partially compensated respiratory acidosis (Table 1). Urinary data suggested the presence of extra-renal loss of Na^+ and K^+ with appropriate increase of urinary water and electrolyte retention (Table 1). The patient was promptly admitted to the intensive care unit of the hospital and intravenous isotonic NaCl solution along with K-lactate supplementation was started (Figure 1). The electrolyte disorder was intensively monitored with blood sample evaluation performed every two hours. However, during the first six hours after admission an excessive rate of correction of serum Na^+ concentration ([Na^+]) occurred (Δ 10 mmol/L). Hence, isotonic solution was replaced with hypotonic solution (5% dextrose, Figure 1); K-lactate supplementation was maintained. However, after 24 hours serum [Na^+] was 124 nmol/L (Δ 17 mmol//L) and at 48 hours 128 nmol/L. The neurological symptoms worsened with the appearance of hypotonia, tremors and involuntary muscle spasms. Hormonal data showed the presence of thyrotoxicosis likely induced by hCG; serum ACTH and cortisol levels showed no abnormalities. In addition, laboratory data (e.g. reduced total proteins, albuminemia, retinol binding protein, creatinine, azotemia) indicated the presence of relatively recent, important malnutrition (Table 1). Electroencephalogram showed a non-specific slow wave activity consistent with the presence of a metabolic disorder. Magnetic resonance imaging (MRI) of the brain revealed, despite a normal pons, bilateral increased signal intensity of the lenticular, claustrum, and caudate cerebral nuclei on axial T2 weighted images (Figure 2, panel A) and FLAIR images (Figure 2, panel B). In addition, the Tl weighted images showed moderate hypointensity in the same nuclei (Figure 2, panel C). These foci did not enhance with GDTPA. The clinical and radiological picture was considered to be consistent with extra-pontine ODS associated with an overly rapid correction of hyponatraemia, which was caused by hyperemesis gravidarum At that point, intravenous steroid infusion and enteral nutrition support were started with slow improvement of biochemical and clinical abnormalities. The gynecological examination and ultrasound fetal monitoring revealed no alterations and were in agreement with the gestational age. The patient and her husband were informed on the possible fetal neurological risks and decided to continue the pregnancy. At the time of discharge, 20 days later, the patient was able to walk and eat autonomously with only minimal external support; serum electrolytes and nutritional parameters were normal. The patient delivered a healthy male at 36 weeks of gestation (caesarean section). At 4 months of age the child is apparently healthy. Unfortunately, only a mild improvement of the neurological alterations of the mother has been obtained despite physical therapy.

The case presented here describes a condition of ODS associated with overly rapid correction of serum [Na^+] in a patient with severe hyponatraemia. ODS was first described in 1959 in a series of alcoholic and malnourished

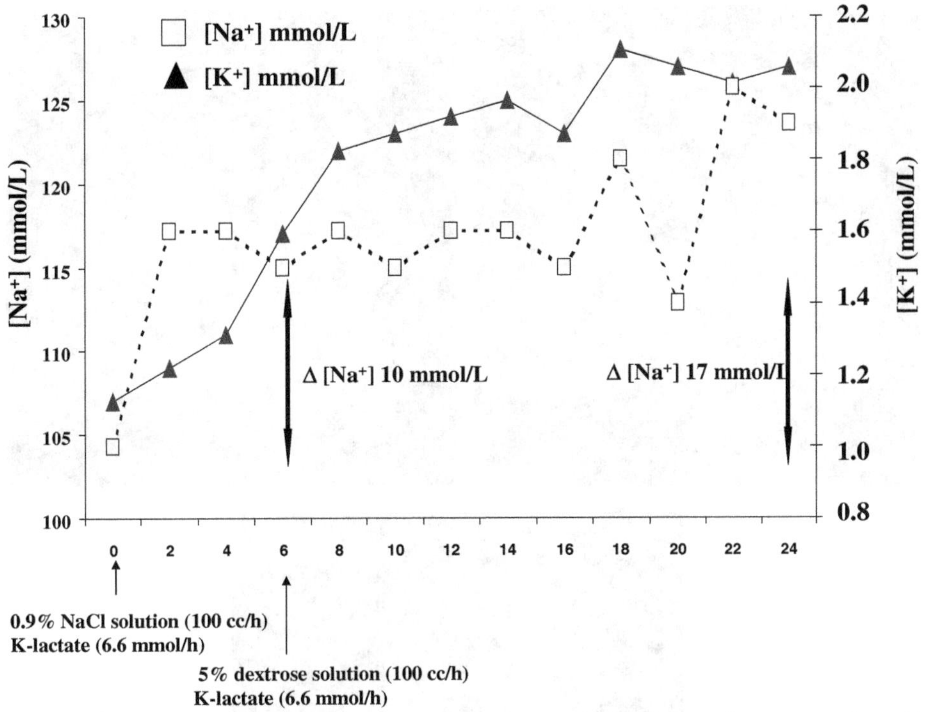

Figure 1 Serum [Na^+] and [K^+] progression during active treatment for the correction of severe hyponatraemia and hypokalemia in the patient.

patients who developed quadriparesis and pseudobulbar palsy. Post-mortem assessment revealed the presence of a demyelinative lesion within the central pons [3]. Its relationship with electrolyte disorders was not apparent, because routine measurement of serum electrolytes was not available at that time. A link between ODS and overly rapid correction of hyponatraemia was established only in the mid-1970s [4]. ODS is recognized as a rather rare disease, although the exact frequency with which occurs is not known. The largest autopsy series indicated a prevalence of 0.25-0.5% in the general population with a peak incidence in males aged 30 to 60 years [1]. From a pathological point of view, ODS is characterized by loss of myelin sheath, whereas axons and neurons are relatively spared [5]. Traditionally, ODS has been associated with rapid correction of hyponatraemia; however, a number of different conditions have been reported in association with the development of this syndrome, independent of serum [Na^+] alterations. The most common predisposing condition is chronic alcoholism, which was not present in our case [6]. Many patients developed ODS during the terminal stage of binge drinking; however, a few case reports of ODS after alcohol withdrawal have been reported [7]. In these instances, the osmotic change due to a decreased intake of food or water that occurs during binge drinking or alcohol withdrawal may be the cause of ODS development.

ODS has been described in patients after liver transplant, after treatment for hyperammonemic disease or with dialysis disequilibrium syndrome. This syndrome is characterized by the occurrence of neurological signs and symptoms attributed to cerebral edema during or following shortly after intermittent hemodialysis and is associated particularly with "aggressive" (high solute removal) dialysis [8,9]. The occurrence of ODS has been also associated with hyperglycemia or with the correction of hyperglycemia [10,11]. Severely burned patients are especially susceptible to ODS, which is tightly associated with serum hyperosmolality resulting from hyperglycemia, azotemia and/or hypernatraemia in these patients [12]. In pregnant women, ODS may occur following rapid correction of hyponatraemia, which may be observed in hyperemesis gravidarum [2], as in the case described here. Furthermore, several cases of ODS in women with post-partum hypernatraemia have been described in India [13]. The authors suggested that a possible cause of hypernatraemia in these patients might be the presence of gestational diabetes insipidus together with the habit to restrict fluid intake during puerperal state in some regions of India.

Overall, these findings strongly suggest that any change in brain cellular volume as the result of a rapid change in serum osmolarity may cause an injury to myelin sheats. In chronic, but not in acute, hypoosmolar states brain cells adapt by decreasing their intracellular solute content. Thus, the risk to develop ODS is substantially associated with chronic hyponatraemia. Noticeably, glial cells have

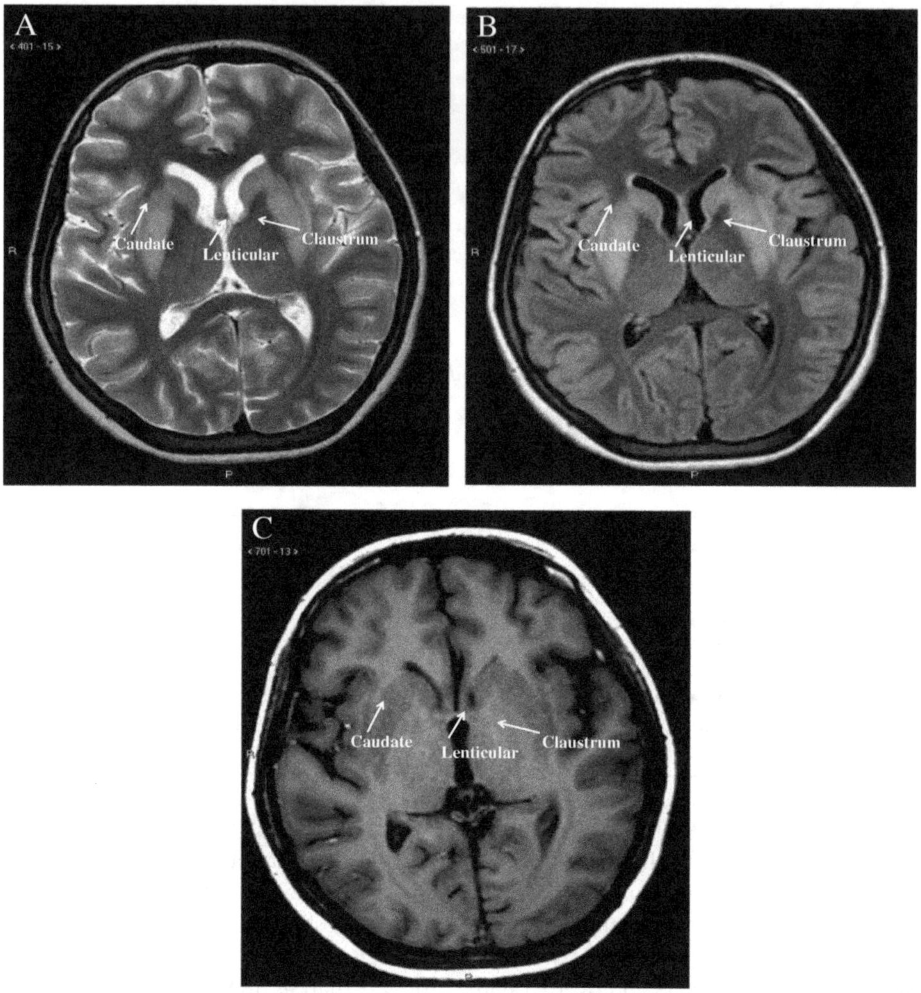

Figure 2 MRI features. Signal intensity of the lenticular, claustrum, and caudate cerebral nuclei on axial T2 weighted images **(A)**, FLAIR images **(B)** and TI weighted images **(C)**.

a critical role in brain water handling. These cells, and not neurons, swell after hypotonic stress, thus suggesting the existence of glia-specific water pores (i.e. aquaporin 1 and 4) [14]. Brain adaptation to cellular swelling requires 24-48 hours and is driven by glial cells, which expel solutes followed by water. This is an energy-dependent phenomenon and requires the activity of the Na^+-K^+-ATPase pump. If a rapid correction of a hypoosmolar state then occurs, glial cells start to increase the production of organic osmolites and the intracellular ion content, in order to reverse the previous modification and regulate cellular volume [15]. However, the synthesis of organic osmolites, as well as the up-regulation of ion pumps, require time and causes energy deprivation. Thus, if an overly rapid correction of a hypotonic state occurs, the cells may not be able to effectively respond to osmotic changes and water moves into the extra-cellular space [15]. Consequently, the resulting shrinkage of glial cells may cause axonal shear damage. Oligodendrocyte apoptosis may also be induced [15], which may lead to disruption of the blood-brain barrier. The latter may cause inflammatory demyelination and further oligodendrocyte damage [15,16].

Besides serum sodium imbalance, other electrolyte alterations, such as hypophosphataemia and hypokalemia, which were also present in our case, have been associated with the development of ODS. Acute hypophosphataemia is a recognized complication of refeeding syndrome when mineral supplementation is inadequate. The phosphate depletion causes failure to convert ADP into ATP leading to an intracellular energy crisis [17], which likely causes altered function of the Na^+-K^+-ATPase pump and consequently brain cells dysfunction. In addition, because phospholipids are a major component of myelin, phosphate depletion may disrupt myelin integrity [18]. With regard to hypokalemia, the mechanism leading to an increased risk of ODS is not completely clear. Nevertheless, different possibilities have been proposed [1]. For instance, a reasonable explanation is that when hyponatraemia is also present, which was the situation of the case reported here, its correction rate may be increased by the simultaneous correction of hypokalemia. This statement is based on the observation that the Na^+-K^+-ATPase pump on the cell membrane expels Na^+ as K^+ enter the cell to replenish depleted intracellular stores. The consequence is a more rapid rate of correction of serum [Na^+], which increases the risk to develop ODS. The simultaneous correction of hypokaliemia may has been therefore an important trigger for the overly rapid correction of hyponatraemia observed in this case and for the further raise occurred also after the replacement of saline infusion with 5% dextrose solution. With this critical aspect in mind, admittedly a more cautious correction of hyponatraemia and a more appropriate intervention aiming to re-lower serum [Na^+], i.e. using also desmopressin, would have likely prevent the onset of ODS.

Clinically, ODS may present with a variety of neurological signs and symptoms, depending on the severity of the involvement and on the affected areas. In about 50% of cases isolated central pontine myelinolysis (CPM) occurs, whereas the remaining cases are more or less equally divided into isolated extra-pontine myelinolysis (EPM) or a combination of CPM and EPM, with a slight prevalence of the latter condition [19]. A number of sites may be involved, besides the pons, and among the most frequently affected sites there are the cerebellum, lateral geniculate bodies, external and extreme capsule and hippocampus. A complete list of affected areas is shown in Table 2 and includes caudate and lenticular nuclei and the claustrum, three extra-pontine areas in which lesions were observed in the patient described here. In CPM usually the clinical presentation includes dysarthria and dysphagia secondary to the involvement of corticobulbar fibres, flaccid quadriparesis followed by spasticity, due to corticospinal tract involvement, oculomotor abnormalities. Changes in mental status and conscious level may occur. In EPM a variety of behavioral changes and movement disorders may be present. These include parkinsonism, dystonia, mutism, catatonia and dysphonia [19]. Usually, these alterations develop several days after the correction of the hypoosmolar condition, although encephalopathy may be already present after a few hours [6]. A possible case of ODS with peripheral nervous system involvement after hyponatraemia correction, causing bilateral and symmetrical motor demyelinating polyneuropathy in the lower and upper extremities in association with central nervous system involvement, has been described [20]. However, admittedly systematic neurophysiological screening of an adequate series of patients with ODS would be required in order to confirm this hypothesis.

Table 2 Cerebral areas involved in CPM and EPM

Common	Rare
Pons	Internal capsula
Cerebellum	Claustrum
Lateral geniculate body	Midbrain
Extreme capsule	Mammillary body
External capsule	Medulla oblongata
Putamen	Internal medullary lamella
Hippocampus	
Thalamus	
Cerebral cortex/subcortex	
Caudate nucleus	

The diagnosis of ODS is based initially on clinical suspicion. Any patient with new onset neurological signs/symptoms and with a recent rise in serum [Na^+] and/or with associated risk factors for ODS, as mentioned previously, should be considered possibly affected by ODS. Clinical findings have to be correlated with radiological assessment. MRI of the brain is the gold standard imaging technique to reveal ODS lesions. These include hypointense T1-weighted lesions and hyperintense lesions demonstrated on T2-weighted and FLAIR images. The lesions are non-contrast enhancing. All these features are in agreement with the findings we observed in our case. The time of appearance may vary and may be delayed; sometimes lesions appeared at MRI even 2 weeks after the onset of clinical alterations [21]. Typically, radiological findings do not improve over time, despite a complete clinical recovery [22].

The prognosis of ODS has been considered very negative for a long time and before the availability of modern imaging techniques usually ODS was a post-mortem diagnosis. The first in-life diagnosis was formulated only 10 years after the first description of ODS. In recent years, the mortality rate has markedly decreased and patients with complete recovery are not rarely observed. In a series of 44 German patients with ODS, for instance, only 6% died during the observation period and 40% recovered without apparent neurological alterations [22].

With regard to treatment, the best therapy for ODS would be...to prevent it to occur! Particular attention should be dedicated to patients presenting conditions known to be associated with a higher risk to develop this condition. As a general rule, the rate of correction should not exceed 12 mmol/L within 24 hours, or 18 mmol/L within 48 hours. These limits should be reduced to 8 mmol/L within 24 hours and 12 mmol/L within 48 hours in patients with chronic hyponatraemia and associated risk factors for developing ODS, which include very low serum [Na^+], hypokalemia, malnutrition and hypophosphataemia, which were present in the case reported here [23,24]. In terms of more prudential approaches, it has also to be considered, as reported by the recently published "expert panel recommendations" on hyponatraemia, that a 4-6 mmol/L increase in serum [Na^+] is already sufficient to reverse the most serious manifestations of acute hyponatraemia [24]. In this patient simultaneous correction of severe hyponatraemia and hypokalemia resulted in a 24-hour increase of serum [Na^+] of 17 mmol/L. In such instances, uncertainty regarding the optimal approach still exists, mostly due to the lack of trials in human subjects. Re-induction of hyponatraemia by using desmopressin, intravenous 5% dextrose solution or a combination of both is usually unnecessary in acute hyponatraemia, may be optional in patients with low to moderate risk of ODS, but it is definitively recommended in patients at high risk of ODS [24]. The occasional use of corticosteroids has been reported in the literature. A possible favorable effect of corticosteroids in ODS, which were administered to the patient described here, is to stabilize the blood-brain barrier [1], although there is no definitive evidence of a clear benefit in humans. Urea or myoinositol have been used in animal studies, aiming to restore intracellular organic osmolites, thus protecting from cellular dehydration [1]. Prompt treatment with minocycline, a selective and potent inhibitor of microglial activation, has been proven to be effective in counteracting the accumulation and the pro-inflammatory activity of microglia, which usually occurs in demyelinative lesions in ODS [25]. Plasmapheresis has been used in a few patients and its beneficial effect has been possibly related to the reduction of inflammatory mediators and consequently to a protective effect on the blood-brain barrier [1]. Similarly, a few cases of successful treatment with intravenous immunoglobulin have been reported [26]. The mechanism of action of immunoglobulin in reversing the effects of demyelination remains to be elucidated, but it includes the possible reduction of myelinotoxic substances and the induction of remyelination [27]. Dopaminergic molecules appear helpful in improving neurological alterations once ODS is fully established [5]. Besides pharmacological treatment, the approach to ODS includes physical therapy, similarly to other neurological disorders.

Conclusions

We reported here a case of ODS occurred in a pregnant woman with hyperemesis gravidarum after an overly rapid correction of low serum [Na^+] in the presence of several concomitant risk factors. The overly rapid increase of serum sodium may has been likely caused by the simultaneous correction of severe hypokalemia and it might have been prevented by a more cautious and thoughtful management of the patient. This case may very well be considered as an appropriate example to reinforce warning among physicians about the care that should be taken in a clinical setting, in order to prevent rapid changes in serum osmolarity, which may lead to dramatic and sometimes irreversible consequences.

Abbreviations

ODS: Osmotic demyelination syndrome; [Na^+]: Serum sodium concentration; MRI: Magnetic resonance imaging; CPM: Central pontine myelinolysis; EPM: Extra-pontine myelinolysis.

Competing interests

AP is on the Otsuka Pharmaceutical advisory board for tolvaptan and has received honoraria from Otsuka Pharmaceutical for speaking at symposia; GC, LS, CG, AS declare that they have no competing interests.

Authors' contributions

Acquisition of medical report of the patient: GC, AS. *Analysis and interpretation of data*: GC, AP, AS. *Drafting of the manuscript*: AP, GC, CG *MRI. examination*: LS. All authors read and approved the final manuscript.

Acknowledgements

Giovanni Corona, Corinna Giuliani and Alessandro Peri wish to thank Prof. Gianni Forti and Prof. Mario Maggi for encouraging and supporting their interest in clinical endocrinology and for their invaluable critical advice.

Author details

[1]Medical Department, Endocrinology Unit, Azienda USL Bologna, Maggiore-Bellaria Hospital, Bologna, Italy. [2]Emergency Interventional Radiology and Neuroradiology Unit, Azienda USL Bologna, Maggiore-Bellaria Hospital, Bologna, Italy. [3]Department of Experimental and Clinical Biomedical Sciences, Endocrine Unit, University of Florence, Florence, Italy.

References

1. King JD, Rosner MH: **Osmotic Demyelination Syndrome.** *Am J Med Sci* 2010, **339**:561–567.
2. Sonkusare S: **The clinical management of hyperemesis gravidarum.** *Arch Gynecol Obstet* 2011, **283**:1183–1192.
3. Adams RD, Victor M, Mancall EL: **Central pontine myelinolysis: a hitherto undescribed disease occurring in alcoholic and malnourished patients.** *Arch Neurol Psychiatry* 1959, **81**:154–172.
4. Tomlinson BE, Pierides AM, Bradley WG: **Central pontine myelinolysis. Two cases with associated electrolyte disturbance.** *Q J Med* 1976, **45**:373–386.
5. Love S: **Demyelinating diseases.** *J Clin Pathol* 2006, **59**:1151–1159.
6. Kleinschmidt-Demasters BK, Rojiani AM, Filley CM: **Central and extrapontine myelinolysis: then…and now.** *J Neuropathol Exp Neurol* 2006, **65**:1–11.
7. Yoon B, Shim YS, Chung SW: **Central pontine and extrapontine myelinolysis after alcohol withdrawal.** *Alcohol Alcohol* 2008, **43**:647–649.
8. Cardenas JF, Bodensteiner JB: **Osmotic demyelination syndrome as a consequence of treating hyperammonemia in a patient with ornithine transcarbamylase deficiency.** *J Child Neurol* 2009, **24**:884–886.
9. Bagshaw SM, Peets AD, Hameed M, Boiteau PJ, Laupland KB, Doig CJ: **Dialysis Disequilibrium Syndrome: brain death following hemodialysis for metabolic acidosis and acute renal failure: a case report.** *BMC Nephrol* 2004, **19**:5–9.
10. Guerrero WR, Dababneh H, Nadeau SE: **Hemiparesis, encephalopathy, and extrapontine osmotic myelinolysis in the setting of hyperosmolar hyperglycemia.** *J Clin Neurosci* 2013, **20**:894–896.
11. O'Malley G, Moran C, Draman MS, King T, Smith D, Thompson CJ, Agha A: **Central pontine myelinolysis complicating treatment of the hyperglycaemic hyperosmolar state.** *Ann Clin Biochem* 2008, **45**:440–443.

12. McKee AC, Winkelman MD, Banker BQ: **Central pontine myelinolysis in severely burned patients: relationship to serum hyperosmolality.** *Neurology* 1988, **38:**1211–1217.
13. Naik KR, Saroja AO: **Seasonal postpartum hypernatremic encephalopathy with osmotic extrapontine myelinolysis and rhabdomyolysis.** *J Neurol Sci* 2010, **15:**5–11.
14. Suzuki R, Okuda M, Asai J, Nagashima G, Itokawa H, Matsunaga A, Fujimoto T, Suzuki T: **Astrocytes co-express aquaporin-1,-4, and vascular endothelial growth factor in brain edema tissue associated with brain contusion.** *Acta Neurochir Suppl* 2006, **96:**398–401.
15. Ashrafian H, Davey P: **A review of the causes of central pontine myelinosis: yet another apoptotic illness?** *Eur J Neurol* 2001, **8:**103–109.
16. Murase T, Sugimura Y, Takefuji S, Oiso Y, Murata Y: **Mechanisms and therapy of osmotic demyelination.** *Am J Med* 2006, **119:**S69–S73.
17. Turnbull J, Lumsden D, Siddiqui A, Lin JP, Lim M: **Osmotic demyelination syndrome associated with hypophosphataemia: 2 cases and a review of literature.** *Acta Paediatr* 2013, **102:**e164–e168.
18. Haglin L: **Phosphate Depletion is the link between growth, stress and diet in the aetiology of MS.** *Med Hypotheses* 2004, **63:**262–267.
19. Martin RJ: **Central pontine and extrapontine myelinolysis: the osmotic demyelination syndromes.** *J Neurol Neurosurg Psychiatry* 2004, **75:**22–28.
20. Serrano-Castro PJ, Alonso-Verdegay G, López-Martínez G, Arjona-Padillo A, Callejón JR, Olmedo VM, Guardado-Santervás P, Huete-Hurtado A, Olivares-Romero J, Naranjo Fernández C: **Possible case of peripheral osmotic demyelination syndrome.** *J Neurol Neurosurg Psychiatry* 2007, **79:**331–332.
21. Miller GM, Baker HL Jr, Okazaki H, Whisnant JP: **Central pontine myelinolysis and its imitators: MR findings.** *Radiology* 1988, **168:**795–802.
22. Menger H, Jorg J: **Outcome of central pontine and extrapontine myelinolysis (n: 44).** *J Neurol* 1999, **246:**700–705.
23. Adrogué HJ, Madias NE: **Hyponatraemia.** *N Engl J Med* 2000, **342:**581–1589.
24. Verbalis JG, Goldsmith SR, Greenberg A, Korzelius C, Schrier RW, Sterns RH, Thompson CJ: **Diagnosis, evaluation, and treatment of hyponatremia: expert panel recommendations.** *Am J Med* 2013, **126:**S1–S42.
25. Suzuki H, Sugimura Y, Iwama S, Suzuki H, Nobuaki O, Nagasaki H, Arima H, Sawada M, Oiso Y: **Minocycline prevents osmotic demyelination syndrome by inhibiting the activation of microglia.** *J Am Soc Nephrol* 2010, **21:**2090–2098.
26. Murthy SB, Izadyar S, Dhamne M, Kass JS, Goldsmith CE: **Osmotic demyelination syndrome: variable clinical and radiologic response to intravenous immunoglobulin therapy.** *Neurol Sci* 2013, **34:**581–584.
27. Rodriguez M, Miller DJ, Lennon V: **Immunoglobulins reactive with myelin basic protein promote CNS remyelination.** *Neurology* 1996, **46:**538–545.

The association of anthropometry indices with gout in Taiwanese men

Wen-Yu Lin[1], Chia-Chi Lung[2,3], Ting-Sung Liu[2], Zhi-Hong Jian[2], Pei-Chieh Ko[2], Jing-Yang Huang[2], Chien-Chang Ho[4], Shih-Chang Chen[5], Yi-Chen Chiang[2,3] and Yung-Po Liaw[2,3*]

Abstract

Background: To examine the association of anthropometry indices with gout and to compare the performance of indices to predict gout in Taiwanese men.

Methods: There were 1443 male subjects aged more than 20 years who participated in the Nutrition and Health Survey in Taiwan (NAHSIT, 1993–1996). Anthropometric evaluation consisted of weight, height, hip and waist circumference (WC) with later body mass index (BMI), waist to height (WHtR) and waist to hip (WHR) estimations. We conducted 4 logistic models to determine the relationships between anthropometric indices and gout. Receiver operating characteristic (ROC) curve were used to compare the predictive performance and to identify the optimal cut-off points, sensitivity and specificity of these indices for gout in men.

Results: After controlling for other covariables, the adjusted odds ratios for the mid and top tertiles of WHtR were 2.55 (95% CI: 1.16, 5.59) and 3.01 (95% CI: 1.13, 7.99), respectively, but no linear association was found for BMI, WHR and WC. In ROC curve, the greatest area under curve was 0.684 for WHtR and the cut-off point of WHtR was 0.57.

Conclusions: WHtR had a significant linear association with gout in Taiwanese men and was superior to BMI, WHR and WC.

Keywords: Gout, Anthropometry, Waist to height ratio

Background

The prevalence of gout has increased in recent years [1]. Twenty-six percent of adult males (≥19 years) and 22% of older males (≥45 years) either had hyperuricemia or were taking medication for it in Nutrition and Health Survey in Taiwan (NAHSIT, 1993–1996) [2]. The data from the Taiwan National Health Insurance Research Database showed that the prevalence of gout was 4.26% and male to female ratio was 3.2:1 [3]. Subjects with high serum uric acid levels are at higher risk for all-cause and cardiovascular mortality [4]. Gout increases the risk of cardiovascular disease, even in young people and those without cardiovascular risk factors [5]. Gout also increases mortality risk in both genders, especially in kidney diseases, endocrine and metabolic diseases, and cardiovascular diseases [6].

Overweight and obesity are epidemic and obese people often have hyperuricemia. Increased serum uric acid [7] and gout occurrence [8] have been known to be closely associated with an increase in visceral fat accumulation. The significance of visceral fat obesity has been found to be associated with chronic metabolic disorders [9]. Insulin resistance plays a key role in the connection between hyperuricemia and metabolic syndrome [10,11]. It is known that body mass index (BMI), triglycerides, hypertension, inflammation and insulin resistance increase the uric acid concentration [12-14]. High plasma urate concentration is associated with articular deposits of urate crystals that cause gout [15]. The predisposing factors such as alcohol consumption, diuretics use, and excess weight gain increase risks of gout attack among patients with hyperuricemia [16]. Gout has also been linked with metabolic syndrome and diabetes [17]. Obesity is positively associated with gout, whereas body weight loss is protective [18].

* Correspondence: Liawyp@csmu.edu.tw
[2]Department of Public Health and Institute of Public Health, Chung Shan Medical University, Taichung City 40201, Taiwan
[3]Department of Family and Community Medicine, Chung Shan Medical University Hospital, Taichung City 40201, Taiwan
Full list of author information is available at the end of the article

Thus, on the basis of these evidences, it is important to find an easy, practical screening index for predicting gout in the general male Taiwanese population. However, the evidence about the correlation of BMI, waist circumference (WC), waist to hip ratio (WHR), or waist to height ratio (WHtR) with gout in the Taiwanese population is scant. We tried to assume that other anthropometric index rather than BMI could more accurately predict gout. Therefore, the aim of this study was to ascertain which anthropometric index can be better at predicting gout in the Taiwanese men.

Methods

Study participants

The data were obtained from the Nutrition and Health Survey in Taiwan that was performed between 1993 and 1996 (NAHSIT, 1993–1996). NAHSIT was a nationwide survey for the nutrition and health status of Taiwanese. All instruments of the NAHSIT 1993–1996 were evaluated for validity and reliability in 3 pilot studies conducted from January to June in 1993 [19]. All subjects were gave written informed consent for participation before enrollment in the study. The database consists of de-identified secondary data and is released for purposes of public researches.

The details of the design and the operational techniques about the survey have been described previously [20]. Briefly, data were drawn from 7 geographical district samples according to their unique dietary patterns of the residents, ancestral origins, geographic location, and degree of urbanization (Hakka people areas, mountainous areas, the East coast area, the Peng-Hu islands, metropolitan cities, urbanization Class I townships, and urbanization Class II townships).

Data collection

After the strata were classified, 3 townships or city districts were selected within each stratum by selection probability proportional to its population size (PPS). Three communities were selected in each township or city district by PPS method. People in each communities were further divided into 7 age groups (4–6, 7–12, 13–15, 16–18, 19–44, 45–64, and ≧ 65 years) and 2 sex groups. Eight or 16 individuals (depending on the available age groups) were sampled in each age group by sex group. A pseudo-Latin square design was used to allocate survey time to balance the effects of season and year in this subtropical land. Demographic and clinical characteristics, and physical examinations were recorded and documented during face-to-face interviews with structured questionnaires. Finally, there were 6464 subjects completed the physical examination and 5843 adequate fasting blood samples. The present study enrolled 1443 Taiwanese males aged ≥20 years with complete questionnaires (sex, age, area, alcohol consumption, and medical history), physical examinations and results of fasting blood samples.

Definitions

Hyperuricemia was defined as serum uric acid ≧ 7.0 mg/dl for males [21]. Taiwan definitions adopted BMI 24 kg/m^2 as the cutpoint for overweight and 27 kg/m^2 for obesity [22]. The definitions of metabolic syndrome in males are WC ≥90 cm and any two of the following: (1) high triglyceride ≥150 mg/dL, (2) low HDL-cholesterol <40 mg, (3) high blood pressure ≥130/85 mg or on medication, (4) raised fasting plasma glucose ≧100 mg/dl or diabetes [23].

Table 1 Demographic, clinical, laboratory and anthropometric characteristics of subjects with and without gout

Variables	Gout (n = 104)	Non gout (n = 1339)	p-value
Age (year)	55.1 ± 13.7	51.1 ± 15.7	0.01
Area (%)			<0.01
Hakka area	13.5	14.3	
Mountainous area	37.5	13.7	
East Coast area	9.6	15.3	
Penghu islands	10.6	14.0	
Metropolitan cities	9.6	14.9	
Provincial class I townships	10.6	13.1	
Provincial class II townships	8.7	14.7	
Lifestyle factors			
Smoking (%)	68.6	70.9	0.63
Alcohol drinking (%)			
Low	17.7	19.7	0.80
Moderate	54.9	51.6	
High	27.5	28.7	
Hypertension medication (%)	21.2	8.2	<0.01
Anthropometric indices			
BMI (kg/m^2)	25.2 ± 2.9	23.5 ± 3.4	<0.01
WC (cm)	86.3 ± 7.6	81.3 ± 9.8	<0.01
WHR	0.90 ± 0.05	0.87 ± 0.07	<0.01
WHtR	0.53 ± 0.04	0.49 ± 0.06	<0.01
Renal disease (%)	4.9	2.5	0.15
Metabolic syndrome (%)	41.4	16.9	<0.01
Triglyceride ≧ 150 mg/dl (%)	45.2	24.1	<0.01
HDL <40 mg/dl (%)	37.5	28.5	0.05
High blood pressure (%)*	71.2	53.6	0.01
High fasting glucose (%)#	15.4	12.0	0.31
Uric acid ≧ 7.0 mg/dl (%)	64.4	40.3	<0.01

Data are expressed as mean ± standard deviation, unless otherwise indicated.
Abbreviations: *BMI* Body mass index, *HDL* High density lipoprotein, *WC* Waist circumference, *WHR* Waist to hip ratio, *WHtR* Waist to height ratio.
*Blood pressure ≧ 130/85 mmHg or participants with medication control.
Fasting glucose ≧ 100 mg/dl or participants with medication control.

We defined gout as reporting gout diagnosed by a physician from questionnaires.

The self-reported alcohol consumption was categorized into low, moderate and high. Anthropometric variables included height, weight, WC and hip circumference. Hip circumference was measured at the level of the greater trochanter. WC was measured at the mid-level between the iliac crest and the last rib. BMI was calculated as weight (kilogram) divided by height (meter) squared, WHR was calculated as WC (centimeter) divided by HC (centimeter), and WHtR was calculated as WC (centimeter) divided by height (centimeter).

Statistical analyses

All analyses were carried out by using the SAS ver. 9.1 software package (SAS Institute, Cary, NC, USA). Comparisons between gout and non-gout subjects' demographic data, laboratory measurements, and anthropometric indices were made using Student's t test and Chi-square tests. Adjusted odds ratios (ORs) with 95% confidence intervals (CIs) for gout were calculated from the multiple logistic regression analysis according to obesity (BMI ≥ 27 kg/m^2 and top tertile of WC, WHR, and WHtR) and the tertiles of the indices. In the current study, the ROC curve analyses were performed by calculating the true positive rate (sensitivity) against the false-positive rate (1 – specificity) to assess and measure the predictive power of each anthropometric index in the association with gout based on the area under the curve (AUC). A p value <0.05 was considered statistically significant.

Results

The basic characteristics of the 104 gout and 1339 non-gout male participants aged ≧ 20 years are shown in Table 1. The age of gout group was older than non-gout Taiwanese. The highest prevalence of gout was found in the mountainous areas. The prevalence of high anthropometric indices, metabolic syndrome, dyslipidemia, high blood pressure and hyperuricemia were significantly higher in gout group than that in non-gout group. There were no significant differences in smoking, alcohol drinking and renal disease between the two groups.

In Table 2, BMI ≥27 kg/m^2 and the top tertile of WC, WHR and WHtR were considered to be obese. It shows the ORs for gout by BMI ≥ 27 kg/m^2 and top tertile of WC, WHR, and WHtR after adjusting for age, smoking, areas and hypertension medications. Hyperuricemia and metabolic syndrome were significantly associated with gout in all models. The adjusted OR for gout was significantly increased in the top tertile of WC (OR, 1.70; 95% CI, 1.04-2.79), WHR (OR, 1.77; 95% CI, 1.07-2.92), and WHtR (OR, 2.28; 95% CI, 1.35-3.86). A non-

Table 2 The ORs for gout in relation to obesity definitions after adjustment for potential confounders

Variables		Model 1		Model 2		Model 3		Model 4	
		OR	95% CI	OR	95% CI	OR	95% CI	OR	95% CI
Hyperuricemia									
	No	1.00		1.00		1.00		1.00	
	Yes	1.90	(1.21, 3.00)	1.92	(1.22, 3.02)	1.87	(1.19, 2.96)	1.92	(1.22, 3.02)
Renal disease									
	No	1.00		1.00		1.00		1.00	
	Yes	1.32	(0.46, 3.77)	1.36	(0.48, 3.85)	1.31	(0.46, 3.74)	1.22	(0.43, 3.50)
Alcohol drinking									
	Low	1.00		1.00		1.00		1.00	
	Moderate	1.05	(0.58, 1.90)	1.07	(0.59, 1.92)	1.03	(0.57, 1.86)	1.08	(0.60, 1.95)
	High	0.83	(0.42, 1.65)	0.81	(0.41, 1.61)	0.81	(0.49, 1.62)	0.89	(0.45, 1.75)
Metabolic syndrome									
	No	1.00		1.00		1.00		1.00	
	Yes	1.85	(1.14, 3.02)	1.84	(1.13, 3.00)	1.71	(1.06, 2.77)	1.88	(1.15, 3.07)
Obesity*									
WC (cm)	≧ 88.1	1.70	(1.04, 2.79)						
WHR	≧ 0.91			1.77	(1.07, 292)				
WHtR	≧ 0.53					2.28	(1.35, 3.86)		
BMI (kg/m^2)	≧ 27							1.59	(0.98, 2.57)

Adjustment for age, smoking, areas and hypertension medication in all models.
Abbreviations: *BMI* Body mass index, *WC* Waist circumference, *WHR* Waist to hip ratio, *WHtR* Waist to height ratio.
*Obesity is defined as BMI ≥ 27 kg/m^2 and top tertile of WC,WHR, and WHtR.

Table 3 The ORs for gout in relation to tertiles of each anthropometric index after adjustment for potential confounders

Variables		Model 1		Model 2		Model 3		Model 4	
		OR	95% CI	OR	95% CI	OR	95% CI	OR	95% CI
Renal disease	No	1.00		1.00		1.00		1.00	
	Yes	1.47	(0.51, 4.19)	1.55	(0.55, 4.39)	1.45	(0.51, 4.13)	1.43	(0.50, 4.10)
Alcohol drinking	Low	1.00		1.00		1.00		1.00	
	Moderate	1.08	(0.60, 1.96)	1.09	(0.60, 1.97)	1.08	(0.59, 1.98)	1.10	(0.61, 2.00)
	High	0.85	(0.42, 1.70)	0.82	(0.41, 1.65)	0.85	(0.42, 1.72)	0.88	(0.44, 1.77)
Metabolic disorders*									
Hypertriglyceridemia	No	1.00		1.00		1.00		1.00	
	Yes	1.70	(1.06, 2.72)	1.65	(1.03, 2.64)	1.64	(1.02, 2.63)	1.70	(1.06, 2.72)
Low HDL	No	1.00		1.00		1.00		1.00	
	Yes	1.13	(0.72, 1.79)	1.11	(0.70, 1.75)	1.10	(0.70, 1.75)	1.13	(0.72, 1.79)
High blood pressure	No	1.00		1.00		1.00		1.00	
	Yes	1.14	(0.69, 1.88)	1.14	(0.69, 1.87)	1.12	(0.68, 1.85)	1.11	(0.68, 1.84)
High fasting glucose	No	1.00		1.00		1.00		1.00	
	Yes	0.78	(0.42, 1.45)	0.75	(0.40, 1.40)	0.78	(0.41, 1.46)	0.76	(0.41, 1.43)
Hyperuricemia	No	1.00		1.00		1.00		1.00	
	Yes	1.78	(1.12, 2.85)	1.77	(1.11, 2.83)	1.78	(1.12, 2.85)	1.77	(1.11, 2.82)
WC (cm)	<81.7	1.00		1.00		1.00		1.00	
	81.7-88.1	1.81	(1.04, 3.14)	1.47	(0.78, 2.75)	0.91	(0.42, 1.98)	1.52	(0.81, 2.86)
	≧ 88.1	1.83	(1.06, 3.18)	1.38	(0.68, 2.81)	0.78	(0.31, 1.95)	1.35	(0.61, 2.99)
	P trend	0.03		0.41		0.61		0.38	
WHR	<0.87			1.00					
	0.87-0.91			1.53	(0.81, 2.88)				
	≧ 0.91			1.57	(0.75, 3.26)				
	P trend			0.21					
WHtR	<0.49					1.00			
	0.49-0.53					2.55	(1.16, 5.59)		
	≧ 0.53					3.01	(1.13, 7.99)		
	P trend					0.03			
BMI (kg/m^2)	<24							1.00	
	24-27							1.42	(0.76, 2.65)
	≧ 27							1.50	(0.64, 3.51)
	P trend							0.42	

Adjustment for age, smoking, areas, and hypertension medication in all models.
Abbreviations: *BMI* Body mass index, *HDL* High density lipoprotein, *WC* Waist circumference, *WHR* Waist to hip ratio, *WHtR* Waist to height ratio.
*Hypertriglyceridemia: triglyceride ≧ 150 mg/dl; low HDL: HDL < 40 mg/dl; high blood pressure: blood pressure ≧ 130/85 mmHg or hypertension medication; high fasting glucose: glucose ≧ 100 mg/dl or diabetic medication; hyperuricemia: uric acid ≧ 7.0 mg/dl.

Table 4 Estimated area under curve (AUC) of the indices in predicting gout in men

Index	Estimated AUC	95% CI	Optimal cut-point	Sensitivity	Specificity
WHtR	0.684	(0.639, 0.729)	0.57	0.67	0.67
BMI	0.659	(0.610, 0.708)	27.12	0.72	0.60
WHR	0.657	(0.608, 0.706)	0.89	0.71	0.62
WC	0.655	(0.607, 0.703)	94	0.69	0.64

Abbreviations: *BMI* Body mass index, *WC* Waist circumference, *WHR* Waist to hip ratio, *WHtR* Waist to height ratio.

significant result was found for BMI (≧27 kg/m^2) (OR, 1.59; 95% CI, 0.98-2.57) in Model 4.

Four multivariable models of gout consisting of variables for renal disease, alcohol drinking, metabolic syndrome, hyperuricemia and anthropometric indices after adjustment for age, smoking, areas and hypertension medication are shown in Table 3. The OR for gout was significantly increased in the mid and top tertiles of WC in Model 1 (p trend = 0.03). We simultaneously adjusted WC into the Model 2, 3, and 4. After the adjustments, the ORs for gout increased significantly for WHtR, but not for BMI and WHR. The adjusted odds ratios for the mid and top tertiles of WHtR were 2.55 (95% CI: 1.16, 5.59) and 3.01 (95% CI: 1.13, 7.99) in Model 3, respectively. The obesity index, WHtR, seemed to have more stable effects on gout than did WC.

Table 4 shows the AUC values of WHtR, BMI, WHR, and WC by using ROC analysis to detect the predictive power of all anthropometric indices for gout. Of the 4 anthropometric indices, WHtR was found to have the largest areas under the ROC curve (0.684). The best combination of sensitivity and specificity for gout was 0.67 and 0.67, respectively. The optimal cut-off values for gout showed WHtR of 0.57.

Discussion

The proxy measures of visceral fat obesity, principally, WC, WHR or WHtR are used as a surrogate of body fat centralization and have been use for cardiovascular risk evaluation because of their association with cardiometabolic parameters and outcome [9,24,25]. In 2001 Chang et al. [2] reported a nationwide survey from Taiwan that showed strong associations of serum uric acid concentrations with mountainous area, age and BMI in men. A cross-sectional study of 2023 military personnel in Taiwan showed positive associations of serum uric acid with BMI, systolic and diastolic blood pressure, and dyslipidemia [26]. Villegas et al. investigated hyperuricemia in a population consisting middle-aged, urban Chinese men and identified graded positive associations of BMI, WHR, WC, and weight gain [27]. A nationwide study in Taiwan demonstrated that WC has the strongest correlation with hyperuricemia for both men and women than BMI and WHR [28].

In a community based epidemiological study in Taiwan, the risk factors for gout among either the general population or subjects with hyperuricemia were serum uric acid level, alcohol drinking and central obesity [21]. Hypertriglyceridemia in men may potentiate the effect of serum uric acid to increase the risk of gout development [29]. In a large prospective cohort of men, higher BMI and weight gain are strong risk factors for gout in men, while weight reduction is protective [18].

WHtR is a more practical anthropometric index to find higher metabolic risks in normal and overweight Japanese men and women than WC and BMI [30]. A hospital based case–control study of 92 gout and 92 non-gout men showed that WHtR had a significant linear effect on gout risk, independent of BMI [31]. In our study, altered WC increased the chances of gout, but this fact occurred only in the first adjustment of the model in Table 3. When the BMI, WHR and WHtR separately were added, the effect of WC was lost. After adjustment by WC, the OR of WHtR remained significant. From our multivariable models, it suggested that the index of central obesity, especially WHtR, was better index for identifying the risk for gout in this population than were WC and WHR.

One of the strengths of our study was the use of a computerized database, which was population-based and highly representative. A number of important limitations warrant discussion. First, NAHSIT was a cross-sectional study and susceptible to unmeasured confounders and reverse causation. Second, as a result of modernization and life style changes globally, the anthropometric variables of the studied population may have changed. The results from data collected between 1993 and 1996 could be established as a reference or model to which future studies could compare. Third, the diagnosis of gout is based on self reported diagnosis by a physician that might be biased. Although gold standard diagnosis of gout is based upon aspiration of joint fluid for the identification of urate crystals [32], it is impractical for epidemiologic research. Gout is often defined by self-report in epidemiologic studies. Previous population-based cohort study suggested that the self-report of physician diagnosed gout has good reliability and sensitivity and is appropriate for epidemiologic studies [33].

Conclusion

We had confirmed the hypothesis that WHtR rather than BMI could more accurately predict gout. Among the 4 anthropometric indices used in the present study, although higher values of WC, WHR, and WHtR were associated with gout, WHtR appears to be an independent and better anthropometric index for identifying individuals with gout.

Abbreviations

AUC: Area under the curve; BMI: Body mass index; CI: Confidence intervals; NAHSIT: Nutrition and Health Survey in Taiwan; OR: Odds ratio; PPS: Probability proportional to population size; ROC: Receiver operating characteristic; WC: Waist circumference; WHtR: Waist to height; WHR: Waist to hip.

Competing interests

All the authors declare that they have no competing interests.

Authors' contributions

YPL designed the study, provided conceptual input and contributed to the final manuscript. TSL, PCK and JYH extracted and analyzed data. WYL, ZHJ and CCL wrote the draft. SCC, YCC and CCH provided conceptual input and contributed to the final manuscript. All authors read and provided feedback on the draft versions of the article. All the authors have read and approved the final version.

Acknowledgments
This study is based on the dataset from Nutrition and Health Survey in Taiwan (NAHSIT, 1993–1996), conducted and provided by the National Health Research Institutes and Department of Health, Taiwan. The descriptions or conclusions herein do not represent the viewpoints of the Department.

Author details
[1]Jen-Ai Hospital, Taichung City 41265, Taiwan. [2]Department of Public Health and Institute of Public Health, Chung Shan Medical University, Taichung City 40201, Taiwan. [3]Department of Family and Community Medicine, Chung Shan Medical University Hospital, Taichung City 40201, Taiwan. [4]Department of Health and Leisure Management, Yuanpei University, Hsinchu City 300, Taiwan. [5]Department of Leisure Industry and Health Promotion, National Ilan University, Yilan City 260, Taiwan.

References

1. Chuang SY, Lee SC, Hsieh YT, Pan WH: **Trends in hyperuricemia and gout prevalence: nutrition and health survey in Taiwan from 1993–1996 to 2005–2008.** *Asia Pac J Clin Nutr* 2011, **20**(2):301–308.
2. Chang HY, Pan WH, Yeh WT, Tsai KS: **Hyperuricemia and gout in Taiwan: results from the nutritional and health survey in Taiwan (1993–96).** *J Rheumatol* 2001, **28**(7):1640–1646.
3. Kok VC, Horng JT, Lin HL, Chen YC, Chen YJ, Cheng KF: **Gout and subsequent increased risk of cardiovascular mortality in non-diabetics aged 50 and above: a population-based cohort study in Taiwan.** *BMC Cardiovasc Disord* 2012, **12:**108.
4. Kuo CF, See LC, Yu KH, Chou IJ, Chiou MJ, Luo SF: **Significance of serum uric acid levels on the risk of all-cause and cardiovascular mortality.** *Rheumatology* 2013, **52**(1):127–134.
5. Kuo CF, Yu KH, See LC, Chou IJ, Ko YS, Chang HC, *et al*: **Risk of myocardial infarction among patients with gout: a nationwide population-based study.** *Rheumatology* 2013, **52**(1):111–117.
6. Kuo CF, Yu KH, See LC, Chou IJ, Tseng WY, Chang HC, *et al*: **Elevated risk of mortality among gout patients: a comparison with the national population in Taiwan.** *Joint Bone Spine* 2011, **78**(6):577–580.
7. Tamba S, Nishizawa H, Funahashi T, Okauchi Y, Ogawa T, Noguchi M, *et al*: **Relationship between the serum uric acid level, visceral fat accumulation and serum adiponectin concentration in Japanese men.** *Intern Med* 2008, **47**(13):1175–1180.
8. Takahashi S, Yamamoto T, Tsutsumi Z, Moriwaki Y, Hada T: **Increased visceral fat accumulation in patients with primary gout.** *Adv Exp Med Biol* 2000, **486:**131–134.
9. Janssen I, Katzmarzyk PT, Ross R: **Waist circumference and not body mass index explains obesity-related health risk.** *Am J Clin Nutr* 2004, **79**(3):379–384.
10. Li C, Hsieh MC, Chang SJ: **Metabolic syndrome, diabetes, and hyperuricemia.** *Curr Opin Rheumatol* 2013, **25**(2):210–216.
11. Chou P, Lin KC, Lin HY, Tsai ST: **Gender differences in the relationships of serum uric acid with fasting serum insulin and plasma glucose in patients without diabetes.** *J Rheumatol* 2001, **28**(3):571–576.
12. de Oliveira EP, Moreto F, Silveira LV, Burini RC: **Dietary, anthropometric, and biochemical determinants of uric acid in free-living adults.** *Nutr J* 2013, **12:**11.
13. Perticone F, Sciacqua A, Perticone M, Arturi F, Scarpino PE, Quero M, *et al*: **Serum uric acid and 1-h postload glucose in essential hypertension.** *Diabetes care* 2012, **35**(1):153–157.
14. So A, Thorens B: **Uric acid transport and disease.** *J Clin Invest* 2010, **120**(6):1791–1799.
15. Roddy E, Doherty M: **Epidemiology of gout.** *Arthritis Res Ther* 2010, **12**(6):223.
16. Lin KC, Lin HY, Chou P: **The interaction between uric acid level and other risk factors on the development of gout among asymptomatic hyperuricemic men in a prospective study.** *J Rheumatol* 2000, **27**(6):1501–1505.
17. Chen SY, Chen CL, Shen ML: **Manifestations of metabolic syndrome associated with male gout in different age strata.** *Clin Rheumatol* 2007, **26**(9):1453–1457.
18. Choi HK, Atkinson K, Karlson EW, Curhan G: **Obesity, weight change, hypertension, diuretic use, and risk of gout in men: the health professionals follow-up study.** *Arch Intern Med* 2005, **165**(7):742–748.
19. Pan WH, Kao MD, Tzeng MS, Yen LL, Hung YT, Li LA, *et al*: **Nutrition and health survey in Taiwan (NAHSIT) 1993–1996: design, contents, and operations.** *Nutr Sci J* 1999, **24**(1):1–10.
20. Pan WH, Chang HY, Yeh WT, Hsiao SY, Hung YT: **Prevalence, awareness, treatment and control of hypertension in Taiwan: results of Nutrition and Health Survey in Taiwan (NAHSIT) 1993–1996.** *J Hum Hypertens* 2001, **15**(11):793–798.
21. Lin KC, Lin HY, Chou P: **Community based epidemiological study on hyperuricemia and gout in Kin-Hu, Kinmen.** *J Rheumatol* 2000, **27**(4):1045–1050.
22. Pan WH, Lee MS, Chuang SY, Lin YC, Fu ML: **Obesity pandemic, correlated factors and guidelines to define, screen and manage obesity in Taiwan.** *Obes Rev* 2008, **9**(Suppl 1):22–31.
23. Alberti KG, Zimmet P, Shaw J: **The metabolic syndrome–a new worldwide definition.** *Lancet* 2005, **366**(9491):1059–1062.
24. Schneider HJ, Glaesmer H, Klotsche J, Bohler S, Lehnert H, Zeiher AM, *et al*: **Accuracy of anthropometric indicators of obesity to predict cardiovascular risk.** *J Clin Endocrinol Metab* 2007, **92**(2):589–594.
25. Schneider HJ, Friedrich N, Klotsche J, Pieper L, Nauck M, John U, *et al*: **The predictive value of different measures of obesity for incident cardiovascular events and mortality.** *J Clin Endocrinol Metab* 2010, **95**(4):1777–1785.
26. Chu NF, Wang DJ, Liou SH, Shieh SM: **Relationship between hyperuricemia and other cardiovascular disease risk factors among adult males in Taiwan.** *Eur J Epidemiol* 2000, **16**(1):13–17.
27. Villegas R, Xiang YB, Cai Q, Fazio S, Linton M, Li H, *et al*: **Prevalence and determinants of hyperuricemia in middle-aged, urban Chinese men.** *Metab Syndr Relat Disord* 2010, **8**(3):263–270.
28. Chen CC, Wang WS, Chang HY, Liu JS, Chen YJ: **Heterogeneity of body mass index, waist circumference, and waist-to-hip ratio in predicting obesity-related metabolic disorders for Taiwanese aged 35–64 y.** *Clin Nutr* 2009, **28**(5):543–548.
29. Chen JH, Pan WH, Hsu CC, Yeh WT, Chuang SY, Chen PY, *et al*: **Impact of obesity and hypertriglyceridemia on gout development with or without hyperuricemia: a prospective study.** *Arthritis Care Res* 2013, **65**(1):133–140.
30. Hsieh SD, Yoshinaga H, Muto T: **Waist-to-height ratio, a simple and practical index for assessing central fat distribution and metabolic risk in Japanese men and women.** *Int J Obes Relat Metab Disord* 2003, **27**(5):610–616.
31. Lyu LC, Hsu CY, Yeh CY, Lee MS, Huang SH, Chen CL: **A case–control study of the association of diet and obesity with gout in Taiwan.** *Am J Clin Nutr* 2003, **78**(4):690–701.
32. Pluta RM, Shmerling RH, Burke AE, Livingston EH: **JAMA patient page. Gout.** *JAMA* 2012, **308**(20):2161.
33. McAdams MA, Maynard JW, Baer AN, Kottgen A, Clipp S, Coresh J, *et al*: **Reliability and sensitivity of the self-report of physician-diagnosed gout in the campaign against cancer and heart disease and the atherosclerosis risk in the community cohorts.** *J Rheumatol* 2011, **38**(1):135–141.

14

Ethinylestradiol$_{30\mu g}$-drospirenone and metformin: could this combination improve endothelial dysfunction in polycystic ovary syndrome?

Ioana Rada Ilie[1*], Ioan Marian[2], Teodora Mocan[3], Razvan Ilie[4], Lucian Mocan[5], Ileana Duncea[1] and Carmen Emanuela Pepene[1]

Abstract

Background: We are hereby investigating for the first time the effect of the association ethinylestradiol$_{30\mu g}$ -drospirenone $_{3mg}$ (DRP/EE$_{30\mu g}$) plus metformin and weight loss on endothelial status and C-reactive protein (hsCRP) levels in polycystic ovary syndrome (PCOS).

Methods: 25 young women with PCOS (mean age 22.76 ± 0.83 years, body mass index (BMI): 28.44 ± 6.23) who completed the study were prospectively evaluated. The oral contraceptive- DRP/EE$_{30\mu g}$ (21 days/month) and metformin (1700 mg daily) were administered for 6 months to the PCOS group. Additionally, the 15 overweight and obese patients (BMI > 25 kg/m2) were instructed in a diet of no more than 1500 cal daily. Primary outcome measures were surrogate markers of cardiovascular disease and included endothelial function, *i.e.* flow-mediated dilatation (FMD) on the brachial artery and endothelin-1 levels, as well as hsCRP concentrations, body composition (measured by whole-body dual-energy X-ray-absorptiometry) and insulin resistance. Variables were assessed at baseline, as well as after our medical intervention.

Results: The combination between DRP/EE$_{30\mu g}$ plus metformin combined with weight loss triggered a significant improvement in the FMD values (FMD-PCOS$_{basal}$ 3.48 ± 1.00 *vs* FMD-PCOS$_{6\ months}$7.43 ± 1.04, p = 0.033), as well as body composition and insulin insensitivity ($p < 0.05$). Regarding hsCRP levels, there was no significant intragroup (PCOS$_{6months}$ − PCOS$_{basal}$) difference.

Conclusion: A 6-month course of metformin- DRP/EE$_{30\mu g}$ (associated with weight loss) improves the endothelial dysfunction in PCOS and shows neutral effects on hsCRP concentrations as an inflammation marker. These data demand for reevaluation of the medical therapy in PCOS, particularly in women with additional metabolic and cardiovascular risk factors (ClinicalTrials.gov Identifier: NCT01459445).

Keywords: Ethinylestradiol$_{30\mu g}$-drospirenone, Flow-mediated dilatation, Endothelial dysfunction, HsCRP, Metformin, Polycystic ovary syndrome

Background

Women with polycystic ovary syndrome (PCOS) frequently cluster several cardiovascular risk markers and early subclinical atherosclerosis which seem to be in relation to their unfavourable endocrine and metabolic milieu [1,2] represented mainly by insulin resistance, central obesity and hyperandrogenemia [3]. Endothelial dysfunction and arterial stiffness are considered early stages of cardiovascular disease development [4]. Previous studies [3,5-7], have shown that endothelial function is impaired in women with PCOS. Moreover, low-grade chronic inflammation plays a major role in inducing endothelial injury, atherosclerosis development and progression in these patients.

Lifestyle modification, diet and weight loss are essential for the cardiovascular disease and diabetes mellitus prevention in overweight and obese PCOS women. In addition to these, and aside from therapeutic strategies directed towards fertility restoration, the current pharmacological treatment of this disease is mainly based on two drug

* Correspondence: ioanamanaila@yahoo.com
[1]Department of Endocrinology, University of Medicine and Pharmacy, 3-5 Louis Pasteur, 400349, Cluj-Napoca, Romania
Full list of author information is available at the end of the article

categories: (combined) oral contraceptives ((C) OC) and insulin sensitizers.

The insulin sensitizer metformin has been shown to ameliorate insulin resistance, reduce hyperandrogenism and triglyceride (TG) levels in PCOS [7-9]. Moreover, some studies also reported endothelial structure and function improvement [7,10] and a decrement of highly sensitive C-reactive protein (hsCRP) concentrations in PCOS after metformin [11,12].

On the other hand, COC have a long history of use in these patients and are prescribed for obtaining a regular menstrual cycle and for improving hyperandrogenism. Because COCs might adversely influence insulin resistance, glucose tolerance, lipid profile [9,11] or aggravate chronic inflammation [11,13] the possibility of worsening the already unfavorable cardiovascular risk profile of PCOS subjects is of concern. However, the metabolic effects of pills are extremely variable; for example estrogens impair insulin action dose-dependently and the associated progestins may modify these effects [14]. It was suggested that when a dose of ethinylestradiol (EE) < 50 μg/day is used, the effects of the COCs on the lipid and glycoinsulinemic metabolism is related to the progestin used in the combination [15]. Drospirenone (DRP) is a progestin with antiandrogenic and antimineralocorticoid activity. However, the studies assessing the effect of the COC containing 30 μg EE + 3mg DRP ($DRP/EE_{30\mu g}$) on surrogate markers of atherosclerosis are few and inconclusive [15,16]. All the hereinabove considered, the present study aimed to assess the effects of $DRP/EE_{30\mu g}$ combined with metformin and weight loss by means of dietary intervention on indices of endothelial dysfunction, *i.e.* flow-mediated dilation (FMD) and serum endothelin-1 (ET-1), serum hsCRP and lipids, and insulin resistance in young women with PCOS.

Methods

Study populations

We prospectively studied 26 women with PCOS who presented to our clinic. The study protocol was conducted with the approval of the local ethics committee (246/09.02.2011), in accordance with the Helsinki Declaration. Participants gave written informed consent before their inclusion in the study protocol. The diagnosis of PCOS was based on Androgen Excess Society 2006 guidelines [17]. Hyperandrogenism was defined as hirsutism and/or as an elevated total testosterone concentration. Menstrual irregularities were defined as oligomenorrhea (eight or fewer menses/ year) or amenorrhea (absence of menstruation for 3 consecutive months). Polycystic ovaries were defined by the ultrasound appearance of 12 or more follicles in each ovary measuring 2–9 mm in diameter and/or ovarian volume greater than 10 ml. Secondary causes of hyperandrogenism such as hyperprolactinemia, thyroid disease, androgen-secreting tumours, Cushing's syndrome and congenital adrenal hyperplasia were excluded in all patients. The presence and extent of hirsutism were quantified using the Ferriman-Gallwey (F-G) score. Exclusion criteria included current or previous use (within 6 months) of oral contraceptives, anti-androgens, ovulation induction medications, drugs known to affect carbohydrate-lipid metabolism, or a personal history of diabetes.

Study design

At the first visit, subjects with PCOS and BMI < 25 kg/m2 and those with BMI > 25 kg/m2 were instructed in a diet of no more than 2000- and respectively 1500 cal daily, composed of 50% carbohydrates, 20% proteins, and 30 % fat –with a polyunsaturated-saturate ratio of 2:1. Dietary adherence was assessed by review with the same investigator (I.I.) at 3 and 6 months after inclusion in the study. The treatment with the monophasic COC- $DRP/EE_{30\mu g}$ (21 days/month) and metformin, given as 850 mg twice per day, was started the fifth day of a spontaneous or progestin-induced menstrual cycle. To reduce metformin gastrointestinal side effects, doses were titrated up over a 20-day period starting at 425 mg up to a final dose of 1700 mg /day (two tablets daily, one before lunch and one before dinner). All women received their medications for 6 months.

A complete history and physical examination, including BMI and waist hip ratio (WHR) were determined by the same physician. Systolic blood pressure (SBP) and diastolic blood pressure (DBP) were measured in the right arm, with the subjects in a seated position, using a mercury sphygmomanometer. More than 5 cigarettes/ day was considered active smoking, while a sustained physical activity (fitness, swimming, jogging etc.) of at least 1h per day, at least 3 times a week, for at least 3 consecutive months was considered significant. None of the study subjects performed significant physical activity before or during the study. All patients were instructed to not modify their physical activity throughout the trial.

PCOS subjects were investigated at baseline, during early follicular phase (days 2–5) of a spontaneous or progestin-induced menstrual cycle, and after six cycles of treatment-during days 5–7 of week 4 (week of placebo pills, no exogenous hormones). Evaluation included anthropometric, laboratory, flow-mediated dilation (FMD) and body composition measurements. In seventeen PCOS subjects (68%) menstruation was induced using dydrogesterone, 20 mg/day for 5 days, a progestin which appears to exert neutral effects on nitric oxide release, as recently demonstrated [18].

Assay methods

All blood samples were obtained between 08.00 and 10.00 h in the morning after overnight fasting. Blood samples were immediately centrifuged and the serum obtained was stored at −80°C until the time of assay. Serum fasting glucose (GLU, mg/dl) was measured by the glucose oxidase colour method (Glucose GOD/PAP; Diagnosticum Zrt, Budapest, Hungary). Total cholesterol (TC, mg/dl) and TG (mg/dl) were measured by an enzymatic, colorimetric method (Diagnosticum Zrt, Budapest, Hungary).

All other measurements were performed using the ELISA TECAN auto-analyzer. Insulin (INS, μU/ml), total testosterone (TT, ng/ml), sex hormone-binding globulin (SHBG, nmol/l), endothelin-1 (ET-1, pg/ml) were all measured using commercial enzyme–linked immunosorbent assay kits from DRG Instruments, Marburg, Germany. The intra-assay coefficients of variation for low and high values for INS, TT, SHBG and ET-1 respectively were as follows: 2.6% and 1.8%, 4.1% and 3.3%, 8.6% and 5.3%, 8.8% and 6.7% respectively. The intra-assay coefficients of variance for hsCRP were 6. 9% for CRP values <1.0 mg/l and 4.1% for CRP values >3.0 mg/l, respectively. The minimal detectable concentrations for ET-1 and hsCRP were 0.41 pg/ml and 0.02 μg/ml.

The free androgen index (FAI) was calculated according to the equation: FAI (%) = TT (ng/ml) x 3.47 X 100/SHBG (nmol/l). Insulin resistance was estimated by the homeostasis model assessment of insulin resistance (HOMA-IR) defined fasting glucose (mg/dl) x insulin (μU/ml)/405 and by the quantitative insulin sensitivity check index (QUICKI) defined as 1/ [log (fasting insulin) + log (fasting glucose)].

Body composition

Body composition was assessed by whole-body dual-energy X-ray-absorptiometry (DXA) with a DPX-NT (GE, Madison, USA) device. Fat-free mass was automatically determined as the difference between total body weight and bone mineral content and fat mass. Both total and segmental fat mass and fat-free mass were expressed as weight percentage. The coefficient of variance, evaluated at 3% for total fat mass, was determined by measurements on 10 patients, each one evaluated 3 times.

Hemodynamic studies

FMD was measured for all subjects by the same cardiologist, who was blinded to PCOS status, using a colour Doppler (AGILENT SONOS 4500) with a high-resolution 10-Mhz linear probe. Each patient was taken into a quiet, temperature-controlled room at 20-25°C. After resting in a supine position for 15 minutes, the right brachial artery was identified and its position marked at about 5 cm above the elbow joint. Diameter (mm) of the artery was measured at end-diastole. After the resting measurement, limb flow occlusion was produced by inflating a standard sphygmomanometer cuff on the upper arm to 50 mmHg above systolic pressure for 5 minutes. This caused ischemia and consequently, dilatation of downstream resistance vessels. Subsequent cuff deflation induced a brief high-flow state through the brachial artery (reactive hyperemia) for endothelial nitric oxide release, to accommodate the dilated resistance vessels. The brachial artery was scanned continuously for 90 seconds after cuff deflation and the measurements were performed during the 30–90 seconds interval. The vessel's diameter was measured at the same point with resting measurement at least twice and the maximal diameter was again defined (diameter during reactive hyperemia). FMD was calculated as the percentage maximum change in vessel size from baseline. The coefficient of variation for repeated measurements of resting arterial diameter was 2.3%.

Statistical analysis

Prospective sample size estimation was performed based on a pilot study data (n = 10 for each group) which showed FMD levels for before and after treatment measurements of 3.37 ± 6.6 and 7.97 ± 4.77, respectively. For alpha = 0.05 and beta = 0.20, we have calculated a sample size of n = 24 patients to be evaluated before and after treatment. An additional estimative 8% was added to the calculated sample size in order to cover patient loss, resulting in a sample size of n = 26. Analysis was performed on the 25 subjects who completed the study. Results are reported as mean values ± SEM. The distribution of continuous variables was tested with Kolmogorov-Smirnov test. Differences among continuous variables before and after treatment were assessed by Wilcoxon test. For this type of analysis additional adjustments for dichotomous weight loss were done using weight loss thresholds of 5% and 10% respectively. Bivariate correlations were performed calculating the Spearman rho coefficient. P values of <0.05 were considered statistically significant. The analysis was performed using SPSS version 17.0 (Chicago, Il, USA) and MedCalc 8.3.1.1.

Results

The study initially included all 26 subjects who were eligible after screening. During the follow-up period, 1 patient withdrew from the study because of some moderate gastrointestinal side effects related to metformin and was, therefore, excluded. This resulted in a final number of n = 25 patients (ages: 15–30, mean age 22.76 ± 0.83 years) completing the study.

Treatment and diet effects on measured parameters

Table 1 illustrates the anthropometric characteristics, the main metabolic and hormonal pattern as well as the endothelial and inflammatory profile of these 25 PCOS patients over the 6 months.

The BMI, total fat mass %, lean mass, fasting insulin and HOMA-IR, the F-G score and both TT and FAI were significantly decreased by the pharmacologic approach

Table 1 PCOS subjects (n=25) characteristics at baseline and at the sixth cycles of treatment. Data as means ± SEM

Variables	Baseline	6 months	p-value
BMI (kg/m^2)	28.44 ± 1.24	26.51 ± 1.00	<0.001‡
WHR	0.83 ± 0.07	0.82 ± 0.01	0.071
Glucose (mg/dl)	85.36 ± 1.43	83.08 ± 1.29	0.192
HOMA-IR	3.67 ± 0.32	2.82 ± 0.23	<0.001‡
QUICKI	0.31 ± 0.003	0.33 ± 0.004	0.001†
Insulin (µU/ml)	17.26 ± 1.37	13.74 ± 1.11	0.001†
TC (mg/dl)	198.00±4.87	215.28 ± 6.42	0.005†
TG (mg/dl)	100.56 ± 6.82	125.40 ± 12.88	0.04*
Total fat mass (%)	44.08 ± 1.54	42.56 ± 1.47	0.018*
Trunk fat mass (%)	45.44 ± 1.81	44.02 ± 1.81	0.065
Lean mass (kg)	39.03 ± 1.38	37.84 ± 1.32	0.009†
TT (ng/ml)	0.84 ± 0.06	0.68 ± 0.02	0.007†
FAI (%)	9.70 ± 1.72	3.55 ±1.02	<0.001‡
SHBG (nmol/l)	44.41 ± 5.34	148.44 ± 16.22	<0.001‡
F-G score	9.72 ± 1.06	8.20 ± 0.92	0.02*
SBP (mmHg)	106.20 ± 2.43	104.00 ±2.39	0.184
DBP (mmHg)	70.80 ± 1.95	72.60 ± 1.68	0.318
hsCRP (mg/l)	5.02 ± 0.72	5.20 ± 0.87	0.518
FMD (%)	3.48 ± 1.00	7.43 ± 1.04	0.033*
Baseline artery diameter (mm)	3.14 ± 0.07	3.03 ± 0.06	0.039*
ET-1 (pg/ml)	2.10 ± 0.59	1.60 ± 0.26	0.179

PCOS, polycystic ovary syndrome; BMI, body mass index; WHR, waist-to-hip ratio; HOMA-IR, homeostasis model assessment of insulin resistance; QUICKI, quantitative insulin sensitivity check index; TC, total cholesterol; TG, triglycerides; TT, total testosterone; FAI, free androgen index; SHBG, sex-hormone binding protein; SBP, systolic blood pressure; DBP, diastolic blood pressure; FMD, flow-mediated dilatation; ET-1, endothelin-1
*$P<0.05$; †$p<0.01$; ‡$p<0.001$.

and diet in the total PCOS group, while WHR and trunk fat mass % declined only borderline. We also noted a significant increment of QUICKI and SHBG concentrations as well as of TC and TG levels over the study.

The combination of diet with metformin + DRP/EE$_{30µg}$ was associated with a higher FMD (Table 1). A trend towards lower ET-1 levels was found after 6-month DRP/EE$_{30µg}$ and metformin therapy. However, the difference failed to reach statistical significance. Moreover, there was no change in hsCRP levels at the end of the follow-up period as compared to baseline ones (Table 1).

HsCRP levels were significantly correlated with BMI (r = 0.554, p = 0.004), TC (r = 0.600, p = 0.002), total fat mass % (r = 0.484, p = 0.014) and trunk fat mass (r = 0.404, p = 0.045) at the beginning of the research whereas at 6 months they significantly correlated with BMI (r = 0.550, p = 0.004), trunk fat mass (r = 0.431, p = 0.032), insulin (r = 0.418, p = 0.038), HOMA-IR (r = 0.411, p = 0.041), QUICKI (r = −0.412, p = 0.041), and TC concentrations (r = 0.403, p = 0.046) but only borderline with total fat mass (r = 0.353, p = 0.091). No other significant correlation between the studied parameters was found.

Influence of obesity and smoking habits on post-therapeutic results

Overall the PCOS women achieved a 6.61% (−5.04 ± 5.31kg) moderate weight loss, whereas the obese- overweight and non-obese PCOS subgroups undergone a weight loss of 8.78% (−7.53 ± 4.92 kg) and 2.1 % (−1.3 ±3.41 kg), respectively.

Compared with their non-obese counterparts, obese and overweight PCOS women had higher WHR (p = 0.02), DBP (p = 0.017), FAI levels (p = 0.035), fasting glucose (p = 0.009), fasting insulin (p = 0.003), HOMA-IR (p = 0.001), total and trunk fat mass % (p < 0.001), hsCRP concentrations (p = 0.045) and a lower QUICKI (p = 0.001) and SHBG concentrations (p = 0.031). Considering non-obese and obese PCOS subjects separately, the insulin resistance indices, total fat mass and lean mass showed a significant improvement after 6 months of therapy associated with diet, compared to baseline in the sub-group of obese and overweight women. However, none of the endothelial dysfunction or inflammatory markers seemed to have significantly improved (Table 2). In contrast, non-obese PCOS patients only noted significant changes in markers of hyperandrogenemia and a borderline increase in QUICK index. Regarding the lipid profile, TG levels significantly rose in the obese sub-group while TC concentrations were significantly increased at the end of the 6-month period in the non-obese subgroup and borderline in the obese one (Table 2).

Even after adjusting for a decline of >5% in BMI, there was still a significant difference between the basal values of HOMA-IR (p = 0.014), QUICKI (p = 0.026), INS (p = 0.016), SHBG (p = 0.003), total fat mass % (p = 0.007), trunk fat mass % (p = 0.033), lean mass (p = 0.016) and a borderline one with respect to FMD (p = 0.093) and their values at 6 months. The adjustment for > 10% decrease in body weight was still accompanied by significant differences in pre-treatment vs post treatment values of total fat mass % (p = 0.043) and SHBG (p = 0.028), respectively. Additionally, the unfavorable increments in TG levels over the 6- month treatment observed in our research were significant after applying the same adjustments (p = 0.012, p = 0.027 respectively).

Eight (32%) PCOS women were currently light smokers (i.e. no more than 10 cigarettes per day, <5 years). There were however no statistically significant differences in any of the studied parameters between PCOS smokers and PCOS non-smokers at baseline. Regarding the smoking influence, the fasting glucose (p = 0.021), both HOMA-IR (p = 0.003) and QUICKI (p = 0.006), SHBG levels (p < 0.001) and FAI (p = 0.003) improved significantly in non-smokers during the study and they

Table 2 Hormonal, metabolic, inflammatory and functional endothelial status in obese and non-obese PCOS women pre- and post-medical intervention. Data as means ± SEM

Variables	Obese PCOS		p-value	Non-Obese PCOS		p-value
	Baseline	6 months		Baseline	6 months	
BMI (kg/m^2)	32.56 ± 1.13	29.71 ± 0.94	0.001†	22.26 ± 0.55	21.72 ± 0.66	0.263
WHR	0.87 ± 0.01	0.86 ± 0.01	0.440	0.77 ± 0.01	0.75 ± 0.01	0.056
Glucose (mg/dl)	88.40 ± 1.62	84.60 ± 3.96	0.117	80.80 ± 1.91	80.80 ± 2.18	0.859
HOMA-IR	4.48 ± 0.42	3.29 ± 0.30	0.002†	2.46 ± 0.17	2.10 ± 0.23	0.139
QUICKI	0.31 ± 0.004	0.32 ± 0.005	0.003†	0.33 ± 0.003	0.34 ± 0.005	0.074
Insulin (μU/ml)	20.48 ± 1.79	15.85 ± 1.49	0.002†	12.43 ± 0.85	10.57 ± 1.11	0.169
TC (mg/dl)	202 ± 20.65	220 ± 37.84	0.057	192 ± 29.24	208.20 ±20.77	0.047*
TG (mg/dl)	103.20 ± 35.41	135 ± 72.67	0.004†	96.60 ± 33.48	111 ± 49.69	1.00
Total fat mass (%)	49.51 ± 3.30	47.43 ± 4.36	0.016*	35.94 ± 4.37	35.26 ± 3.71	0.508
Trunk fat mass (%)	51.82 ± 3.56	50.39 ± 4.00	0.173	35.86 ± 5.44	34.46 ± 5.00	0.203
Lean mass (kg)	40.54 ± 8.52	38.72 ± 8.27	0.006†	36.75 ± 2.38	36.51 ± 2.56	0.721
TT (ng/ml)	0.86 ± 0.08	0.68 ± 0.03	0.009†	0.80 ± 0.09	0.68 ± 0.01	0.241
FAI (%)	12.33 ± 2.64	4.56 ± 1.64	0.011*	5.74 ± 0.82	2.04 ± 0.41	0.007†
F-G score	10.40 ± 1.42	8.67 ±1.21	0.007†	8.70 ± 1.64	7.50 ± 1.45	0.016*
SHBG (nmol/l)	35.98 ± 6.10	144.03 ± 23.03	0.001†	57.05 ± 8.59	155.06 ± 22.53	0.013*
SBP (mmHg)	109.67 ± 3.02	104.67 ±3.29	0.042*	101.00 ± 3.63	103.00 ± 3.59	0.732
DBP (mmHg)	74.67 ± 2.41	74.67 ± 1.91	0.886	65.00 ± 2.35	69.50 ± 2.93	0.098
HsCRP (mg/l)	6.10 ± 0.91	6.88 ± 1.14	0.307	3.40 ± 1.03	2.69 ± 0.95	0.646
FMD (%)	4.57 ± 1.31	8.58 ± 1.29	0.133	1.65 ± 1.44	5.55 ± 1.65	0.161
Baseline artery diameter (mm)	3.15 ± 0.11	3.06 ± 0.09	0.402	3.12 ± 0.08	2.99 ± 0.09	0.779
ET-1 (pg/ml)	2.36 ± 0.92	1.80 ± 0.42	0.198	1.71 ± 0.55	1.32 ± 0.20	0.508

PCOS, polycystic ovary syndrome; BMI, body mass index; WHR, waist-to-hip ratio; HOMA-IR, homeostasis model assessment of insulin resistance; QUICKI, quantitative insulin sensitivity check index; TC, total cholesterol; TG, triglycerides; TT, total testosterone; FAI, free androgen index; SHBG, sex-hormone binding protein; SBP, systolic blood pressure; DBP, diastolic blood pressure; FMD, flow-mediated dilatation; ET-1, endothelin-1;
*$P < 0.05$; $^†p < 0.01$.

showed no changes or only borderline modifications towards a better status in smoker PCOS subjects. BMI, insulin levels and F-G score decreased significantly regardless of the smoking status ($p < 0.05$). Neither FMD nor ET-1 or hsCRP significantly changed during the study as a function of smoking.

Discussions

We report for the first time that the 6-month treatment with metformin 1700mg/day and the antiandrogenic COC-DRP/EE $_{30\mu g}$ combined with diet has an overall beneficial effect on endothelial function and shows a neutral effect on hsCRP levels in obese and non-obese women with PCOS.

A novel finding here was the significant improvement of FMD with the medical intervention. However, it is difficult to determine which of the three interventions are responsible for this improvement, especially because when individually assessed, the weight loss, metformin and particularly DRP/EE$_{30\mu g}$ effects on the endothelial function are not settled. Likewise, several recent studies have demonstrated either the favourable impact of lifestyle modifications such as caloric restriction and increased physical activity in improving endothelial function [19-21] or, on the contrary, no improvement of FMD with weight loss [22,23]. However, in PCOS, metformin seems to have improved endothelial function in both obese and non-obese subjects [7,8,10,11,24,25], although not constantly [9]. FMD appears to increase when circulating levels of estrogens augment naturally or synthetically [26-29] and this beneficial vasodilator effect of estrogens on the arterial function might be antagonized by some certain types of progestins [30,31], but not by DRP [32]. Regarding the DRP/EE$_{30\mu g}$, there are very few researches investigating its effect on endothelial function and none evaluating the effect in combination with metformin. Therefore, in PCOS the DRP/EE$_{30\mu g}$ combination administered for 6 months has been shown not to modify the levels of ET-1 which, however, were found to be similar to those of controls and within normal limits [15] or the normal basal vascular reactivity of these women [16]. Others concluded that, while in lean patients with PCOS, the DRP/EE$_{30\mu g}$ does not seem to affect endothelial function, in overweight PCOS women it does not counteract the loss of weight due to healthier lifestyle changes, which is associated with an improvement of insulin sensitivity and FMD [15]. Of note, FMD did not report a significant improvement when evaluating non-obese and obese PCOS subjects separately and this can be accounted for by the small number of subjects in the two groups.

The present results also show that the combination of metformin + DRP/$EE_{30\mu g}$ associated with lifestyle changes has overall beneficial effects on body composition and carbohydrate metabolism in the whole study population and in the obese subjects. The milder metabolic abnormalities in non-obese PCOS women (Table 2) and the small number of subjects may explain the lack of significant effect of medical intervention on body composition and the only borderline improvement of insulin sensitivity in these subjects. However, our results are similar to those of Ibanez et al. who demonstrated that a 3-month treatment with metformin 850 mg/day + DRP/$EE_{30\mu g}$ does not influence the insulin resistance in another group of young non-obese patients with PCOS but with increased adiposity [33]. Nevertheless, the decrease in body weight explains part of our results as a modest weight reduction of 5-10% was demonstrated to be enough to improve insulin resistance [34]. However, we have shown that differences in several parameters persisted after the adjustment for a decrease of > 5% or >10% of body weight thus suggesting that the drug combination used displays an improvement in the insulin sensitivity and can attenuate the central and total body adiposity of young PCOS women. Previous results showed that the increased adiposity found in non-obese adolescents with PCOS diverged further from the norm in subjects on DRP/$EE_{30\mu g}$ alone [35,36] and that the same OC increased TG levels in both overweight and non-obese women with this disease as well as in young, non-obese but hyperinsulinemic PCOS patients [36-38]. Moreover, in a subsequent research by the same authors, the addition of small doses of metformin- 850mg/day to the treatment with DRP/$EE_{30\mu g}$ for 3 months failed to attenuate body adiposity of PCOS subjects and was accompanied by a further deterioration of TG and interleukin-6 (IL-6) levels from the norm [33]. In contrast, others observed that DRP/$EE_{20\mu g}$ + metformin 1500mg/day improved insulin sensitivity, increased HDL-cholesterol concentrations and did not significantly change TG levels in a group of young but non-obese and non-insulin resistant women with PCOS [39]. However, a valid comparison between the study findings of Ibanez et al. and Fruzzetti et al., as well as a further one between their results and ours cannot be performed since the doses of metformin and EE used as well as the basal metabolic profile were different between the populations of these reports. Regarding lipid metabolism, although TG levels rose significantly over the study period in the whole study population as well as in the obese subgroup, most probably as a result of the medical therapy, they remained within the normal range. In other words, it can be hypothesized that metformin clearly does not outperform DRP/$EE_{30\mu g}$ in increasing TG concentrations. Unfortunately, we did not undertake the analysis of cholesterol fraction in our study. Likewise, we do not know if the increase in the total cholesterol is due to a rise in HDL-cholesterol fraction, or to an increase in LDL-cholesterol or both.

Most published data, yet not all [6,40,41], demonstrate increased levels of hsCRP in women with PCOS [5,12,42,43], which may be associated with increased central fat excess rather than PCOS status per se [41,44]. The change in hsCRP levels in our study was not significant by the end of the 6-month follow-up. However, the dosage of metformin and the duration of our study assured the detection of the effects of the medical intervention on hsCRP levels. Therefore, we can conclude that even though moderate weight loss (6–8 %) definitely conferred significant metabolic benefits, it was not sufficient to improve the low-grade chronic inflammation in the total PCOS group and obese subgroup. The following results at the end of the study are noteworthy: both insulin resistance and body adiposity were still abnormal, particularly in the total PCOS group and the obese sub-group, on the one hand and the hsCRP concentrations correlated with trunk fat mass, BMI, TC and insulin resistance indices on the other hand. Therefore, it appears that a more aggressive therapeutic approach and a greater degree of weight loss may be required to achieve metabolic benefits, such as reductions in insulin resistance and body adiposity and consequent decrease of low-grade chronic inflammation. Sustaining our results, it was shown that a 4–5% weight loss improved lipid, glucose, and insulin profiles in women with and without PCOS, but was not effective in lowering CRP concentrations in PCOS women [45] whereas a 15% weight loss in a 2-yr dietary and exercise intervention study was associated with hsCRP reduction [46]. The results obtained in the non-obese subgroup of PCOS women and also those resulted after the adjustment for a decrease >5 % and 10% in body weight showed that the drug combination used in this study did not affect hsCRP levels. It could be hypothesized that metformin and DRP/$EE_{30\mu g}$ may have either different or even opposing effects on chronic inflammation that may balance the risk out and neutralize it overall or may both have neutral effects on hsCRP. Our hypothesis is based on previous results showing that metformin either decreased [11-13] or, used in lower doses (1000-1500mg/day) and for shorter period of time (3 months), caused no change in hsCRP [8,47], as well as on the fact that the effect of DRP/$EE_{30\mu g}$ on chronic inflammation and especially on hsCRP has not been settled. As far as we know, there are no reports evaluating the influence of DRP/$EE_{30\mu g}$ monotherapy on hsCRP levels in PCOS or in other populations. What has been previously observed, though, is that, DRP/$EE_{30\mu g}$ further increased the abnormal levels of IL-6 found in young women with hyperinsulinemic hyperandrogenism [36]. Previous reports suggested that metformin may have direct actions on vascular cells [10,48]. Additionally, metformin might decrease angiogenesis via nuclear factor-κB and Erk1/Erk5 pathways by increasing the antiangiogenic trombospondin-1, an adipokine, preferentially produced by visceral adipose tissue and highly expressed in obese insulin-resistant subjects [49]. However, it is uncertain whether metformin exerts direct effects on hsCRP levels or whether its beneficial changes on the concentration of this inflammation marker are only the result of improved glycemia, insulin resistance, abdominal fat excess and weight loss. Complex interactions and mechanisms might be implied. On the contrary, the serum CRP levels have been shown to increase after a 6-month treatment with COC in young overweight and obese women with PCOS, even if the COC contains an anti-androgen [11,13]. Both estrogens and progestin content and dosage appear to be implicated in CRP regulation [50-52], even though the role of oestrogen might be more important than that of progestin [52]. As far as the mechanism of action is concerned, the literature has been sustaining the direct role of COCs in hsCRP determination by affecting the latter's metabolic and genetic regulation [52]. Hence, a direct estrogen action on the liver was proposed since it is the oral estrogen, and not transdermal estradiol (the latter avoiding the first pass liver effect), which leads to increased serum CRP levels [50,53]. Moreover, COCs have been demonstrated to increment CRP concentrations, without increasing IL-6 ones, suggesting that COCs stimulate hepatocytes to synthesize CRP in a direct way and not via IL-6 mediated inflammation [52]. Regarding anti-androgens, even though their mechanisms of action are not settled, they also appear to modulate and decrease inflammation in PCOS. Hence, low-dose flutamide added to metformin and a fourth-generation OC has been identified to attenuate the hypoadiponectinemia, lean mass deficit as well as central adiposity in young women with PCOS [33]. Up-regulated in states of insulin resistance, IL-6 differentially regulates androgen receptor transactivation via three distinct signaling transduction pathways, the overall effect depending on the balance among these pathways and the androgen concentrations. For instance, at androgen concentration above normal female range and below normal male range, IL-6 and androgens could act synergistically on the androgen receptor [54,33], hereby increasing androgen action. On the other hand, androgen excess in women favors an adipose body composition, including in the abdominal region. A vicious circle amplifying chronic inflammation is thus established. Moreover, adiponectin, which exerts insulin-sensitizing effects, is reversibly down-regulated by androgens and IL-6, but not by estrogens [55]. Therefore, the mechanism of action of flutamide might be at least partly explained by restoration of the androgen receptor transactivation balance and counteraction of the androgen – and IL-6- induced down-regulation of adiponectinemia [33]. Additionally, the mineralocorticoid and the androgen receptor antagonist spironolactone has been shown to inhibit the production of proinflammatory cytokines in patients with congestive heart failure, acting at the transcriptional level and independent of its antimineralocorticoid and antiandrogen activities [56]. We found no data on the effect of the combination metformin-DRP/$EE_{30\mu g}$ on hsCRP, only that Ibanez et al. showed that the treatment with flutamide-metformin plus DRP/ $EE_{30\mu g}$ is associated with a consistent fall in CRP and TNF-α levels, especially in patients with the most abnormal values [57].

In conclusion, our results suggest that the association metformin- DRP/$EE_{30\mu g}$ with lifestyle changes has positive impact on clinical and biochemical hyperandrogenemia, carbohydrate metabolism, body composition and endothelial function-increasing FMD and neutral effects on hsCRP levels. ET-1 levels were not significantly altered by DRP/$EE_{30\mu g}$ and metformin in this follow-up study; however, analyses for ET-1 were significantly underpowered in our set of data. Future revaluation of ET-1 on larger sample size groups is needed for a proper characterization of this marker in relationship with the association metformin- DRP/$EE_{30\mu g}$ and weight loss in PCOS. Although our study is limited by the lack of a weight loss control group, the results obtained, after adjusting for body weight loss, further suggest that the medical treatment used might have neutral/mild positive effects on hsCRP levels, body adiposity and endothelial function, but it might worsen TG levels. Hence, a thorough assessment of the benefits of metformin- DRP/$EE_{30\mu g}$ therapy on vascular function require further trials that should include a weight loss group as a control arm. Concerning the subgroup of non-obese PCOS women, the findings of our study suggest that the use of the association metformin- DRP/$EE_{30\mu g}$ in these women does not seem to affect endothelial function. It can also be considered safe, as no further deterioration of cardiovascular risk factors was noted in this population. Furthermore, the specific effects of the individual components of therapy: metformin and EE/DRP as well as those of the individual COC components on cardiovascular risk markers cannot be ascertained from this study. Nevertheless, these are only cardiovascular risk surrogate markers and we do not know the clinical relevance of our results, which do not provide comprehensive explanations but rather encourage further investigations.

Abbreviations

(BMI),: Body mass index; ((C) OC): (Combined) oral contraceptives; (DBP): Diastolic blood pressure; (DRP): Drospirenone; (ET-1): Endothelin-1;

(EE): Ethinylestradiol; (F-G): scoreFerriman-Gallwey; (FMD): Flow-mediated dilation; (FAI): Free androgen index; (HOMA-IR): Homeostasis model assessment of insulin resistance; (IL-6): Interleukin-6; (PCOS): Polycystic ovary syndrome; (QUICKI): Quantitative insulin sensitivity check index; (SHBG): Sex hormone-binding globulin; (SBP): Systolic blood pressure; (TC): Total cholesterol; (TG): Triglycerides; (TT): Total testosterone; (WHR): Waist hip ratio.

Competing interests

There is no conflict of interest that would prejudice the impartiality of this scientific work. The authors alone are responsible for the content and writing of the article.

Acknowledgements

Funding:
This work was supported by academic grants CNCSIS 552/2007, PN-II-RU-PD-2011-3-0287 and PNCDI II 41_068/2007.

Author details

[1]Department of Endocrinology, University of Medicine and Pharmacy, 3-5 Louis Pasteur, 400349, Cluj-Napoca, Romania. [2]Department of Internal Medicine-Cardiology, University of Medicine and Pharmacy, Cluj-Napoca, Romania. [3]Departmen of Physiology, University of Medicine and Pharmacy, Cluj-Napoca, Romania. [4]Department of Obstetrics and Gynecology, University of Medicine and Pharmacy, Cluj-Napoca, Romania. [5]3-rd Department of Surgery, University of Medicine and Pharmacy, Cluj-Napoca, Romania.

Authors' contributions

IRI has contributed to the design of this study; she was directly implicated in conducting the research, in collecting, analyzing and interpreting data as well as in editing the manuscript and critically revising it. IM has contributed to the design of this study, the measurement of FMD and the data analysis and interpretation. TM participated in the design of the study and performed the statistical analysis. RI has contributed to the design of this study; data collection and interpretation, gynecological ultrasound examination. LM analyzed the data and acquired funding. ID participated in the design of the study and helped to draft the manuscript. CEP has contributed to the design of this study; she was directly implicated in conducting the research, in interpreting data and editing the manuscript as well as in acquiring funding. All authors read and approved the final manuscript.

References

1. Pepene CE, Ilie IR, Marian I, Duncea I: **Circulating osteoprotegerin and soluble receptor activator of nuclear factor {kappa}B ligand in polycystic ovary syndrome: relationships to insulin resistance and endothelial dysfunction.** *Eur J Endocrinol* 2011, **164:**61–8.
2. Shaw LJ, Bairey Merz CN, Azziz R, Stanczyk FZ, Sopko G, Braunstein GD, Kelsey SF, Kip KE, Cooper-Dehoff RM, Johnson BD, Vaccarino V, Reis SE, Bittner V, Hodgson TK, Rogers W, Pepine CJ: **Postmenopausal women with a history of irregular menses and elevated androgen measurements at high risk for worsening cardiovascular event-free survival: results from the National Institutes of Health--National Heart, Lung, and Blood Institute sponsored Women's Ischemia Syndrome Evaluation.** *J Clin Endocrinol Metab* 2008, **93:**1276–84.
3. Ilie IR, Pepene CE, Marian I, Mocan T, Hazi G, Dragotoiu G, Ilie R, Mocan L, Duncea I: **The polycystic ovary syndrome [pcos] status and cardiovascular risk in young women.** *Cent Eur J Med* 2011, **6:**64–75.
4. Buzdugan E, Crisan S, Campean R, Donca V, Radulescu D, Duncea C: **Cardiovascular event risk in relation to arterial stiffness in patients with subclinical peripheral atherosclerosis.** *HVM Bioflux* 2009, **1:**45–54.
5. Diamanti-Kandarakis E, Alexandraki K, Piperi C, Protogerou A, Katsikis I, Paterakis T, Lekakis J, Panidis D: **Inflammatory and endothelial markers in women with polycystic ovary syndrome.** *Eur J Clin Invest* 2006, **36:**691–697.
6. Meyer C, McGrath BP, Teede HJ: **Overweight women with polycystic ovary syndrome have evidence of subclinical cardiovascular disease.** *J Clin Endocrinol Metab* 2005, **90:**5711–5716.
7. Diamanti-Kandarakis E, Spina G, Kouli C, Migdalis I: **Increased endothelin-1 levels in women with polycystic ovary syndrome and the beneficial effect of metformin therapy.** *J Clin Endocrinol Metab* 2001, **86:**4666–73.
8. Agarwal N, Rice SP, Bolusani H, Luzio SD, Dunseath G, Ludgate M, Rees DA: **Metformin reduces arterial stiffness and improves endothelial function in young women with polycystic ovary syndrome: a randomized, placebo-controlled, crossover trial.** *J Clin Endocrinol Metab* 2010, **95:**722–30.
9. Meyer C, McGrath BP, Teede HJ: **Effects of medical therapy on insulin resistance and the cardiovascular system in polycystic ovary syndrome.** *Diabetes Care* 2007, **30:**471–8.
10. Diamanti-Kandarakis E, Alexandraki K, Protogerou A, Piperi C, Papamichael C, Aessopos A, Lekakis J, Mavrikakis M: **Metformin administration improves endothelial function in women with polycystic ovary syndrome.** *Eur J Endocrinol* 2005, **152:**749–756.
11. Teede HJ, Meyer C, Hutchison SK, Zoungas S, McGrath BP, Moran LJ: **Endothelial function and insulin resistance in polycystic ovary syndrome: the effects of medical therapy.** *Fertil Steril* 2010, **93:**184–91.
12. Diamanti-Kandarakis E, Paterakis T, Alexandraki K, Piperi C, Aessopos A, Katsikis I, Katsilambros N, Kreatsas G, Panidis D: **Indices of low-grade chronic inflammation in polycystic ovary syndrome and the beneficial effect of metformin.** *Hum Reprod* 2006, **21:**1426–1431.
13. Morin-Papunen L, Rautio K, Ruokonen A, Hedberg P, Puukka M, Tapanainen JS: **Metformin reduces serum C-reactive protein levels in women with polycystic ovary syndrome.** *J Clin Endocrinol Metab* 2003, **88:**4649–54.
14. Nader S, Diamanti-Kandarakis E: **Polycystic ovary syndrome, oral contraceptives and metabolic issues: new perspectives and a unifying hypothesis.** *Hum Reprod* 2007, **22:**317–22.
15. Mancini F, Cianciosi A, Persico N, Facchinetti F, Busacchi P, Battaglia C: **Drospirenone and cardiovascular risk in lean and obese polycystic ovary syndrome patients: a pilot study.** *Am J Obstet Gynecol* 2010, **202(169):**e1–8.
16. Battaglia C, Mancini F, Fabbri R, Persico N, Busacchi P, Facchinetti F, Venturoli S: **Polycystic ovary syndrome and cardiovascular risk in young patients treated with drospirenone-ethinylestradiol or contraceptive vaginal ring. A prospective, randomized, pilot study.** *Fertil Steril* 2010, **94:**1417–1425.
17. Azziz R, Carmina E, Dewailly D, Diamanti-Kandarakis E, Escobar-Morreale HF, Futterweit W, Janssen OE, Legro RS, Norman RJ, Taylor AE, Witchel SF: **Positions statement: criteria for defining polycystic ovary syndrome as a predominantly hyperandrogenic syndrome: an Androgen Excess Society guideline.** *J Clin Endocrinol Metab* 2006, **91:**4237–4245.
18. Simoncini T, Caruso A, Giretti MS, Scorticati C, Fu XD, Garibaldi S, Baldacci C, Mannella P, Fornari L, Genazzani AR: **Effects of dydrogesterone and of its stable metabolite, 20-alpha-dihydrodydrogesterone, on nitric oxide synthesis in human endothelial cells.** *Fertil Steril* 2006, **86:**1235–1242.
19. Maeda S, Jesmin S, Iemitsu M, Otsuki T, Matsuo T, Ohkawara K, Nakata Y, Tanaka K, Goto K, Miyauchi T: **Weight loss reduces plasma endothelin-1 concentration in obese men.** *Exp Biol Med (Maywood)* 2006, **231:**1044–1047.
20. Raitakari M, Ilvonen T, Ahotupa M, Lehtimäki T, Harmoinen A, Suominen P, Elo J, Hartiala J, Raitakari OT: **Weight reduction with very-low-caloric diet and endothelial function in overweight adults: role of plasma glucose.** *Arterioscler Thromb Vasc Biol* 2004, **24:**124–128.
21. Hamdy O, Ledbury S, Mullooly C, Jarema C, Porter S, Ovalle K, Moussa A, Caselli A, Caballero AE, Economides PA, Veves A, Horton ES: **Lifestyle modification improves endothelial function in obese subjects with the insulin resistance syndrome.** *Diabetes Care* 2003, **26:**2119–2125.
22. Clifton PM, Keogh JB, Foster PR, Noakes M: **Effect of weight loss on inflammatory and endothelial markers and FMD using two low-fat diets.** *Int J Obes (Lond)* 2005, **29:**1445–51.
23. Keogh JB, Brinkworth GD, Clifton PM: **Effects of weight loss on a low-carbohydrate diet on flow-mediated dilatation, adhesion molecules and adiponectin.** *Br J Nutr* 2007, **98:**852–9.
24. Orio F Jr, Palomba S, Cascella T, De Simone B, Manguso F, Savastano S, Russo T, Tolino A, Zullo F, Lombardi G, Azziz R, Colao A: **Improvement in endothelial structure and function after metformin treatment in young normal-weight women with polycystic ovary syndrome: results of a 6-month study.** *J Clin Endocrinol Metab* 2005, **90:**6072–6076.

25. Palomba S, Falbo A, Giallauria F, Russo T, Tolino A, Zullo F, Colao A, Orio F: **Effects of metformin with or without supplementation with folate on homocysteine levels and vascular endothelium of women with polycystic ovary syndrome.** *Diabetes Care* 2010, **33**:246–251.
26. English JL, Jacobs LO, Green G, Andrews TC: **Effect of the menstrual cycle on endothelium-dependent vasodilation of the brachial artery in normal young women.** *Am J Cardiol* 1998, **82**:256–8.
27. Williams MR, Westerman RA, Kingwell BA, Paige J, Blombery PA, Sudhir K, Komesaroff PA: **Variations in endothelial function and arterial compliance during the menstrual cycle.** *J Clin Endocrinol Metab* 2001, **86**:5389–5395.
28. Rickenlund A, Eriksson MJ, Schenck-Gustafsson K, Hirschberg AL: **Oral contraceptives improve endothelial function in amenorrheic athletes.** *J Clin Endocrinol Metab* 2005, **90**:3162–3167.
29. Rickenlund A, Eriksson MJ, Schenck-Gustafsson K, Hirschberg AL: **Amenorrhea in female athletes is associated with endothelial dysfunction and unfavorable lipid profile.** *J Clin Endocrinol Metab* 2005, **90**:1354–9.
30. Wakatsuki A, Okatani Y, Ikenoue N, Fukaya T: **Effect of medroxyprogesterone acetate on endothelium-dependent vasodilation in postmenopausal women receiving estrogen.** *Circulation* 2001, **104**:1773–1778.
31. Faludi AA, Aldrighi JM, Bertolami MC, Saleh MH, Silva RA, Nakamura Y, Pereira IR, Abdalla DS, Ramires JA, Sousa JE: **Progesterone abolishes estrogen and/or atorvastatin endothelium dependent vasodilatory effects.** *Atherosclerosis* 2004, **177**:89–96.
32. Meendering JR, Torgrimson BN, Miller NP, Kaplan PF, Minson CT: **A combined oral contraceptive containing 30 mcg ethinyl estradiol and 3.0 mg drospirenone does not impair endothelium-dependent vasodilation.** *Contraception* 2010, **82**:366–372.
33. Ibanez L, Valls C, Cabre S, De Zegher F: **Flutamide-metformin plus ethinylestradiol-drospirenone for lipolysis and antiatherogenesis in young women with ovarian hyperandrogenism: the key role of early, low-dose flutamide.** *J Clin Endocrinol Metab* 2004, **89**:4716–4720.
34. Holte J, Bergh T, Berne C, Wide L, Lithell H: **Restored insulin sensitivity but persistently increased early insulin secretion after weight loss in obese women with polycystic ovary syndrome.** *J Clin Endocrinol Metab* 1995, **80**:2586–2593.
35. Ibanez L, de Zegher F: **Low-dose flutamide-metformin therapy for hyperinsulinemic hyperandrogenism in non-obese adolescents and women.** *Hum Reprod Update* 2006, **12**:243–252.
36. Ibanez L, de Zegher F: **Ethinylestradiol-drospirenone, flutamide-metformin, or both for adolescents and women with hyperinsulinemic hyperandrogenism: opposite effects on adipocytokines and body adiposity.** *J Clin Endocrinol Metab* 2004, **89**:1592–1597.
37. Palep-Singh M, Mook K, Barth J, Balen A: **An observational study of Yasmin in the management of women with polycystic ovary syndrome.** *J Fam Plann Reprod Health Care* 2004, **30**:163–165.
38. Guido M, Romualdi D, Giuliani M, Suriano R, Selvaggi L, Apa R, Lanzone A: **Drospirenone for the treatment of hirsute women with polycystic ovary syndrome: a clinical, endocrinological, metabolic pilot study.** *J Clin Endocrinol Metab* 2004, **89**:2817–2823.
39. Fruzzetti F, Perini D, Lazzarini V, Parrini D, Gambacciani M, Genazzani AR: **Comparison of effects of 3 mg drospirenone plus 20 mug ethinyl estradiol alone or combined with metformin or cyproterone acetate on classic metabolic cardiovascular risk factors in nonobese women with polycystic ovary syndrome.** *Fertil Steril* 2010, **94**:1793–1798.
40. Mohlig M, Spranger J, Osterhoff M, Ristow M, Pfeiffer AF, Schill T, Schlösser HW, Brabant G, Schöfl C: **The polycystic ovary syndrome per se is not associated with increased chronic inflammation.** *Eur J Endocrinol* 2004, **150**:525–532.
41. Shroff R, Kerchner A, Maifeld M, Van Beek EJ, Jagasia D, Dokras A: **Young obese women with polycystic ovary syndrome have evidence of early coronary atherosclerosis.** *J Clin Endocrinol Metab* 2007, **92**:4609–4614.
42. Tarkun I, Arslan BC, Canturk Z, Turemen E, Sahin T, Duman C: **Endothelial dysfunction in young women with polycystic ovary syndrome: relationship with insulin resistance and low-grade chronic inflammation.** *J Clin Endocrinol Metab* 2004, **89**:5592–5596.
43. Orio F Jr, Palomba S, Cascella T, Di Biase S, Manguso F, Tauchmanovà L, Nardo LG, Labella D, Savastano S, Russo T, Zullo F, Colao A, Lombardi G: **The increase of leukocytes as a new putative marker of low-grade chronic inflammation and early cardiovascular risk in polycystic ovary syndrome.** *J Clin Endocrinol Metab* 2005, **90**:2–5.
44. Puder JJ, Varga S, Kraenzlin M, De Geyter C, Keller U, Muller B: **Central fat excess in polycystic ovary syndrome: relation to low-grade inflammation and insulin resistance.** *J Clin Endocrinol Metab* 2005, **90**:6014–6021.
45. Moran LJ, Noakes M, Clifton PM, Wittert GA, Belobrajdic DP, Norman RJ: **C-reactive protein before and after weight loss in overweight women with and without polycystic ovary syndrome.** *J Clin Endocrinol Metab* 2007, **92**:2944–2951.
46. Esposito K, Pontillo A, Di Palo C, Giugliano G, Masella M, Marfella R, Giugliano D: **Effect of weight loss and lifestyle changes on vascular inflammatory markers in obese women: a randomized trial.** *JAMA* 2003, **289**:1799–1804.
47. Jakubowska J, Bohdanowicz-Pawlak A, Milewicz A, Szymczak J, Bednarek-Tupikowska G, Demissie M: **Plasma cytokines in obese women with polycystic ovary syndrome, before and after metformin treatment.** *Gynecol Endocrinol* 2008, **24**:378–384.
48. Caballero AE, Delgado A, Aguilar-Salinas CA, Herrera AN, Castillo JL, Cabrera T, Gomez-Perez FJ, Rull JA: **The differential effects of metformin on markers of endothelial activation and inflammation in subjects with impaired glucose tolerance: a placebo-controlled, randomized clinical trial.** *J Clin Endocrinol Metab* 2004, **89**:3943–8.
49. Tan BK, Adya R, Chen J, Farhatullah S, Heutling D, Mitchell D, Lehnert H, Randeva HS: **Metformin decreases angiogenesis via NF-kappaB and Erk1/2/Erk5 pathways by increasing the antiangiogenic thrombospondin-1.** *Cardiovasc Res* 2009, **83**:566–74.
50. Lacut K, Oger E, Le Gal G, Blouch MT, Abgrall JF, Kerlan V, Scarabin PY, Mottier D, SARAH Investigators: **Differential effects of oral and transdermal postmenopausal estrogen replacement therapies on C-reactive protein.** *Thromb Haemost* 2003, **90**:124–131.
51. Puder JJ, Freda PU, Goland RS, Wardlaw SL: **Estrogen modulates the hypothalamic-pituitary-adrenal and inflammatory cytokine responses to endotoxin in women.** *J Clin Endocrinol Metab* 2001, **86**:2403–8.
52. Haarala A, Eklund C, Pessi T, Lehtimäki T, Huupponen R, Jula A, Viikari J, Raitakari O, Hurme M: **Use of combined oral contraceptives alters metabolic determinants and genetic regulation of C-reactive protein.** *The Cardiovascular Risk in Young Finns Study. Scand J Clin Lab Invest* 2009, **69**:168–174.
53. Lowe GD, Upton MN, Rumley A, McConnachie A, O'Reilly DS, Watt GC: **Different effects of oral and transdermal hormone replacement therapies on factor IX, APC resistance, t-PA, PAI and C-reactive protein–a cross-sectional population survey.** *Thromb Haemost* 2001, **86**:550–6.
54. Yang L, Wang L, Lin HK, Kan PY, Xie S, Tsai MY, Wang PH, Chen YT, Chang C: **Interleukin-6 differentially regulates androgen receptor transactivation via PI3K-Akt, STAT3, and MAPK, three distinct signal pathways in prostate cancer cells.** *Biochem Biophys Res Commun* 2003, **305**:462–9.
55. Fasshauer M, Kralisch S, Klier M, Lossner U, Bluher M, Klein J, Paschke R: **Adiponectin gene expression and secretion is inhibited by interleukin-6 in 3T3-L1 adipocytes.** *Biochem Biophys Res Commun* 2003, **301**:1045–50.
56. Hansen PR, Rieneck K, Bendtzen K: **Spironolactone inhibits production of proinflammatory cytokines by human mononuclear cells.** *Immunol Lett* 2004, **91**:87–91.
57. Ibanez L, Valls C, de Zegher F: **Discontinuous low-dose flutamide-metformin plus an oral or a transdermal contraceptive in patients with hyperinsulinaemic hyperandrogenism: normalizing effects on CRP, TNF-alpha and the neutrophil/lymphocyte ratio.** *Hum Reprod* 2006, **21**:451–6.

15

Association of blood manganese level with diabetes and renal dysfunction: a cross-sectional study of the Korean general population

Eun Sil Koh[1,2], Sung Jun Kim[1,3], Hye Eun Yoon[1,3], Jong Hee Chung[4], Sungjin Chung[1,2], Cheol Whee Park[1,5], Yoon Sik Chang[1,2] and Seok Joon Shin[1,3*]

Abstract

Background: The purpose of this study was to evaluate the association between blood manganese levels and the prevalence of chronic diseases in the Korean population.

Methods: This was a cross-sectional study based on the Korean National Health and Nutrition Examination Survey (KNAHNES). The study included 3996 participants 20 years of age or older whose blood manganese levels had been measured. The participants were also evaluated for the presence of five chronic diseases: diabetes, renal dysfunction, hypertension, ischemic heart disease, and stroke.

Results: Blood manganese levels were significantly lower in the diabetes group compared with the non-diabetes group (1.26 ± 0.02 vs. 1.35 ± 0.01 μg/dL; $p = 0.001$) and the renal dysfunction group compared with those with normal renal function (1.28 ± 0.03 vs. 1.35 ± 0.01 μg/dL; $p = 0.04$). There was no significant association between blood manganese levels and the presence of ischemic heart disease or stroke. A multivariate logistic regression analysis adjusted for age, sex, and body mass index was performed; the odds ratio was 0.652 (95% CI: 0.46–0.92) for diabetes and 0.589 (95% CI: 0.39–0.88) for renal dysfunction when comparing the higher quartiles (Q2-4) with the lowest quartile (Q1) of blood manganese level. The prevalence of diabetes was 7.6% in Q1 and 5.3% in Q2-4 ($p = 0.02$). Similarly, the prevalence of renal dysfunction was 6.8% in Q1, compared with 4.6% in Q2-4 ($p = 0.02$).

Conclusion: The prevalence of diabetes and renal dysfunction increased in participants with low blood manganese levels, suggesting that blood manganese may play a role in glucose homeostasis and renal function.

Keywords: Manganese, Diabetes, Renal dysfunction

Background

Manganese (Mn) is an essential trace metal with insufficient intake in virtually all diets. It has been reported that Mn is involved in normal immune functions, regulation of blood sugar and cellular energy, and the defense mechanisms against free radicals [1,2]. Experimentally induced Mn deficiency caused a number of detrimental effects, such as impaired bone formation, abnormal glucose tolerance, low levels of high-density lipoprotein (HDL) cholesterol, and skin abnormalities in both animals and humans [3]. Conversely, excess occupational inhalation of Mn may be neurotoxic to humans, producing effects such as psychosis and Parkinsonism. Mn deficiency and intoxication are both associated with adverse metabolic and neuropsychiatric effects [4,5]. Nevertheless, little is known about the optimal blood Mn levels for maintaining homeostasis in humans.

One study found that Mn inhalation in adult animal models markedly down-regulated the gene expression of proteins critical to inflammatory responses or possessing pro-oxidant properties (e.g. tumor growth factor (TGF)-β and neuronal nitric oxide synthase (nNOS)) [6]. These results suggested that a certain amount of Mn exposure may attenuate the inflammatory response to stressful environments. In contrast, Mn is an essential cofactor for metalloenzyme superoxide dismutase, which protects cells

* Correspondence: imkidney@catholic.ac.kr
[1]Department of Internal Medicine, College of Medicine, The Catholic University of Korea, 222 Banpo-daero, Seoul 137-701, Republic of Korea
[3]Division of Nephrology, The Catholic University of Korea Incheon St. Mary's Hospital, 56, Dongsu-ro, Bupyeong-gu, Incheon 403-720, Republic of Korea
Full list of author information is available at the end of the article

against antioxidant processes [3]. Malecki *et al.* demonstrated that Mn deficiency and the resultant decrease in manganese superoxide dismutase (MnSOD) activity caused heart mitochondria to be more sensitive to *in vivo* oxidative damage [7]. This study proposed that subclinical Mn deficiency might also contribute to excess oxidative stress.

Oxidative stress and inflammation are the main pathophysiology behind most chronic diseases. Therefore, we hypothesized that blood Mn levels could be related to the prevalence of chronic diseases. We conducted a cross-sectional analysis on the associations of blood Mn level with five chronic diseases (diabetes, renal dysfunction, hypertension, ischemic heart disease, and stroke) in a representative sample of the adult Korean population from the Korean National Health and Nutritional Examination Survey (KNHANES).

Methods

Study population

The KNHANES was performed to examine the general health and nutritional status of the civilian, non-institutionalized Korean population. KNHANES is a cross-sectional and nationally representative survey composed of a health questionnaire, a health examination, and a nutrition survey. The fourth KNHANES (KNHANES IV) was conducted from 2007 to 2009 using a stratified, multistage probability sampling design. We used data from the second (2008) to third year (2009) of the KNHANES IV. Of the 8641 individuals who participated during this time, we analyzed those who were 20 years of age or older and tested for blood Mn. We excluded participants who were pregnant or had missing values and yielded a final sample size of 3996 adults. The Catholic University of Korea Incheon St. Mary's Hospital Institutional Review Board and the Korea Centers for Disease Control and Prevention approved the study protocol, and written informed consent was obtained from all participants before the study began.

Laboratory measurements

Blood Mn was measured using whole blood at the Neodin Medical Institute (certified by the Korean Ministry of Health and Welfare) in Seoul, Korea, following a standardized protocol. Blood Mn was analyzed by graphite furnace atomic absorption spectrometry with Zeeman background correction (Perkin Elmer AAS800, Perkin Elmer, Turku, Finland). The limit of detection was 0.016 μg/dL for blood Mn. For internal quality assurance and control, standard reference materials were obtained from Bio-Rad (Lyphochek® Whole Blood Metals Control). The inter-assay coefficients of variation ranged from 0.95% to 4.82% for blood Mn samples (reference values were 0.98, 1.18, 2.46, and 3.28 μg/dL). During the survey, overnight fasting venous blood samples were collected. The collected blood samples were properly processed, refrigerated, and transported in cold storage to the Neodin Medical Institute in Seoul, Korea.

Chronic diseases

Diabetes was defined as having one of the following: a fasting blood glucose ≥ 126 mg/dL, a self-reported physician's diagnosis, medication use, or insulin administration at the time of interview. Serum creatinine level was measured using a Hitachi Automatic Analyzer 7600 (Hitachi, Japan) and a modified kinetic Jaffe reaction. The level of kidney function was attained using an abbreviated equation developed from the data from the Chronic Kidney Disease-Epidemiologic Collaboration Group (CKD-EPI) study to estimate the glomerular filtration rate (GFR) [8]. We defined renal dysfunction as an estimated GFR (eGFR) of < 65 mL/min/1.73 m^2 [9]. Hypertension was defined as having one of the following: a mean systolic blood pressure of ≥ 140 mmHg, a mean diastolic blood pressure of ≥ 90 mmHg, a self-reported physician's diagnosis, or antihypertensive medication use at the time of interview. Ischemic heart disease and stroke were based on a self-reported physician's diagnosis.

Other variables

Information on age, sex, residential area, educational status, smoking exposure and alcohol consumption, occupation, body mass index (BMI), and nutritional intake were based on a health questionnaire. Residential area was categorized as either urban or rural. Seoul (the capital city of South Korea) and six other metropolitan cities were grouped as urban areas, and the remaining regions were defined as rural areas. Educational status was divided into ≥ college or ≤ high school. Alcohol consumption was indicated as positive for participants who had consumed at least 30 g per day over the last year. The participants' occupations were categorized as services (which included students, housewives, and the unemployed), agriculture, fishery, or industry. BMI was calculated as weight in kilograms divided by height in meters squared.

Statistical analysis

All statistical analyses and calculations were performed using SAS V9.2 (SAS Institute). We used the stratification variables and sampling weights designated by the Korean Centers for Disease Control and Prevention.

The baseline characteristics were presented as mean ± standard error (SE), median and range, or frequency and proportions. Comparisons of each variable between the two groups were performed using Student's *t*-test or modified Rao-Scott chi-square test. Demographic characteristics were analyzed according to eGFR (< 65 or ≥

65 mL/min/1.73 m^2), the presence of chronic diseases (diabetes, hypertension, ischemic heart disease, or stroke), and quartiles of blood Mn levels (first lowest quartile vs. other quartiles). The odds ratios (OR) and 95% confidence intervals (95% CI) of the associated factors for reduced eGFR and blood Mn quartiles were estimated using logistic regression. A p-value of < 0.05 was considered statistically significant.

Results

The total number of participants was 3996, and the weighted number was 36,990,120. The mean participant age was 45 ± 0.2 years. The mean blood Mn level in the Korean adult population was 1.34 ± 0.01 μg/dL, and the mean eGFR as calculated by the CKD-EPI equation was 95.1 ml/min/1.73 m^2. The mean systolic blood, diastolic blood, and arterial pressures were 116.9 ± 0.4 mmHg, 76.7 ± 0.3 mmHg and 88.7 ± 0.2 mmHg, respectively. The baseline clinical characteristics of the participants were shown in Table 1. Blood Mn levels were significantly different in the baseline characteristics of the following variables: sex, smoking exposure, the history of alcohol drinking, and residential area (data not shown). Mn levels were also different according to the presence of chronic disease (Table 2). Participants with diabetes had significantly lower blood Mn levels than those without diabetes ($p < 0.05$). Renal dysfunction and hypertension presented similarly ($p < 0.05$). There was no significant difference in the blood Mn levels of participants with or without ischemic heart disease or stroke.

We also evaluated the association of blood Mn level with eGFR and blood pressure. In a linear regression analysis adjusted for age, sex, and BMI, there was no statistically significant association between blood Mn levels and eGFR. However, blood Mn levels were positively associated with systolic blood (β coefficient =1.52, $p = 0.01$), diastolic (β coefficient =1.01, $p = 0.02$), and mean arterial blood pressures (β coefficient =1.26, $p = 0.004$) after adjusting for age, sex, BMI, and presence of diabetes.

We divided blood Mn level into quartiles (Q1–Q4) and analyzed the risk for chronic disease. In a multivariate logistic regression analysis, after adjusting for age, sex, and BMI, participants with blood Mn levels in the higher quartiles had a tendency to have lower odds ratios (OR) for the presence of diabetes with a significant test for trend ($p =$ 0.02; Table 3). When the higher quartiles (Q2–4, blood Mn ≥1.060 μg/dL) were compared with the lowest quartile (Q1, blood Mn ≤1.059 μg/dL), the OR for diabetes was 0.652 (95% CI: 0.46–0.92) and 0.589 for renal dysfunction (95% CI: 0.39–0.88, $p < 0.05$) (Table 4). It was well known that diabetes and hypertension were significant risk factors for renal dysfunction; therefore, when adjusted for the presence of diabetes and hypertension, the OR for renal dysfunction was 0.617 (95% CI: 0.41–0.92, $p < 0.05$).

Table 1 Demographic and clinical characteristics of participants (n = 3996)[a]

Characteristics	% (SE)
Age, y[b]	45.2 ± 0.2
< 65	86.2 (0.6)
≥ 65	13.8 (0.6)
Sex	
Male	49.5 (0.5)
Female	50.5 (0.5)
BMI, kg/m^2	
< 25	68.9 (0.9)
≥ 25	31.1 (0.9)
Smoking exposure	
Never	74.3 (0.7)
Former or current	25.7 (0.7)
Alcohol drinking, g/day	
< 30	90.1 (0.6)
≥ 30	9.9 (0.6)
Residence area	
Rural	20.2 (1.8)
Urban	79.8 (1.8)
Education	
≤ High school	70.4 (1.0)
≥ College	29.6 (1.0)
Occupation	
Agriculture & fishery	5.6 (0.6)
Industry	9.2 (0.5)
Services	85.3 (0.8)
GFR, ml/min/1.73 m^2[b]	95.1 ± 0.5
Blood pressure[b]	
SBP, mmHg	116.9 ± 0.4
DBP, mmHg	76.7 ± 0.3
MAP, mmHg	88.7 ± 0.2

BMI = body mass index; GFR = glomerular filtration rate; SBP = systolic blood pressure; DBP = diastolic blood pressure; MAP = mean arterial pressure.
[a]Data are given as% (SE) unless otherwise indicated.
[b]Data as the mean ± SE.

The prevalence of diabetes was significantly higher in the lowest quartile (Q1) when compared with the higher quartiles Q2–4 (7.6% *vs.* 5.3%, $p = 0.02$). Similarly, the prevalence of renal dysfunction showed a significantly higher value in the lowest quartile (Q1) than in the higher quartiles (6.8% *vs.* 4.6%, $p = 0.02$; Table 4).

Discussion

This study was the first to examine the effects of blood Mn on chronic diseases in the general population and determine that blood Mn levels affected the morbidity of chronic diseases. It was found that low blood Mn levels

Table 2 Characteristics of participants and blood Mn levels according to the presence of chronic diseases[a]

	Diabetes			Renal dysfunction			Hypertension			IHD			Stroke		
	Yes (n = 255)	No (n = 3735)	*P* value	Yes (n = 200)	No (n = 3796)	*P* value	Yes (n = 1056)	No (n = 2921)	*P* value	Yes (n = 49)	No (n = 3941)	*P* value	Yes (n = 43)	No (n = 3947)	*P* value
Age (≥ 65 yrs)	39.1 (3.7)	12.2 (0.6)	< .001	61.6 (4.0)	11.2 (0.5)	< .001	30.8 (1.6)	7.7 (0.6)	< .001	48.7 (8.8)	13.3 (0.6)	< .001	42.8 (9.2)	13.5 (0.6)	< .001
Sex (male)	46.0 (3.4)	49.7 (0.6)	0.31	46.4 (3.6)	49.7 (0.5)	0.38	55.0 (1.5)	47.4 (0.7)	< .001	54.6 (8.0)	49.4 (0.5)	0.52	62.0 (9.4)	49.3 (0.5)	0.19
BMI (≥ 25 kg/m^2)	49.7 (3.6)	29.9 (0.9)	<.001	47.4 (4.2)	30.2 (0.9)	< .001	46.2 (1.7)	25.8 (0.9)	< .001	49.6 (8.0)	30.9 (0.9)	0.01	35.1 (8.3)	31.1 (0.9)	0.62
Smoking exposure	23.0 (2.8)	25.8 (0.8)	0.34	9.2 (2.2)	26.6 (0.8)	< .001	24.9 (1.5)	26.0 (0.9)	0.54	17.3 (7.7)	25.8 (0.7)	0.92	21.3 (6.5)	25.7 (0.7)	0.53
Alcohol (≥ 30 g/day)	6.3 (1.7)	10.2 (0.6)	0.08	5.7 (1.9)	10.2 (0.6)	0.07	13.5 (1.3)	8.7 (0.6)	< .001	2.1 (2.1)	10.1 (0.6)	0.07	2.8 (2.8)	10.0 (0.6)	0.16
Residence (rural)	20.6 (3.4)	20.2 (1.8)	0.89	20.9 (4.1)	20.1 (1.8)	0.83	22.2 (2.2)	19.5 (1.8)	0.07	29.2 (7.7)	20.1 (1.8)	0.17	24.0 (6.7)	20.2 (1.8)	0.54
Education (≥ college)	16.4 (2.5)	30.4 (1)	< .001	9.3 (2.3)	30.7 (1.0)	< .001	18.7 (1.5)	33.5 (1.1)	< .001	12.1 (5.3)	29.8 (1.0)	0.02	3.7 (2.5)	29.8 (1.0)	< .001
Occupation			0.02			0.93			< .001			< .001			0.95
Services & others	6.1 (1.8)	5.6 (0.6)		5.2 (1.6)	5.6 (0.6)		7.4 (1.1)	5.0 (0.6)		19.0 (7.1)	5.4 (0.6)		5.9 (3.4)	5.6 (0.6)	
Industry	15.2 (3.1)	8.8 (0.5)		8.6 (2.2)	9.2 (0.5)		11.7 (1.1)	8.2 (0.6)		4.2 (2.7)	9.2 (0.5)		7.9 (4.4)	9.2 (0.5)	
Agriculture & fishery	78.8 (3.4)	85.6 (0.8)		86.2 (2.7)	85.2 (0.8)		81.0 (1.5)	86.8 (0.8)		76.8 (7.3)	85.3 (0.8)		86.2 (5.3)	85.2 (0.8)	
Blood Mn (μg/dL)[b]	1.26 ± 0.02	1.35 ± 0.01	0.001	1.28 ± 0.03	1.35 ± 0.01	0.04	1.32 ± 0.01	1.35 ± 0.01	0.04	1.25 ± 0.05	1.34 ± 0.01	0.09	1.35 ± 0.08	1.34 ± 0.01	0.94

IHD = ischemic heart disease; BMI = body mass index; Mn = Manganese.

[a]Data are given as the percentage (SE) of each category in participants with or without chronic disease unless otherwise indicated.

[b]Data as the mean ± SE.

Table 3 Odds ratio and 95% confidence interval values of chronic disease presence with blood Mn level after adjusting covariates

Mn level quartile (µg/dL)	Diabetes		Renal dysfunction		Hypertension		IHD		Stroke	
	Unadjusted	Adjusted[a]	Unadjusted	Adjusted[b]	Unadjusted	Adjusted[c]	Unadjusted	Adjusted[b]	Unadjusted	Adjusted[b]
Q1 (≤ 1.059)	1 (reference)	1 (reference)	1 (reference)	1 (reference)	1 (reference)	1 (reference)	1 (reference)	1 (reference)	1 (reference)	1 (reference)
Q2 (1.060 - 1.277)	0.66 (0.45, 0.97)	0.65 (0.43, 0.99)	0.52 (0.34, 0.81)	0.51 (0.31, 0.84)	1.09 (0.86, 1.37)	1.21 (0.93, 1.57)	1.03 (0.41, 2.57)	1.04 (0.38, 2.80)	0.92 (0.37, 2.30)	0.91 (0.35, 2.39)
Q3 (1.278 - 1.559)	0.86 (0.57, 1.30)	0.75 (0.49, 1.15)	0.78 (0.50, 1.20)	0.64 (0.39, 1.07)	1.15 (0.92, 1.44)	1.16 (0.90, 1.50)	1.49 (0.62, 3.59)	1.41 (0.55, 3.62)	1.22 (0.50, 3.00)	1.21 (0.48, 3.07)
Q4 (≥ 1.560)	0.53 (0.35, 0.80)	0.53 (0.34, 0.84)	0.67 (0.43, 1.05)	0.72 (0.43, 1.20)	0.86 (0.69, 1.07)	1.07 (0.83, 1.39)	0.47 (0.17, 1.36)	0.55 (0.18, 1.65)	0.94 (0.30, 2.94)	1.22 (0.39, 3.80)
P value	0.01	0.04	0.03	0.06	0.07	0.49	0.11	0.26	0.93	0.92
P for trend	0.02	0.02	0.22	0.28	0.28	0.65	0.41	0.60	0.94	0.62

IHD = ischemic heart disease; Mn = manganese.
[a]adjusted for age, sex, body mass index and hypertension.
[b]adjusted for age, sex, body mass index, diabetes and hypertension.
[c]adjusted for age, sex, body mass index and diabetes.

Table 4 Odds ratio, 95% confidence interval and prevalence of chronic diseases comparing the higher quartiles with the lowest quartile of blood Mn level after adjusting covariates (Q1 vs Q2-4)[a]

Parameter	Odds ratio (95% confidence interval)		Prevalence (%, SE)		
	Unadjusted	Adjusted	Q1	Q2-4	*P* value
Diabetes	0.68 (0.50, 0.94)	0.65 (0.46, 0.92)[b]	7.6 (0.9)	5.3 (0.5)	0.02[b]
Renal dysfunction	0.65 (0.46, 0.92)	0.62 (0.41, 0.92)[c]	6.8 (1.0)	4.6 (0.5)	0.02[c]
Hypertension	1.03 (0.85, 1.24)	1.15 (0.93, 1.42)[d]	25.6 (1.6)	26.2 (1.0)	0.77[d]
IHD	1.00 (0.46, 2.16)	1.04 (0.45, 2.40)[c]	1.2 (0.4)	1.2 (0.2)	0.99[c]
Stroke	1.03 (0.48, 2.20)	1.11 (0.51, 2.42)[c]	0.8 (0.2)	0.8 (0.2)	0.94[c]

IHD = ischemic heart disease.
[a]Blood manganese quartiles (μg/dL): Q1 ≤ 1.059, Q2 1.060 - 1.277, Q3 1.278 - 1.559, Q4 ≥ 1.560.
[b]adjusted for age, sex, body mass index and hypertension.
[c]adjusted for age, sex, body mass index, diabetes and hypertension.
[d]adjusted for age, sex, body mass index and diabetes.

increased the risk and prevalence of diabetes and renal dysfunction, suggesting that blood Mn deficiency might be involved in the pathophysiological processes of diabetes and renal dysfunction.

Mn is stored primarily in skeletal bones and tissues rich in mitochondria. However, no existing biomarker can reliably determine the exact level of Mn accumulated in the body. Because there is a discrepancy in the half-life of Mn in the tissues and blood, Mn levels in red blood cells or whole blood are believed to be more reliable than plasma Mn for measuring Mn accumulation in the body [3]. For practical reasons, whole blood samples have been used as an exposure biomarker of Mn inhalation in most epidemiological studies [3] and were used accordingly in the present study to measure blood Mn.

The importance of Mn in animals was first reported in 1931, but there has been little evidence of its deficiency in humans [1]. In animal models, some of the abnormalities seen in Mn deficiency relate to skeletal abnormalities, changes in circulating HDL cholesterol, and reproductive failure [4]. Some studies have proposed that Mn may influence high glucose conditions. A relationship between Mn and pancreatic function was first seen in 1962 when the blood glucose level dropped in a diabetic patient orally administered Mn. It was postulated that Mn might accelerate cellular glucose uptake by potentiating insulin action and that Mn might act on the pancreas by stimulating the release of stored insulin into the bloodstream or by inhibiting the release of glucagon [10]. In addition, Baly *et al.* demonstrated that Mn deficiency resulted in decreased synthesis of pancreatic insulin, enhanced insulin degradation, and lowered insulin secretion in an Mn-deficient animal model [11]. It was also suggested that Mn deficiency could affect glucose transport and metabolism in adipose cells [12]. A recent experiment demonstrated *in vitro* and *in vivo* that Mn^{2+} supplementation lowered the risk of endothelial dysfunction in diabetes [13].

In the present study, we found a statistically significant relationship between blood Mn levels and diabetes in a representative Korean population. Blood Mn levels were lower in participants with diabetes but not in participants with ischemic heart disease or stroke. Furthermore, the prevalence of diabetes significantly increased in participants with blood Mn levels in the lowest quartile. The pathophysiological mechanism of these results remained unclear. However, the present findings were consistent with previous reports of hypoglycemia induced by low-dose Mn intake in diabetic patients, as well as changes in insulin metabolism in Mn-deficient animal models [10,11,14]. Further studies into the association of blood Mn and insulin metabolism or glucose control status (such as hemoglobin A1c) are needed.

Prior to this study, no clear relationship between Mn and diabetes had been found, and the few epidemiologic studies that addressed this issue in humans were controversial. With limited comparable data, one study into the general elderly population of the Czech Republic found no association between blood Mn and diabetes; instead, seniors with atherosclerosis had higher Mn levels than those without [15]. Three other studies linked low Mn levels with diabetes. Kazi *et al.* showed that diabetic patients of both genders in Pakistan had significantly lower blood and hair levels of Mn than those in the controls [16]. Ekmekcioglu *et al.* found decreased Mn levels in the whole blood and erythrocytes of diabetic individuals [17]. The most recent study revealed Mn deficiency in both type 1 and type 2 diabetic patients with respect to control subjects [18].

Many studies have focused on environmental Mn toxicity rather than on its deficiency and metabolism. Mn toxicity in humans primarily occurs as a consequence of chronic inhalation of high concentrations of airborne Mn-containing particles, linking symptoms of Mn toxicity mainly to miners as well as ferroalloy and battery manufacturing workers [5]. In Korea, Mn may be exposed occupationally or environmentally. Typical toxicity symptoms resemble those of idiopathic Parkinson's disease and include tremor, rigidity, bradykinesia, and posture instability. Patients may also display neuropsychological difficulties that include apathy and even psychosis as Mn affects the dopaminergic systems with a neuropathology that closely resembles Parkinson's disease [19]. Most studies have examined outcomes following relatively high-level acute or chronic exposure to Mn. Less is known about the effects of chronic exposure to lower levels of Mn or the threshold levels sufficient for altering cognitive and motor function [19].

Oxidative stress and inflammation play a major role in the progression of renal damage in chronic kidney disease (CKD). Mn is a potent antioxidant and cofactor of the enzyme MnSOD, which is the main antioxidant enzyme in the mitochondria responsible for protecting the cell from reactive oxygen species (ROS) by scavenging mitochondrial superoxides. Various studies using Mn^{2+} have linked its effects with the function and role of MnSOD. The results in this study showed a significant association of blood Mn level with the prevalence and risk of renal dysfunction after adjusting for diabetes and hypertension in logistic regression analysis, although not in linear regression. Because the KNAHNES was conducted in the general population of Koreans, we projected that including too small a size of subjects with moderate to advanced renal dysfunction may influence the statistical result. Thus, we cautiously postulated that subgroups with lower blood Mn levels may have lower MnSOD activities, possibly making them more sensitive to oxidative stress. Further studies are needed to verify this hypothesis.

High blood Mn levels were found, in this study, to be consistently associated with high systolic, diastolic, and mean arterial blood pressures after adjustment, although no differences in the prevalence of hypertension were found between the lower and higher blood Mn quartile subgroups. These results may have been conflicting as hypertension was partially dependent on self-reported data. Nevertheless, these findings were somewhat compatible with a previous study based on the KNHANES 2008, which reported that blood Mn levels may have been associated with an increased risk of hypertension [20]. The study assumed that chronic Mn accumulation in the mitochondria affected MnSOD activity, resulting in an abnormal response to the mechanism that blocked oxidative stress in the mitochondria and protected against endothelial dysfunction. The exact pathophysiology of Mn on blood pressure is unclear and remains to be elucidated.

This study had some limitations. First, it was cross-sectional, making it difficult to establish a cause-and-effect relationship. Diabetes appeared to have caused lower Mn based on data showing low stores of albumin and other binding proteins in diabetic patients [21], suggesting that Mn and diabetes may affect each other. Further analysis with a longer follow-up period is needed to support the clinical importance of blood Mn levels in diabetes. Second, our regression models were not fully adjusted for potential confounders, such as serum iron or albumin levels, which are the main Mn-binding proteins in the blood. Furthermore, we did not adjust for other metals with the same valence states as Mn, including copper and calcium, which may affect blood Mn levels and other chronic diseases. There may have been participants with chronic diseases without Mn readings, which may explain the lack of a significant association between blood Mn levels and ischemic heart disease or stroke. Last, insufficient information was available to specify whether the diabetes subgroups were type I or II. Despite these limitations, the study presented solid findings as it was performed on a representative sample of the general Korean population with strict quality control of the study procedures of the KNHANES.

Conclusion

The prevalence of diabetes and renal dysfunction decreased in participants with high blood Mn levels, suggesting that blood Mn may have some role in glucose homeostasis and renal function. Further studies are needed to determine any protective effects of Mn on diabetes and renal dysfunction.

Competing interests

The authors declare that they have no competing interests.

Authors' contributions

SJS had full access to all the data in the study and took responsibility for the integrity of the data and accuracy of the data analysis. Study concept and design: SJS, SC, and JHC. Acquisition of data: SJS, ESK, HEY, and SJK. Statistical analysis and interpretation of data: SJS, SC, and JHC. Draft of the manuscript: SJS and ESK. Critical revision of the manuscript for important intellectual content: CWP and YSC. All authors read and approved the final manuscript.

Author details

[1]Department of Internal Medicine, College of Medicine, The Catholic University of Korea, 222 Banpo-daero, Seoul 137-701, Republic of Korea. [2]Division of Nephrology, The Catholic University of Korea Yeouido St. Mary's Hospital, 10, 63-ro, Yeongdeungpo-gu, Seoul 150-713, Republic of Korea. [3]Division of Nephrology, The Catholic University of Korea Incheon St. Mary's Hospital, 56, Dongsu-ro, Bupyeong-gu, Incheon 403-720, Republic of Korea. [4]Department of Statistics, The Graduate School of Ewha Womans University, 52, Ewhayeodae-gil, Seodaemun-gu, Seoul 120-750, Republic of Korea. [5]Division of Nephrology, The Catholic University of Korea Seoul St. Mary's Hospital, 222, Banpo-daero, Seoul 137-701, Republic of Korea.

References

1. Aschner JL, Aschner M: **Nutritional aspects of manganese homeostasis.** *Mol Aspects Med* 2005, **26**(4–5):353–362.
2. Malecki EA, Huttner DL, Greger JL: **Manganese status, gut endogenous losses of manganese, and antioxidant enzyme activity in rats fed varying levels of manganese and fat.** *Biol Trace Elem Res* 1994, **42**(1):17–29.
3. Rucker D, Thadhani R, Tonelli M: **Trace element status in hemodialysis patients.** *Seminars in dialysis* 2010, **23**(4):389–395.
4. Greger JL: **Nutrition versus toxicology of manganese in humans: evaluation of potential biomarkers.** *Neurotoxicology* 1999, **20**(2–3):205–212.
5. **Manganese deficiency in humans: fact or fiction?** *Nutrition reviews* 1988, **46**(10):348–352.
6. HaMai D, Rinderknecht AL, Guo-Sharman K, Kleinman MT, Bondy SC: **Decreased expression of inflammation-related genes following inhalation exposure to manganese.** *Neurotoxicology* 2006, **27**(3):395–401.

7. Malecki EA, Greger JL: **Manganese protects against heart mitochondrial lipid peroxidation in rats fed high levels of polyunsaturated fatty acids.** *J Nutr* 1996, **126**(1):27–33.
8. Levey AS, Stevens LA, Schmid CH, Zhang YL, Castro AF 3rd, Feldman HI, Kusek JW, Eggers P, Van Lente F, Greene T, Coresh J: **A new equation to estimate glomerular filtration rate.** *Ann Intern Med* 2009, **150**(9):604–612.
9. Greenberg A: **Urinalysis.** In *Primer on Kidney Diseases.* 5th edition. Edited by Greenberg A, Cheung AK, Coffman TM, Falk RJ, Jennette JC. Philadelphia: Saunders; 2009:24–32.
10. Rubenstein AH, Levin NW, Elliott GA: **Manganese-induced hypoglycaemia.** *Lancet* 1962, **2**(7270):1348–1351.
11. Baly DL, Curry DL, Keen CL, Hurley LS: **Dynamics of insulin and glucagon release in rats: influence of dietary manganese.** *Endocrinology* 1985, **116**(5):1734–1740.
12. Baly DL, Schneiderman JS, Garcia-Welsh AL: **Effect of manganese deficiency on insulin binding, glucose transport and metabolism in rat adipocytes.** *J Nutr* 1990, **120**(9):1075–1079.
13. Burlet E, Jain SK: **Manganese supplementation reduces high glucose-induced monocyte adhesion to endothelial cells and endothelial dysfunction in Zucker diabetic fatty rats.** *J Biol Chem* 2013, **288**(9):6409–6416.
14. Baly DL, Curry DL, Keen CL, Hurley LS: **Effect of manganese deficiency on insulin secretion and carbohydrate homeostasis in rats.** *J Nutr* 1984, **114**(8):1438–1446.
15. Rambouskova J, Krskova A, Slavikova M, Cejchanova M, Wranova K, Prochazka B, Cerna M: **Trace elements in the blood of institutionalized elderly in the Czech Republic.** *Arch Gerontol Geriatr* 2013, **56**(2):389–394.
16. Kazi TG, Afridi HI, Kazi N, Jamali MK, Arain MB, Jalbani N, Kandhro GA: **Copper, chromium, manganese, iron, nickel, and zinc levels in biological samples of diabetes mellitus patients.** *Biol Trace Elem Res* 2008, **122**(1):1–18.
17. Ekmekcioglu C, Prohaska C, Pomazal K, Steffan I, Schernthaner G, Marktl W: **Concentrations of seven trace elements in different hematological matrices in patients with type 2 diabetes as compared to healthy controls.** *Biol Trace Elem Res* 2001, **79**(3):205–219.
18. Forte G, Bocca B, Peruzzu A, Tolu F, Asara Y, Farace C, Oggiano R, Madeddu R: **Blood metals concentration in type 1 and type 2 diabetics.** *Biol Trace Elem Res* 2013, **156**(1–3):79–90.
19. Aschner M, Guilarte TR, Schneider JS, Zheng W: **Manganese: recent advances in understanding its transport and neurotoxicity.** *Toxicol Appl Pharmacol* 2007, **221**(2):131–147.
20. Lee BK, Kim Y: **Relationship between blood manganese and blood pressure in the Korean general population according to KNHANES 2008.** *Environ Res* 2011, **111**(6):797–803.
21. Folsom AR, Ma J, Eckfeldt JH, Nieto FJ, Metcalf PA, Barnes RW: **Low serum albumin. Association with diabetes mellitus and other cardiovascular risk factors but not with prevalent cardiovascular disease or carotid artery intima-media thickness. The Atherosclerosis Risk in Communities (ARIC) Study Investigators.** *Ann Epidemiol* 1995, **5**(3):186–191.

16

Serum levels of pancreatic stone protein (PSP)/reg1A as an indicator of beta-cell apoptosis suggest an increased apoptosis rate in hepatocyte nuclear factor 1 alpha (HNF1A-MODY) carriers from the third decade of life onward

Siobhan Bacon[1], Ma Peyh Kyithar[1], Jasmin Schmid[2], Syed R Rizvi[1], Caroline Bonner[2], Rolf Graf[3], Jochen HM Prehn[2] and Maria M Byrne[1,4*]

Abstract

Background: Mutations in the transcription factor hepatocyte nuclear factor-1-alpha (HNF1A) result in the commonest type of maturity onset diabetes of the young (MODY). HNF1A-MODY carriers have reduced pancreatic beta cell mass, partially due to an increased rate of apoptosis. To date, it has not been possible to determine when apoptosis is occurring in HNF1A-MODY.We have recently demonstrated that beta cell apoptosis stimulates the expression of the pancreatic stone protein/regenerating (PSP/reg) gene in surviving neighbour cells, and that PSP/reg1A protein is subsequently secreted from these cells. The objective of this study was to determine whether serum levels of PSP/reg1A are elevated during disease progression in HNF1A-MODY carriers, and whether it may provide information regarding the onset of beta-cell apoptosis.

Methods: We analysed serum PSP/reg1A levels and correlated with clinical and biochemical parameters in subjects with HNF1A-MODY, glucokinase (GCK-MODY), and type 1 diabetes mellitus. A control group of normoglycaemic subjects was also analysed.

Results: PSP/reg1A serum levels were significantly elevated in HNF1A-MODY ($n = 37$) subjects compared to controls ($n = 60$) (median = 12.50 ng/ml, IQR = 10.61-17.87 ng/ml versus median = 10.72 ng/ml, IQR = 8.94-12.54 ng/ml, $p = 0.0008$). PSP/reg1A correlated negatively with insulin levels during OGTT, (rho = −0.40, $p = 0.02$). Interestingly we noted a significant positive correlation of PSP/reg1A with age of the HNF1A-MODY carriers (rho = 0.40 $p = 0.02$) with an age of 25 years separating carriers with low and high PSP/reg1A levels. Patients with type 1 diabetes mellitus also had elevated serum levels of PSP/reg1A compared to controls, however this was independent of the duration of diabetes.

Conclusion: Our data suggest that beta cell apoptosis contributes increasingly to the pathophysiology of HNF1A-MODY in patients 25 years and over. PSP/reg1A may be developed as a serum marker to detect increased beta-cell apoptosis, or its therapeutic response.

Keywords: Maturity onset diabetes of the young (MODY), Apoptosis, Serum biomarker, Beta-Cell, Type 1 diabetes, Pancreatic stone protein (PSP), Regenerating gene 1A (reg1A)

* Correspondence: mbyrne@mater.ie
[1]Department of Diabetes, Mater Misericordiae University Hospital, Dublin 7, Ireland
[4]Department of Endocrinology, Mater Misericordiae University Hospital, 30 Eccles Street, Dublin 7, Ireland
Full list of author information is available at the end of the article

Background

Maturity-onset diabetes of the young (MODY), is a monogenic form of diabetes characterized by autosomal dominant mode of inheritance including a three-generation family history of diabetes, age at diagnosis of diabetes of 25 years or less in at least one family member and reduced glucose-stimulated insulin secretion [1]. MODY can result from mutations in at least six different genes [2]. The two most common forms are HNF1A-MODY and glucokinase (GCK)-MODY in all populations studied accounting for approximately 70% of all cases [3].

Insulin secretory defects have been observed in carriers of HNF1A-MODY and GCK-MODY with and without diabetes [4,5]. HNF1A encodes a transcription factor important for pancreatic development, beta cell differentiation and function. HNF1A-MODY subjects with pre-diabetes have defective glucose-induced beta cell insulin secretion indicative of reduced beta cell mass [4]. Homozygous *hnf-1a/tcf-1* knockout mice likewise have a reduced beta cell mass [6]. HNF1A-MODY is associated with a severe and progressive clinical course with up to 50% of patients requiring insulin. The decline in functional beta cell mass may be attributed to increased beta cell apoptosis [7-9]. Mutations in HNF1A are usually detected later in life when they are incidentally discovered through a screening programme or if subjects become symptomatic. Diabetes usually becomes manifest when additional superimposed environmental factors supervene such as a physiological decrease in insulin sensitivity with puberty and pregnancy. The decline in beta cell mass therefore, is progressive but gradual. The possible contribution of apoptosis to this decrease in beta cell mass however, has not been investigated due to a lack of accessible, specific biomarkers for beta cell apoptosis.

In contrast to HNF1A-MODY carriers, patients with GCK-MODY do not show a comparably progressive decrease in beta cell mass. Glucokinase is a key regulatory enzyme in the pancreatic beta cell catalyzing the conversion of glucose to glucose-6-phosphate, the first step in glycogen storage and glycolysis. GCK-MODY is often subclinical but can be detected at any stage of life [10,11]. GCK-MODY carriers have mild fasting and post-prandial hyperglycaemia from birth, lack of progression, and absence of insulin requirement and vascular complications [10-12]. Patients with GCK mutations, in contrast to HNF1A-MODY rarely require any pharmacological intervention and the majority are managed with diet alone.

One of the challenges in evaluating the contribution of beta cell apoptosis in human disease development is the lack of appropriate tools to evaluate the extent of beta cell apoptosis in patients other than *post mortem* studies [13]. Another complicating factor is that the actual process of apoptosis execution is very rapid and occurs within minutes [14], and apoptosing cells can rapidly detach from the extracellular matrix, and are subsequently phagocytised [15], thereby limiting the chance of detecting apoptosis by *in-vivo* imaging techniques. An alternative strategy therefore, is to detect signals that are generated directly or indirectly from apoptosing beta cells. Previous studies from our laboratory have demonstrated that beta cells undergoing apoptosis induce the expression of the PSP/*reg* gene in neighbouring beta cells. This paracrine gene induction occurs in a caspase-dependent manner, and is mediated by the shedding of microparticles from apoptosing cells. PSP/reg1A protein is subsequently secreted from neighbouring cells, and provides a regenerative cue to the microenvironment. We also demonstrated elevated serum levels of PSP/reg1A, the human homologue of PSP/reg, in human subjects with HNF1A-MODY and in subjects with type 1 diabetes mellitus, suggesting that the endocrine pancreas is the primary source of this signal [16].

In the present study, we sought to clinically validate this finding with a larger group and to investigate whether elevated PSP/reg1A levels in HNF1A-MODY correlated with a clinical phenotype and progression of disease. We also investigated whether PSP/reg1A was upregulated in GCK-MODY.

Methods

Subjects

37 HNF1A-MODY and 13 patients with GCK-MODY participated in the study. The HNF1A-MODY group consisted of 13 different families and the GCK-MODY group represented 6 different families. HNF1A mutations included L17H, G207D, P291finsC, S352fsdelG, F426X, P379T, and IVS7-6 G > A, and R200Q/N. GCK mutations included D160N, Y61X, A378V, L146fs, Ile293Arg, and p.Asp311fs. A historic value for PSP/reg1A was also available based on data from 60 normoglycaemic subjects (median = 10.72 ng/ml, IQR = 8.94-12.54 ng/ml). In addition, 27 patients with antibody positive (GAD and or Islet cell antibody) type 1 diabetes mellitus were recruited from the diabetes outpatients in the Mater Misericordiae University Hospital. Clinically, on presentation, all subjects with type 1 diabetes mellitus had osmotic symptoms with ketosis requiring insulin from diagnosis. There was no significant family history recorded in any of the subjects with type 1 diabetes mellitus. All subjects were BMI-matched. The clinical characteristics of all groups analyzed are presented in Table 1 and Table 2 contains the glucose levels during OGTT in HNF1A-MODY subjects. Ethics approval was attained from the ethics committee at the Mater

Table 1 Clinical characteristics of subjects

Subject group	HNF1A-MODY	Glucokinase Mutations	Type 1 diabetes mellitus
Number of subjects	37	13	27
Age (yrs)	43 (21–52)	38 (27–60)	41 (23–52)
Diabetes duration (yrs)	6 (3–19)	From birth	21 (3–34)
BMI (kg/m^2)	24.4 (22.0-26.3)	24.0 (21.6-26.4)	24.4 (22.3-28.6)
Fasting plasma glucose (mmol/l)	6.8 (5.4-9.0)	6.5 (6.0-7.0)	9.6 (8.5-11.1)
Fasting C peptide (ng/ml)	1.5 (1.0-1.8)	1.3 (1.0-1.7)	<0.5[a]
HbA_{1c} (%)	7.0 (6.3-7.9)	6.3 (6.1-6.6)	7.7 (7.2-9.2)

Clinical characteristics of subjects with HNF1A-MODY, GCK-MODY, type 1 diabetes mellitus,
[a] = median is below detection limit. Data are given as median (IQR).

Misericordiae University Hospital. All study subjects gave written informed consent to participate in the study.

Clinical and laboratory measurements

All subjects underwent a full clinical assessment, including a full medical history and physical examination. Anthropometric measurements including weight, height, and body mass index (BMI) were obtained. Blood samples were drawn for the measurement of HBA_{1c}, fasting lipids, full blood count, thyroid function, renal and liver profiles, glutamic acid decarboxylase (GAD65) auto antibodies, and pancreatic islet cell auto antibodies (ICA). In addition a blood sample for PSP/reg1A was drawn.

A 75 g OGTT was performed on subjects (excluding subjects with type 1 diabetes mellitus) after a 12-h overnight fast with measurement of glucose, insulin and C-peptide at baseline and at 30 minute intervals for 120 minutes to determine the degree of glucose tolerance and insulin secretory response. In patients with diabetes, oral hypoglycaemic agents were stopped at least 48 h before the OGTT while, in those taking insulin, long-acting insulin therapy was stopped for 24-h and short-acting insulin stopped for 12-h prior to OGTT. The diagnostic criteria for the American Diabetes Association was used to define the degree of glucose tolerance.

Assays

All laboratory analyses were performed with commercially available standardized methods. The plasma glucose concentration was measured using Beckman Synchron DXC800 (Beckman Instruments Inc, Brea, USA). HbA_{1c} was determined using high performance liquid chromatography (Menarini HA81-10, Rome, Italy). Insulin and C-peptide were analyzed using Immulite 2000 immunoassay (Siemens Healthcare Diagnostics, Deerfield, IL, USA). GAD antibodies were analysed using competitive fluid-phase radioimmunoassay by the neurosciences group in John Radcliffe Hospital in Oxford, and ICA by indirect immunofluoresence test by the Supra-Regional Protein Reference Unit and Department of Immunology in Sheffield, UK.

Table 2 Glucose levels during OGTT in HNF1A-MODY subjects

Time (mins)	Glucose (mmol/l)
0	7.6 ± 0.5
30	13.3 ± 0.9
60	17.7 ± 1.5
90	18.3 ± 1.5
120	18.6 ± 1.9

Data are presented as mean and standard error of the mean (SEM).

The ELISA to quantify human PSP/reg was performed using the anti-sera from rabbits and guinea pigs immunized with recombinant human PSP/reg protein as previously described [17,18]. Patient serum PSP/reg levels were compared with standard amounts of protein of recombinant human PSP/reg. The technical specificity of the PSP/reg assay has been determined: addition of 0.5 ng/ml to diluted serum from different individuals gave a recovery of 101 +/− 20% (n = 19). The intra-plate and inter-plate variability is less than 5% and 10% respectively.

Statistical analysis

Data are presented as median and interquartile range (IQR). Areas under the curve (AUCs) for insulin were calculated using the trapezoidal rule. Statistical analysis was performed using MATLAB (Mathworks, Natick, Massachusetts, USA). Differences between groups were determined by two-sided Mann–Whitney/Wilcoxon rank sum test. The Spearman correlation test was used for correlation analysis. Differences and correlations were considered to be significant at $P < 0.05$.

Results

PSP/reg1A serum levels are elevated in HNF1A-MODY subjects and correlate negatively with AUC insulin

We determined the fasting serum PSP/reg1A levels in the HNF1A-MODY group using a previously described ELISA assay [17,18]. The levels of PSP/reg1A were significantly elevated in subjects with HNF1A-MODY compared to historic controls (median = 12.5 ng/ml, IQR = 10.61-17.87 ng/ml versus median = 10.72 ng/ml, IQR = 8.94-12.54 ng/ml, p = 0.0008, Figure 1). These results validate our previous finding that PSP/reg1A, produced in response to beta cell apoptosis, is elevated in HNF1A-MODY [16].

We next sought to ascertain the presence or absence of a correlation between levels of PSP/reg1A and insulin levels determined using a 120 minute OGTT and calculated AUC insulin using trapezoidal rule in subjects with HNF1A-MODY. We found a negative correlation between AUC insulin and PSP/reg1A (rho = −0.40, p = 0.02, Figure 2A).

PSP/reg1A levels do not correlate with HbA_{1c}, triglyceride levels or clinical infectious/inflammatory markers

Potential factors leading to beta cell death in diabetes include high concentrations of glucose [19]. Surprisingly, however, we did not find a correlation between PSP/reg1A and HbA_{1c} (rho = −0.09, p = 0.62, Figure 2B). There was, likewise no correlation noted with total cholesterol (rho = 0.11, p = 0.58), HDL cholesterol (rho = 0.12, p = 0.54), LDL cholesterol (rho = 0.05, p = 0.78) or triglycerides (rho = −0.21, p = 0.25). It has also been postulated that PSP may be increased during infection/inflammation [20]. However, we did not detect any correlation with common markers of inflammation such as total white cell count (rho = 0.30, p = 0.09) or neutrophil count (rho = 0.30, p = 0.09).

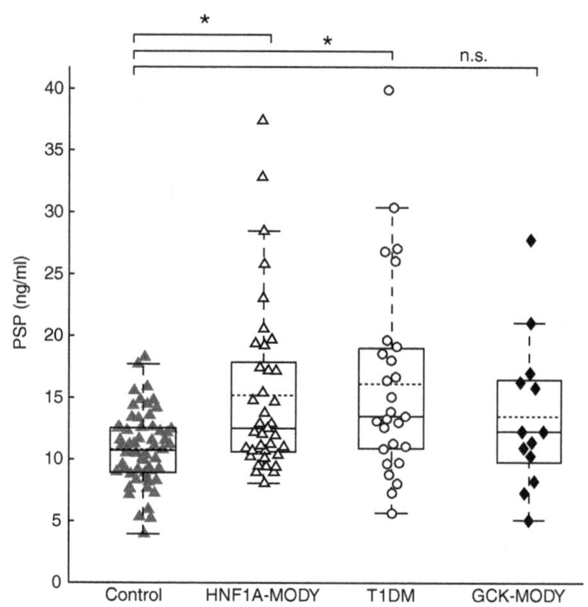

Figure 1 Serum levels of PSP/reg1A in HNF1A-MODY(Δ), T1DM (○) and GCK-MODY (♦) versus non-diabetic controls (▲). Solid lines/box plot showing median and interquartile range (IQR) and dotted line showing mean. Serum levels of PSP/reg1A in HNF1A-MODY are at a median of 12.50 ng/ml showing an IQR of 10.61 to 17.87 ng/ml in n = 37 patients. The median in n = 27 type 1 diabetes mellitus (T1DM) patients is 13.52 ng/ml with IQR of 10.91 to 19.01 ng/ml and the median in n = 60 control subjects is 10.72 ng/ml and IQR is 8.94-12.54 ng/ml. A Mann–Whitney *U*-test of the groups resulted in (*) p = 0.0008 for differences between HNF1A-MODY and controls and (*) p = 0.0007 for comparison of T1DM versus controls. The median of GCK-MODY is 12.27 ng/ml with an IQR of 9.79 to 16.47 ng/ml in n = 13 patients, which resulted in (n.s.) p = 0.164 when compared to controls.

PSP/reg1A serum level increase with age in HNF1A-MODY subjects

As beta cell dysfunction progresses in HNF1A-MODY patients [21], we next explored whether there was a correlation between PSP/reg1A serum levels and age. We found a positive correlation between age and PSP/reg1A (r = 0.40, p = 0.02). Further analysis of the data demonstrated that those diagnosed with HNF1A-MODY under 25 years of age had significantly lower levels of PSP/reg1A than those diagnosed at the age of 25 years or over (median = 10.85 ng/ml, IQR = 9.41-12.12 ng/ml versus median = 15.40 ng/ml, IQR = 11.05-19.91 ng/ml, p = 0.0039, Figure 3).

PSP/reg1A serum levels are elevated in autoantibody-type 1 diabetes mellitus, but independent of age and disease onset

We next wished to confirm these data in a second group of patients with the principal pathogenic factor being beta cell destruction. A cohort of auto-antibody positive, BMI-matched type 1 diabetes mellitus patients were compared with the (n = 60) historic controls. We found that PSP/reg1A levels were significantly higher in the type 1 diabetes mellitus population (median = 13.52 ng/ml, IQR = 10.91-19.01 ng/ml versus median = 10.72 ng/ml, IQR = 8.94-12.54 ng/ml, p = 0.0007, Figure 1). Interestingly, we did not detect any correlation between age (rho = 0.27, p = 0.18) or disease onset (rho = 0.33, p = 0.09) and PSP/reg1A serum levels in this cohort of patients, suggesting that beta cell apoptosis occurs during disease independent of these factors. As with the subjects with HNF1A-MODY there was no correlation between PSP/reg1A levels and HbA_{1c} (rho = −0.08, p = 0.68). There was likewise, no correlation with total cholesterol (rho = −0.08, p = 0.75), HDL cholesterol (rho = 0.24, p = 0.32), LDL cholesterol (rho = −0.31, p = 0.19), triglycerides (rho = −0.07, p = 0.77), or white cell count (rho = −0.22, p = 0.39).

PSP/reg1A serum levels are not significantly elevated in GCK-MODY

We next tested whether patients with GCK-MODY also showed a pronounced increase in PSP/reg1A levels. Although there was a tendency towards elevated PSP/reg1A levels, we did not find a statistically significant

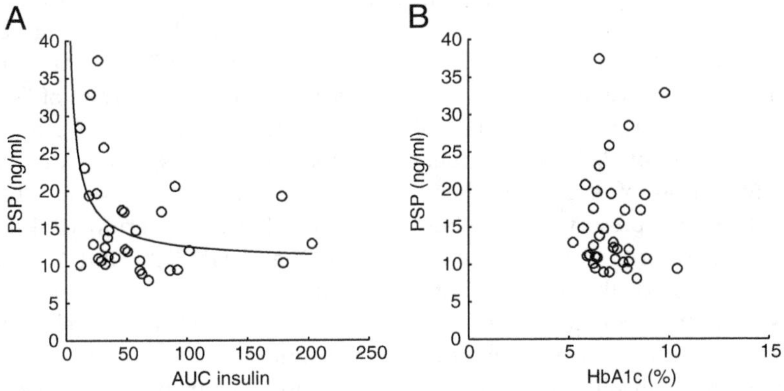

Figure 2 Correlations of PSP/reg1A in HNF1A-MODY. (**A**) PSP/reg1A correlation with AUC of insulin (Spearman r = −0.40, p = 0.02, n = 34). The regression curve highlights the negative correlation ($R^2 = 0.17$). (**B**) No correlation was found between PSP/reg1A and HbA_{1c} (Spearman r = −0.09, p = 0.62, n = 37).

elevation of PSP/reg1A level when compared to historic controls (median = 12.27 ng/ml, IQR = 9.79-16.47 ng/ml versus median = 10.72 ng/ml, IQR = 8.94-12.54 ng/ml, p = 0.16, Figure 1). There was also no correlation noted with AUC insulin (r = 0.21, p = 0.55) or HbA_{1c} (r = 0.52, p = 0.07). There was no statistically significant difference between serum PSP/reg1A levels of GCK-MODY and HNF1A-MODY or type 1 diabetes mellitus patients (p = 0.55/p = 0.34 respectively).

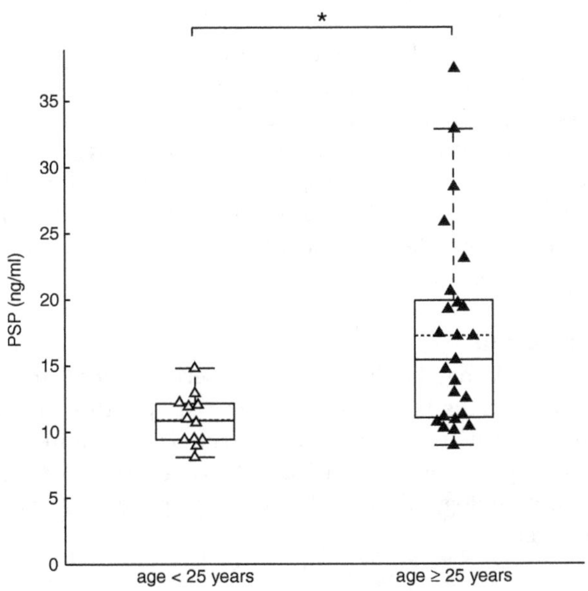

Figure 3 Serum levels of PSP/reg1A at age < 25 years (Δ) versus older (▲) in HNF1A-MODY subjects. Solid lines/box plot showing median and interquartile range and dotted line showing mean. The medians of PSP/reg1A are demonstrated between young HNF1A-MODY (median = 10.85 ng/ml, IQR = 9.41-12.12 ng/ml, n = 12) and older subjects (median = 15.40 ng/ml, IQR = 11.05-19.91 ng/ml, n = 25), Mann–Whitney *U*-test (*) p = 0.004.

Discussion

The Irish HNF1A-MODY cohort investigated in this study has been recently characterized [22]. This study reported on a mutation identification rate of 30.5% among Irish adults clinically selected for HNF1A-MODY from attendees at the diabetes clinic. In the present study, we report that PSP/reg1A levels are significantly elevated in human subjects with HNF1A-MODY when compared to controls. Higher levels of circulating PSP/reg1A in HNF1A-MODY were associated with increased age suggesting that the rate of beta cell apoptosis increases during disease progression and within the third life decade. PSP/reg1A did not correlate with HbA_{1c} nor did it correlate with the common clinical infectious/inflammatory markers. Patients with type 1 diabetes mellitus also showed elevated PSP/reg1A levels independent of age or disease onset. Together these data suggest that PSP/reg1A may be a clinical indicator of beta cell apoptosis.

We have previously provided biological evidence in insulinoma cell lines and transgenic mice models of HNF1A-MODY, that beta cells undergoing apoptosis induce the expression of the PSP/reg gene in neighbouring beta cells [16]. The induction of PSP/reg during apoptosis was inhibited in cells treated with caspase inhibitors. Paraffin embedded pancreatic sections from 5 month old diabetic mice expressing HNF1A-MODY in beta cells also demonstrated elevated expression of PSP/reg throughout the islets compared with wild-type mice, with PSP/reg positive cells positioned in the vicinity of cells displaying apoptotic nuclear morphology. These earlier findings demonstrated that PSP/reg1A gene expression was induced during apoptosis in in vitro and animal models of diabetes. One of the core findings of the present study is that PSP/reg1A serum levels may be used as a non-invasive marker to evaluate the extent of beta cell apoptosis during disease progression in human subjects.

The development and implementation of non-invasive techniques for the quantitative measurement of beta cell apoptosis would help in the early diagnosis of beta cell dysfunction in pre-clinical phases of diabetes. Furthermore, it would enable evaluation of emerging therapeutic approaches which focus on preservation of beta cell mass through stimulation of anti-apoptotic signalling. Currently, only indirect methods that evaluate total beta cell mass through secretory responses of islet cells are available, such as arginine-induced insulin secretion [23,24]. These rely on measuring insulin secretion following different metabolic stimuli. Direct visualization of either native or transplanted pancreatic islets was unsuccessful due to their small size, the little difference in physical characteristics from the surrounding tissue, and their relatively low number dispersed over a large area of the pancreas or the liver as the most common site of transplantation [25]. However, modern diagnostic equipment may provide very high sensitivity by positron emission tomography (PET) and single photon emission computed tomography (SPECT), spatial resolution by magnetic resonance imaging (MRI), or both (by PET/CT) [26]. Despite these advances in imaging devices, the main problem is the lack of a specific structural or molecular marker to enable differentiation between scattered islets or single beta cells, and surrounding tissue. Moreover, these techniques require dedicated imaging centres and are costly.

A previously reported paper hypothesized as to whether serum reg protein levels could be representative of the regenerative process at the beta cell level during the early phases of type 1 diabetes mellitus in humans [27]. We have found that PSP/reg1A levels are higher in type 1 diabetes mellitus but independent of disease onset or age. This finding should be considered in the context of recent investigations suggesting that beta cell regeneration may occur even in patients with long standing type 1 diabetes mellitus [28-31]. Our study indicates that this regeneration may be accompanied by continuing beta cell apoptosis, even in patients with long standing type 1 diabetes mellitus. Therefore, therapeutic interventions that boost beta cell survival could be a valuable therapeutic approach even in long standing type 1 diabetes mellitus.

In contrast to type 1 diabetes mellitus patients who have a rapid disease onset, HNF1A-MODY carriers represent an interesting and important study group for the study of beta cell apoptosis during disease progression as carriers will ultimately develop diabetes [1]. As demonstrated in HNF1A-MODY subjects' beta cell apoptosis appeared to correlate with age, but not with HbA_{1c} suggesting that aging is an important risk factor, and that young islets have an increased resistance towards mutant HNF1A-induced apoptosis. Although patients with a GCK-MODY mutation did not have significantly elevated levels of serum PSP/reg1A when compared to controls, we cannot draw any conclusions in relation to this group due to the limited numbers available. There was also no statistically significant difference between serum PSP/reg1A levels of GCK-MODY and HNF1A-MODY or type 1 diabetes mellitus patients.

The pancreatic acinar cells are considered to be the most important source of PSP/reg under normal conditions however in pathological conditions other cells/tissues may contribute to elevated levels of the protein. PSP has been shown to be elevated in liver/pancreatic disease and in chronic renal failure [32]. When originally discovered, PSP/reg was proposed to be a marker of pancreatic injury in pancreatitis [33,34] however; subsequent studies have failed to demonstrate elevated levels even after severe pancreatitis [35]. In this study the subjects had normal liver and renal function. Furthermore, PSP/reg1A levels did not correlate with infection/inflammation markers such as white cell count.

As a result of the growing interest in beta cell preservation as a potential cure for diabetes, a number of different treatments aimed at protecting the beta cell and maintaining beta cell mass have been evaluated. Insulinotropic agents such as repaglinide or GLP-1 have been shown to be cytoprotective *in-vitro* and in animal models of diabetes [36,37]. From a clinical aspect, beta cell protection may also be induced by reducing the peripheral insulin demand by either improving sensitivity e.g. through physical exercise, pharmacologically using metformin/glitazones, or by lowering blood glucose through the administration of exogenous insulin [38-40]. Our study suggests that PSP/reg1A serum levels may be useful as a biomarker for such potentially cytoprotective treatment paradigms.

Conclusion

PSP/reg1A may be developed as a serum marker to detect alterations in the rate of beta cell apoptosis during disease or in response to treatment. Furthermore, our data suggests that beta cell apoptosis contributes to the pathophysiology of HNF1A-MODY in patients 25 years and over.

Abbreviations

AUC: Area under the curve; GCK: Glucokinase; GAD65: Glutamic acid decarboxylase; HNF: Hepatocyte nuclear factor; ICA: Islet cell antibodies; OGTT: Oral glucose tolerance test; PSP: Pancreatic stone protein; TG: Triglycerides.

Competing interests

The authors declare that they have no competing interests.

Authors' contributions

SB coordinated and contributed to the recruitment of subjects, carried out functional studies, interpreted results and wrote manuscript, PMK contributed to the recruitment of subjects and carried out functional studies, JS performed statistical analysis of data, SRR contributed to the recruitment of subjects and carried out functional studies. RG carried out the PSP/reg assay. CB contributed to the writing of the manuscript and performed initial basic studies, JHM contributed to the interpretation of the results, the writing and the critical review of the manuscript. MMB coordinated and designed the study, contributed to the interpretation of the results, the writing and the critical review of the manuscript. All authors read and approved the final manuscript.

Acknowledgements

The authors would like to acknowledge the patients and their referring clinicians. This work was supported by grants from the Health Research Board (HRB RP2004/220), the Mater Foundation (MRCG/HRB Co-funded Grant Scheme 06-01) and the Mater College Grant 2008 to Dr M. M. Byrne. We thank the research nurses Eilish Donnelly, Hazel Little and Mary Joyce for helping with the data collection, and Mark Kilbane and Jennifer Brady in the Endocrine Laboratory at the Mater Misericordiae University Hospital Dublin for analyzing blood samples. IntegraGen GmbH (Bonn, Germany 2006–2007) and Prof Sian Ellard and Dr Kevin Colclough (Department of Molecular Genetics, Exeter, Devon, UK 2008–2010) for genetic testing.

Author details

[1]Department of Diabetes, Mater Misericordiae University Hospital, Dublin 7, Ireland. [2]Department of Physiology and Medical Physics, Centre for Systems Medicine, Royal College of Surgeons in Ireland, Dublin 2, Ireland. [3]Department of Visceral and Transplantation Surgery, University Hospital Zurich, Zurich, Switzerland. [4]Department of Endocrinology, Mater Misericordiae University Hospital, 30 Eccles Street, Dublin 7, Ireland.

References

1. Fajans SS, Bell GI, Polonsky KS: **Molecular mechanisms and clinical pathophysiology of maturity-onset diabetes of the young.** *N Engl J Med* 2001, **345**:971–980.
2. Fajans SS, Bell GI: **MODY: history, genetics, pathophysiology, and clinical decision making.** *Diabetes Care* 2011, **34**:1878–1884.
3. Ellard S, Bellanne-Chantelot C, Hattersley AT: **Best practice guidelines for the molecular genetic diagnosis of maturity-onset diabetes of the young.** *Diabetologia* 2008, **51**:546–553.
4. Byrne MM, Sturis J, Menzel S, Yamagata K, Fajans SS, Dronsfield MJ, Bain SC, Hattersley AT, Velho G, Froguel P, *et al*: **Altered insulin secretory responses to glucose in diabetic and nondiabetic subjects with mutations in the diabetes susceptibility gene MODY3 on chromosome 12.** *Diabetes* 1996, **45**:1503–1510.
5. Byrne MM, Sturis J, Clement K, Vionnet N, Pueyo ME, Stoffel M, Takeda J, Passa P, Cohen D, Bell GI, *et al*: **Insulin secretory abnormalities in subjects with hyperglycemia due to glucokinase mutations.** *J Clin Invest* 1994, **93**:1120–1130.
6. Pontoglio M, Sreenan S, Roe M, Pugh W, Ostrega D, Doyen A, Pick AJ, Baldwin A, Velho G, Froguel P, *et al*: **Defective insulin secretion in hepatocyte nuclear factor 1alpha-deficient mice.** *J Clin Invest* 1998, **101**:2215–2222.
7. Wobser H, Dussmann H, Kogel D, Wang H, Reimertz C, Wollheim CB, Byrne MM, Prehn JH: **Dominant-negative suppression of HNF-1 alpha results in mitochondrial dysfunction, INS-1 cell apoptosis, and increased sensitivity to ceramide-, but not to high glucose-induced cell death.** *J Biol Chem* 2002, **277**:6413–6421.
8. Wobser H, Bonner C, Nolan JJ, Byrne MM, Prehn JH: **Downregulation of protein kinase B/Akt-1 mediates INS-1 insulinoma cell apoptosis induced by dominant-negative suppression of hepatocyte nuclear factor-1alpha function.** *Diabetologia* 2006, **49**:519–526.
9. Yamagata K, Nammo T, Moriwaki M, Ihara A, Iizuka K, Yang Q, Satoh T, Li M, Uenaka R, Okita K, *et al*: **Overexpression of dominant-negative mutant hepatocyte nuclear fctor-1 alpha in pancreatic beta-cells causes abnormal islet architecture with decreased expression of E-cadherin, reduced beta-cell proliferation, and diabetes.** *Diabetes* 2002, **51**:114–123.
10. Froguel P, Vaxillaire M, Sun F, Velho G, Zouali H, Butel MO, Lesage S, Vionnet N, Clement K, Fougerousse F, *et al*: **Close linkage of glucokinase locus on chromosome 7p to early-onset non-insulin-dependent diabetes mellitus.** *Nature* 1992, **356**:162–164.
11. Stoffel M, Patel P, Lo YM, Hattersley AT, Lucassen AM, Page R, Bell JI, Bell GI, Turner RC, Wainscoat JS: **Missense glucokinase mutation in maturity-onset diabetes of the young and mutation screening in late-onset diabetes.** *Nat Genet* 1992, **2**:153–156.
12. Cuesta-Munoz AL, Tuomi T, Cobo-Vuilleumier N, Koskela H, Odili S, Stride A, Buettger C, Otonkoski T, Froguel P, Grimsby J, *et al*: **Clinical heterogeneity in monogenic diabetes caused by mutations in the glucokinase gene (GCK-MODY).** *Diabetes Care* 2010, **33**:290–292.
13. Butler AE, Janson J, Bonner-Weir S, Ritzel R, Rizza RA, Butler PC: **Beta-cell deficit and increased beta-cell apoptosis in humans with type 2 diabetes.** *Diabetes* 2003, **52**:102–110.
14. Rehm M, Dussmann H, Janicke RU, Tavare JM, Kogel D, Prehn JH: **Single-cell fluorescence resonance energy transfer analysis demonstrates that caspase activation during apoptosis is a rapid process. Role of caspase-3.** *J Biol Chem* 2002, **277**:24506–24514.
15. Fuchs Y, Steller H: **Programmed cell death in animal development and disease.** *Cell* 2011, **147**:742–758.
16. Bonner C, Bacon S, Concannon CG, Rizvi SR, Baquie M, Farrelly AM, Kilbride SM, Dussmann H, Ward MW, Boulanger CM, *et al*: **INS-1 cells undergoing caspase-dependent apoptosis enhance the regenerative capacity of neighboring cells.** *Diabetes* 2010, **59**:2799–2808.
17. Graf R, Schiesser M, Lussi A, Went P, Scheele GA, Bimmler D: **Coordinate regulation of secretory stress proteins (PSP/reg, PAP I, PAP II, and PAP III) in the rat exocrine pancreas during experimental acute pancreatitis.** *J Surg Res* 2002, **105**:136–144.
18. Bimmler D, Angst E, Valeri F, Bain M, Scheele GA, Frick TW, Graf R: **Regulation of PSP/reg in rat pancreas: immediate and steady-state adaptation to different diets.** *Pancreas* 1999, **19**:255–267.
19. Robertson RP, Harmon J, Tran PO, Poitout V: **Beta-cell glucose toxicity, lipotoxicity, and chronic oxidative stress in type 2 diabetes.** *Diabetes* 2004, **53**(Suppl 1):S119–S124.
20. Keel M, Harter L, Reding T, Sun LK, Hersberger M, Seifert B, Bimmler D, Graf R: **Pancreatic stone protein is highly increased during posttraumatic sepsis and activates neutrophil granulocytes.** *Crit Care Med* 2009, **37**:1642–1648.
21. Shepherd M, Shields B, Ellard S, Rubio-Cabezas O, Hattersley AT: **A genetic diagnosis of HNF1A diabetes alters treatment and improves glycaemic control in the majority of insulin-treated patients.** *Diabet Med* 2009, **26**:437–441.
22. Kyithar MP, Bacon S, Pannu KK, Rizvi SR, Colclough K, Ellard S, Byrne MM: **Identification of HNF1A-MODY and HNF4A-MODY in Irish families: phenotypic characteristics and therapeutic implications.** *Diabetes Metab* 2011, **37**:512–519.
23. Teuscher AU, Kendall DM, Smets YF, Leone JP, Sutherland DE, Robertson RP: **Successful islet autotransplantation in humans: functional insulin secretory reserve as an estimate of surviving islet cell mass.** *Diabetes* 1998, **47**:324–330.
24. Ryan EA, Lakey JR, Paty BW, Imes S, Korbutt GS, Kneteman NM, Bigam D, Rajotte RV, Shapiro AM: **Successful islet transplantation: continued insulin reserve provides long-term glycemic control.** *Diabetes* 2002, **51**:2148–2157.
25. Evgenov NV, Medarova Z, Dai G, Bonner-Weir S, Moore A: **In vivo imaging of islet transplantation.** *Nat Med* 2006, **12**:144–148.
26. Malaisse WJ: **On the track to the beta-cell.** *Diabetologia* 2001, **44**:393–406.
27. Christofilis MA, Carrere J, Atlan-Gepner C, Zevaco-Mattei C, Thivolet C, Baeza N, Figarella C, Vialettes B: **Serum reg protein level is not related to the beta cell destruction/regeneration process during early phases of diabetogenesis in type I diabetes.** *Eur J Endocrinol* 1999, **141**:368–373.
28. Meier JJ, Bhushan A, Butler AE, Rizza RA, Butler PC: **Sustained beta cell apoptosis in patients with long-standing type 1 diabetes: indirect evidence for islet regeneration?** *Diabetologia* 2005, **48**:2221–2228.
29. Keenan HA, Sun JK, Levine J, Doria A, Aiello LP, Eisenbarth G, Bonner-Weir S, King GL: **Residual insulin production and pancreatic ss-cell turnover after 50 years of diabetes: Joslin Medalist Study.** *Diabetes* 2010, **59**:2846–2853.
30. Lohr M, Kloppel G: **Residual insulin positivity and pancreatic atrophy in relation to duration of chronic type 1 (insulin-dependent) diabetes mellitus and microangiopathy.** *Diabetologia* 1987, **30**:757–762.

31. Madsbad S, Kehlet H, Hilsted J, Tronier B: **Discrepancy between plasma C-peptide and insulin response to oral and intravenous glucose.** *Diabetes* 1983, **32**:436–438.
32. Tatemichi N, Takahashi C, Hayakawa S, Hayakawa T, Shibata T, Kitagawa M, Sobajima H, Nakae Y: **Enzyme immunoassay and characterization of pancreatic stone proteins in human urine.** *J Clin Lab Anal* 1993, **7**:365–370.
33. Hayakawa T, Naruse S, Kitagawa M, Nakae Y, Harada H, Ochi K, Kuno N, Kurimoto K, Hayakawa S: **Pancreatic stone protein and lactoferrin in human pancreatic juice in chronic pancreatitis.** *Pancreas* 1995, **10**:137–142.
34. Schmiegel W, Burchert M, Kalthoff H, Roeder C, Butzow G, Grimm H, Kremer B, Soehendra N, Schreiber HW, Thiele HG, *et al*: **Immunochemical characterization and quantitative distribution of pancreatic stone protein in sera and pancreatic secretions in pancreatic disorders.** *Gastroenterology* 1990, **99**:1421–1430.
35. Jin CX, Hayakawa T, Ko SB, Ishiguro H, Kitagawa M: **Pancreatic stone protein/regenerating protein family in pancreatic and gastrointestinal diseases.** *Intern Med* 2011, **50**:1507–1516.
36. Farilla L, Bulotta A, Hirshberg B, Li Calzi S, Khoury N, Noushmehr H, Bertolotto C, Di Mario U, Harlan DM, Perfetti R: **Glucagon-like peptide 1 inhibits cell apoptosis and improves glucose responsiveness of freshly isolated human islets.** *Endocrinology* 2003, **144**:5149–5158.
37. Chen D, Liao J, Li N, Zhou C, Liu Q, Wang G, Zhang R, Zhang S, Lin L, Chen K, *et al*: **A nonpeptidic agonist of glucagon-like peptide 1 receptors with efficacy in diabetic db/db mice.** *Proc Natl Acad Sci U S A* 2007, **104**:943–948.
38. DeFronzo RA, Tripathy D, Schwenke DC, Banerji M, Bray GA, Buchanan TA, Clement SC, Henry RR, Hodis HN, Kitabchi AE, *et al*: **Pioglitazone for diabetes prevention in impaired glucose tolerance.** *N Engl J Med* 2011, **364**:1104–1115.
39. Weng J, Li Y, Xu W, Shi L, Zhang Q, Zhu D, Hu Y, Zhou Z, Yan X, Tian H, *et al*: **Effect of intensive insulin therapy on beta-cell function and glycaemic control in patients with newly diagnosed type 2 diabetes: a multicentre randomised parallel-group trial.** *Lancet* 2008, **371**:1753–1760.
40. Kahn SE, Haffner SM, Heise MA, Herman WH, Holman RR, Jones NP, Kravitz BG, Lachin JM, O'Neill MC, Zinman B, Viberti G: **Glycemic durability of rosiglitazone, metformin, or glyburide monotherapy.** *N Engl J Med* 2006, **355**:2427–2443.

Central precocious puberty in a 3 year-old girl with Phenylketonuria: a rare association?

Laura Lucaccioni[1,3], Bernd C Schwahn[2], Malcolm Donaldson[3] and Claudio Giacomozzi[3,4*]

Abstract

Background: Central precocious puberty (CPP) and phenylketonuria (PKU) are two rare conditions, the latter being the rarer. To date, only one case featuring both these conditions has been reported, and hyperphenylalaninemia was assumed triggering CPP.

Case presentation: We present a 3.2 years old girl referred with a 12 months history of breast and pubic hair development, and vaginal discharge. Hyperphenylalaninemia had been identified by newborn screening and PKU subsequently confirmed by plasma amino acid and genetic analysis. Early dietary control of plasma phenylalanine had been excellent afterwards, resulting in phenylalanine concentrations consistently within the recommended range. Clinical scenario, hormonal assessment and imaging were in keeping with true idiopathic central precocious puberty. Treatment with long lasting gonadotropin-releasing hormone analogue led to regression of secondary sexual characteristics.

Conclusion: We describe for the first time CPP in a girl affected with PKU but with persistently well controlled blood phenylalanine concentrations. This finding is in contrast to a previous report which suggested persistently high phenylalaninemia levels as potential trigger for CPP in PKU patients. Our report, together with the lack of evidence in published cohort studies of children with PKU, strongly suggests this rare association is coincidental and independent of the presence of severe hyperphenylalaninemia.

Keywords: Precocious puberty, Phenylketonuria, Hyperphenylalaninaemia, Gonadotropin-realising hormone agonist treatment

Background

True Central Precocious puberty (TCPP), also called GnRH-dependent precocious puberty, can be defined as true puberty, mediated by the hypothalamus, with the onset of secondary sexual characteristics before the age of eight in girls and nine in boys [1-4]. The estimated incidence of TCPP is 1:5.000-10.000 throughout the world [2] with a female:male ratio of between 3:1 and 23:1 [3]. It is less common than, and should be differentiated from, other forms of sexual precocity such as premature thelarche and exaggerated adrenarche. Early activation of the hypothalamic-pituitary-gonadal axis (HPGA) in TCPP is mostly idiopathic, especially in girls [1-4]. However TCPP may be secondarily related to brain tumors (hamartoma especially), brain infections, congenital brain defects, cranial irradiation, insults and injuries to the brain or spinal cord (including cerebral palsy, hydrocephalus and brain ischemia) [4]. Moreover TCPP has been widely described in association with learning disability syndromes, including Angelman, Kabuki make-up syndrome and other genetic conditions in which mental retardation is a key clinical feature [5-8]. Phenylketonuria (PKU) is an autosomal recessive disease caused by a deficient activity of Phenylalanine Hydroxylase (PAH), the enzyme which metabolizes Phenylalanine (Phe) to Tyrosine (Tyr). Deficiency of PAH results in tyrosine deficiency, hyperphenylalaninemia (HP) and accumulation of Phe in other body fluids [9]. If left untreated or not appropriately controlled, patients may develop mental retardation, microcephaly and epilepsy due to the high sensitivity of the immature brain to pathological Phe concentrations. Insufficiently treated patients can also have behavioural problems and some

* Correspondence: dr.giacomozzi@gmail.com
[3]Paediatric Endocrinology Unit, Royal Hospital for Sick Children, Dalnair St, Yorkhill, G3 8SJ Glasgow, UK
[4]Dipartimento di Medicina Pediatrica, Bambino Gesù Children's Hospital, Piazza S. Onofiro 4, 00165 Rome, Italy
Full list of author information is available at the end of the article

may suffer from psychiatric illnesses [10]. To our knowledge only one girl affected by HP has been described in the medical literature with associated TCPP [11]. In their paper the authors highlight the poor control of serum Phe level due to their patient's inadequate adherence to the low Phe diet and hypothesized that chronically elevated Phe concentrations were the trigger of TCPP. Since then, no other data supporting or rejecting this conjecture have been reported. We present the case of a three-year-old girl affected by severe PAH deficiency who was diagnosed with TCPP, and have compared her to the single case previously reported, pointing out differences and similarities.

Case presentation

A girl was referred to our endocrinology outpatient clinic at 3.2 years with a one year history of increasing breast enlargement followed by the development of pubic hair, body odour and brown vaginal discharge. She had been born at 38 weeks gestation by caesarean section due to maternal pre-eclampsia, birth weight 2.7 kg (−0.72 SD). Her family history was negative for developmental anomalies. Newborn screening revealed HP with a Phe level of 435 μmol/L on day 5 and she was started on dietary treatment from day 9 of life once severe isolated hyperphenylalaninaemia had been confirmed with plasma amino acid analysis (975 μmol/L). Bi-directional sequence analysis of the PAH gene identified two heterozygote mutations: p.Phe39Leu which is associated with a variably severe phenotype, as well as a second well-characterised null mutation, p.Pro281Leu. Her phenylalanine tolerance remained around 200 mg per day throughout the first 2.5 years of life. She showed normal neurodevelopment but for transitory mild speech delay. From infancy to the time of referral the girl underwent weekly Phe measurements with median (range) values of 194 μmol/L (63–527) and thus almost exclusively within the target range of 120-360 micromol/l for children from 0 to 5 years of age in the UK (Figure 1).

On examination in the endocrine clinic the girl was tall in comparison to her parents' height, 0.8 SDS according to normal reference [12], while her mid parental height (MPH) was −1.2 SDS, with a height corrected for MPH of 2.0 SDS. Pubertal staging according to Tanner's method [13] was assessed at B4, P2, A1.

Results

Bone age was advanced by over one year at 4.62 years using the TW2 (RUS) method [14] leading to a predicted final height below the cut-off of −2.5 SDS. An LHRH stimulation test was arranged and showed a pattern which was diagnostic for TCPP (Table 1). Pelvic ultrasound scan showed a bulky uterus of 4.75 cm length with a fundo-cervical-ratio of 1.17 and endometrial thickness of 5.7 mm. Ovaries were 1.70 and 0.78 ml in volume, both within the normal volume range for age although large follicles were evident. Brain and pituitary MRI showed a normal pituitary gland with a mild convexity presentation compatible with the HPGA activation, but no other organic causes for TCPP were detected. Treatment with the GnRH agonist (Triptorelin) was started at the dosage of 11.25 mg every twelve weeks. After nine months, because of persistent breast enlargement and increased height velocity, the interval between injections was reduced to ten weeks. Subsequently the girl showed regression of breast development and a decrease in height velocity. Now aged 4.6 years the patient remains on treatment, showing reduced height velocity and regression of secondary sexual characteristics (Table 1). Throughout treatment her dietary management had been adjusted. Phenylalanine tolerance remains elevated at around 350 mg per day on GnRH agonist treatment and Phe concentrations have been maintained within the target range with median (range) values of 194 μmol/L (63–527).

Conclusions

Phenylketonuria was first described by Asbjørn Følling in 1934 as one of the most common inherited metabolic

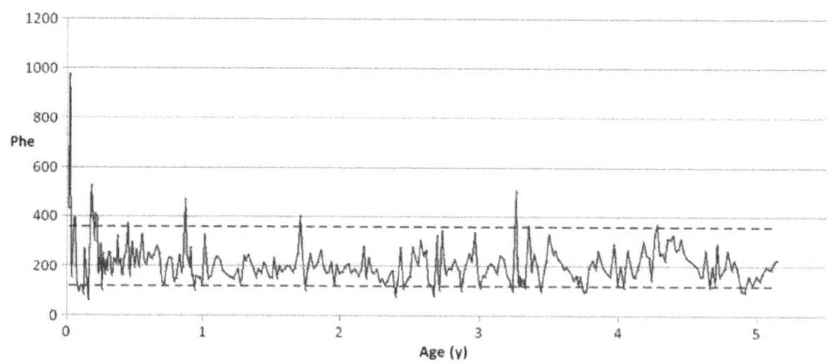

Figure 1 Patient serum Phe concentration from birth. The area within dotted line represents the treatment target range. Phe concentration is in μmol/l.

Table 1 Clinical and biochemical features in a girl with phenylketonuria presenting with sexual precocity aged 3 years

Age	3.2 yr	3.9 yr	4.2 yr	4.6 yr
Height, cm	98.8 (0.8)	107.5 (1.5)	109.7 (1.4)	111 (1.2)
Weight, Kg	16.1 (0.8)	18.54 (1.1)	18.76 (0.9)	19.44 (0.8)
BMI, Kg/m^2	16.43 (0.4)	16.0 (0.2)	15.6 (0.0)	15.7 (0.1)
MPH, cm	156.0 (−1.2)			
Ht corrected for MPH, SDS	2.0	2.7	2.6	2.4
Bone age, yr	4.62	-	5.37	-
Ht velocity, cm/y	14.3 (5.3)	10.6 (2.9)	7.1 (0.1)	4.3 (−2.2)
Pubertal status	B_4,P_2,A_1	B_2,P_2,A_1	B_{1-2},P_1, A_1	B_{1-2},P_1, A_1
Basal/Peak LH, U/l	1.9/33.1			
Basal/Peak FSH, U/l	2.4/6.5			
Triptorelin dose	11.25 mg/12 weeks	11.25 mg/10 weeks	11.25 mg/10 weeks	11.25 mg/10 weeks

SDS is presented in brackets. Height velocity assessed according to Tanner et al. [13].

disorders. The overall incidence of PKU in Europe and North America is 1:10.000-15.000 live births [15]. It occurs, however, more frequently in certain areas such as Turkey (1:3.500-1:5.000), Ireland (1:4.500) or the West of Scotland (1:7.500) [16]. Patients can be classified on the basis of residual enzyme activity as judged by peak blood Phe levels or, better, long-term phenylalanine tolerance. Phe-restricted diets with amino acid and micronutrient supplementation are highly effective in preventing irreversible brain damage and allow for a normal physical and cognitive development [10]. The recommendations for acceptable safe blood Phe concentrations are to some extent age specific [17]. Our patient has a severe enzyme deficiency with a low phenylalanine tolerance, increasing the risk for neurocognitive anomalies. Her parents achieved an excellent dietary control of Phe concentrations with subsequent normal neurodevelopment. To our knowledge, there is only one previous case reported in the literature [11] describing TCPP in a Turkish girl aged 7.5 years with severe PAH deficiency. While most countries represented in the medical literature have universal neonatal screening programs in place to avoid symptomatic PKU, classical PKU was diagnosed late in this patient at 2.5 years of age, indicating that she had been exposed to elevated Phe concentrations from birth. Moreover, satisfactory Phe concentrations could not be achieved in the girl because of poor adherence to dietary recommendations. The authors assumed that persistent poor dietary control could have prompted TCPP due to a premature activation of the HPGA by a toxic effect on the brain. Concerning this latter conjecture, there are currently insufficient data in the literature as to the incidence of TCPP in untreated or insufficiently treated individuals with PAH deficiency. However, expert opinion corroborated by a poll of the metabolic listserv "metab-l" suggests that this is an extremely rare occurrence. Our patient is the first case where idiopathic TCPP occurred under conditions of perfect dietary control. Since encountering TCPP in our patient we have performed a literature search to identify studies that describe the growth pattern of patients with PKU, but none of them focused on the timing of pubertal onset. Recent studies of larger cohorts of individuals on PKU diets have identified an increased prevalence of obesity and overweight towards adolescence in female subjects, with no specific records about precocious or early pubertal progression [17,18]. Lack of evidence for different timing of pubertal onset in PKU patients compared with the general population corroborates our observation, and strongly supports the notion of a co-incidental association between PKU and TCPP. We can not entirely exclude, however, that significant anomalies in the onset and tempo of puberty in PKU patients might have been overlooked by previous population studies.

We conclude that TCPP is a rare coincidental event in children with PKU and can occur independently by the persistently high phenylalanine concentrations.

Abbreviations

CPP: Central precocious puberty; PKU: Phenylketonuria; TCPP: True central precocious puberty; HPGA: Hypothalamic-pituitary-gonadal axis; PAH: Phenylalanine hydroxylase; Phe: Phenylalanine; Tyr: Tyrosine; HP: hyperphenylalaninemia; LH: Luteinizing hormone; FSH: Follicle stimulating hormone; Cr: Creatinine.

Competing interests

The authors declare they have no competing interests.

Authors' contributions

LL reviewed the case note and performed the first draft of the manuscript. CG and MD followed the patient from and Endocrine Point of view, while BS from a metabolic point of view. CG supervised the draft of the manuscript and reviewed it with MD and BS. All authors read and approve the final manuscript.

Acknowledgements
The authors would like to thank the patient's family.

Author details
[1]Paediatric Unit, Department of Medical and Surgical Sciences for the Children and Adults, University of Modena & Reggio Emilia, via del Pozzo n. 71, 41125 Modena, Italy. [2]Metabolic Unit, Royal Hospital for Sick Children, Dalnair St, Yorkhill, G3 8SJ Glasgow, UK. [3]Paediatric Endocrinology Unit, Royal Hospital for Sick Children, Dalnair St, Yorkhill, G3 8SJ Glasgow, UK. [4]Dipartimento di Medicina Pediatrica, Bambino Gesù Children's Hospital, Piazza S. Onofiro 4, 00165 Rome, Italy.

References

1. Grumbach MM, Styne DM: **Puberty: Ontogeny, neuroendocrinology, physiology, and disorders.** In *Williams Textbook of Endocrinology.* 9th edition. Edited by Wilson JD, Foster DW, Kronenberg HM, Larsen PR. Philadelphia: W.B. Saunders; 1998:1509–1625.
2. González ER: **For puberty that comes too soon, new treatment highly effective.** *JAMA* 1982, **248:**1149–1151. 1155.
3. Bridges NA, Christopher JA, Hindmarsh PC, Brook CG: **Sexual precocity: sex incidence and etiology.** *Arch Dis Child* 1994, **70:**116–118.
4. Fahmy JL, Kaminsky CK, Kaufman F, Nelson MD Jr, Parisi MT: **The radiological approach to precocious puberty.** *Br J Radiol* 2000, **73:**560–567.
5. Raphaelson MI, Stevens JC, Elders J, Comite F, Theodore WH: **Familial spastic paraplegia, mental retardation and precocious puberty.** *Arch Neurol* 1983, **40:**809–810.
6. Kurosawa K, Kawame H, Okamoto N, Ochiai Y, Akatsuka A, Kobayashi M, Shimohira M, Mizuno S, Wada K, Fukushima Y, Kawawaki H, Yamamoto T, Masuno M, Imaizumi K, Kuroki Y: **Epilepsy and neurological findings in 11 individuals with 1p36 deletion syndrome.** *Brain Dev* 2005, **27:**378–382.
7. Ito N, Ihara K, Tsutsumi Y, Miyake N, Matsumoto N, Hara T: **Hypothalamic pituitary complications in Kabuki syndrome.** *Pituitary* 2013, **16:**133–138.
8. Young C, Wang PJ, Tsai WY, Shen YZ: **Precocious puberty in a case with probable Angelman syndrome.** *Brain Dev* 1994, **16:**249–252.
9. Waisbren SE, Noel K, Fahrbach K, Cella C, Frame D, Dorenbaum A, Levy H: **Phenylalanine blood levels and clinical outcomes in phenylketonuria: a systematic literature review and meta-analysis.** *Mol Genet Metab* 2007, **92:**63–70.
10. Brenton DP, Pietz J: **Adult care in phenylketonuria and hyperphenylalaninaemia: the relevance of neurological abnormalities.** *Eur J Pediatr* 2000, **159**(Suppl 2):114–120.
11. Büyükgebiz B, Eroğlu Y, Büy ukgebiz A: **True precocious puberty associated with phenylketonuria.** *J Pediatr Endocrinol* 1994, **7:**361–363.
12. Freeman JV, Cole TJ, Chinn S, Jones PR, White EM, Preece MA: **Cross sectional stature and weight reference curves for the UK, 1990.** *Arch Dis Child* 1995, **73:**17–24.
13. Marshall WA, Tanner JM: **Variations in pattern of pubertal changes in girls.** *Arch Dis Child* 1969, **44:**291–303.
14. Tanner JM, Whitehouse RH, Marshall WA, Healy MJR, Goldstein H: *Assessment of skeletal maturity and prediction of adult height (TW2 method).* 2nd edition. London: Academic; 1983.
15. Christ SE: **Asbjørn Følling and the discovery of phenylketonuria.** *J Hist Neurosci* 2003, **12:**44–54.
16. Woolf LI: **Phenylketonuria in Turkey, Ireland and West Scotland.** *J Inherit Metab Dis* 1994, **17:**246–247.
17. Belanger-Quintana A, Martínez-Pardo M: **Physical development in patients with phenylketonuria on dietary treatment: a retrospective study.** *Mol Genet Metab* 2011, **104:**480–484.
18. Burrage LC, McConnell J, Haesler R, O'Riordan MA, Sutton VR, Kerr DS, McCandless SE: **High prevalence of overweight and obesity in females with phenylketonuria.** *Mol Genet Metab* 2012, **107:**43–48.

18

Differential effects of vitamin D2 and D3 supplements on 25-hydroxyvitamin D level are dose, sex, and time dependent

Muhammad M. Hammami[1,2*] and Ahmed Yusuf[1]

Abstract

Background: Vitamin D (D) supplements are indispensable for its world-wide deficiency. Controversy continues on ergocalciferol (D2) and cholecalciferol (D3) relative potency as well as on dosing-schedule and sex role in raising 25-hydroxy D (25(OH)D) level, the best indicator of D status.

Methods: We randomized 279 adults to daily D2, D3, D2/D3, or placebo; 2-weekly D2 or D3; or 4-weekly D2 or D3 (250,000 IU over/140 days). Randomization sequence, stratified by body-mass-index (BMI) and sex, was concealed from study coordinators and participants who were then blinded to capsules' content. D2, D3, 25(OH)D2, and 25(OH)D3 Serum levels were determined blindly on days 0,1,2,3,4,7,14, and 2-weekly thereafter by high performance liquid chromatography assay. The results of 269 participants were available for analysis. Primary endpoint was area-under-the-curve (AUC) of 25(OH)D (25(OH)D2 + 25(OH)D3) adjusted for sex, BMI, and baseline 25(OH)D level.

Results: Mean(SD) age was 33.0(8.5) year, 41% were males, and 85% completed follow-up. Baseline 25(OH)D level was 39.8(11.9) and increased by 3.3(11.6) and 28.6(16.3) nmol/L, in the placebo and active-treatment groups, respectively. AUC from day 0 to 140 (AUC_{140}) of 25(OH)D was 40% (D3 daily) to 55% (D3 2-weekly) higher with active-treatment than placebo ($p < 0.001$). 25(OH)D2 AUC_{140} was higher in daily than 2-weekly (17%, $p = 0.006$) and 4-weekly (20%, $p = 0.001$) D2-treated groups. 25(OH)D3 AUC_{140} was lower in daily than 2-weekly (11%, $p = 0.002$) and 4-weekly D3-treated groups (10%, $p = 0.008$). In D2-treated groups, there was 16.4 nmol/L decrease in 25(OH)D3 level that correlated ($p < 0.001$) with 25(OH)D2 level increase ($r = 0.48$) and baseline 25(OH)D level ($r = 0.58$), in one participant with measurable baseline 25(OH)D2 level, D3 caused a similar decrease in 25(OH)D2 level, while in the D2/D3-treated group, 25(OH)D3 level didn't increase. Incremental AUC from day 0 to 7 (AUC_7) of D3 and 25(OH)D3 in D3-treated groups were 118–243% higher and 31–39% lower, respectively, than incremental AUC_7 of D2 and 25(OH)D2 in D2-treated groups. Incremental AUC_7 of D3 and 25(OH)D3 in D3-treated groups and D2 and 25(OH)D2 in D2-treated groups were higher in females than males (55, 13, 64, and 28%, respectively). Baseline 25(OH)D level predicted response to D2 and D3 ($p < 0.001$), whereas, BMI was significant predictor only for early response to D2.

Conclusions: Effects of D2 and D3 supplements on 25 (OH)D level may be dosing-schedule and sex-dependent. D2-associated reduction in 25(OH)D3 level may be related to total 25(OH)D level rather than being D2-specific. D2 may be 25-hydroxylated faster than D3.

(Continued on next page)

* Correspondence: Muhammad@kfshrc.edu.sa
[1]Clinical Studies and Empirical Ethics Department, King Faisal Specialist Hospital and Research Center, P O Box # 3354 (MBC 03), Riyadh 11211, Saudi Arabia
[2]Alfaisal University College of Medicine, Riyadh, Saudi Arabia

(Continued from previous page)

Keywords: Cholecalciferol supplement, Ergocalciferol supplement, Sex effect, Dose effect, D2 level, D3 level, 25-hydroxyvitamin D2 level, 25-hydroxyvitamin D3 level, Creatinine production, BMI

Background

The increasingly recognized effects of vitamin D (D) on skeletal and extra-skeletal tissues [1, 2] together with worldwide D deficiency have amplified attention to D supplementation. Nevertheless, the relative potency of ergocalciferol (D2) vs cholcalciferol (D3), and the preferable dosing strategy continue to be controversial [3].

The same unit is used for both D2 and D3, suggesting biological equivalence in terms of raising serum total 25-hydroxy D (25(OH)D) level, [4] the best current biomarker of D status. However, published studies have yielded mixed results [4–13]. This may be due in part to the facts that supplement-induced increase in 25(OH)D level may be related to baseline level, [9, 11, 13–16] body mass index (BMI), [12–14, 16–21] sex, [13, 22, 23] dosing strategy, [24] meal content, [25] and duration of follow up, which have not been systematically controlled for. A meta-analysis found that D3 is significantly more potent than D2 as bolus dosing but not as daily dosing [24]. Further, the dose–response curve may be curvilinear rather than linear [13, 20, 21, 26, 27].

D2 and D3 differ in their side chain structure, conversion to 25(OH)D by hepatic 25-hydroxylase, affinity (and affinity of their metabolites) to circulating D binding protein, inactivation by 24-hydroxylation, and plasma half-life [24, 28]. However, in respect to binding to D receptor, the active dihydroxyvitamin D forms, $1,25(OH)_2D2$ and $1,25(OH)_2D3$, appear to be comparable [1]. Further, 25(OH)D2 and 25(OH)D3 appear to be equally recognized by the kidney 1-alpha hydroxylase [29–31].

Equivalent oral doses of D given daily compared to less frequently may result in differing increments in 25(OH)D [32] and D [2] levels. Circulating D has better general cellular accessibility than 25(OH)D due to its lower affinity to circulating D binding protein and may play an important physiological role as a substrate for many tissues [2].

It has been noticed that D2 supplementation is associated with reduction in 25(OH)D3 [5, 8, 33–35] and $1,25(OH)_2D3$ [36] levels. The underlying mechanism has not been elucidated; it is possible that the reduction is not specific to D2 supplementation and merely reflects a response to increasing 25(OH)D levels.

The primary aim of this study was to systematically evaluate the relative efficacy of various dosing strategies of D2 and D3 oral supplements in raising 25(OH)D levels.

Methods

Design

The study was randomized, placebo-controlled, partially blinded trial to compare the effect of seven D oral regimens on 25(OH)D level. Participants were randomly allocated to daily D2, D3, combination of D2 and D3, or placebo; 2-weekly D2 or D3; or 4-weekly D2 or D3. Total D dose in the active treatment groups was 250,000 IU over 140 days.

Participants

Volunteers were recruited via advertisement throughout the King Faisal Specialist Hospital and Research Center (KFSH&RC) and other medical centers in the City of Riyadh, Saudi Arabia. We enrolled healthy non-pregnant adults (age 18–60 years) living in Riyadh area who don't consume more than one serving of milk daily, don't take vitamin supplements, habitually have less than 10 h of sun exposure weekly, don't suffer from granulomatous, liver, or kidney diseases, don't take anticonvulsants, barbiturates, or steroids, and have 25(OH)D level between 20 and 50 nmol/L. Potential participants were screened by obtaining medical history and the following tests: complete blood count, serum creatinine, calcium, phosphorous, albumin, bilirubin, and alanine aminotransferase, and spot urine calcium, phosphate, and creatinine. The study was conducted at KFSH&RC from February 2013 through April 2016 after obtaining approval of the KFSH&RC Research Ethics Committee. All participants gave written informed consent and were compensated based on the Wage-Payment model [37] in a prorated manner.

Procedures and interventions

Ergocalciferol and cholecalciferol crystals (40,000,000 IU/g) were purchased from AGD Nutrition, LLC (Lewisville, TX, USA) and manufactured together with a matching placebo by Jamjoom Pharma (Jeddah, Saudi Arabia) into green soft gelatin capsules containing 2000, 25,000, or 50,000 IU of either D2 or D3 or a combination of 1000 IU D2 and 1000 IU D3. The content of the capsules was confirmed by in-house laboratory analysis (Jamjoom Pharma, accuracy 98–102%, coefficient of variation (CV) <2%) at manufacturing date and yearly thereafter. On average, the recovered content ranged from 89.33% (D3 2000 IU) to 91.91% (D2 25,000 IU) of the label claim and showed no trend of decrease over study period.

Daily doses (D2 2000 IU, D3 2000 IU, combined D2 1000 IU and D3 1000 IU, or placebo) on days 0, 1, 2, 3, 4, 7, and 14 and 2-weekly thereafter and all of the 2-weekly (D2 25,000 IU or D3 25,000 IU) and 4-weekly (D2 50,000 IU or D3 50,000 IU) doses were administered by study coordinators in the research clinic after blood samples were obtained and a standardized meal was given. The rest of the daily doses were dispensed to participants on a 2-weekly basis to self-administer with the first meal of the day; compliance was emphasized and checked by capsule counting at each research clinic visit. Participants on daily doses were asked to skip the dose on three Saturdays every 4 weeks so that their 4-weekly dose totals 50,000 IU. All participants were asked to report any more than habitual sun exposure or new medication/supplement. All of the seven active-treatment groups were given the same total D dose (250,000 IU over 140 days) and followed up for 140 days.

D2, D3, 25(OH)D2, and 25(OH)D3 serum levels were simultaneously and blindly measured by a locally validated reversed-phase high performance liquid chromatography assay (HPLC) [38] on days 0, 1, 2, 3, 4, 7, and 14, and 2-weekly thereafter. The intra-assay and inter-assay CVs were, respectively, 4.9 and 7.5% for D2, 4.8 and 6.0% for D3, 5.0 and 6.7% for 25(OH)D2, and 6.3 and 6.9% for 25(OH)D3. Limits of detection and quantification were, respectively, 7.5 and 12.5 nmol/L for D2 and D3 and 5 and 12.5 nmol/L for 25(OH)D2 and 25(OH)D3 [38]. Serum calcium and phosphorous and spot urine calcium, phosphate, and creatinine levels were determined by the clinical laboratory at KFSH&RC on days 0 and 140.

Randomization and blinding

Blocked (block size = 8) randomization sequences, stratified by body mass index (BMI $\leq$ 30, $\geq$30 kg/m^2) and sex were generated (by MMH) using an online program [39]. Assignment was concealed from potential participants and recruiting coordinators. Participants and study coordinators continued to be blinded to the content of individual assignments (D2, D3, D2 and D3, or placebo for daily doses; D2 or D3 for 2-weekly and 4-weekly doses).

Outcome measures and analysis

The primary outcome measure was the area-under-the-curve from day 0 to 140 (AUC_{140}) of 25(OH)D. Predetermined secondary outcome measures were AUC_{140} of 25(OH)D2, 25(OH)D3, D2, and D3 as well as incidence of hypercalcemia and hypercalciuria. AUC from day 0 to 7, day 0 to 14 and day 0 to 28 (AUC_7, AUC_{14}, and AUC_{28}) were also calculated. AUCs were analyzed using analysis of covariance (ANCOVA). The model included treatment group, BMI, sex, and the corresponding day zero level. One way ANOVA was used to compare baseline continuous variables among groups and t test was used to compare day zero and day 140 continuous variables as well as estimated effect sizes. Analyses were performed (by MMH) with IBM SPSS Statistics version 21 software. Two-tailed p-values and 95% confidence intervals (CI) are reported.

Results

Two hundred seventy nine participants were randomized to 8 groups (D2 daily, D3 daily, combined D2/D3 daily, placebo daily, D2 2-weekly, D3 2-weekly, D2 4-weekly, or D3 4-weekly). Ten participants withdrew within the first week of the study and were not included in the analysis. Two hundred twenty nine participants completed the study and 40 (15%) lost to follow up, including one who became pregnant (Fig. 1).

Table 1 summarizes the main characteristics per treatment group of the 229 participants who completed the study and of the entire cohort of 269 participants. There were no statistically significant differences among the eight groups in the listed characteristics ($p = 0.32–0.90$ for the 229 participants, $p = 0.41–0.90$ for the entire cohort). The 269 participants had a mean (SD) age of 33.0 (8.5) years and baseline 25(OH)D level of 39.8 (11.9) nmol/L, and 41% were males. All were of Middle Eastern or East Asian ethnicity.

Incompliance with self-administered daily doses as determined by capsule counting was 1.6% for the D2, 1.3% for the D3, 1.0% for the combined D2/D3, and 1.3% for the placebo group (9,8,7, and 6 participants missed a total of 56, 52, 40, and 46 doses, respectively). None of the participants reported more than habitual sun exposure or taking supplements containing vitamin D during enrollment. At day 140, there was no incidence of hypercalcemia and mean (SD) changes in urinary calcium/creatinine ratio and phosphate/creatinine ratio in the seven active-treatment groups were 0.013 (0.259) and −0.183 (1.164) mol/mol, respectively ($p = 0.48$ and $p = 0.03$, respectively). In the placebo group, they were −0.061 (0.270) and −0.236 (1.035) mol/mol, respectively. These changes were the results of significant increase in urinary calcium and creatinine levels with a mean (95% confidence interval, CI) of 0.90 mmol/L (CI, 0.34 to 1.47, $p = 0.002$) and 1.75 mmol/L (CI, 0.56 to 2.94, $p = 0.004$), respectively, and insignificant increase in urinary phosphate of 0.37 mmol/L (−2.11 to 2.85, $p = 0.77$) in the 7 active treatment groups. There were no significant changes in the corresponding parameters in the placebo group ($p = 0.23$ to 0.95). No adverse events were reported.

Differential effects of vitamin D regimens on 25(OH)D level

Figure 2a to c depicts mean 25(OH)D level from day 0 to day 140 in the eight groups. The concentration-time curve in the placebo group was rather flat with a maximum

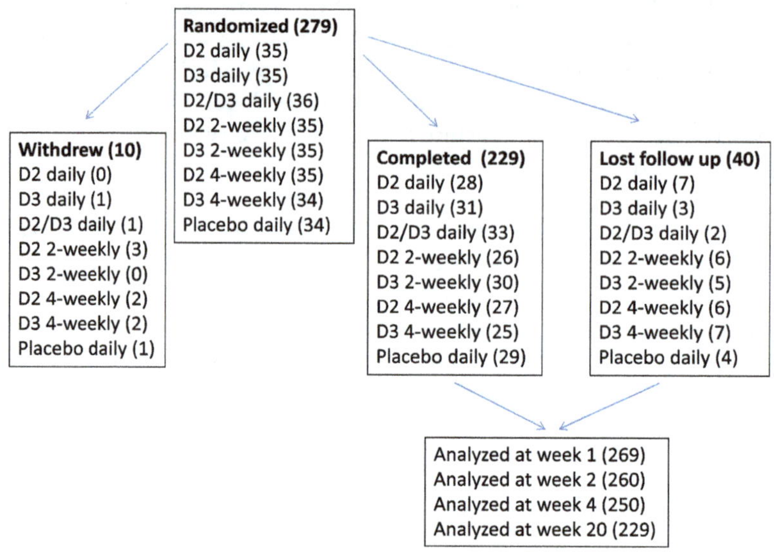

Fig. 1 Participants flow chart. "Withdrew" indicates participants who did not complete the first week of the study and who were excluded from analysis

mean increase in 25(OH)D level of 6.2 compared to 27.5 to 37.3 nmol/L in the seven active-treatment groups. At day 140, the mean increase in in the active-treatment groups was 28.6 (16.3) compared to 3.3 (11.6) nmol/L in the placebo group. The curve flattened around day 70 in the daily groups and around day 112 in the 2-weekly groups. In the 4-weekly groups, it showed consistent fluctuation (mean differences around 6.6 and 5.2 nmol/L in D2 and D3 groups, respectively) with peaks and troughs, 2 weeks and 4 weeks after dosing, respectively. Interestingly, there was no further increase in peak 25(OH)D level after day 70 in the D2 4-weekly group, however, peak

Table 1 Baseline characteristics of study participants

	D2 daily	D3 daily	D2/D3 daily	D2 2-weekly	D3 2-weekly	D2 4-weekly	D3 4-weekly	Placebo daily
Number	28	31	33	26	30	27	25	29
	35	34	35	32	35	33	32	33
Age, year	34.4 (10.2)	34.5 (9.7)	33.1 (6.8)	31.5 (6.1)	33.5 (10.5)	32.3 (7.2)	32.6 (8.5)	32.8 (7.3)
	34.7 (9.4)	33.7 (9.7)	32.8 (7.1)	31.5 (7.8)	33.4 (10.5)	33.5 (8.0)	31.4 (8.1)	32.4 (7.3)
Male, number (%)	13 (46)	13 (42)	15 (45)	12 (46)	13 (43)	11 (41)	10 (40)	13 (45)
	14 (40)	14 (41)	14 (40)	14 (44)	14 (40)	13 (39)	14 (44)	13 (39)
BMI, kg/m^2	24.6 (2.9)	26.1 (5.1)	26.2 (3.8)	24.1 (4.0)	24.8 (5.1)	25.3 (5.2)	25.6 (3.4)	23.9 (4.3)
	25.3 (3.3)	25.9 (4.9)	26.0 (3.6)	24.3 (3.9)	24.8 (4.7)	25.4 (4.8)	25.9 (3.7)	24.1 (4.4)
Sun exposure, hour/week	2.0 (2.2)	2.2 (2.1)	2.3 (2.3)	2.3 (2.7)	3.0 (2.9)	2.5 (2.5)	3.2 (3.1)	2.3 (2.3)
	2.3 (2.6)	2.2 (2.0)	2.3 (2.3)	2.7 (3.0)	2.8 (2.7)	2.4 (2.5)	3.1 (3.0)	2.2 (2.2)
Serum 25(OH)D, nmol/L	39.5 (12.2)	41.3 (10.7)	40.7 (14.5)	38.2 (10.5)	39.5 (12.5)	40.9 (12.0)	40.9 (12.2)	42.9 (10.2)
	38.8 (12.1)	40.9 (10.3)	40.8 (14.5)	37.6 (10.5)	39.4 (13.0)	39.5 (12.7)	39.4 (12.3)	41.8 (10.3)
Serum 25(OH)D3, nmol/L	39.1 (12.1)	41.3 (10.7)	38.0 (12.1)	38.2 (10.5)	38.0 (11.5)	40.4 (12.2)	40.9 (12.2)	42.9(10.2)
	37.2 (12.3)	40.3 (10.9)	37.8 (12.3)	37.6 (10.5)	38.2 (12.2)	38.7 (12.8)	39.4 (12.3)	41.8 (10.3)
Urinary calcium/creatinine, mol/mol	0.30 (0.19)	0.39 (0.21)	0.32 (0.22)	0.33 (0.19)	0.37 (0.26)	0.42 (0.24)	0.32 (0.20)	0.40 (0.24)
	0.34 (0.23)	0.39 (0.20)	0.29 (0.17)	0.32 (0.18)	0.37 (0.26)	0.38 (0.24)	0.31 (0.20)	0.38 (0.23)
Urinary phosphate, creatinine, mol/mol	1.69 (0.80)	1.83 (1.02)	1.57 (0.91)	1.70 (0.67)	1.75 (0.76)	2.08 (1.74)	1.47 (0.78)	1.79 (1.06)
	1.66 (0.83)	1.79 (1.01)	1.53 (0.78)	1.62 (0.66)	1.81 (0.74)	2.00 (1.59)	1.60 (1.18)	1.68 (1.04)

Data are means (SD), unless indicated otherwise. The first raw of each entry describes the 229 participants who completed the study; the second raw describes the entire cohort of 269 participants. BMI, body mass index. 25(OH)D, total 25-hydroxyvitamin D. 25(OH)D3, 25-hydroxyvitamin D3

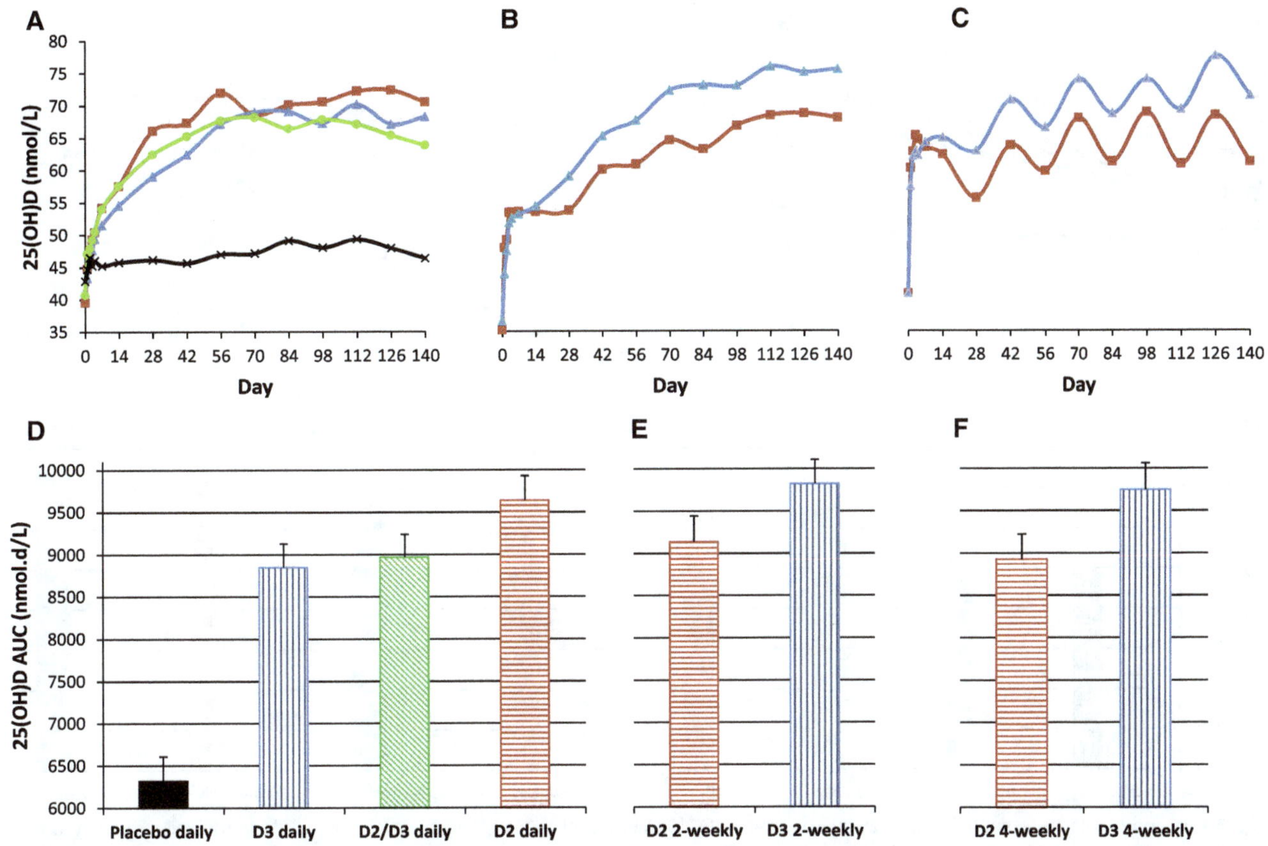

Fig. 2 **a**, **b**, and **c**, data represent mean total 25-hydroxyvitamin D (25(OH)D) level over 140 days, in the daily, 2-weekly, and 4-weekly groups, respectively. *Squares* and *triangles* represent D2 and D3 groups, respectively. *Circles* and *cross marks* represent combined D2/D3 and placebo groups, respectively. **d**, **e**, and **f**, data represent adjusted mean (SE) 25(OH)D AUC_{140} in the daily, 2-weekly, and 4-weekly groups, respectively

25(OH)D level appeared to continue to increase over the duration of the study. The curves were not grossly separable in the three daily active treatment groups; however, they were clearly separable in the two 2-weekly groups and the two 4-weekly groups, with the groups assigned to D3 maintaining higher levels than the groups assigned to D2.

Analysis of 25(OH)D AUC_{140} showed significant effect of treatment group ($p < 0.001$) and baseline 25(OH)D level ($p < 0.001$) but not sex ($p = 0.38$) or BMI ($p = 0.14$). Figure 2d to f shows adjusted mean (SE) 25(OH)D AUC_{140} in the eight groups. All active treatment groups had significantly higher 25(OH)D AUC_{140} than the placebo group (40 to 55%) with mean difference ranging from 2530.4 nmol.d/L (CI, 1741.3 to 3319.6) in D3 daily group to 3503.3 nmol.d/L (CI, 2711.9 to 4294.6) in D3 2-weekly group. Adjusted mean 25(OH)D AUC_{140} was significantly lower in D3 daily group compared to D3 2-weekly group (mean difference −972.8 nmol.d/L (CI, −1751.1 to −194.6, $p = 0.02$) and D3 4-weekly group (mean difference −896.4 nmol.d/L (CI, −1710.2 to −82.6, $p = 0.03$). It was significantly higher in D3 2-weekly group compared to daily D2/D3 (mean difference 852.4 nmol.d/L (CI, 85.9 to 1618.9, $p = 0.03$) and D2 4-weekly group (mean difference 897.5 nmol.d/L (CI, 93.9 to 1701.1, $p = 0.03$). The increase in 25(OH)D level between days 0 and 140 correlated negatively with day zero 25(OH)D level ($r = -0.21$, $p = 0.001$). There was no significant difference in day 140 serum calcium level or urinary calcium, phosphate, or creatinine levels among the 8 groups ($p = 0.58$, to 0.98, adjusted for day zero value and sex).

Figure 3a to c depicts mean 25(OH)D level from day 0 to day 28 in the eight groups. Adjusted mean 25(OH)D level was not significantly different from the placebo group until day 2 in the D2 daily ($p = 0.005$) and until day 3 in the D3 daily ($p = 0.02$) and the D2/D3 daily ($p = 0.001$) groups. However, it was significantly different from day 1 in the D2 and D3 2-weekly and 4-weekly groups ($p < 0.001$ to 0.005). At day 4, adjusted mean 25(OH)D level was significantly lower in the D2 and D3 daily groups compared to the corresponding 2-weekly groups ($p = 0.02$ and 0.006, respectively) and in the D2 and D3 2-weekly groups compared to the corresponding 4-weekly groups ($p = 0.03$ and $p = 0.004$, respectively). At day 28, adjusted mean 25(OH)D level was higher in D3 4-weekly group compared to D2 4-weekly group

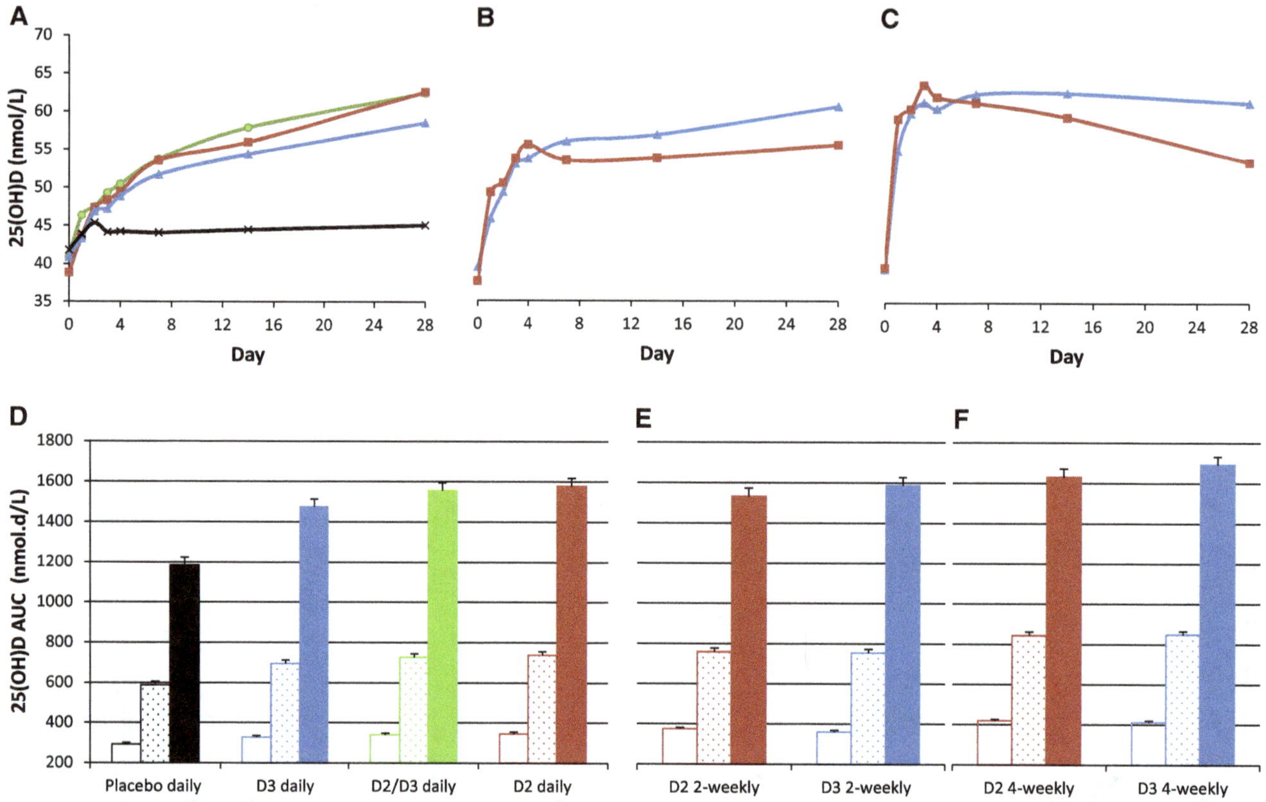

Fig. 3 a, **b**, and **c**, data represent mean total 25-hydroxyvitamin D (25(OH)D) level over the first 28 days of the study, in the daily, 2-weekly, and 4-weekly groups, respectively. *Squares* and *triangles* represent D2 and D3 groups, respectively. *Circles* and *cross marks* represent combined D2/D3 and placebo groups, respectively. **d**, **e**, and **f**, data represent adjusted mean (SE) 25(OH)D AUC_7 (*open bars*), AUC_{14} (*dotted bars*), and AUC_{28} (*closed bars*) in the daily, 2-weekly, and 4-weekly groups, respectively

(mean difference 6.4 nmol/L (CI, 1.5 to 11.3, $p = 0.01$)) and in D3 2-weekly group compared to D2 2-weekly group (mean difference 4.5 nmol/L (CI, −0.4 to 9.5, $p = 0.07$)). On the other hand, 25(OH)D level was significantly higher in D2 daily group compared to D3 daily group (mean difference 6.2 nmol/L (CI, 1.4 to 11.0, $p = 0.01$)).

Analysis of 25(OH)D AUC_7, AUC_{14}, and AUC_{28} showed significant effect of treatment group ($p < 0.001$), baseline 25(OH)D level ($p < 0.001$), and BMI ($p = 0.002$ to 0.004) but not sex ($p = 0.55$ to 0.85). Figure 3d to f depicts adjusted mean (SE) 25(OH)D AUC_7, AUC_{14}, and AUC_{28} in the eight groups. Adjusted mean 25(OH)D AUC_7 was significantly ($p < 0.001$) higher in the active-treatment groups compared to the placebo group (mean difference ranging from 36.0 nmol.d/L (CI, 13.2 to 58.7) to 126.9 nmol.d/L (CI, 104.0 to 149.7). In the D3 treated groups, adjusted means of 25(OH)D AUC_7, AUC_{14}, and AU_{28} were significantly lower in the daily group compared to the 2-weekly ($p = 0.005$ to 0.04) and the 4-weekly ($p < 0.001$) groups. In contrast, in the D2 treated groups, although adjusted mean 25(OH)D AUC_7 was significantly lower in the daily group compared to the 2-weekly and 4-weekly groups ($p = 0.02$ and $p < 0.001$, respectively), adjusted mean 25(OH)D AUC_{14} was significantly lower only in the daily group compared to the 4-weekly group, and adjusted mean 25(OH)D AUC_{28} was not significantly different in the daily group compared to the 2-weekly or 4-weekly groups ($p = 0.42$ and $p = 0.36$, respectively). There was significant negative correlation between 25(OH)D AUC_7, AUC_{14}, and AUC_{28} and BMI in the D2 treated groups ($r = -0.25$, $p = 0.01$ for all) but not in D3 treated groups ($r = -0.10$, $p = 0.32$ to 0.36). In summary, the data suggest that in the long term (20 weeks), D3 2-weekly followed by D3 4-weekly and D2 daily regimens may be superior in raising 25(OH)D level. However, in the first few weeks of treatment, the 4-weekly regimens followed by 2-weekly regimens appear to be superior to all daily regimens. Further, D3 2-weekly and 4-weekly regimens appear to be consistently superior to the corresponding D2 regimens, and D2 daily regimen appears to be consistently superior to D3 daily regimen. Finally, the increase in 25(OH)D level appears to be inversely related to BMI (mainly short term after D2 treatment) and to baseline 25(OH)D level.

Differential effects of vitamin D regimens on 25(OH)D2 and 25(OH)D3 levels

Figure 4a shows mean 25(OH)D2 level from day 0 to day 140 in the eight groups. Analysis of 25(OH)D2 AUC_{140} showed significant effect of treatment group ($p < 0.001$) and baseline 25(OH)D2 level ($p < 0.001$) but not BMI ($p = 0.18$) or sex ($p = 0.28$). Figure 4b depicts adjusted mean (SE) 25(OH)D2 AUC_{140} in the three D2 treated groups. Adjusted mean 25(OH)D2 AUC_{140} was significantly higher (17 and 20%) in D2 daily group compared to D2 2-weekly group (mean difference 881.5 nmol.d/L (CI, 257.0 to 1506.1, $p = 0.006$)) and D2 4-weekly group (mean difference 1029.2 nmol.d/L (CI, 410.5 to 1648.0, $p = 0.001$)), with no significant difference between the 2-weekly and 4-weekly groups ($p = 0.65$). In contrast, adjusted mean 25(OH)D2 AUC_7 and AUC_{14} were significantly lower in the D2 daily group compared to D2 2-weekly group (mean difference −42.0 nmol.d/L (CI, −56.5 to −27.6, $p < 0.001$) and −38.5 nmol.d/L (CI, −70.6 to −6.5, $p = 0.02$), respectively) and to D2 4-weekly group (mean difference −91.4 nmol.d/L (CI, −105.7 t0 -77.2, $p < 0.001$) and −136.9 nmol.d/L (CI, −168.0 to −105.8, $p < 0.001$), respectively). Further, 25(OH)D2 AUC_7, AUC_{14}, and AUC_{28} were significantly higher in D2 4-weekly group compared to 2-weekly group ($p < 0.001$, $p < 0.001$, and $p = 0.01$, respectively). Furthermore, 25(OH)D2 AUC_7, AUC_{14}, and AUC_{28} were significantly associated with BMI ($p < 0.001$, $p < 0.001$, $p = 0.001$, respectively) and sex ($p = 0.003$, $p = 0.02$, $p = 0.046$, respectively).

Figure 4c shows mean 25(OH)D3 level from day 0 to day 140 in the eight groups. Analysis of 25(OH)D3 AUC_{140} showed significant effect of treatment group ($p < 0.001$), baseline 25(OH)D3 level ($p < 0.001$), but not sex or BMI ($p = 0.55$). Figure 4d depicts adjusted mean (SE) 25(OH)D3 AUC_{140} in the three D3 treated groups. Adjusted mean 25(OH)D3 AUC_{140} was significantly lower in the D3 daily group compared to D3 2-weekly group (mean difference −1002.2 nmol.d/L (CI, −1641.4 to −363.0, $p = 0.002$)) and D3 4-weekly group (mean difference −910.5 nmol.d/L (CI, −1577.4 to −243.5, $p = 0.008$)), with no significant difference between the 2-weekly and 4-weekly groups ($p = 0.79$). These differences started early

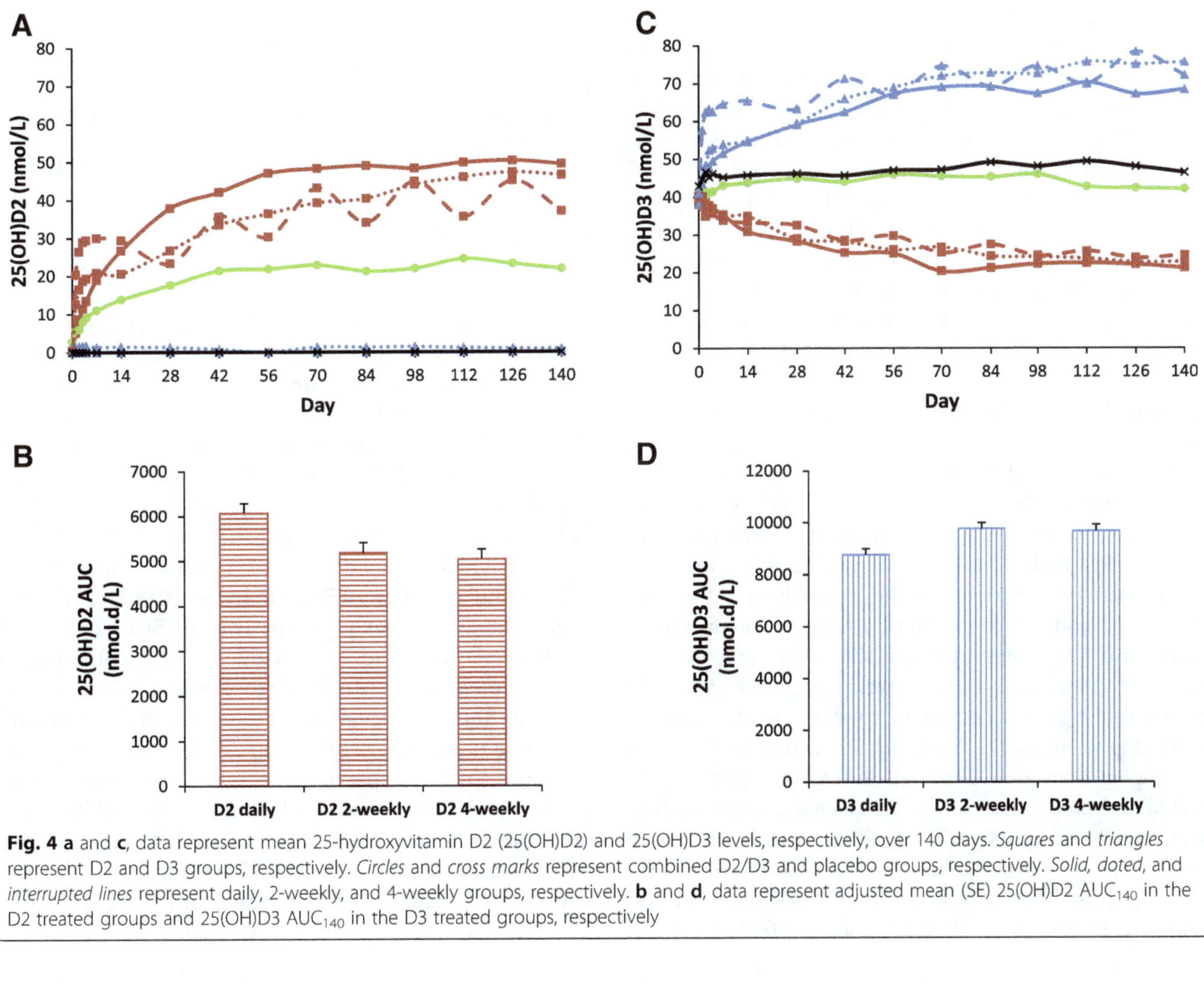

Fig. 4 **a** and **c**, data represent mean 25-hydroxyvitamin D2 (25(OH)D2) and 25(OH)D3 levels, respectively, over 140 days. *Squares* and *triangles* represent D2 and D3 groups, respectively. *Circles* and *cross marks* represent combined D2/D3 and placebo groups, respectively. *Solid, doted*, and *interrupted lines* represent daily, 2-weekly, and 4-weekly groups, respectively. **b** and **d**, data represent adjusted mean (SE) 25(OH)D2 AUC_{140} in the D2 treated groups and 25(OH)D3 AUC_{140} in the D3 treated groups, respectively

on; adjusted mean 25(OH)D3 AUC_7, AUC_{14}, and AUC_{28} were significantly lower in D3 daily group compared to D3 2-weekly group ($p < 0.001$, $p = 0.003$, and $p = 0.01$, respectively) and D3 4-weekly group ($p < 0.001$, $p < 0.001$, and $p < 0.001$, respectively), and adjusted mean 25(OH)D3 AUC_7, AUC_{14}, and AUC_{28} were significantly higher in the D3 4-weekly group compared to 2-weekly group ($p < 0.001$, $p = 0.001$, and $p = 0.046$, respectively). Further, 25(OH)D3 AUC_7, AUC_{14}, and AUC_{28} were not associated with BMI ($p = 0.32$ to 0.61) or sex ($p = 0.18$ to 0.34).

Interestingly, in the D2/D3 group, 25(OH)D2 level increased to about one third to one half the levels in the three D2 treated groups (Fig. 4a, however, 25(OH)D3 did not increase (Fig. 4c. Further, in the three D2 treated groups, 25(OH)D3 level progressively and consistently decreased over the course of the study (Fig. 4c. It declined from a mean of 39.2 nmol/L at day 0 to 33.0, 31.6, 28.6, and 22.9 at days 7, 14, 28, and 140, respectively. To further explore the effect of D2 treatment on 25(OH)D3 level, we examined the correlation between the changes (day 140 minus day 0) in 25(OH)D3 level and 25(OH)D2 level in the three D2 treated groups. As shown in Fig. 5a, there was significant negative correlation ($r = -0.48$, $p < 0.001$). However, the change in 25(OH)D3 level also correlated negatively with day zero 25(OH)D3 level ($r = -0.58$, $p < 0.001$) and with day 140 25(OH)D levels ($r = -0.32$, $p = 0.003$). Of note, in one participant who started with measurable 25(OH)D2 level and received D3 2-weekly, 25(OH)D2 level decreased by 16.4 nmol/L between days 0 and 140 (Fig. 5b). In comparison, the mean decrease in 25(OH)D3 level in the three D2 treated groups was 16.4 nmol/L (CI, 14.0 to 18.7, $p < 0.001$), suggesting that D3 treatment may also induce a decline in 25(OH)D2 level of the same magnitude.

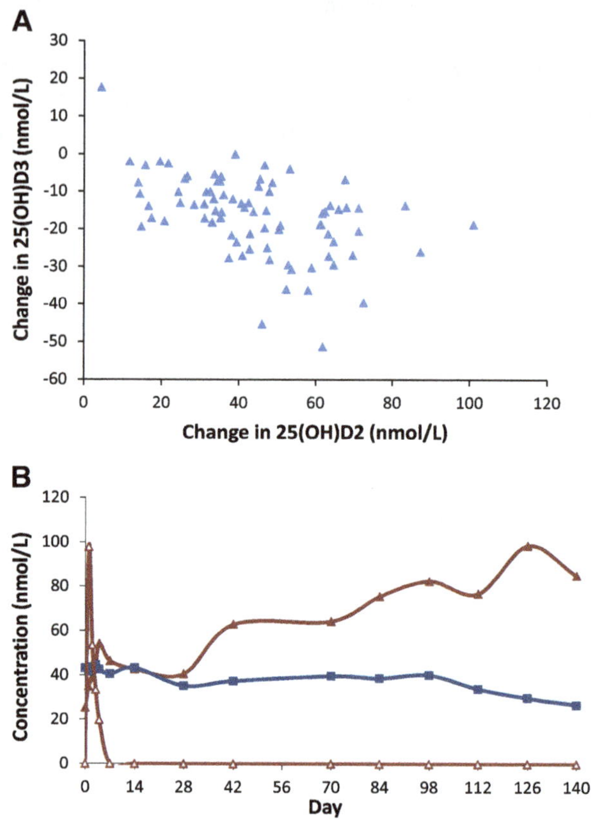

Fig. 5 a, Data show correlation between the changes (day 140 - day 0) in 25(OH)D3 levels and 25(OH)D2 levels in the three D2 treated groups ($r = -0.48$, $p < 0.001$). **b**, levels of D3 (*open triangles*), 25(OH)D2 (*closed squares*), and 25(OH)D3 (*closed triangles*) are depicted over 140 days in one participant from the D3 2-weekly group who happened to have measurable 25(OH)D2 at day zero

Differential effects of vitamin D regimens on D2 and D3 levels

At day zero, D2 and D3 levels were undetectable or only traceable in all the 8 groups. D2 and D3 levels were quantifiable only during the first week of treatment in the 2-weekly and 4-weekly groups. The following analysis is therefore restricted to the 2-weekly and 4-weekly groups. D2 and D3 concentration-time curves in the 2-weekly and 4-weekly groups are shown in Fig. 6a and b. As expected mean D2 and D3 levels were twice as high in the 4-weekly groups compared to the 2-weekly groups. Interestingly, mean D3 levels in the D3 treated groups were higher than mean D2 levels in the corresponding D2 treated groups (Fig. 6a). In the D2 treated groups, analysis of D2 AUC_7 showed significant effect of treatment group ($p < 0.001$), sex ($p = 0.01$), and BMI ($p = 0.001$). In the D3 treated groups, analysis of D3 AUC_7 showed significant effect of treatment group ($p < 0.001$), sex ($p < 0.001$), but not BMI ($p = 0.06$). Adjusted mean D2 AUC_7 was 200% higher in the 4-weekly group compared to 2-weekly group with a mean difference of 100.2 nmol.d/L (CI, 62.3 to 138.0, $p < 0.001$), and adjusted mean D3 AUC_7 was 90% higher in the 4-weekly group compared to 2-weekly group with a mean difference of 155.7 nmol.d/L (CI, 109.8 to 201.6, $p < 0.001$). Adjusted mean D3 AUC_7 was 243% higher than D2 AUC_7 in the 2-weekly groups (mean (SE) 172.2 (16.1) vs 50.2 (13.5) nmol.d/L) with a mean difference of 122.0 nmol.d/L (CI, 79.8 to 164.1, $p < 0.001$) and 118% higher in the 4-weekly groups (mean (SE) 327.9 (16.4) vs 150.4 (13.4) nmol.d/L) with a mean difference of 177.5 nmol.d/L (CI, 135.3 to 219.8, $p < 0.001$). Figure 6b shows that mean D2 levels in D2 treated groups and mean D3 levels in D3 treated groups are (64 and 55%, respectivlely) higher in females than males. Adjusted mean difference in AUC_7 was 48.5 nmol.d/L (CI, 10.3 to 86.6, $p = 0.01$) for D2 and 107.7 nmol.d/L (CI, 61.5 to 154.0, $p < 0.001$) for D3. Interestingly, BMI correlated significantly with D2 AUC_7 ($r = -0.27$, $p = 0.03$) but not D3 AUC_7 ($r = -0.05$, $p = 0.67$).

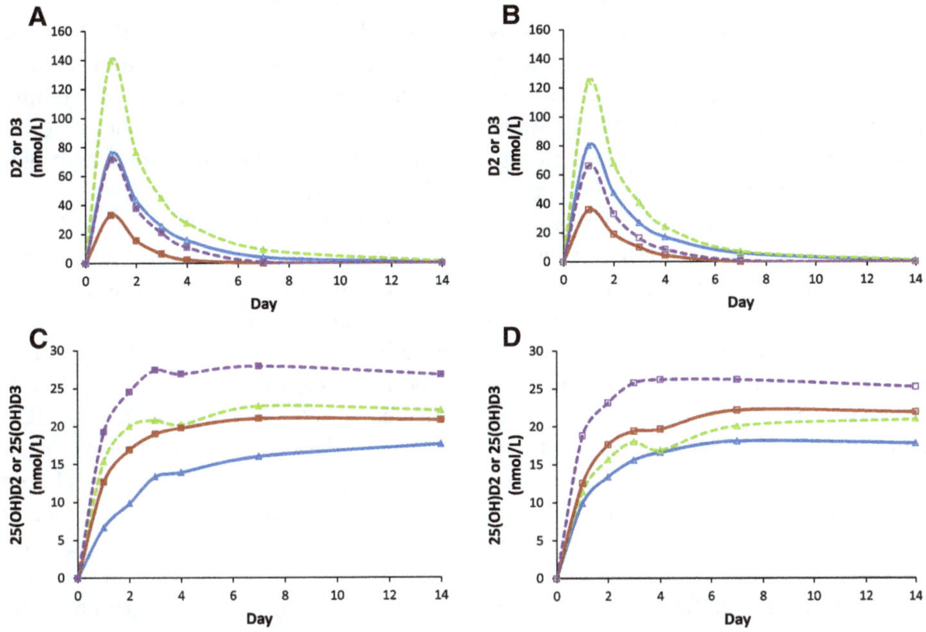

Fig. 6 a, data represent mean D3 (*closed triangles*) and D2 (*closed squares*) levels in the 4-weekly (interrupted lines) and 2-weekly (*solid lines*) groups. **b**, data represent mean D3 (*open triangles*) and D2 (*open squares*) levels in females (*interrupted line*) and males (*solid lines*) in the 2-weekly and 4-weekly groups. C, data represent mean 25(OH)D3 (*closed triangles*) and 25(OH)D2 (*closed squares*) levels in the 4-weekly (*interrupted lines*) and 2-weekly (*solid lines*) groups after subtracting day zero levels. D, data represent mean 25(OH)D3 (*open triangles*) and 25(OH)D2 (*open squares*) levels in females (*interrupted lines*) and males (*solid lines*) in the 2-weekly and 4-weekly groups after subtracting day zero levels

To explore the reasons for the differential effects of sex and D-type on D2 and D3 levels, we examined 25(OH)D2 levels in the D2 treated groups and 25(OH)D3 levels in the D3 treated groups after subtracting the corresponding baseline levels. As shown in Fig. 6c, mean 25(OH)D2 levels in the D2 treated groups were higher than mean 25(OH)D3 levels in the corresponding D3 treated groups. Adjusted mean (SE) 25(OH)D2 AUC_7 was 39% higher than adjusted mean 25(OH)D3 AUC_7 in the 2-weekly groups (mean (SE) 107.9 (8.9) vs 77.4 (7.7) nmol.d/L) with a mean difference of 30.5 nmol.d/L (CI, 7.2 to 53.9, $p = 0.01$) and 31% higher in the 4-weekly groups (mean (SE) 163.2 (8.9) vs 124.5 (8.0) nmol.d/L) with a mean difference of 38.7 nmol.d/L (CI, 14.8 to 62.5, $p < 0.002$). This together with higher D3 levels in the D3 treated groups compared to D2 levels in the D2 treated groups as shown above, suggest faster 25-hydroxylation of D2 compared to D3. However, faster 25-hydroxylation could not account for all the observed difference between D2 and D3 levels.

As shown in Fig. 6d, mean 25(OH)D2 levels in the D2 treated groups and mean 25(OH)D3 levels in the D3 treated groups were higher in females compared to males. Adjusted mean (SE) 25(OH)D2 AUC_7 was 28% higher in females compared to males (152.2 (8.1) vs 118.9 (9.6) nmol.d/L) with a mean difference of 33.4 nmol.d/L (CI, 8.2 to 58.5, $p = 0.01$). Adjusted mean (SE) 25(OH)D3 AUC_7 was 13% higher in females compared to males (106.9 (7.2) vs 95.0 (8.6) nmol.d/L) with a mean difference of 11.9 nmol.d/L (CI, −10.8 to 34.6, $p = 0.3$). In retrospect, the significant difference between females and males in 25(OH)D2 levels in the 2-weekly and 4-weekly groups was found to be present at day 140; mean (SE) 25(OH)D2 AUC_{140} was 5509.0 (274.2) vs 4526.5 (313.5) nmol.d/L with a mean difference of 982.5 nmol.d/L (CI, 137.6 to 1827.3, $p = 0.02$). This together with higher D2 levels in D2 treated groups and D3 levels in the D3 treated groups in females compared to males as shown above, suggest higher D2 and D3 circulation availability in females compared to males. Finally, BMI correlated significantly with 25(OH)D2 AUC_7 ($r = -0.34$, $p = 0.006$) but not 25(OH)D3 AUC_7 ($r = -0.11$, $p = 0.38$).

Discussion

The primary aim of this randomized placebo-controlled, partially-blinded study on 269 healthy adults with mean 25(OH)D of 39.8 (11.9) nmol/L was to evaluate the relative efficacy of equi-unit D2 and D3 oral supplements given daily, 2-weekly, or 4-weekly in raising 25(OH)D level over 20 weeks. Predetermined secondary aims included comparing D2, D3, 25(OH)D2, and 25(OH)D3 levels. The primary outcome measure was adjusted area-under-the-curve between days 0 and 140 (AUC_{140}). The main results were: 1) in the long term (20 weeks), the D3 2-weekly followed by D3 4-weekly and D2 daily regimens were superior in raising 25(OH)D levels. In the first few weeks of treatment, however, the 4-weekly followed by 2-weekly regimens were superior to all daily regimens. 2) D3 2-weekly and 4-weekly regimens were consistently superior to the corresponding D2 regimens; however, D2 daily regimen was consistently superior to D3 daily regimen. 3) 25(OH)D2 level was significantly higher in the daily compared to the 2-weekly and 4-weekly D2-treated groups, whereas, 25(OH)D3 level was lower in the daily compared to the 2-weekly and 4-weekly D3-treated groups 4) The increase in 25(OH)D level was inversely related to baseline level, however, its inverse relation to BMI appeared to be D-type and time dependent (mainly short time after D2 treatment). 5) Daily, 2-weekly, and 4-weekly D2 regimens were associated with a similar and significant decrease in 25(OH)D3 level that correlated with the increase in 25(OH)D2 level and baseline 25(OH)D level, in one participant with measurable baseline 25(OH)D2 level, D3 caused a similar decrease in 25(OH)D2 level, while in the D2/D3-treated group, 25(OH)D3 level didn't increase. 6) The increases in D3 level in the 2-weekly and 4-weekly D3 treated groups were higher than the increases in D2 level in the corresponding D2 treated groups, the opposite was true for 25(OH)D2 and 25(OH)D3 levels. 7) Females had higher increases in D3, D2, 25(OH)D2, and 25(OH)D3 levels than males. 8) D treatment was associated with significant increases in urinary calcium and creatinine levels but not calcium/creatinine ratio.

All of the seven D supplement regimens in our study significantly increased 25(OH)D. At day 140, mean increase was 3.3 nmol/L in the placebo group and 28.6 nmol/L in the active-treatment groups. Although comparison is difficult because the dose–response curve is curvilinear, with an average of 1786 IU/day, this translates into an increase of about 16 nmol/L per 1000 IU, which is consistent with previous observations [8, 21, 26, 27, 36, 40]. In men with baseline 25(OH)D of 70 nmol/L, it was estimated that the increase in 25(OH)D level is about 17.5 nmol/L per 1000 IU daily D3 dose [40]. A review of recordings of 17,614 healthy adults participating in a preventive health program found an average increase of 12 nmol/L per 1000 IU for daily dosing interval of 0 to 1000 IU [21]. In a multicenter, retrospective data extraction study, an average daily dose of 2700 IU D3 increased 25(OH)D by 11.8 nmol/L per 1000 IU [27]. It is to be noted that the recovered content of the capsules in our study was about 90% of the label claim and that compliance with study medication was 98.4 to 100%. In our study, the increase in 25(OH)D level plateaued around days 70 and 112 in the daily and 2-weekly groups, respectively. Time to plateau ranged from 5 weeks to five months in previous studies [40, 41]. Due to our relatively frequent sampling, we were able to observe clear fluctuations in 25(OH)D levels when measured 2 weeks and 4 weeks after dosing, which may have clinical implication in term of monitoring response to therapy. Interestingly, the fluctuations were more pronounced with D2 dosing, consistent with shorter half life of 25(OH)D2 [4, 7, 42].

Our finding that D3 is superior to D2 in raising 25(OH)D level when given 2-weekly or 4-weekly is consistent with the published literature. The superiority of D3 was seen in studies that used 50,000 IU daily [5] or weekly, [4] a bolus of 300,000 [42] or 50,000 IU, [7] and a bolus of 10,000,000 IU in cows, [43] but not in studies that used 400 IU daily, [8, 9] 1000 IU daily, [29, 36] or 2000 IU daily [10]. Nevertheless, it was also reported with daily doses of 4000 IU for 14 days [11]. A 2012 meta-analysis found that D3 is more potent than D2, interestingly the difference was significant in the 4 RCTs (48 patients) that used bolus oral or intramuscular doses but not in the 6 RCTs (146 patients) that used daily supplements [24]. The interaction between D-type and dosing schedule was clearly shown in this study; while daily D3 was less efficient than 2-weekly and 4-weekly D3 in raising 25(OHD3, daily D2 was superior to 2-weekly and 4-weekly D2 in raising 25(OH)D2 levels. It is to be noted that the formulation of the capsules in our study was based on the common unitage that 1 IU equals 25 ng crystalline D2 or D3. Since the molecular weights of D2 and D3 are 384 and 396, respectively, 25 ng D3 would be equivalent to 25.78 ng, [28] thus the potency of D2 may have been underestimated by about 3% if one considers molar equivalence rather than weight equivalence in determining potency in IUs. Our results suggest that for long term results, D2 is best given daily while D3 is best given 2-weekly. However, the 4-weekly followed by the 2-weekly (D2 or D3) regimens are clearly superior in in rapidly raising 25(OH)D levels.

We observed consistent decrease in 25(OH)D3 levels in D2 treated groups. This was observed in most [8, 33, 44] but not all [29] previous studies that fractionated 25(OH)D levels. In a meta-analysis of RCTs on the effect of UV-exposed mushrooms consumption, the increase in 25(OH)D2 level was associate with a decrease in 25(OH)D3 level [35]. Further, 1000 IU D3 daily for 11 week did not change $1,25(OH)_2D3$ level, while 1000 IU D2 daily increased $1,25(OH)_2D2$ level by 7.4 pg/ml and decreased $1,25(OH)_2D3$ level by 9.9 pg/ml [36]. A similar decrease in $1,25(OH)_2D3$ was seen in response to 4000 IU D2 daily for 8 weeks [44]. Several observations from our study may shed light on the mechanism(s) underlying these observations. We found that the D2-induced decrease in 25(OH)D3 level was similar in the daily, 2-weekly, and 4-weekly groups, that it was correlated with the increase in 25(OH)D2 level, baseline

25(OH)D level, and day 140 25(OH)D level, that there was no change in 25(OH)D3 level in the group treated with a combination of D2 and D3, and that when 25(OH)D2 level is measurable (one case), D3 treatment resulted in a similar decrease in 25(OH)D2 level. These observations suggest that the D2-induced decrease in 25(OH)D3 level may more related to the resulting 25(OH)D level rather than being specific to D2 treatment. In fact, in one study, 400 and 1000 IU D3 daily for one year resulted in an increase in 25(OH)D3 level with a concomitant decrease in 25(OH)D2 level [34]. Interestingly, in a crossover study on high-yielding dairy cows, pre-administration of 10,000,000 IU of D3 significantly reduced 25(OH)D2 response to 10,000,000 IU of D2 [43]. It may be that there is a regulatory mechanism that increases the disposal of 25(OH)D in response to increases in its level [20] and that it has been observed with D2 treatment mainly because study participants commonly don't have measurable 25(OH)D2 levels. Since there was essentially no change in 25(OH)D3 level in the group that received combination of 1000 IU D2 and 1000 IU D3, it appears that, in a setting similar to our study (baseline 25(OH)D level around 40 nmol/L and average dose of 1800 IU daily), an amount of 25(OH)D that can be produced by 1000 IU intake is disposed daily. If such a mechanism really exists it can be exploited in defining normal 25(OH)D levels.

Consistent with the above interpretation and with previous studies, [9, 11–16, 26, 35] we found significant negative correlation between baseline 25(OH)D level and response to treatment. A recent review found that 17 out of 20 studies documented such correlation (3 studies had inadequate sample size and variation in baseline level), which may explain up to 20% of response variation [13]. A recent systematic review of studies that used modest daily doses of D3 (200 to 800 IU), also found negative correlation, albeit not significant [26]. The negative correlation together with the non-linear response in 25(OH)D level to increasing doses of D [6, 16, 20, 21] again suggest a regulatory step mechanism [20]. In our study, the significant negative correlation between baseline and increment 25(OH)D level was first seen at day 28 (when 25(OH)D level was 59.1 (14.7) nmol/L), suggesting a threshold effect. Interestingly, pooling data of 3 RCTs, subjects with single nucleotide polymorphisms (linked to D binding proteins and 25-hydroxylase) that are associated with the lowest baseline 25(OH)D level had the smallest increase in 25(OH)D level (32). Thus in some subjects, low baseline 25(OH)D level may reflect a genetic potential rather than lifestyle influence and may be associated with lower rather than higher increment in 25(OH)D level.

Higher BMI/body fat percentage was associated with smaller response to D supplement in several studies [12–14, 18–21, 45]. BMI may be a better predictor than absolute weight [21] and was suggested as the most powerful response predictor to D supplement [19]. Up to 34.5% of response variation may be related to BMI, more apparently with higher D doses [13]. In a large retrospective study, mean increases in 25(OH)D level were 28.7, 23.6, and 20.1 nmol/L with BMI <25, 25–29, or ≥ 30 kg/m2, respectively [18]. Nevertheless, not all studies showed such negative association [13]. This may be due to the fact that higher BMI is also associated with baseline lower 25(OH)D levels, [17, 45] which is itself positively associated with response to D supplement. In our study, BMI was a significant response predictor to D2 but not D3 and only during the first 4 weeks of treatment, suggesting two additional potential modifiers of the relationship between BMI and 25(OH)D response to D supplement, D-type and time of assessment. The mechanisms underlying the association between BMI and response to D supplement are not clear. It was suggested that D and 25(OH)D may be trapped in access adipose tissue, as 25(OH)D is released with weight loss 1–6 months following bariatric surgery [46, 47]. However, total body fat storage may account for only 17% of the administered dose (extrapolated from subcutaneous fat), [4] and D and 25(OH)D may be also deposited in liver, muscle, and skin as shown in animal studies, suggesting that volume dilution may play a role [20]. The relatively lower affinity of D binding protein to D2 and 25(OH)D2 [24, 28] makes them more accessible to extra-vascular tissues, which may explain our finding.

We found that the increase in D3 level was 2–3 fold higher than the increase in D2 level (in the 2-weekly and 4-weekly treated groups). Few studies examined D2 and D3 after D2 and D3 supplementation [4, 43]. After similar doses of D2 and D3 (50,000 IU weekly for 12 weeks), subcutaneous fat D3 storage was 2 times higher than D2 storage [4]. Equivalent pharmaceutical doses of D3 and D2 in cows increased D3 level more than D2 level, respectively [43]. The difference may be related to the different structure of D2 and D3 side chains, theoretically causing differential absorption, binding to D binding proteins, inactivation by 24-hydroxylation, or activation by 25-hydroxylation. Absorption is not likely to be involved as studies of tritium-labeled D2 and D3 in healthy subjects found similar recoveries after oral dosing, however, D binding protein has double association constant to D3 compared to D2, and in vitro, mitochondrial 25-hydroxylase is 5 times faster for D3 compared to D2 [11, 24, 28]. It is to be noted that most of the ingested D is not converted to 25(OH)D; an RCT found that oral 25(OH)D3 is 4–5 more potent than D3 in raising 25(OH)D3 levels, [41] Interestingly, in our study, 25(OH)D2 levels were higher than 25(OH)D3 levels, suggesting that the lower D2 levels were due, at least in part, to higher D2 accessibility to the 25-hydroxylase enzyme because of lower affinity to D binding proteins. It is of note that the combination of D3 AUC_7 and 25(OH)D3 AUC_7 was about 50% higher than the combination of D2 AUC_7 and 25(OH)D2 AUC_7; indicating that a mechanism other than faster 25-hydroxylation (such as higher accessibility of D2 and 25(OH)D2 to extra-vascular tissues and faster degradation) is also involved. These mechanisms may apply only for schedules using high doses as 25(OH)D AUC_{140} was higher in D2 daily than D3 daily treatment.

The higher levels of D3 compared to D2 may have important implication regardless of their impact on serum 25(OH)D level. Because of lower affinity to D binding protein, D2 and D3 have more cellular accessibility than 25(OH)D2 and 25(OH)D3 (except for the kidney, parathyroid gland, and placenta, where the megalin-cubulin system is expressed) and may have important physiological roles in breast milk and as substrates for many tissues [2].

We found that females had significantly larger (60, 55, 28%) adjusted AUC_7 than males for D2, D3, and 25(OH)D2 levels (and larger 13%,but not significant increase in 25(OH)D3 level). Females also had significantly 22% larger adjusted 25(OH)D2 AUC_{140}.

The results suggest about 49% better bioavailability of both D2 and D3 in females. Sex effect on response to D supplement has not been directly studied before. However, it is of note that D binding proteins are higher in females than males, in premenopausal women compared to postmenopausal women, in pregnant women, in women on oral contraceptives, [22] and in postmenopausal women hormone replacement therapy [23]. Further, estrogens increase hepatic 25-hydroxylation of D and the impact of D binding protein on response to D treatment may be partly D-type dependent [13]. The observed sex differences may be related to higher D binding protein and faster 25-hydroxyaltion in females; although a sex difference in D absorption rate cannot be excluded. It is also possible that higher body fat and lower baseline 25(OH)D levels in females may play a role.

In agreement with previous studies using even higher doses of D, [6, 48, 49] none of our participants developed hypercalcemia or hypercalciuria. In fact, the increase in urinary calcium/creatinine ratio was not significant. Nevertheless, the calcium/creatinine ratio may be misleading as there was significant increase in both calcium and creatinine urinary excretion. An increase in creatinine generation and urinary excretion has been described in patients with chronic kidney disease treated with vitamin D receptor activator, paricacitol [50]. The increase in creatinine excretion associated with D treatment casts doubt on the usefulness of ratios that include urinary creatinine (such as albumin/creatinine and calcium/creatinine) in evaluating the effect of D treatment on kidney function [51, 52] or D intoxication [53].

The strengths of this study include using repeated measurements, having a placebo arm, and ability to study several active-treatment regimens simultaneously, which enabled observing small changes and uncovering mechanistic insights. They also include effective randomization and concealment, partial blinding, frequent follow up to strengthen and verify compliance and verification of D capsule content across the study period.

Limitations

The interpretation of the results of this study may be limited by its sample size, 15% follow up loss, lower compliance with daily compared to 2-weekly and 4-weekly regimens, capsule content that is lower than label claim, and capsule formulation based on weight equipotency of D2 and D3. The rate of follow up loss was similar across the groups, the characteristics of participants who completed the study were similar to those of the entire cohort, incompliance rate was 1 to 1.6% in the daily groups, and the discrepancy between capsule content and label claim was similar across the capsules; thus these factors would not be expected to affect the main findings of the study. Although the incompliance rate was low, it was measured by capsule count, which may not be reliable. Thus the lower dose–response observed with daily D3 treatment compared to 2-weekly and 4-weekly D3 treatments could be explained at least in part by incompliance. However, such explanation is not likely given our observation that the dose–response was higher with daily D2 treatment compared to 2-weekly and 4-weekly D2 treatments and the fact that assignment to daily D2 or D3 treatment was random and blinded. The lower capsule content implies that the observed increments in D and 25(OH)D levels may have been up to 10% higher. Further, the fact that the molecular weight of D2 is about 3% higher compared to D3 indicates that our study may have underestimated response to D2 treatment. Nevertheless, such difference would not be expected to change the conclusions of the study. Further, the strength (in terms of IU) of most currently available D supplements is based on the assumption of weight rather than molar equipotency of D2 and D3. Another limitation of the study is that our findings may not be generalizable to lower or higher doses of vitamin D, or to subjects with different baseline 25 (OH)D levels, with different demographics, or with co-morbidities. Also, since the study was exploratory in nature, we have conducted multiple comparisons (including ad hoc comparisons), which would increase the rate of type 1 error. Further, the study examined surrogate endpoints (vitamin D and hydroxyvitamin D levels) rather than clinical endpoints. Finally, due to our assay sensitivity, we were not able to measure D2 and D3 levels in the daily treated groups.

Conclusions

We conclude that: 1) the effects of D2 and D3 supplements on 25(OH)D level may be dosing-schedule, time and sex dependent. In the long term, D2 appears to be most effective when given daily and D3 appears to be most effective when given 2-weekly. Further, females appear to mount larger 25(OH)D response to D2 than males. 2) The D2-associated reduction in 25(OH)D3 level appears to be related to the increase in 25(OH)D level rather than being D2-specific, as it is related to baseline 25(OH)D level and D3 treatment may be also associated with a reduction in 25(OH)D2 level. This together with the well known association between baseline 25(OH)D level and response to D treatment suggest a regulatory mechanism that may be exploited in fine tuning determination of normal 25(OH)D level. 3) D2 appears to be 25-hydroxylated faster than D3. 4) The association between BMI and response to D supplement may be more pronounced with D2 and during the first few weeks of treatment. 5) D2 and D3 level in response to treatment are higher in females compared to males. 6) D treatment is associated with an increase in urinary creatinine level, which makes assessment of D effect using ratios that include creatinine misleading.

Abbreviations

1,25(OH)$_2$D2: 1,25 diydroxyvitamin D2; 1,25(OH)$_2$D3: 1,25 diydroxyvitamin D3; 25(OH)D: Total 25-hydroxyvitamin D (25(OH)D2 + 25(OH)D3); 25(OH)D2: 25-hydroxyvitamin D2; 25(OH)D3: 25-hydroxyvitamin D3; ANCOVA: Analysis of co-variance; AUC_{14}: Area-under-the-curve from day 0 to day 14; AUC_{140}: Area-under-the-curve from day 0 to day 140; AUC_{28}: Area-under-the-curve from day 0 to day 28; AUC_7: Area-under-the-curve from day 0 to day 7; BMI: Body mass index; CI: Confidence interval; CV: Coefficient of variation (standard deviation/mean); D: Vitamin D; D2: Vitamin D2 or ergocalcifrol; D3: Vitamin D3 or cholecaciferol; HPLC: High performance liquid chromatography; KFSH&RC: King Faisal Specialist Hospital and Research Center

Acknowledgments

Jamjoom Pharmaceuticals, Jeddah, Saudi Arabia manufactured the vitamin D and placebo capsules. Special thanks to participants of the study for their dedication and contribution to research. The superb assistance by the research staff at the Clinical Studies and Empirical Ethics Department is gratefully acknowledged.

Funding

This study was funded by a research grant to MMH from the King Abdul-Aziz City for Science and Technology (KACST), under National Comprehensive Plan for Science and Technology, Riyadh, Saudi Arabia (Biotech:10-MED 1362-20). The funder had no role in the design and conduct of the study; in the collection, management, analysis, and interpretation of the data; or in the preparation, review, or approval of the manuscript.

Authors' contributions

MMH had full access to all of the data in the study and takes responsibility for the integrity of the data and the accuracy of the data analysis. Study concept and design: MMH. Acquisition, analysis, or interpretation of data: both authors. Vitamin D and 25(OH)D measurements: AY. Statistical analysis: MMH. Manuscript writing: MMH. Critical revision of the manuscript for important intellectual content: both authors read and approved the final manuscript.

Competing interests

The authors declare that they have no competing interests.

References

1. Bikle D. Nonclassic actions of vitamin D. J Clin Endocrinol Metab. 2009;94(1): 26–34. doi:10.1210/jc.2008-1454.
2. Hollis BW, Wagner CL. The role of the parent compound vitamin D with respect to metabolism and function: why clinical dose intervals can affect clinical outcomes. J Clin Endocrinol Metab. 2013;98(12):4619–28. doi:10.1210/jc.2013-2653.
3. Romagnoli E, Carnevale V, Biondi P, Minisola S. Vitamin D supplementation: when and how? J Endocrinol Invest. 2014;37:603–7.
4. Heaney RP, Recker RR, Grote J, Horst RL, Armas LA. Vitamin D(3) is more potent than vitamin D(2) in humans. J Clin Endocrinol Metab. 2011;96(3): E447–52. doi:10.1210/jc.2010-2230.
5. Melhem SJ, Aiedeh KM, Hadidi KA. Effects of a 10-day course of a high dose calciferol versus a single mega dose of ergocalciferol in correcting vitamin D deficiency. Ann Saudi Med. 2015;35(1):13–8. doi:10.5144/0256-4947.2015.13.
6. Drincic A, Fuller E, Heaney RP, Armas LA. 25-Hydroxyvitamin D response to graded vitamin D3 supplementation among obese adults. J Clin Endocrinol Metab. 2013;98(12):4845–51. doi:10.1210/jc.2012-4103.
7. Armas LA, Hollis BW, Heaney RP. Vitamin D2 is much less effective than vitamin D3 in humans. J Clin Endocrinol Metab. 2004;89(11):5387–91.
8. Nimitphong H, Saetung S, Chanprasertyotin S, Chailurkit LO, Ongphiphadhanakul B. Changes in circulating 25-hydroxyvitamin D according to vitamin D binding protein genotypes after vitamin D3 or D2 supplementation. Nutr J. 2013;12:39. doi:10.1186/1475-2891-12-39.
9. Gallo S, Phan A, Vanstone CA, Rodd C, Weiler HA. The change in plasma 25-hydroxyvitamin D did not differ between breast-fed infants that received a daily supplement of ergocalciferol or cholecalciferol for 3 months. J Nutr. 2013;143(2):148–53.
10. Gordon CM, Williams AL, Feldman HA, May J, Sinclair L, Vasquez A, Cox JE. Treatment of hypovitaminosis D in infants and toddlers. J Clin Endocrinol Metab. 2008;93(7):2716–21. doi:10.1210/jc.2007-2790.
11. Trang HM, Cole DE, Rubin LA, Pierratos A, Siu S, Vieth R. Evidence that vitamin D3 increases serum 25-hydroxyvitamin D more efficiently than does vitamin D2. Am J Clin Nutr. 1998;68(4):854–8.
12. Didriksen A, Grimnes G, Hutchinson MS, Kjærgaard M, Svartberg J, Joakimsen RM, Jorde R. The serum 25-hydroxyvitamin D response to vitamin D supplementation is related to genetic factors, BMI, and baseline levels. Eur J Endocrinol. 2013;169(5):559–67. doi:10.1530/EJE-13-0233.
13. Mazahery H, von Hurst PR. Factors affecting 25-hydroxyvitamin D concentration in response to vitamin D supplementation. Nutrients. 2015; 7(7):5111–42. doi:10.3390/nu7075111.
14. Waterhouse M, Tran B, Armstrong BK, Baxter C, Ebeling PR, English DR, Gebski V, Hill C, Kimlin MG, Lucas RM, Venn A, Webb PM, Whiteman DC, Neale RE. Environmental, personal, and genetic determinants of response to vitamin D supplementation in older adults. J Clin Endocrinol Metab. 2014; 99(7):E1332–40. doi:10.1210/jc.2013-4101.
15. Shab-Bidar S, Bours S, Geusens PP, Kessels AG, van den Bergh JP. Serum 25(OH)D response to vitamin D3 supplementation: a meta-regression analysis. Nutrition. 2014;30(9):975–85. doi:10.1016/j.nut.2013.12.020.
16. Mazahery H, Stonehouse W, von Hurst PR. The effect of monthly 50,000 IU or 100,000 IU vitamin D supplements on vitamin D status in premenopausal Middle Eastern women living in Auckland. Eur J Clin Nutr. 2015;69(3):367–72. doi:10.1038/ejcn.2014.264.
17. McKibben RA, Zhao D, Lutsey PL, Schneider AL, Guallar E, Mosley TH, Michos ED. Factors associated with change in 25-hydroxyvitamin D levels over longitudinal follow-up in the ARIC study. J Clin Endocrinol Metab. 2016;101(1):33–43. doi:10.1210/jc.2015-1711.
18. Saliba W, Barnett-Griness O, Rennert G. The relationship between obesity and the increase in serum 25(OH)D levels in response to vitamin D supplementation. Osteoporos Int. 2013;24(4):1447–54. doi:10.1007/s00198-012-2129-0.
19. Tepper S, Shahar DR, Geva D, Ish-Shalom S. Predictors of serum 25(Oh)D increase following bimonthly supplementation with 100,000IU vitamin D in healthy, men aged 25–65 years. J Steroid Biochem Mol Biol. 2014;144(Pt A): 163–6. doi:10.1016/j.jsbmb.2013.12.005.

20. Gallagher JC, Yalamanchili V, Smith LM. The effect of vitamin D supplementation on serum 25(OH)D in thin and obese women. J Steroid Biochem Mol Biol. 2013;136:195–200. doi:10.1016/j.jsbmb.2012.12.003.
21. Ekwaru JP, Zwicker JD, Holick MF, Giovannucci E, Veugelers PJ. The importance of body weight for the dose response relationship of oral vitamin D supplementation and serum 25-hydroxyvitamin D in healthy volunteers. PLoS One. 2014;9(11):e111265. doi:10.1371/journal.pone.0111265.
22. Yousefzadeh P, Shapses SA, Wang X. Vitamin D binding protein impact on 25-hydroxyvitamin D levels under different physiologic and pathologic conditions. Int J Endocrinol. 2014;2014:981581. doi:10.1155/2014/981581. 6 pages.
23. Møller UK, Streym S, Jensen LT, Mosekilde L, Schoenmakers I, Nigdikar S, Rejnmark L. Increased plasma concentrations of vitamin D metabolites and vitamin D binding protein in women using hormonal contraceptives: a cross-sectional study. Nutrients. 2013;5(9):3470–80. doi:10.3390/nu5093470.
24. Tripkovic L, Lambert H, Hart K, Smith CP, Bucca G, Penson S, Chope G, Hyppönen E, Berry J, Vieth R, Lanham-New S. Comparison of vitamin D2 and vitamin D3 supplementation in raising serum 25-hydroxyvitamin D status: a systematic review and meta-analysis. Am J Clin Nutr. 2012;95(6): 1357–64. doi:10.3945/ajcn.111.031070.
25. Mulligan GB, Licata A. Taking vitamin D with the largest meal improves absorption and results in higher serum levels of 25-hydroxyvitamin D. J Bone Miner Res. 2010;25(4):928–30. doi:10.1002/jbmr.67.
26. Whiting SJ, Bonjour J-P, Payen FD, Rousseau B. Moderate amounts of vitamin D3 in supplements are effective in raising serum 25-hydroxyvitamin D from low baseline levels in adults: a systematic review. Nutrients. 2015; 7(4):2311–23. doi:10.3390/nu7042311.
27. Aterrado S, Ono G, Kanehira-Mar S, Meier J, Swislocki A. Evaluating vitamin D repletion regimens and effects in veteran patients. Ann Pharmacother. 2015;49(9):969–77.
28. Houghton LA, Vieth R. The case against ergocalciferol (vitamin D2) as a vitamin supplement. Am J Clin Nutr. 2006;84(4):694–7.
29. Holick MF, Biancuzzo RM, Chen TC, Klein EK, Young A, Bibuld D, Reitz R, Salameh W, Ameri A, Tannenbaum AD. Vitamin D2 is as effective as vitamin D3 in maintaining circulating concentrations of 25-hydroxyvitamin D. J Clin Endocrinol Metab. 2008;93(3):677–81.
30. Clemens TL, Zhou XY, Myles M, Endres D, Lindsay R. Serum vitamin D2 and vitamin D3 metabolite concentrations and absorption of vitamin D2 in elderly subjects. J Clin Endocrinol Metab. 1986;63:656–60.
31. Hartwell D, Hassager C, Christiansen C. Effect of vitamin D2 and vitamin D3 on the serum concentrations of 1,25(OH)2D2 in normal subjects. Acta Endocrinol (Copenh). 1987;115:378–84.
32. Chel V, Wijnhoven HA, Smit JH, Ooms M, Lips P. Efficacy of different doses and time intervals of oral vitamin D supplementation with or without calcium in elderly nursing home residents. Osteoporos Int. 2008;19(5):663–71.
33. Demetriou ET, Travison TG, Holick MF. Treatment with 50,000 IU vitamin D2 every other week and effect on serum 25-hydroxyvitamin D2, 25-hydroxyvitamin D3, and total 25-hydroxyvitamin D in a clinical setting. Endocr Pract. 2012;18(3):399–402. doi:10.4158/EP11268.OR.
34. Macdonald HM, Wood AD, Tang JCY, Fraser WD. Comparison of vitamin D2 and vitamin D3 supplementation in increasing serum 25-hydroxyvitamin D status: a systematic review and meta-analysis. Am J Clin Nutr. 2012;96(5):1152–3.
35. Cashman KD, Kiely M, Seamans KM, Urbain P. Effect of ultraviolet light–exposed mushrooms on vitamin D status: liquid chromatography–tandem mass spectrometry reanalysis of biobanked sera from a randomized controlled trial and a systematic review plus meta-analysis. J Nutr. 2016; 146(3):565–75.
36. Biancuzzo RM, Clarke N, Reitz RE, Travison TG, Holick MF. Serum concentrations of 1,25-dihydroxyvitamin D2 and 1,25-dihydroxyvitamin D3 in response to vitamin D2 and vitamin D3 supplementation. J Clin Endocrinol Metab. 2013;98(3):973–9. doi:10.1210/jc.2012-2114.
37. Dickert N, Grady C. What's the price for a research subject? Approaches to payment for research participation. N Engl J Med. 1999;341(3):198–203.
38. Alvi SN, Yusuf A, Hammami MM. Simultaneous quantification of vitamin D-2, vitamin D-3, and their 25-hydroxy metabolites in human plasma by high performance liquid chromatography. J Bioequiv Availab. 2012;S14:1–5.
39. Randomization.com. Dallal GE. http://www.randomization.com/. Accessed 1 Feb 2017.
40. Heaney RP, Davies KM, Chen TC, Holick MF, Barger-Lux MJ. Human serum 25-hydroxycholecalciferol response to extended oral dosing with cholecalciferol. Am J Clin Nutr. 2003;77(1):204–10.
41. Cashman KD, Seamans KM, Lucey AJ, Stöcklin E, Weber P, Kiely M, Hill TR. Relative effectiveness of oral 25-hydroxyvitamin D3 and vitamin D3 in raising wintertime serum 25-hydroxyvitamin D in older adults. Am J Clin Nutr. 2012;95(6):1350–6.
42. Romagnoli E, Mascia ML, Cipriani C, Fassino V, Mazzei F, D'Erasmo E, Carnevale V, Scillitani A, Minisola S. Short and long term variations in serum calciotropic hormones after single very large dose of ergocalciferol (vitamin D2) or cholecalciferol (vitamin D3) in the elderly. J Clin Endocrinol Metab. 2008;93:3015–20.
43. Hymøller L, Jensen SK. Vitamin D2 impairs utilization of vitamin D3 in high-yielding dairy cows in a cross-over supplementation regimen. J Dairy Sci. 2011;94(7):3462–6. doi:10.3168/jds.2010-4111.
44. Tjellesen L, Hummer L, Christiansen C, Rødbro P. Serum concentration of vitamin D metabolites during treatment with vitamin D2 and D3 in normal premenopausal women. Bone Miner. 1986;1(5):407–13.
45. Samuel L, Borrell LN. The effect of body mass index on adequacy of serum 25-hydroxyvitamin D levels in US adults: the National Health and Nutrition Examination Survey 2001 to 2006. Ann Epidemiol. 2014;24(10):781–4.
46. Lin E, Armstrong-Moore D, Liang Z, Sweeney JF, Torres WE, Ziegler TR, Tangpricha V, Gletsu-Miller N. Contribution of adipose tissue to plasma 25-hydroxyvitamin D concentrations during weight loss following gastric bypass surgery. Obesity (Silver Spring). 2011;19(3):588–94.
47. Aasheim ET, Björkman S, Søvik TT, Engström M, Hanvold SE, Mala T, Olbers T, Bøhmer T. Vitamin status after bariatric surgery: a randomized study of gastric bypass and duodenal switch. Am J Clin Nutr. 2009;90(1):15–22. doi: 10.3945/ajcn.2009.27583.
48. Heaney RP. The Vitamin D requirement in health and disease. J Steroid Biochem Mol Biol. 2005;97(1–2):13–9.
49. Hathcock JN, Shao A, Vieth R, Heaney R. Risk assessment for vitamin D. Am J Clin Nutr. 2007;85(1):6–18.
50. Agarwal R, Hynson JE, Hecht TJ, Light RP, Sinha AD. Short-term vitamin D receptor activation increases serum creatinine due to increased production with no effect on the glomerular filtration rate. Kidney Int. 2011;80(10): 1073–9. doi:10.1038/ki.2011.207.
51. Kim MJ, Frankel AH, Donaldson M, Darch SJ, Pusey CD, Hill PD, Mayr M, Tam FW. Oral cholecalciferol decreases albuminuria and urinary TGF-β1 in patients with type 2 diabetic nephropathy on established renin-angiotensin-aldosterone system inhibition. Kidney Int. 2011;80(8):851–60. doi:10.1038/ki.2011.224.
52. Michelle P, Kayode JB, Hong F, Laurence SM. Increase in vitamin D improves urine protein/creatinine ratio and complement in systemic lupus erythematosus. Arthritis Rheum. 2011;63 Suppl 10:596 [abstract].
53. Battista C, Viti R, Minisola S, Chiodini I, Frusciante V, Scillitani A, Carnevale V. Over-supplementation of vitamin D in two patients with primary hyperparathyroidism. Hormones. 2013;12(4):598–601. doi:10.14310/horm. 2002.1449.

19

Agenesis of internal carotid artery associated with isolated growth hormone deficiency

Stefano Stagi[1*], Giovanna Traficante[2], Elisabetta Lapi[2], Marilena Pantaleo[2], Sabrina Becciani[1], Marzia Mortilla[3], Salvatore Seminara[1] and Maurizio de Martino[1]

Abstract

Background: Agenesis of the internal carotid artery (ICA) is a rare congenital abnormality, sporadically reported to be associated with a combined congenital hypopituitarism. Nevertheless, only a few cases have been extensively described, and none of these have been characterized by an isolated growth hormone (GH) deficiency.

Case presentation: Here, we describe a 17-year old boy referred to our hospital for fatigue, decreased muscle strength and severe headache reported after the cessation of rhGH treatment for a GH deficiency diagnosed at the age of 2 years and 3 months. Magnetic resonance imaging (MRI) showed an adenohypophyseal hypoplasia with a lack of posterior pituitary hyperintensity, whereas MRI angiography indicated the absence of a normal flow void in the left ICA. Endocrinological tests confirmed the GH deficiency (GH peak after growth-hormone-releasing hormone (GHRH) + arginine: 2.42 ng/mL) with a very low IGF-I value (31 ng/mL) and normal function of other pituitary axes.

Conclusion: To the best of our knowledge this is the first confirmed case of an isolated GH deficiency in a patient with ICA agenesis. The presence of an isolated pituitary deficit is unlike to be considered only as an effect of hemodynamic mechanism, suggesting a role for genetic factor(s) as a common cause of these two rare birth defects. Further studies could clarify this issue and the underlying mechanisms to better understand the etiopathogenetic characteristics of this disorder.

Background

Agenesis, aplasia and hypoplasia of the internal carotid artery (ICA) are rare congenital vascular malformations [1]. Of these, agenesis of the ICA is an extremely rare vascular anomaly occurring in less than 0.01 % of the population [2]. A 3:1 left side predominance in the ICA agenesis has been reported [1].

Agenesis of the ICA is rarely associated with congenital hypopituitarism (CH) [3]. CH is also a very rare congenital manifestation presenting either as an isolated hormone deficiency—the most common of which is isolated growth hormone deficiency (IGHD)—or multiple pituitary hormone involvement (combined pituitary hormone deficiencies (CPHD)) [4].

* Correspondence: stefano.stagi@yahoo.it
[1]Paediatric Endocrinology Unit, Health Sciences Department, University of Florence, Anna Meyer Children's University Hospital, Viale Pieraccini 24, 50139 Florence, Italy
Full list of author information is available at the end of the article

The etiology of this association is not clear: even if the blocking of a unilateral blood supply might cause the pituitary hypoplasia, a possible genetic cause, such as complex neural crest differentiation and/or migration disorders, cannot be excluded.

To the best of our knowledge, no more than 12 cases of CPHD associated with ICA have been reported [2, 5–14] (Table 1). However, a case of transient IGHD has been also described even though it may be caused by a reduced flow because of a focal stenosis in the right distal internal carotid artery and right middle cerebral artery due to a moyamoya [15]. Given the rarity of these two conditions, the association is unlikely to be causal, although this possibility cannot be excluded. In this report, we describe for the first time a 17-year-old boy with a confirmed diagnosis of IGHD and we review the literature and discuss the etiology of this association.

Case report

The patient was a 17-year-old boy on rhGH therapy for 14 years because of a GH deficiency that was diagnosed at the age of 2 years and 3 months. Therapy was stopped 9 months before the beginning of symptoms—fatigue, decreased muscle strength and severe headache. However, the patient had not come for retesting one month after discontinuation of rhGH treatment.

The propositus was the first child of non-consanguineous Italian parents. The mother was in treatment for postpartum depression. The maternal grandfather was in treatment for autoimmune hyperthyroidism.

The mother's height was 152 cm and she had menarche at the age of 13; the father's height was 168 cm and he had a normal development. The target height was 166.0 ± 6.0 cm (−1.70 SDS). All auxological data were normalized for chronological age by conversion to standard deviation scores (SDS) that were calculated according to the following formula: patient value - mean of age-related reference value/standard deviation of the age-related reference value [16].

The child was born at 40 weeks of gestation with an uncomplicated delivery. The birth weight was 2970 g (−1.15 SDS), length at birth was 50 cm (−0.30 SDS), and his occipito-frontal head circumference (OFC) was 34 cm (−0.61 SDS). He had neonatal jaundice requiring phototherapy. The child's neuromotor development was normal: he sat at 6 months, walked independently at 12 months, and began to use language at 14 months.

At 6 months, the patient exhibited very deficient growth (Fig. 1a and b). At 2 years and 3 months, he was admitted to our Paediatric Endocrine Unit for an endocrinological evaluation. His height, evaluated according the growth charts compiled by Cacciari *et al.* [17], was 78.6 cm (−2.79 SDS). His weight was 9.830 kg (−2.78 SDS), and his BMI was 15.91 (−0.28 SDS) (Fig. 1a-d). Extensive biochemical, endocrinological and metabolic examinations did not reveal any abnormalities with the exception of plasma concentrations of IGF-I and IGFBP-3 that were low for his age and sex: 27 ng/mL and 1.38 μg/mL, respectively. Thus, GH stimulation tests were performed and showed a reduced response after the clonidine (GH peak of 5.2 ng/mL) and insulin (glucose nadir 2.0 mmol/L at 30 min; GH peak of 3.9 ng/mL) tests. This revealed a GH deficiency (GHD). Bone age was assessed according to the Greulich and Pyle method [18], and it was delayed (1 year and 2 months versus a chronological age of 2 years and 3 months). Brain MRI of the hypophyseal region showed the presence of a pituitary hypoplasia (height 1.8 mm and width 2.7 mm). Consequently, hGH therapy (0.22 mg/kg/wk) was started.

The child responded very well to rhGH treatment (Fig. 1c) and at 3 years and 4 months old, his height was 94.5 cm (−1.14 SDS), weight 12.450 kg (−2.10 SDS), height velocity 15.06 cm/yr (5.05 SDS), and BMI 13.94 (−1.75 SDS). At 4 years and 3 months old, his height was 101.9 cm (−0.82 SDS), his weight was 15.300 kg (−1.24 SDS), his height velocity was 8.05 cm/yr (1.12 SDS), and his BMI was 14.73 (−0.82 SDS).

The onset of puberty occurred at 12 years old with normal onset, timing, tempo, and magnitude of pubertal changes [19]. He stopped rhGH treatment at 16 years and 3 months old when he reached the definitive stature [16]: his height was 170.8 cm (−0.64 SDS) and his weight was 51.800 kg (−1.56 SDS) with a BMI of 17.76 (−1.63 SDS) (Fig. 1c and d).

At 17 years old, his GH secretion was re-tested by the growth-hormone-releasing hormone (GHRH) + arginine test, which is a reliable test of ITT in retesting patients who had undergone GH treatment in childhood [20]. The test confirmed a severe GH deficiency (basal GH value of 0.18 ng/mL; GH peak of 2.42 ng/mL).

MRI angiography was performed because of the severe growth hormone deficiency (GHD) and headache; it confirmed the presence of adenohypophyseal hypoplasia (height 2.5 mm and width 3.5 mm) with a lack of posterior pituitary hyperintensity. The MRI angiography also showed the absence of a normal flow void in the left ICA (Fig. 2).

No abnormal findings were noted in the electrocardiogram. Chromosomal studies of the peripheral lymphocyte cultures revealed a 46,XY normal male karyotype. An array of CGH analyses on the patient's DNA was performed with an Agilent 60 K array platform with a resolution of approximately 100 kb. No genomic imbalances were detected. A complete examination was performed with particular attention to neurology, metabolism, and endocrinology (Table 2). The only abnormal result was a very low IGF-I value (31 ng/mL). In light of these results, the patient restarted rhGH therapy, and his symptoms at the time of referral disappeared.

Discussion

ICA agenesis is a rare congenital abnormality that is very rarely associated with CH. All reported cases refer to patients with CPHD and ICA agenesis although many of these reports did not describe—or only poorly described—the possible associated endocrinological abnormalities and treatments. This had led many to hypothesize a vascular cause of pituitary disorders. Two different theories involving the hemodynamic mechanisms or disorders of differentiation and/or migration of the neural crest have been reported [2].

The ICA originates from the third aortic arch during embryogenesis. However, it is controversial whether the common and external carotids really originate from the same third aortic arch or from the aortic sac [21]. In

Table 1 Review of endocrinological and anatomical characteristics of patients with congenital hypopituitarism and internal carotid malformations

	Sex	Age	Pituitary MRI	Internal carotid RMI	Other characteristics	Molecular studies	References
1	N	N	Not specified (except for normal posterior pituitary).	Absence of ICA and carotid canal.	Not specified.	NP	[14]
2	M	18 m	Pituitary hypoplasia.	Anomaly of right ICA.	TSH, GH, ACTH deficiency. Central diabetes insipidus. Possible hypogonadism.	NP	[13]
3	F	5 m	Absence of anterior pituitary and ectopic pituitary posterior lobe.	Absence of right common carotid artery, right ICA, right anterior cerebral artery.	TSH, ACTH and GH deficiency. No evidence of diabetes insipidus. Genitalia were normal. Single central maxillary incisor.	NP	[7]
4	M	23 year	Absence of anterior pituitary and ectopic pituitary posterior lobe.	Absence of right ICA and carotid canal and A1 segment of the right anterior cerebral artery.	Congenital microphthalmia with cataract and coloboma of the right eye, encephalocele. Hormonal substitution treatments not specified.	NP	[5]
5	M	37 year	Absence of anterior pituitary.	Hypoplasia of right ICA and carotid canal.	Amblyopia of the left eye caused by an optic nerve coloboma, encephalocele. Hormonal substitution treatments not specified.	NP	[5]
6	F	29 year	Pituitary hypoplasia and ectopic pituitary posterior lobe.	Absence of right ICA, carotid canal, and A1 segment of the right anterior cerebral artery.	TSH, ACTH, and GH deficiency. No evidence of diabetes insipidus. Hypogonadism. Chiari I malformation with syringomyelia.	NP	[9]
7	M	5 year	Absence of anterior pituitary and ectopic pituitary posterior lobe.	Absence of left ICA and carotid canal, A1 segment of the left anterior cerebral artery and the anterior communicating artery.	Retrognathia, microphallus, and cryptorchidism. TSH, ACTH, GH deficiency, but no evidence of diabetes insipidus. Possibile hypogonadism.	NP	[10]
8	M	11 year	Pituitary hypoplasia	Absence of left ICA and carotid canal; hypoplasia of A1 segment of left anterior cerebral artery	TSH, ACTH, GH deficiency. Central diabetes insipidus. Microphallus with possible hypogonadism.	NP	[6]
9	F	10 year	Hypoplastic anterior pituitary, flat sella turcica, absent pituitary stalk	Agenesis of the left ICA and the left carotid canal	GH, TSH, gonadotropin deficiency. No evidence of diabetes insipidus. Born out of a consanguineous marriage.	No *HESX1*, *LHX4*, *OTX2* mutations	[8]
10	F	7 month	Adenohypophyseal hypoplasia with a lack of posterior pituitary hyperintensity	Absence of the left ICA	Desaturation episodes, recurrent respiratory infections. Short hands and feet. GH, ACTH and TSH deficiency.	17q24.2 deletion	[3]
11	F	2 year	Adenohypophyseal hypoplasia with a lack of posterior pituitary hyperintensity	Absence of the right ICA	GH, TSH, and gonadotropin deficiency. No clinical evidence of diabetes insipidus.	NP	[11]
12	M	3 week	Absence of anterior pituitary with ectopic posterior pituitary	Absence of the left ICA and carotid canal	GH, TSH, ACTH and gonadotropin deficiency. Microphallus.	NP	[12]
13	M	17 year	Adenohypophyseal hypoplasia with a lack of posterior pituitary hyperintensity	Agenesis of the left ICA	GH deficiency. No other pituitary deficiencies. No clinical evidence of diabetes insipidus.	Normal array-CGH	Our case

NP not performed

patients presenting a vascular anomaly of the ICA, the blood supply of the affected side is partially or completely compensated by the vertebrobasilar or contralateral ICA system. This is characterized by the enlargement of a normally existing segment or presence of abnormal or persisting fetal arteries [22]. In most patients, this vascular anomaly is asymptomatic [23], and the rarity of a pediatric ICA agenesis diagnosis suggests that the arterial collateral pathways are initially sufficient to support cerebral perfusion [24]. However, some patients may experience recurrent headaches, blurred vision, hemiparesis, and hypopituitarism [25, 26] likely due to cerebrovascular insufficiency, compression by collateral vessels, or associated cerebral aneurysms [21]. Moreover, the symptoms

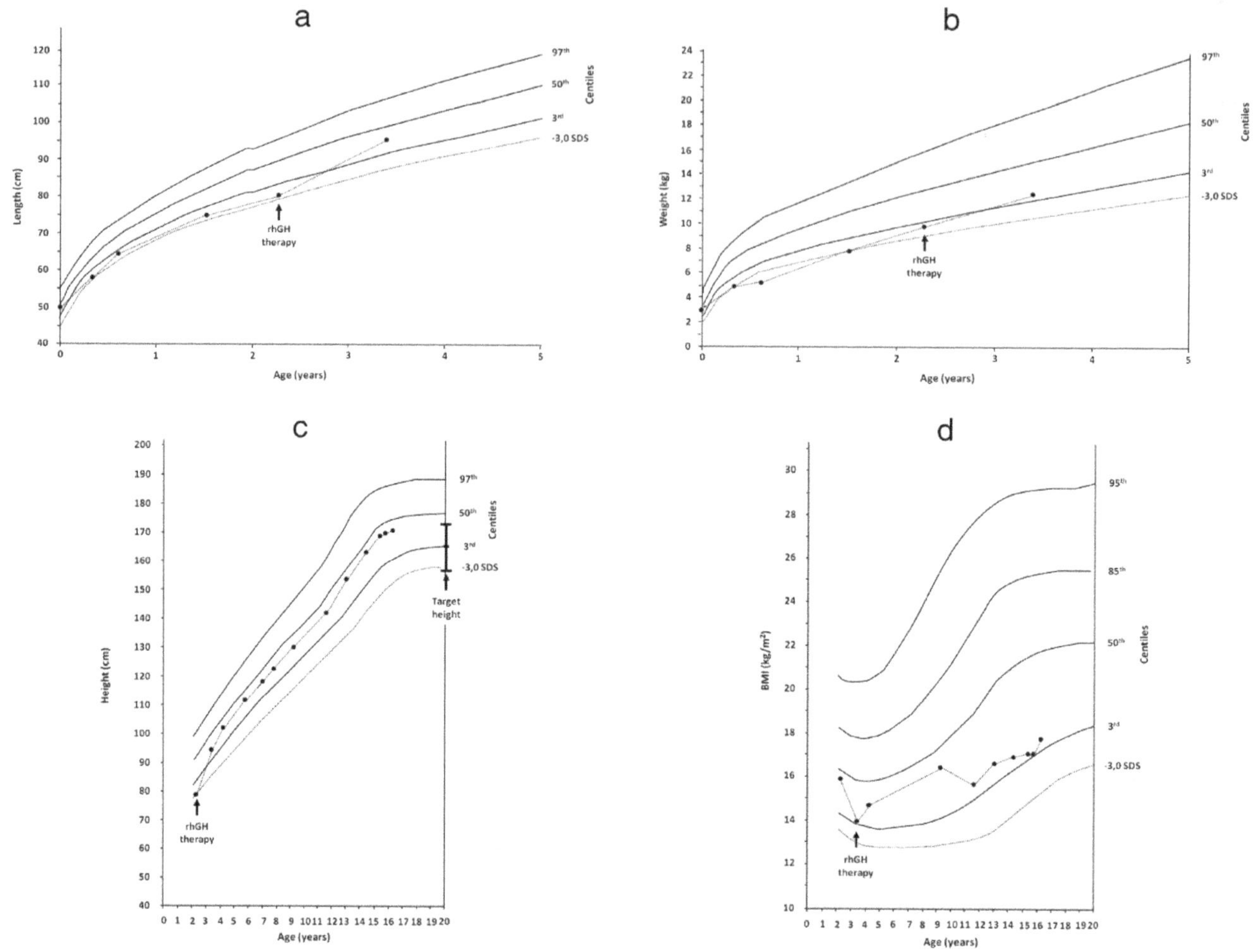

Fig. 1 Length (**a**), weight (**b**), height (**c**) and body mass index (BMI; **d**) growth charts of the patient. The growth charts of the length and weight refer to the first 3 years 4 months of life. The arrows indicate the age at which growth hormone treatment was initiated (black arrow). The length and the weight were evaluated according the growth charts compiled by de Onis et al. [37]. The height and BMI were evaluated according the growth charts compiled by Cacciari et al. [17]

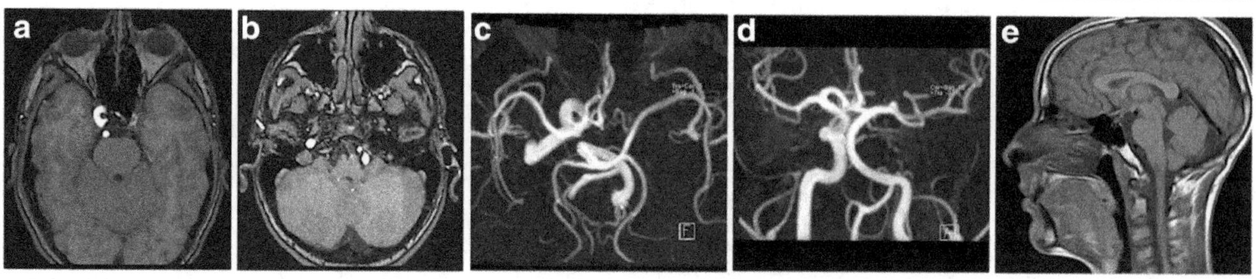

Fig. 2 A MRI angiography time-of-flight (TOF) three-dimensional (3D) technique through the circle of Willis revealed agenesis of the intracranial portion of the left internal carotid artery (ICA). **a**. 3D TOF in the axial plane at the carotid siphon level shows agenesis of the left ICA. **b**. 3D TOF in the axial plane for the vertebrobasilar system shows the left vertebral artery and the compensatory hypertrophy. **c**. MRI angiography maximum intensity projection (MIP) reconstruction in the axial plane reveals agenesis of the intracranial portion of the left ICA. **d**. MRI angiography MIP reconstruction in the coronal plane highlights hypertrophy in the left vertebral collateral blood flow. **e**. Sagittal T1W TSE sequence shows adenohypophyseal hypoplasia (height 2.5 mm and width 3.5 mm) with a lack of posterior pituitary hyperintensity

Table 2 Laboratory results at left ICA agenesis diagnosis

	Value	Reference values		Value	Reference values
FreeT4, pmol/L	12.4	10.3–19.4	HbA1c, %	4.4	<5.5
TSH, mIU/L	1.20	0.40–4.0	Na^+, mEq/L	138	135–145
Cortisol, μg/dL	16.8	5.0–19.0	K^+, mEq/L	4.2	3.5–5.0
ACTH, ng/L	25.7	9.0–52.0	Cl^-, mEq/L	101	95–105
Prolactin, mIU/L	271	87.0–392.0	Plasma osmolality, mOsm/kg	295	280–300
Total testosterone, ng/mL	378	270.0–1070.0	Urine Osmolality, mOsm/kg	1037	400–1100

TSH thyroid-stimulating hormone, *ACTH* adrenocorticotrophic hormone

reported by our patient were probably the result of both GHD (fatigue, decreased muscle strength, etc.) and ICA agenesis (headache).

Only one of the 13 patients previously described in the literature had MRI evidence of associated vascular defects. This patient had transient GH deficiency and was described by Quah *et al.* [15]. This patient's pituitary defects and neurological symptoms may have been caused by reduced flow due to a focal stenosis of the other distal internal carotid artery and right middle cerebral artery due to a moyamoya [15]. However, the presence of a defect in the vascular perfusion is difficult to reconcile with the pituitary anatomical abnormalities and with the variability of the endocrinological defects reported including isolated GH deficiency or central diabetes insipidus (described only rarely) [6, 15].

The ICA is formed in embryos during the fourth week from the third aortic arch arteries and during the fifth and sixth weeks from the terminal segments of the dorsal aorta [27]. Conversely, the pituitary gland fully develops due to merging of the Rathke pouch and the infundibulum by the eighth week of gestation. The blood supply of the anterior and posterior pituitary gland comes from the bilateral superior and inferior hypophyseal arteries arising from the ICA [28]. It is not clear why pituitary hypoplasia would result from blocking of a unilateral blood supply and from abnormalities of the hypophyseal anatomy such as adenohypophysis hypoplasia and aplasia. However, the presence of ectopic neurophypophysis, which has been described in some patients, or other hypophyseal abnormalities, may also suggest a genetic etiology.

Pituitary gland development and function depend on the sequential temporal and spatial expression of multiple transcription factor genes such as *POU1F1* (*POU class 1 homeobox 1*; OMIM 173110), *PROP1* (*prophet of PIT1*; OMIM 601538), *HESX1* (*homeobox gene expressed in ES cells*; OMIM 601802), *LHX3* (*LIM homeobox gene 3*; OMIM 600577), *LHX4* (*LIM homeobox gene 4*; OMIM 602146), *SOX3* (*SRY-related HMG-box gene 3*; OMIM 313430), and *OTX2* (*orthodenticle homolog 2*; OMIM 600037) [4]. However, these defects may cause a deficiency in one or more pituitary hormones. Its clinical features vary in both severity and time of presentation, and onset may occur in the neonatal period or develop later in life [29–31]. In some patients, the hormonal deficiencies may present as a part of a syndrome with patients manifesting abnormalities in structures that share a common embryological origin with the pituitary gland [29–31].

In our review 6 patients, in addition to our, had a pituitary hypoplasia [3, 6, 8, 9, 11, 13]. This abnormality was isolated in two cases [6, 13], associated with ectopic neurohypophysis [9], absent pituitary stalk [8], or associated with a lack of posterior pituitary hyperintensity [3, 11]. However 5 patients had an absent adenohypophysis [5, 7, 10, 12] and 4 associated of these showed an ectopic neurohypophysis [5, 7, 10, 12].

Moreover, ectopic neurohypophysis may be accompanied by midline brain defects [32] supporting an embryological defect due to genetic factors [32, 33]. This has been reported in idiopathic GH deficiency or in subjects with *HESX1*, *LHX4*, and *SOX3* gene mutations [34]. For example, both the *SOX3* under- and over-expression may result in CPHD or IGHD in males, associated with infundibular hypoplasia, ectopic/undescended posterior pituitary, and abnormalities of the corpus callosum [35]. In these patients, congenital abnormalities of the ICA or other vessels have not been reported [35]. However, the associated midline anomalies (coloboma, single central maxillary tooth, transsphenoidal encephalocele, and Chiari I malformation) reported in some cases [5, 7, 9, 15] may support this hypothesis.

Of the patients in our review, one case had unilateral agenesis of the internal carotid artery associated with CPHD without *HESX1*, *LHX4*, or *OTX2* mutations [8]. Moreover, Savasta *et al.* [3] recently reported a CNV (copy number variant) i.e. a paternally inherited 200-kb deletion in 17q24.2. Thus, we performed array-CGH in our patient, but discovered no genomic imbalances. However, we indicate the need for further molecular analysis by NGS techniques to discover possible molecular abnormalities associated with this syndrome.

Given the rarity of the two conditions, the association is unlikely to be causal, although this cannot be excluded [36]. So, we hypothesize that an unknown gene mutation is the most likely explanation for the anatomical defects seen in these patients, suggesting a role for genetic factor(s) as a common cause of these two birth defects.

Conclusions

Here were report the first case of a confirmed isolated GH deficiency in a patient with ICA agenesis. Our experience suggests the opportunity to carefully evaluate possible vascular abnormalities in case of IGHD or CPHD. The presence of an isolated pituitary deficit, and the rare association between the two conditions, suggest a genetic rather than a hemodynamic mechanism. Further studies, especially with NGS-based molecular analysis, could clarify this issue and the underlying mechanisms to better understand the etiopathogenetic characteristics of this disorder.

Abbreviations

ACTH: Adrenocorticotrophic hormone; CH: Congenital hypopituitarism; CPHD: Combined pituitary hormone deficiencies; GH: Growth hormone; GHD: Growth hormone deficiency; GHRH: Growth-hormone-releasing hormone; ICA: Internal carotid artery; IGHD: Isolated growth hormone deficiency; MRI: Magnetic resonance image; TSH: Thyroid-stimulating hormone.

Competing interests

Stefano Stagi (SStagi), Giovanna Traficante (GT), Elisabetta Lapi (EL), Marilena Pantaleo (MP), Sabrina Becciani (SB), Marzia Mortilla (MM), Salvatore Seminara (SSeminara) and Maurizio de Martino (MdM) have no financial interests to disclose and no conflict of interest to declare.

Authors' contributions

SStagi carried out the endocrinological evaluation, conceived of the study, and participated in its design. GT performed the clinical genetic evaluation, conceived of the study, and participated in its design. EL performed the clinical genetic evaluation, and revised critically the manuscript. MP performed the molecular genetic studies, participated in the acquisition of data, and was involved in drafting the manuscript. SB performed the endocrinological evaluation, participated in the acquisition of data, and was involved in drafting the manuscript. MM performed the neuroradiological evaluation, was involved in drafting, and revised critically the manuscript. SSeminara performed the endocrinological evaluation and revised critically the manuscript. MdM participated in the endocrinological evaluation and participated in its coordination. All authors read and approved the final manuscript.

Acknowledgements

The authors would like to thank the patient's family.

Author details

[1]Paediatric Endocrinology Unit, Health Sciences Department, University of Florence, Anna Meyer Children's University Hospital, Viale Pieraccini 24, 50139 Florence, Italy. [2]Genetics and Molecular Medicine Unit, Anna Meyer Children's University Hospital, Florence, Italy. [3]Radiology Unit, Anna Meyer Children's University Hospital, Florence, Italy.

References

1. Clarós P, Bandos R, Gilea I, Clarós Jr A, Capdevila A, García Rodríguez J, et al. Major congenital anomalies of the internal carotid artery: agenesis, aplasia and hypoplasia. Int J Pediatr Otorhinolaryngol. 1999;49:69–76.
2. Lee JH, Oh CW, Lee SH, Han DH. Aplasia of the internal carotid artery. Acta Neurochir (Wien). 2003;145:117–25.
3. Savasta S, Merli P, Introzzi F, Strocchio L, Lanati G, Incorpora G, et al. Agenesis of internal carotid artery and hypopituitarism: case report and review of literature. J Clin Endocrinol Metab. 2012;97:3414–20.
4. Kelberman D, Rizzoti K, Lovell-Badge R, Robinson IC, Dattani MT. Genetic regulation of pituitary gland development in human and mouse. Endocr Rev. 2009;30:790–829.
5. Blustajn J, Netchine I, Frédy D, Bakouche P, Piekarski JD, Meder JF. Dysgenesis of the internal carotid artery associated with transsphenoidal encephalocele: a neural crest syndrome? AJNR Am J Neuroradiol. 1999;20:1154–7.
6. Inamo Y, Harada K. Agenesis of the internal carotid artery and congenital pituitary hypoplasia: proposal of a cause of congenital hypopituitarism. Eur J Pediatr. 2003;162:610–2.
7. Kjellin IB, Kaiserman KB, Curran JG, Geffner ME. Aplasia of right internal carotid artery and hypopituitarism. Pediatr Radiol. 1999;29:586–8.
8. Lamine F, Kanoun F, Chihaoui M, Saveanu A, Menif E, Barlier A, et al. Unilateral agenesis of internal carotid artery associated with congenital combined pituitary hormone deficiency and pituitary stalk interruption without HESX1, LHX4 or OTX2 mutation: a case report. Pituitary. 2012;15 Suppl 1:S81–6.
9. Mellado JM, Merino X, Ramos A, Salvadó E, Saurí A. Agenesis of the internal carotid artery with a trans-sellar anastomosis: CT and MRI findings in late-onset congenital hypopituitarism. Neuroradiology. 2001;43:237–41.
10. Moon WJ, Porto L, Lanfermann H, Weis R, Zanella FE. Agenesis of internal carotid artery associated with congenital anterior hypopituitarism. Neuroradiology. 2002;44:138–42.
11. Seixas D, Ayres-Basto M, Fontoura M, Silva ML, Fonseca J. Agenesis of the internal carotid artery and hypogenesis of the pituitary gland: cause, consequence or coincidence? Neuroradiol J. 2006;19:629–32.
12. Shulman DI, Martinez CR. Association of ectopic posterior pituitary and anterior pituitary hypoplasia with absence of the left internal carotid. J Pediatr Endocrinol Metab. 1996;9:539–42.
13. Tanaka R, Tokuda M, Shinakawa S, Okasora K, Suzuki S, Konishi K. A multiple pituitary hormone deficiency patient with anomaly of internal carotid artery, Proc 21st International Symposium on Growth Hormone and Growth Factors in Endocrinology and Metabolism, Venice. 1996.
14. Triulzi F, Scotti G, di Natale B, Pellini C, Lukezic M, Scognamiglio M, et al. Evidence of a congenital midline brain anomaly in pituitary dwarfs: a magnetic resonance imaging study in 101 patients. Pediatrics. 1994;93:409–16.
15. Quah BL, Hamilton J, Blaser S, Héon E, Tehrani NN. Morning glory disc anomaly, midline cranial defects and abnormal carotid circulation: an association worth looking for. Pediatr Radiol. 2005;35:525–8.
16. Stagi S, Galli L, Cecchi C, Chiappini E, Losi S, Gattinara CG, et al. Final height in patients perinatally infected with the human immunodeficiency virus. Horm Res Paediatr. 2010;74:165–71.
17. Cacciari E, Milani S, Balsamo A, Spada E, Bona G, Cavallo L, et al. Italian cross-sectional growth charts for height, weight and BMI (2 to 20 year). J Endocrinol Invest. 2006;29:581–93.
18. Greulich WW, Pyle SI. Radiographic Atlas of Skeletal Development of the Hand and Wrist. Stanford, CA: Stanford University Press; 1959.
19. Tanner JM, Whitehouse RH. Clinical longitudinal standards for height, weight, height velocity, weight velocity, and stages of puberty. Arch Dis Child. 1976;51:170–9.
20. Aimaretti G, Baffoni C, Bellone S, Di Vito L, Corneli G, Arvat E, et al. Retesting young adults with childhood-onset growth hormone (GH) deficiency with GH-releasing-hormone-plus-arginine test. J Clin Endocrinol Metab. 2000;85:3693–9.
21. Quint DJ, Boulos RS, Spera TD. Congenital absence of the cervical and petrous internal carotid artery with intercavernous anastomosis. AJNR Am J Neuroradiol. 1989;10:435–9.
22. Midkiff RB, Boykin MW, McFarland DR, Bauman JA. Agenesis of the internal carotid artery with intercavernous anastomosis. AJNR Am J Neuroradiol. 1995;16:1356–9.
23. Elazab NE, Riel-Romero RM, Gonzalez-Toledo E. Internal carotid artery agenesis and basilar artery aneurysm with third nerve palsy. Pediatr Neurol. 2010;42:451–4.

24. Mayer PL, Leon Kier E. The ontogenetic and phylogenetic basis of cerebrovascular anomalies and variants. In: Apuzzo MLJ, editor. Brain Surgery: Complications, avoidance and management. 1st ed. New York: Churchill and Livingstone; 1993. p. 741–7.
25. Florio F, Balzano S, Nardella M, Strizzi V, Cammisa M, Bozzini V, et al. Congenital absence of the internal carotid artery. Cardiovasc Intervent Radiol. 1999;22:74–8.
26. Harps E, Helmke K. Diagnosis of congenital absence of internal carotid artery by power angio sonography. Eur Radiol. 1998;8:1245–7.
27. Padget DH. The development of the cranial arteries in the human embryo. Contrib Embryol Carnegie Inst. 1948;32:205–61.
28. Lasjaunias P, Santoyo-Vazquez A. Segmental agenesis of the internal carotid artery: angiographic aspects with embryological discussion. Anat Clin. 1984;6:133–41.
29. Kelberman D, Dattani MT. Hypopituitarism oddities: congenital causes. Horm Res. 2007;68 Suppl 5:138–44.
30. Alatzoglou KS, Dattani MT. Genetic forms of hypopituitarism and their manifestation in the neonatal period. Early Hum Dev. 2009;85:705–12.
31. Romero CJ, Pine-Twaddell E, Radovick S. Novel mutations associated with combined pituitary hormone deficiency. J Mol Endocrinol. 2011;46:R93–R102.
32. Ultmann MC, Siegel SF, Hirsch WL, Finegold DN, Foley Jr TP. Pituitary stalk and ectopic hyperintense T1 signal on magnetic resonance imaging. Implications for anterior pituitary dysfunction. Am J Dis Child. 1993;147:647–52.
33. Chen S, Léger J, Garel C, Hassan M, Czernichow P. Growth hormone deficiency with ectopic neurohypophysis: anatomical variations and relationship between the visibility of the pituitary stalk asserted by magnetic resonance imaging and anterior pituitary function. J Clin Endocrinol Metab. 1999;84:2408–13.
34. di Iorgi N, Secco A, Napoli F, Calandra E, Rossi A, Maghnie M. Developmental abnormalities of the posterior pituitary gland. Endocr Dev. 2009;14:83–94.
35. Stagi S, Lapi E, Pantaleo M, Traficante G, Giglio S, Seminara S, et al. A SOX3 (Xq26.3-27.3) duplication in a boy with growth hormone deficiency, ocular dyspraxia, and intellectual disability: a long-term follow-up and literature review. Hormones (Athens). 2014;13:552–60.
36. Thomas M, Massa G, Craen M, de Zegher F, Bourguignon JP, Heinrichs C, et al. Prevalence and demographic features of childhood growth hormone deficiency in Belgium during the period 1986–2001. Eur J Endocrinol. 2004;151:67–72.
37. de Onis M, Onyango AW, Borghi E, Garza C, Yang H, WHO Multicentre Growth Reference Study Group. Comparison of the World Health Organization (WHO) Child Growth Standards and the National Center for Health Statistics/WHO international growth reference: implications for child health programmes. Public Health Nutr. 2006;9:942–7.

20

Splicing analysis of *CYP11B1* mutation in a family affected with 11β-hydroxylase deficiency

Pattaranatcha Charnwichai[1,2], Patra Yeetong[2,3], Kanya Suphapeetiporn[2,4], Vichit Supornsilchai[5], Taninee Sahakitrungruang[5*] and Vorasuk Shotelersuk[2,4]

Abstract

Background: Congenital adrenal hyperplasia (CAH) due to steroid 11β-hydroxylase deficiency (11β-OHD) is a rare form of CAH associated with low renin hypertension, hypokalemia, hyperandrogenemia and ambiguous genitalia in affected females. Herein we describe the clinical, hormonal and molecular characteristics of two Uzbekistan siblings with 11β-OHD and analyze the effects of a splicing mutation.

Case presentation: A 46,XX girl presented with genital ambiguity and low renin hypertension; her 46,XY brother presented with precocious puberty. Hormonal studies suggested 11β-OHD. Mutation analysis was performed by PCR followed by Sanger sequencing of the entire coding regions and their flanking introns of the *CYP11B1* gene. Mutation analysis showed that both patients were compound heterozygous for IVS7 + 1G > A, and c.421C > T. Although the identified mutations have been previously described, this is, to our knowledge, the first report of these mutations in compound heterozygotes. A minigene assay was used to determine the effects of the splicing mutation. The constructs containing either the wild-type or the splice-site mutant *CYP11B1* genomic DNA of exons-introns 6–9 were transfected into COS-7 cells; subsequently, RNA splicing was assessed by reversed transcribed-PCR of *CYP11B1* complementary DNA. The minigene assay revealed that the IVS7 + 1G > A mutation resulted in two shorter incorrectly spliced products; one skipping the exon 7 and the other skipping the exons 7–8. The c.421C > T mutation leads to the introduction of a premature stop codon at residue 141 (p.R141X). These mutations are expected to code non-functional proteins.

Conclusion: Compound heterozygous mutations (IVS7 + 1G > A and p.R141X) in the *CYP11B1* gene were found to cause 11β-OHD. The IVS7 + 1G > A mutation causes aberrant splicing of *CYP11B1* leading to exon skipping. This finding could facilitate the future novel therapies targeted on splicing modulation to treat human disease.

Keywords: *CYP11B1*, Splicing, Mutation, 11β-hydroxylase deficiency, Congenital adrenal hyperplasia, Case report

Background

11β-hydroxylase deficiency (11β-OHD) caused by mutations in the *CYP11B1* gene accounts for approximately 5–8 % of congenital adrenal hyperplasia (CAH) in non-consanguineous populations, but accounts for ~15 % of cases in both Muslim and Jewish Middle Eastern populations [1]. Steroid 11β-hydroxylase (P450c11β, *CYP11B1*) converts 11-deoxycortisol to cortisol, representing the final step in cortisol biosynthesis, and 11-deoxycorticosterone (DOC) to corticosterone. Thus, deficient P450c11β activity results in impaired cortisol synthesis and accumulation of 11-deoxycortisol and the mineralocorticoid precursor DOC, which leads to significant hypertension, a hallmark feature of this CAH variant [1]. Accumulated steroid precursors are shunted into the androgen synthesis pathway, leading to androgen excess. Classic 11β-OHD results in virilization of the external genitalia in affected females (46,XX disorders of sex development) as well as precocious puberty, accelerated growth and bone maturation in both sexes. Patients with 11β-OHD can have elevated concentrations of 17-hydroxyprogesterone (17OHP), which accumulates two steps behind the enzymatic block, so that 11β-

* Correspondence: Taninee.P@chula.ac.th
[5]Division of Pediatric Endocrinology, Department of Pediatrics, Faculty of Medicine, Chulalongkorn University, Bangkok 10330, Thailand
Full list of author information is available at the end of the article

OHD may be detected by 17OHP newborn screening program [2]. The diagnosis is established by elevated basal concentrations of DOC and 11-deoxycortisol, which hyper respond to ACTH stimulation.

CYP11B1 is located on the long arm of chromosome 8 (8q21), consisting of 9 exons, and encodes 503 amino acids. To date, over 80 mutations in *CYP11B1* gene are described. Most are missense and nonsense mutations, but splice-site mutations, small or gross deletions/insertions, and complex rearrangements with *CYP11B2* have also been identified [3–5]. The majority of *CYP11B1* mutations are associated with classic 11β-OHD, and only a few mutations causing non-classic 11β-OHD which can manifest later in otherwise asymptomatic women with hirsutism, and menstrual irregularities [6, 7].

In this report, we describe two siblings with the clinical and hormonal phenotypes of 11β-OHD and identified compound heterozygous mutations in the *CYP11B1* gene. The splicing mutation was studied in vitro for its functional consequences with a minigene experiment and showed exon-skipping which confirmed the clinical diagnosis.

Case presentation

The patients were siblings from a non-consanguineous Uzbekistan family. *Patient 1* was a 3-yr-old 46,XX female with ambiguous genitalia. She was previously evaluated for her abnormal genital development and underwent first genital surgery in Turkey. On an initial evaluation at age 2 y 8 m, her height was 100 cm (+2.1 SD), her weight was 15.8 kg, (+1.4 SD), blood pressure (BP) was 110/70 mmHg ($94^{th}/96^{th}$ percentiles). The physical examination revealed that the phallus was 5 cm long and 2 cm wide (Prader grade IV); no gonads were palpable in the inguinal region. The areola and palmar creases were pigmented bilaterally. An ACTH stimulation test (250 μg) showed grossly elevated baseline ACTH (238 pg/mL) and basal cortisol of 4.7 μg/dL with non-response to ACTH and moderately elevated progesterone and 17OHP after 60 min; 11-deoxycortisol and androstenedione concentrations were markedly high (Table 1). The serum sodium was 136 mmol/L, potassium 3.1 mmol/L, plasma renin activity (PRA) was very low at 15 ng/dL/h (nl, 171–1115), and aldosterone 2 ng/dL (nl, 3–35). Her total testosterone levels were 132 ng/dL (nl, <3–10) and dehydroepiandrosterone sulfate (DHEAS) 165.2 μg/dL (nl, <5-57). She was followed up at the King Chulalongkorn Memorial Hospital (Bangkok, Thailand) due to the family relocation at age 3 yr for further management. After receiving the results of an ACTH stimulation test, she was started treatment with hydrocortisone, 5 mg thrice daily (10 $mg/m^2/d$) which improved BP into the normal range (90/60 mmHg), suppressed testosterone, and PRA became measurable (200–496 ng/dL/h).

Patient 2 is the younger brother of Patient 1. He presented at 2 years of age with acne and masculinization (isosexual precocious puberty). Physical examination revealed an advanced maturation of external genitalia as well as a low-pitched voice. His Tanner stages were G3 and PH1, and each of his testes was 3 mL in volume. His height was 97 cm (+3.2 SD) and weight was 17 kg (+2.9 SD). Height gain was accelerated from 12-month-old on the growth chart (from +2.6 SD to +3.2 SD). Skin pigmentation appeared consistent with his ethnicity, but no evident mucosal pigmentation. His BP was 110/65 mmHg ($92^{th}/95^{th}$ percentiles). Labs revealed serum Na 136 mmol/L, K 4.3 mmol/L, bicarbonate 24 mmol/L, BUN 12 and Cr 0.3 mg/dL, respectively. An ACTH stimulation test showed elevated baseline ACTH, a low basal cortisol (2.3 μg/dL) with non-response to ACTH and moderately elevated 17OHP after 60 min (Table 1). 11-deoxycortisol concentrations were not measured. PRA was low at 106 ng/dL/h (nl, 171–1115), and low aldosterone 0.2 ng/dL (nl, 3–35). He was then treated with hydrocortisone 2.5 mg thrice daily (11 $mg/m^2/d$). His blood pressure was well controlled, and PRA was increased up to 738 ng/dL/h.

DNA sequencing

Genomic DNA from peripheral blood leucocytes of the patients and their parents was extracted by using the QIAamp® DNA Blood Mini Kit (Qiagen, Valencia, CA) after taking informed consent. The coding sequence of

Table 1 Basal and 60 min post ACTH (250 μg) stimulated adrenal steroid profile

Steroids	Patient 1		Patient 2		Reference values	
	(age 2 y 8 m)		(age 2 y)			
	Basal	Stimulated	Basal	Stimulated	Basal	Stimulated
ACTH (pg/mL)	238	-	150	-	10–65	-
Cortisol (μg/dL)	4.72	4.65	2.3	2.3	3–22	27–50
17-OHP (ng/dL)	2880	2730	1310	2380	13–173	85–250
Progesterone (ng/dL)	464	499	-	-	[a]	[a]
Androstenedione (ng/dL)	2750	2710	-	-	<10-48	<10–87
11-deoxycortisol (ng/dL)	15100	-	-	-	7-210	95–323

[a]*Note*: Reference values are unavailable

CYP11B1 gene including exon-intron boundaries was amplified in eight fragments using specific primers (Table 2). PCR products were treated with *ExoSAP-IT* (USP Corporation, Cleveland, OH), and sent for direct sequencing at Macrogen Inc. (Seoul, Korea). Analyses were performed by Sequencher 4.2 (Gene Codes Corporation, Ann Arbor, MI).

Minigene construction and splicing analysis

We performed a minigene in vitro experiment of the *CYP11B1* splicing mutation. A segment of the wild-type (WT) and mutant (IVS7 + 1G > A) genomic DNA (gDNA) of *CYP11B1* gene consisting of exons 6 to 9 and their in-between introns was amplified by PCR using the oligonucleotides listed in Table 2. We used the gDNA of a normal control and the patient with IVS7 + 1G > A *CYP11B1* mutation as a template of minigene constructs. PCR reactions were carried out in a 20 μl volume containing 50 ng gDNA, 10xPCR buffer, 25 mM $MgCl_2$, 10 μM dNTPs, 5 U/μl *Taq polymerase* and 10 μM of each primer, using the following parameters: 30s at 94 °C, 30s at 60 °C and 1.30 min at 72 °C. The PCR product was cleaved with *BamHI-HF* and *XbaI* enzymes and cloned into the corresponding sites of pcDNA™3.1/myc-His B mammalian expression vector (Invitrogen, Carlsbad, CA) using *T4 DNA ligase* (New England BioLabs, UK). The wild-type and mutant vectors were confirmed by direct sequencing using NCBI Reference Sequences (RefSeq) NG_007954.1 as the genomic reference and NM_000497.3 as the mRNA reference.

COS-7 cells were cultured in Dulbecco's Modified Eagles Medium, High Glucose (HyClone Laboratories, Logan, UT) supplemented with 10 % fetal bovine serum (Sigma-Aldrich, Singapore) and 0.01 % penicillin/streptomycin (HyClone Laboratories) at 37 °C in a humidified 5 % CO_2 incubator. Cells were grown on 6-well plates and transiently transfected with the wild-type and mutant minigene constructs (1 μg) using Effectene® Transfection Reagent (Qiagen). Cells incubated for 48 h after transfection and then were washed 3 times with PBS and kept frozen at − 20 °C. Total cellular RNA was extracted using QIAamp® RNA Blood Mini Kit (Qiagen) and treated with *DNaseI* (Qiagen). The RNAs were then used as template for cDNA synthesis using ImProm-II™ Reverse Transcription System (Promega Corporation, Madison, WI). Finally, both the WT and mutant cDNAs were amplified by PCR using the same primers and conditions as used for the minigene construction. The PCR products were analyzed by electrophoresis on a 1 % agarose gel followed by staining with ethidium bromide. Each PCR product was confirmed by Sanger sequencing after subcloning into pGEM®-T Easy vectors (Promega).

Results

Mutation analysis

DNA sequencing of the entire coding regions and their flanking introns of the *CYP11B1* gene showed that both siblings were compound heterozygous for a nonsense mutation c.421C > T in its exon 3 (NCBI RefSeq NG_007954.1), causing the introduction of a premature stop codon at residue 141 (p.R141X); and a splice site mutation, c.1200 + 1G > A which is at the 5' donor splice site of the intron 7 (IVS7 + 1G > A). These identified mutations were reported previously [8–10], but their pathogenic mechanisms have not clearly been elucidated. Sequence analysis of the parental gDNA demonstrated that the mother was heterozygous for the c.421C > T mutation and the father, heterozygous for the c.1200 + 1G > A mutation (Fig. 1).

Minigene analysis of the splice site mutation

We hypothesized that the c.1200 + 1G > A (IVS7 + 1G > A) mutation located at the splicing donor site of intron 7 would create an abnormal splicing of the mRNA. To examine this possibility, we constructed expression vectors containing the WT and the mutant c.1200 + 1G > A *CYP11B1* minigene sequence from exons 6 to 9 (Fig. 2a). The resultant minigenes were transfected into COS-7 cells. Then, total RNA was isolated and analyzed by the RT-PCR method. We found that the mutant c.1200 + 1G > A *CYP11B1* minigene was processed to two major incorrectly spliced products which were shorter than the WT minigene (Fig. 2b). Sequence analysis of the RT-PCR products after subcloning into pGEM®-T Easy vector revealed that one of the mutant

Table 2 Sequences of oligonucleotide primers used for PCR amplification and minigene construction

Primer	Sense Strand	Antisense Strand
CYP11B1_Exon 1	5'- GTTCTCCCATGACGTGATCCCTCT – 3'	5'- TCCAAAGGATGCAGAGTGCC – 3'
CYP11B1_Exon 2	5' – TGGACAGGAGACACTTTGGAT – 3'	5' – TCGCCGCTTACAGCAAGAAC – 3'
CYP11B1_Exon 3–4	5' – TGGGGACAAGGAGGATGGGATAC – 3'	5' – TGGTGGAGAGGGAGAAATTGGG – 3'
CYP11B1_Exon 4	5' – CGTGGGAAGATCCAGCCTCAG – 3'	5' – GGAAGGTGAGGAATCCCCGAC – 3'
CYP11B1_Exon 5	5' – AGGAGGAGGACACTGAAGGATG – 3'	5' – AGGCAGGCTTGGCATCACC – 3'
CYP11B1_Exon 6	5' – GGCTCTGTCGTTCTCAGGGTATGC – 3'	5' – GGCGTTGAAGAGGGATTCCAGAG – 3'
CYP11B1_Exon 7–8	5' – AGAGAGCACAGGAAGCCCCATC – 3'	5' – CAGTCCCACATTGCTCAAGC – 3'
CYP11B1_Exon 9	5' – GTTCCCCCTTCAGCATAATCTC – 3'	5' – GCCCTCGGGAGTTCCATTT – 3'
CYP11B1_IVS7_construct	5' - AGTCGGATCCCTTGCTGATGACGCTCTTTG - 3'	5'- GTACTCTAGAATGGCTCTGAAGGTGAGGAG - 3'

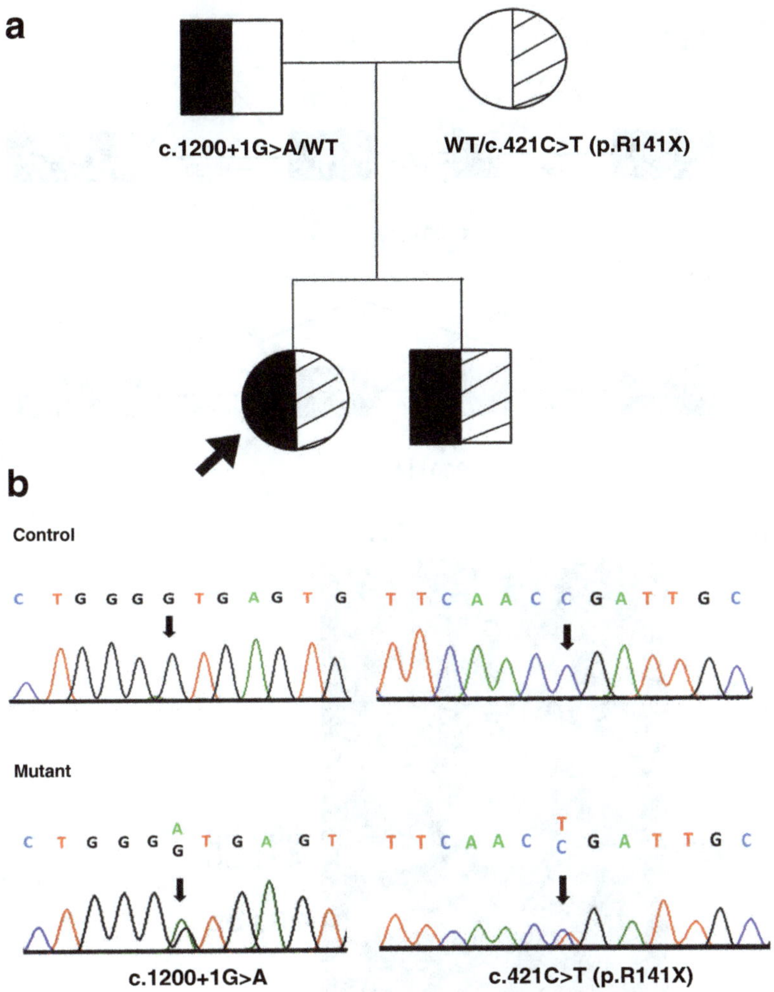

Fig. 1 Mutation analysis by direct DNA sequencing. **a** Family tree. The arrow indicates our proband. Both siblings carried compound heterozygous mutations; the point mutation at position bp 421 (c.421C > T) leads to the substitution of arginine to stop at amino acid position 141 (p.R141X), and the base change from G to A at the first position in intron 7 (c.1200 + 1G > A or IVS7 + 1G > A). The father is heterozygous for the c.1200 + 1G > A mutation and the mother is heterozygous for p.R141X. **b** Electropherograms of the patient and a healthy control

fragments skipped the entire exon 7, while containing the full-length sequences of exons 6, 8, 9. The other mutant PCR product skipped the exons 7 and 8, while retaining full-length sequences of exons 6 and 9 (Fig. 2c).

Discussion

In this study, we have described two severe *CYP11B1* mutations found in two siblings diagnosed with classic 11β-OHD in a family from Uzbekistan. Virilization and hypertension are the main clinical features of the classic 11β-OHD. Despite inability of aldosterone synthesis, overproduction of DOC, which is a less potent mineralocorticoid, causes salt retention and hypertension. However, affected newborns may have mild, transient salt loss presumably due to relatively high mineralocorticoids resistance in the newborn period [11]. Signs of mineralocorticoid excess generally correlate poorly with the degree of virilization in affected girls [3]. Blood pressure is usually normal during infancy and hypertension is often identified later in toddlerhood or in childhood, although its presence in infancy was demonstrated [12].

Most of the *CYP11B1* mutations described to date result in the classic form of 11β-OHD. Unlike 21-hydroxylase deficiency, molecular-genetic studies of 11β-OHD are relatively fewer, and a number of identified *CYP11B1* mutations have not been functionally characterized [5, 13]. Therefore, the exact genotype-phenotype prediction of 11β-OHD has not been well established. Previous studies showed that in vitro activities less than 5 % were considered severe and consistent with classic 11β-OHD [5, 13]. In this present study, we describe two siblings suffering from classic 11β-OHD who were compound heterozygous for a nonsense and a splice-site *CYP11B1* mutations. The nonsense p. R141X is expected

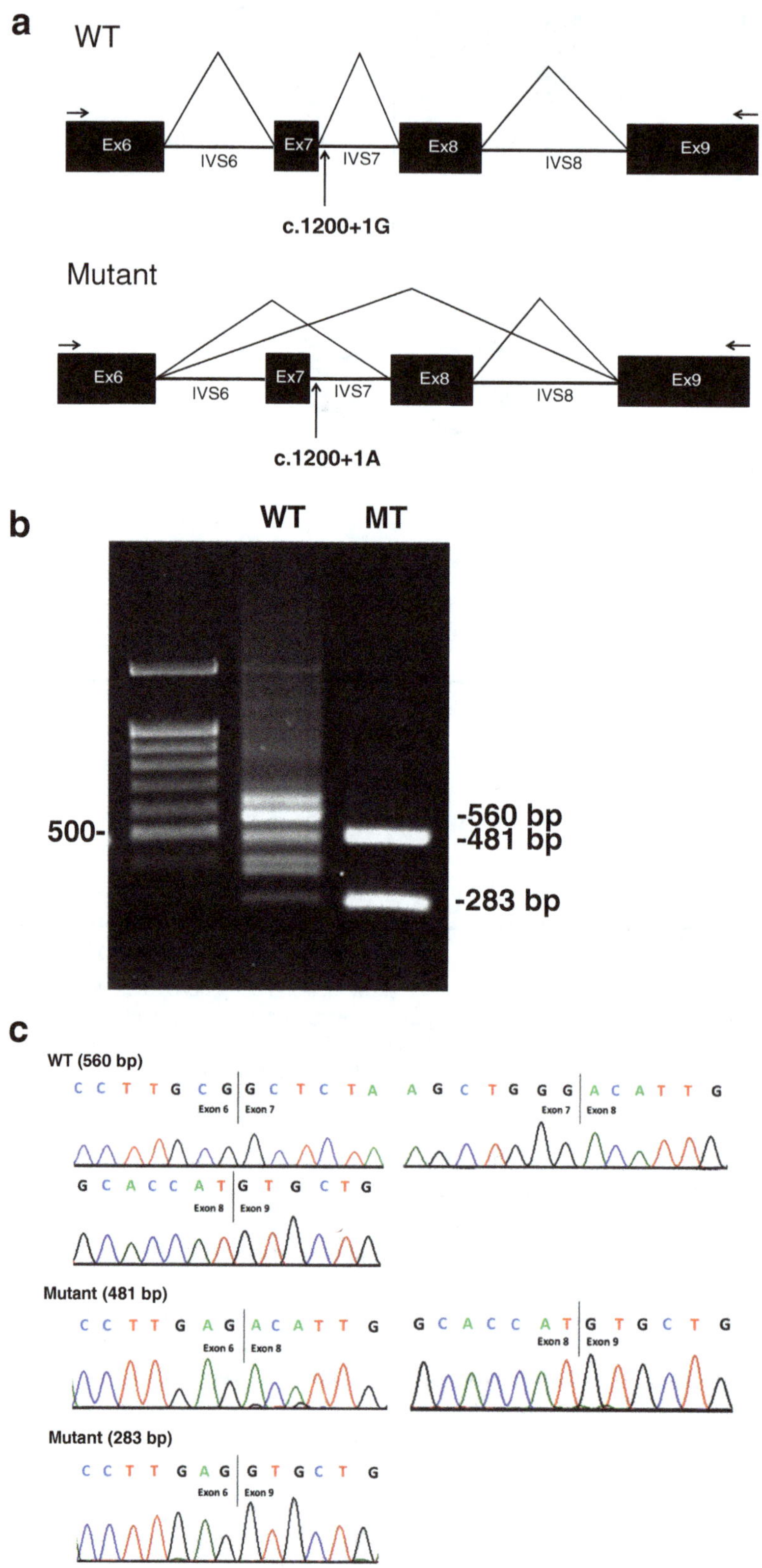

Fig. 2 (See legend on next page.)

(See figure on previous page.)
Fig. 2 Minigene experiment. **a** The scheme shows the set-up of the minigene constructs for the splicing analysis in the WT and mutant expression vectors containing c.1200 + 1G > A mutation (arrows). **b** COS-7 cells were transfected with the wild-type (WT) or mutant (MT) minigene constructs. Total RNA from the transfected cells were used for RT-PCR of *CYP11B1* cDNA. The figure shows the expected 560-bp PCR product from the WT construct and two shorter incorrectly spliced products from the mutant, sized 481 and 283 bp on an agarose gel. **c** Electropherograms of the minigene PCR products. The 481 bp mutant fragments skipped the entire exon 7, while containing the full-length sequences of exons 6, 8, 9. The 283 bp mutant PCR product skipped the exons 7 and 8, while retaining full-length sequences of exons 6 and 9. Black lines indicated exon–exon boundaries

to lead to a premature stop in the exon 3 and yields a truncated enzyme lacking the essential residues for heme binding domain, consistent with our patients' clinical phenotypes and near-completely abolished in vitro CYP11B1 activity in a recent study [14].

In addition, we identified a previously described IVS7 + 1G > A mutation in *CYP11B1* affecting the consensus slice donor site of the exon 7. The minigene experiment confirmed that this splice site mutation caused exon skipping (either a complete loss of the exon 7 or both exons 7 and 8). Most reported *CYP11B1* mutations are located in exons 6, 7, and 8 and 70 % of amino acid sequences in these exons are identical in human, ox, rat, and mouse, suggesting that exons 6–8 are essential for the enzymatic activity of CYP11B1 [15]. Recently, Nguyen et al. [9] studied a minigene experiment of this same mutation. Nonetheless, the authors designed a shorter minigene construct which had only exon 7, intron 7, and exon 8. They found that the IVS7 + 1G > A mutation caused an intron retention.

Splicing errors are well recognized causes of genetic diseases. Previous data point to an estimated frequency of sequence variations affect pre-mRNA splicing up to 50 % of the alleles causing human disease [16, 17]. Splice site nucleotide substitutions may result in skipping of the involved exon, intron retention, creation of a pseudo-exon within intron, usage of a cryptic splice site, or a combination of several of these [18, 19]. Hence, the design of minigene constructs is important to correctly identify the splicing effect of specific splice site mutations. Recent data have suggested that cassette exon skipping is the most common alternative splicing event in humans [19, 20]. To date, a +1G > A substitution at the 5'-splice donor site has been identified in a number of human diseases [21]. Functional studies of other +1G > A 5'-splice site mutations have shown either recognition of a 5'-cryptic splice site or exon skipping [22]. Therefore, we have designed the minigene constructs including exons 6–9 and introns 6–8 and our results confirmed that the IVS7 + 1G > A mutant construct results in exon skipping. To date, the therapies to modulate RNA mis-splicing using antisense oligonucleotide or small molecules are emerging [19]. The understanding of definite genetic mechanism could expand opportunities for gene therapy. Modulation of aberrant splicing transcripts can become a novel therapeutic approach for many diseases caused by splice site defects.

Conclusions

In summary, we describe two compound heterozygous *CYP11B1* mutations that severely affect normal protein structure explaining a severe phenotype of classic 11β-hydroxylase deficiency. Our findings suggest the mutation IVS7 + 1G > A causes aberrant splicing of *CYP11B1* leading to exon skipping. Our findings may help for better understanding of splice site mutation mechanism and facilitate the future new therapies targeted on splicing modulation to treat human disease.

Abbreviations

11β-OHD, 11β-hydroxylase deficiency; 17OHP, 17-hydroxyprogesterone; ACTH, adrenocorticotropic hormone; CAH, congenital adrenal hyperplasia; DHEAS, dehydroepiandrosterone sulfate; DOC, 11-deoxycorticosterone; gDNA, genomic DNA; mRNA, messenger RNA; MT, mutant; nl, normal; PCR, polymerase chain reaction; PRA, plasma renin activity; RT-PCR, reverse transcription polymerase chain reaction; WT, wild-type

Funding

This study was supported by the Thailand Research Fund grant no.RSA5780054 (to T.S.), RTA56800003 (to V.S.), and the Chulalongkorn Academic Advancement into Its 2nd Century Project. P.C. was supported by the scholarship from the Graduate Scholarship to commemorate the 72nd Anniversary of His Majesty King Bhumibol Adulyadej, Chulalongkorn University.

Authors' contributions

PC carried out the molecular genetic studies and drafted the manuscript. The patients were under the care of VS[5]. TS conceived the idea of the report and drafted the manuscript. PY, KS, TS, and VS[2] participated in the writing, review of the literature, text editing and finalization of the manuscript. All authors read and approved the final manuscript.

Competing interests

The authors declare that they have no competing interests.

Author details

[1]Department of Bioscience, Faculty of Science, Chulalongkorn University, Bangkok 10330, Thailand. [2]Excellence Center for Medical Genetics, Department of Pediatrics, Faculty of Medicine, Chulalongkorn University, Bangkok 10330, Thailand. [3]Department of Botany, Faculty of Science, Chulalongkorn University, Bangkok 10330, Thailand. [4]Center of Excellence for Medical Genetics, King Chulalongkorn Memorial Hospital, Bangkok 10330, Thailand. [5]Division of Pediatric Endocrinology, Department of Pediatrics, Faculty of Medicine, Chulalongkorn University, Bangkok 10330, Thailand.

References

1. Miller WL, Auchus RJ. The molecular biology, biochemistry, and physiology of human steroidogenesis and its disorders. Endocr Rev. 2011;32:81–151.

2. Peter M, Janzen N, Sander S, Korsch E, Riepe FG, Sander J. A case of 11β-hydroxylase deficiency detected in a newborn screening program by second-tier LC-MS/MS. Horm Res. 2008;69:253–6.
3. Nimkarn S, New MI. Steroid 11β-hydroxylase deficiency congenital adrenal hyperplasia. Trends Endocrinol Metab. 2008;19:96–9.
4. Zhu YS, Cordero JJ, Can S, Cai LQ, You X, Herrera C, et al. Mutations in CYP11B1 gene: phenotype-genotype correlations. Am J Med Genet A. 2003; 122A:193–200.
5. Zhao LQ, Han S, Tian HM. Progress in molecular-genetic studies on congenital adrenal hyperplasia due to 11β-hydroxylase deficiency. World J Pediatr. 2008;4:85–90.
6. Joehrer K, Geley S, Strasser-Wozak EM, Azziz R, Wollmann HA, Schmitt K, et al. CYP11B1 mutations causing nonclassic adrenal hyperplasia due to 11β-hydroxylase deficiency. Hum Mol Genet. 1997;6:1829–34.
7. Reisch N, Högler W, Parajes S, Rose IT, Dhir V, Götzinger J, et al. A diagnosis not to be missed: nonclassic steroid 11β-hydroxylase deficiency presenting with premature adrenarche and hirsutism. J Clin Endocrinol Metab. 2013;98:E1620–25.
8. Matsubara K, Kataoka N, Ogita S, Sano S, Ogata T, Fukami M, et al. Uniparental disomy of chromosome 8 leading to homozygosity of a CYP11B1 mutation in a patient with congenital adrenal hyperplasia: implication for a rare etiology of an autosomal recessive disorder. Endocr J. 2014;61:629–33.
9. Nguyen HH, Eiden-Plach A, Hannemann F, Malunowicz EM, Hartmann MF, Wudy SA, et al. Phenotypic, metabolic, and molecular genetic characterization of six patients with congenital adrenal hyperplasia caused by novel mutations in the CYP11B1 gene. J Steroid Biochem Mol Biol. 2016; 155(Pt A):126–34.
10. Sólyom RK, Péter F, Homoki J, Sippell WG, Peter M. Clinical, hormonal and molecular genetic characterization of Hungarian patients with 11β-hydroxylase deficiency. J Pediatr Endocrinol. 2001;2:37–44.
11. Holcombe JH, Keenan BS, Nichols BL, Kirkland RT, Clayton GW. Neonatal salt loss in the hypertensive form of congenital adrenal hyperplasia. Pediatrics. 1980;65:777–81.
12. Mimouni M, Kaufman H, Roitman A, Morag C, Sadan N. Hypertension in a neonate with 11β-hydroxylase deficiency. Eur J Pediatr. 1985;143:231–3.
13. Parajes S, Loidi L, Reisch N, Dhir V, Rose IT, Hampel R, et al. Functional consequences of seven novel mutations in the CYP11B1 gene: four mutations associated with nonclassic and three mutations causing classic 11β-hydroxylase deficiency. J Clin Endocrinol Metab. 2010;95:779–88.
14. Zhang M, Liu Y, Sun S, Zhang H, Wang W, Ning G, et al. A prevalent and three novel mutations in CYP11B1 gene identified in Chinese patients with 11β-hydroxylase deficiency. J Steroid Biochem Mol Biol. 2013;133:25–9.
15. Curnow KM, Slutsker L, Vitek J, Cole T, Speiser PW, New MI, et al. Mutations in the CYP11B1 gene causing congenital adrenal hyperplasia and hypertension cluster in exons 6, 7, and 8. Proc Natl Acad Sci U S A. 1993;90:4552–6.
16. Lopez-Bigas N, Audit B, Ouzounis C, Parra G, Guigo R. Are splicing mutations the most frequent cause of hereditary disease? FEBS Lett. 2005;579:1900–3.
17. Ward AJ, Cooper TA. The pathobiology of splicing. J Pathol. 2009;220:152–63.
18. Desviat LR, Pérez B, Ugarte M. Minigenes to confirm exon skipping mutations. Methods Mol Biol. 2012;867:37–47.
19. Scotti MM, Swanson MS. RNA mis-splicing in disease. Nat Rev Genet. 2016;17:19–32.
20. Gerstein MB, Rozowsky J, Yan KK, Wang D, Cheng C, Brown JB, et al. Comparative analysis of the transcriptome across distant species. Nature. 2014;512:445–8.
21. Merke DP, Tajima T, Chhabra A, Barnes K, Mancilla E, Baron J, et al. Novel CYP11B1 mutations in congenital adrenal hyperplasia due to steroid 11β-hydroxylase deficiency. J Clin Endocrinol Metab. 1998;83:270–3.
22. Samaranch L, Lorenzo-Betancor O, Arbelo JM, Ferrer I, Lorenzo E, Irigoyen J, et al. PINK1-linked parkinsonism is associated with Lewy body pathology. Brain. 2010;133(Pt4):1128–42.

21

Severe hyperkalemia following adrenalectomy for aldosteronoma: prediction, pathogenesis and approach to clinical management

A. Tahir[1*], K. McLaughlin[2] and G. Kline[3]

Abstract

Background: As the field of Primary Aldosteronism (PA) becomes ever expanded, diagnosis of PA is increasingly diagnosed by endocrinologists. With increased PA screening, many of the cases are now found in patients with complex co-morbidities in addition to their hypertension. Post adrenalectomy renal impairment with hyperkalemia is now increasingly seen in these complex patients, as evidenced by the numerous reports on this issue that have appeared within the past 3 years. We present a small case series to illustrate the breadth of the problem, along with a discussion about how such CKD/hyperkalemic events may be predicted.

Case presentation: We present three cases of primary aldosteronism with long standing hypertension (more than 10 years) hypokalemia (2.0–3.0 mmol/l). Serum aldosterone was high with low renin activity leading to high aldosterone to renin ratio (ARR). They underwent abdominal CT scan revealing adrenal mass and adrenal vein sample confirmed lateralization. None of the patients had evidence of renal disease before surgery (as evident by normal eGFR and serum creatinine). Post adrenalectomy they had reduction in the blood pressure and became eukalemic. Serum aldosterone and renin activity were low leading to a low ARR. Case 1 developed hyperkalemia and increased serum creatinine 6 weeks post operatively which resolved with initiation of fludrocortisone and every attempt to discontinue fludrocortisone resulted in hyperkalemia and rising creatinine. Her hyperkalemia is under control with oral sodium bicarbonate. Case 2 developed hyperkalemia and increasing creatinine 2 months post operatively transiently requiring fludrocortisone and later on managed with furosemide for hyperkalemia. Case 3 developed renal impairment and hyperkalemia 2 weeks post operatively requiring fludrocortisone.

Conclusion: Post APA resection severe hyperkalemia may be a common entity and screening should be actively considered in high risk patients. Older age, longer duration of hypertension, impaired pre-op and post-op GFR and higher levels of pre-op aldosterone and are all risk factors which predict the likelihood of developing post-operative hyperkalemia. Fludrocortisone, sodium bicarbonate, loop diuretics and potassium binders can be used for treatment. Treatment choice should be tailored to patient characteristics including fluid status, blood pressure and serum creatinine. Potassium binders should be avoided in patients with history of recent abdominal surgery, opioid use and constipation. Serum electrolytes and creatinine should be monitored every 1–2 weeks after starting treatment to ensure an adequate response. Prolonged management may be necessary in some cases and at-risk patients should be counselled as to the meaning and importance of post-operative changes in measured renal function and potassium.

Keywords: Case report, Adrenalectomy, Hyperkalemia, Aldosteronoma

* Correspondence: Taffan01@gmail.com
[1]Department of Internal Medicine, Cummings School of Medicine- University of Calgary, Alberta, Canada
Full list of author information is available at the end of the article

Background

Primary aldosteronism (PA) is characterized by hypertension, suppressed plasma renin levels, inappropriately high aldosterone secretion and in some cases hypokalemia. PA accounts for about 10 % of hypertensive patients [1, 2] who are known to have a higher risk of cardiovascular disease as compared to patients with essential hypertension. For those with an Aldosterone producing adenoma (APA), adrenalectomy offers a high rate of possible cure.

Moderate-to-severe hyperkalemia post adrenalectomy has been described in the literature but the risk factors and outpatient management is not very well delineated. We describe three cases of severe post adrenalectomy hyperkalemia requiring complex and long term therapy and discuss the known risk factors for developing post APA-resection hyperkalemia and suggest an approach to outpatient endocrinology management.

Case 1

A 51 year old woman with a 12 year history of hypertension developed hypokalemia (as low as 2.2 mmol/L). Her blood pressure was controlled with amlodipine 10 mg once daily and she received potassium supplements to maintain eukalemia. Her serum aldosterone was 2832 pmol/l with undetectable plasma renin activity. Her aldosterone to renin ratio (ARR) was therefore estimated at greater than 28,000 pmol/l/ng/ml/h (normal less than 2000 using renin activity of 0.1 ng/ml/h to avoid over-inflation). Her serum creatinine was 75 umol/l with eGFR of 85 ml/min. Abdominal CT showed a 3.5 cm low density left adrenal mass and adrenal vein sampling confirmed left lateralization with lateralization index values of 23:1 and 28:1 pre and post cosyntropin infusion. She underwent left adrenalectomy for what was reported as a 15.6 g adrenocortical adenoma on pathology. The post-operative biochemical course is presented in Table 1. At 2 weeks post-operative follow up, her blood pressure was 124/80, serum potassium 4.5 mmol/L and serum creatinine 52 umol/l without any medications. Her serum aldosterone was less than 70 pmol/l and renin activity of 0.36 ng/ml/h yielding ARR less than 194. However, at 6 weeks post-operative, she presented with serum potassium of 6.7 mmol/l, serum creatinine of 152 umol/l associated with persistent diarrhea (determined to be non-infectious) and clinical volume depletion. After fluid resuscitation she was started on fludrocortisone 0.1 mg daily and up-titrated to 0.1 mg bid over a 1-week period. At the higher fludrocortisone dose she became normokalemic and her serum creatinine decreased to 134 umol/l (Table 1). One month later, her serum potassium continued to be 4.8 mmol/l and serum creatinine 112 umol/l and so a dose reduction in fludrocortisone was attempted but at 0.1 mg per day, her potassium promptly rose to 5.6 mmol/l with creatinine 140 umol/l. Hyperkalemia persisted in the fluid replete state. She was not on any medications causing hyperkalemia. In the context for fludrocortisone responsive hyperkalemia we did not calculate TTKG (trans tubular potassium gradient). The fludrocortisone dose was increased again with similar normalization of potassium and drop in serum creatinine but her resultant blood pressures rose to 160/100.

Another attempt was made to decrease the fludrocortisone to 0.1 mg daily which was initially tolerable but by 2 months on this dose, her serum potassium was again found to be 6.4 mmol/l with creatinine 152 umol/l. This was transiently treated with higher dose fludrocortisone but the patient felt unwell on the medication, complaining of abdominal pain and so the drug was stopped in favour of furosemide 20 mg daily. Off of the fludrocortisone, her blood pressures were 135/88 but there was resultant hyponatremia, mild hyperkalemia and a sharp rise in serum creatinine to 188 umol/l and so the furosemide was stopped in favour of a return to fludrocortisone once more. Again, her potassium normalized to 4.5 mmo/l with drop in serum creatinine to 127 umol/l. Nephrology was consulted and the patient started on sodium bicarbonate 650 mg tid with cessation of fludrocortisone. During the last 8 months of such

Table 1 (Case1) Changes in Serum creatinine, potassium and blood pressure relative to medications. (Abbreviations: Bicarb- Bicarbonate)

Follow up period	Drugs	Creatinine umol/l	Potassium mmol/l	Blood pressure
2 weeks	None	52	4.5	124/80
6 weeks	None	152	6.7	-
10 weeks	Fludrocortisone 0.1 mg bid	112	4.8	140/96
14 weeks	Fludrocortisone 0.1 mg daily	140	5.6	-
5 months	Fludrocortisone 0.1 mg bid	121	4.7	160/100
6 months	Fludrocortisone 0.1 mg daily	152	6.4	-
7 months	Furosemide 20 mg daily	188	5.1	-
8 months	Sodium bicarb. 650 mg tid	160	5.5	-
16 months	Sodium bicarb. 650 mg tid	160	5.2	122/88

therapy, her blood pressures have been normal (122/88), potassium levels have been near-normal (5.2 mmol/l) with stable renal function (creatinine 160 umol/l, eGFR 31 ml/min).

Case 2

A 60 year old man with a 30 year history of hypertension and serum potassium as low as 2.9 mmol/l was referred for assessment. At presentation he required five antihypertensive agents to control his blood pressure which ranged from 130-150/80-100. His medications were perindopril 8 mg once daily, irbesartan/hydrochlorothiazide 300/25 mg once daily, nifedipine 60 mg twice daily and carvedilol 6.25 mg twice daily. After temporarily stopping carvedilol, irbesartan/hydrochlorothiazide and perindopril, his serum aldosterone was 1041 pmol/l with plasma renin activity of 0.2 ng/l/s yielding an aldosterone to renin ratio (ARR) of 5205 pmol/l/ng/ml/h (normal less than 2000). CT abdomen showed a multinodular left adrenal gland with a 1.3 cm dominant nodule. Adrenal vein sampling (AVS) showed left lateralization with lateralization indices of 4:1 and 12:1 pre and post cosyntropin infusion. Preoperative serum creatinine and GFR were 77 umol/l and 60 ml/min respectively. He underwent left adrenalectomy for 1.5 cm adrenocortical adenoma in the setting of background adrenal hyperplasia. At 4 weeks follow up his blood pressure was 128/80, serum creatinine 77 umol/l, serum aldosterone less than 70 pmol/l with renin activity of 0.31 ng/l/s yielding ARR of less than 225 pmol/l/ng/ml/h. At that time his irbesartan/hydrochlorothiazide was discontinued and nifedipine was reduced to 60 mg daily instead of twice daily and he continued to take carvedilol and perindopril. At 2 months follo up his serum potassium was found to be 6.0 mmol/l and serum creatinine 141 umol/l. He admitted using four pills of Ibuprofen for a fall related injury. At that visit his ACE inhibitor was stopped. A day later his serum creatinine came down to 121 umol/l but potassium remained at 5.9 mmol/l. He was started on fludrocortisone 0.05 mg daily. Two months later his serum creatinine was 115 umol/l and potassium 5.3 mmol/l. He did not have clinical signs of volume depletion and no other apparent reason for high potassium was found; therefore he was switched to furosemide 20 mg once daily. He required loop diuretic to normalize his serum potassium for 6 months after which it was stopped as his serum potassium remained 4.5–4.9 mmol/l without further intervention. At that time his only medications were nifedipine 60 mg daily and carvedilol 6.25 mg daily. At 15 months post-operative, he was successfully weaned off of carvedilol and his only continuing medication was nifedipine 30 mg daily with average blood pressures of 136/90.

Case 3

A 52 year old woman with type 2 diabetes and congenital right kidney aplasia was referred with a 12 year history of hypertension and hypokalemia as low as 2.3 mmol/l. At presentation she required amlodipine 10 mg once daily, telmisartan 80 mg once daily and spironolactone 25 mg once daily to maintain normotension and eukalmeia. Off of spironolactone, her aldosterone was 1157 pmol/l and direct renin was 3 ng/l yielding ARR of 368 pmol/l/ng/l (normal < 60 using the newer direct renin assay). CT abdomen showed 1.5 cm hypodense left adrenal mass. AVS showed left lateralization with lateralization index of 20:1 pre and post stimulation. Preoperative GFR was 69 ml/min and serum creatinine of 80 umol/l. She underwent adrenalectomy for what was reported as 2 cm adrenal cortical mass with no surrounding hyperplasia. Two weeks after the surgery she presented to emergency department with intermittent nausea and vomiting. Her serum potassium was 6.3 mmol/l and serum creatinine was 150 umol/l. After fluid resuscitation her serum potassium dropped to 5.1 mmol/l but creatinine persisted at 160 umol/l. She was started on sodium bicarbonate 650 mg bid. At 2 weeks follow up her serum creatinine was 208 umol/l and potassium remained at 5.1 mmol/l. She did not require any more antihypertensive medications and her blood pressure was 140/70. She was started on fludrocortisone 0.05 mg once daily and at 1 week follow up lab work her serum creatinine reduced to 170 umol/l with serum potassium of 5.2. She is currently on fludrocortisone 0.05 mg once daily.

Discussion

Post APA resection hyperkalemia is a well-documented entity, however the incidence and prevalence is not definitively known given the predominant reliance upon case reports and case series for its reporting. As the number of PA diagnoses increase with increasing visibility of the PA literature, it is possible that post APA-resection hyperkalemia will become a more common problem and endocrinologists will need to be familiar with the management options as severe hyperkalemia may be life-threatening.

Three retrospective studies have attempted to define the incidence and risk factors for post-operative hyperkalemia. Chiang et al. studied 55 post-operative APA patients through weekly blood testing and 16 (29.1 %) out of those developed hyperkalemia with serum potassium levels 5.3–6.2 mmol/l within 1 to 3 weeks of surgery [3]. In most cases, the hyperkalemia was transient, resolving by 2 months post-operative but in several cases, the high potassium persisted for longer than 9 months. Results from the German Conn's Registry [4] showed that of 110 patients, 18 (16 %) developed post-operative hyperkalemia, of whom 12 patients had transient hyperkalemia while in six patients hyperkalemia persisted beyond 11 months. Three out of the six patients required emergency room treatment for serum potassium greater than 6.8 mmol/l. A third study [5] described an incidence of post-operative hyperkalemia approximating 10.5 % (13 out of 124 patients). In that series, 3.2 % had transient hyperkalemia and 7.3 % had hyperkalemia that was prolonged beyond 3 months. Together, these studies from diverse populations demonstrate that hyperkalemia is not rare following APA resection and in a small but meaningful proportion it can be severe and prolonged.

Risk factors for post-adrenalectomy hyperkalemia

Older aged patients

Older age seems to correlate with the propensity to develop post-operative hyperkalemia in patients with primary hyperaldosteronism. Subjects aged more than 53 years old had greater odds of developing post-op hyperkalemia than those aged less than 53 years (OR = 15.6) as described in the Korean study [5]. Fischer et al. noted that patients who developed hyperkalemia were significantly older as compared to normokalemic population (65 ± 9 vs. 50 ± 12 years. $P = 0.026$) [4]. This theme is consistent in the study by Chiang et al.: Patients who developed hyperkalemia were older (56.4 ± 4 vs. 46.5 ± 10.0 year. $P = 0.002$). However, in the same study risk factors were analyzed further using multivariate regression and after backward elimination, older age was not one of the independent risk factors [3]. It is possible that older patients had longer duration of hypertension with more advanced hypertensive comorbidities including hypertensive nephropathy.

Duration of hypertension

Duration of pre-operative hypertension has been shown to be another potentially important risk factor for developing post adrenalectomy hyperkalemia. In the study by Chiang et al. [3], post-op hyperkalemics had longer duration of hypertension (12.8 ± 9.3 vs. 6.7 ± 5.0 year. $P = 0.013$). Park [5] found that subjects with duration of hypertension greater than 9.5 years had 10 times higher risk of developing hyperkalemia than those with less than 9.5 years of hypertension in an age adjusted model. All of the three subjects presented in our report had a lengthy duration of hypertension (> 10 years) prior to diagnosis and surgery.

Impaired renal function

Impaired renal function is an important risk factor in predicting post-operative hyperkalemia. The Chiang paper demonstrated that CKD (Stages III to–V) was 30 % more prevalent in patients who ultimately developed hyperkalemia [3]. Park took a more formal approach performing a ROC analysis to determine the most likely cut off values for pre-operative eGFR's ability to predict post-operative hyperkalemia; an eGFR of < 58.2 ml/min was associated with increased risk of developing hyperkalemia (OR = 26.6 $p < 0.05$) [5]. Fisher found that post-op hyperkalemics had significantly worse pre-operative renal function (creatinine: 91umol/l [76; 114 umol/l] vs. 61umol/l [53; 76 umol/l], $P = 0.001$; GFR: 56 ± 17 vs. 84 ± 21 ml/min, $P = 0.024$) [4].

While overt pre-existing renal impairment may be a strong factor in predicting post-operative hyperkalemia, there is now evidence that PA itself may induce a hyperfiltration injury that may mask renal impairment until the operative reversal of aldosterone mediated hyperfiltration [6]. In the first case presented above, the patient did not have any evidence of renal impairment pre operatively but after APA resection her eGFR decreased until it plateaued at 30–40 ml/min. Thus it may be that a "normal" eGFR (60–100 ml/min) in the PA pre-operative state may actually portend underlying nephropathy that will become evident and clinically relevant in the post-operative period.

Ribstein et al. [7] studied 25 patients with tumoral PA. Renal studies (urinary excretion of proteins, GFR, and effective renal plasma flow [ERPF] were performed both before and 6 months after adrenalectomy. A control group consisting of patients with essential hypertension (EH) was studied before and after 6 months of antihypertensive therapy. At baseline, PA and EH patients were similar with respect to demographic data, duration and level of hypertension, and GFR and ERPF. Urinary excretion of albumin and β2 microglobulin (a marker of glomerular filtration) was higher in PA than EH. Adrenalectomy was followed by a decrease in arterial urinary excretion of albumin and β2 microglobulin, and GFR and ERPF. In EH, a similar decrease in pressure was associated with a decrease in albuminuria but no change in GFR or ERPF. In patients who received a 6 months treatment of spironolactone, both GFR and ERPF decreased in parallel with BP, similar to what was observed after surgery. This data suggests that PA was associated with relative hyperfiltration, unmasked after suppression, removal or blockade of aldosterone excess.

A few studies have attempted to identify predictors of decreasing eGFR after APA resection. Tanase-Nakao et al. [8] studied patients with PA who underwent unilateral adrenalectomy and were followed for 1 month post operatively. Patients who underwent non-PA adrenalectomy were studied as control. Of PA patients, 37.8 % "developed CKD" (defined as eGFR < 60 ml/min/ 1.73 m2). None of non-PA group developed CKD post op. Of the pre op variables, logistic regression analysis showed that lower pre-surgical eGFR and higher aldosterone-to-renin ratios (ARR) were the independent predictors of post-op CKD in PA. Another Japanese study [6] prospectively described 120 patients with APA who underwent adrenalectomy while 111 patients with bilateral adrenal hyperplasia (BAH) received MR antagonists. Urine albumin excretion (UAE), blood pressure and eGFR decreased significantly at 1 month after treatment in both arms but did not decrease further at 12 months. Multivariate regression analysis revealed that higher UAE and lower serum potassium at initial visit were independent predictors of decreasing eGFR after intervention.

Ribstein et al. [7] showed that baseline serum potassium correlated with the post-operative change in GFR by univariate analysis. Rossi [2] in the PAPY study provided evidence that low serum potassium at baseline predicts albuminuria. Renicke [9] described that hypokalemic PA tended to be associated with renal impairment. Initial potassium concentration (odds ratio, 1.3; 95 % confidence interval, 1.0–5.2; $P < 0.01$), plasma aldosterone concentrations ($P < 0.05$), and presence or absence of the hypokalemic variant of PA ($P < 0.05$) were independent predictors of higher creatinine.

While hypokalemia may simply be a marker of more severe aldosteronism, it must also be considered that hypokalemia could actually play a pathophysiologic role in renal impairment. Low potassium itself can cause functional and structural defects in kidneys, such as cyst formation, tubular vacuolization, interstitial inflammation and gradual loss of renal function [10].

Post-operative hypoaldosteronism

Connell et al. [11] described a case of a 50 year old woman who developed hyperkalemia and acute kidney injury 1 month after resection of APA. Her aldosterone level was inappropriately low, given hypovolaemia and hyperkalaemia, suggesting hypoaldosteronism (plasma aldosterone 100 pmol/l; plasma renin activity 4.4 pg/ml/h). Gadallah [12] reported a case in which unilateral adrenalectomy for adrenal adenoma was followed by severe hyperkalemia, marked volume depletion and undetectable plasma renin activity and serum aldosterone suggesting chronic suppression of the renin-aldosterone axis. One year later, a gradual return to normokalemia, normotension, and normal plasma renin activity and aldosterone levels was achieved, indicating resolution of the suppression of the renin-aldosterone axis.

In the German Conn's registry post-operative hyperkalemia caused by suppression of the zona glomerulosa (ZG) insufficiency was examined. They measured serum potassium, post-operative aldosterone and trans-tubular potassium gradient (TTKG) to determine ZG insufficiency which was defined as was defined as undetectable plasma aldosterone level (< 97pmol/l) in the presence of hyperkalemia (K > 5.0). Of the 18 patients who developed hyperkalemia 14 had undetectable and four had low aldosterone levels (aldosterone level < 138 pmol/l). In all six patients who developed persistent hyperkalemia, serum aldosterone level was less than 97pmol/l. The calculation of the TTKG showed decreased values of less than 6, in three of four evaluated hyperkalemic patients, showing inappropriate renal response to hyperkalemia. The normal response to hyperkalemia is an increase in aldosterone secretion leading to an increased urinary potassium excretion, with an increase of TTKG to greater than 10 [13]. A result of less than 6 in a hyperkalemic patient indicates inadequate aldosterone concentration or effect [14]. They also assessed the contralateral gland suppression index in those patients who had selective adrenal vein sampling (AVS) prior to surgery ($n = 77$). Five of five investigated patients with persistent hyperkalemia demonstrated a contralateral aldosterone/cortisol ratio suppression index of aldosterone in the non-dominant gland less than 1 versus inferior vena cava [4].

Taniguchi et al. [15] reported a case of a 46-year-old woman who underwent unilateral adrenalectomy and developed episodes of severe hyperkalemia for 4 months. Plasma aldosterone concentration (PAC) was low (102.5 pmol/l) and undetectable renin activity. Serum potassium levels gradually decreased with concomitant increase in PAC (162pmol/l).

It is plausible that aldosterone synthesis of adjacent and contralateral adrenal glands is severely impaired in some cases with primary hyperaldosteronism, as is glucocorticoid synthesis in Cushing syndrome. Since many instances of hyperkalemia may go undetected post operatively, a larger series with prospective, standardized, sequential potassium measures may be needed in order to better determine if contralateral suppression might predict hyperkalemia.

Pre-operative mineralocorticoid receptor (MR) antagonists

MR antagonists are often administered in APA patients to control hypokalemia. Reversal of hyperaldosteronism after long term treatment with spironolactone (SP) has been reported in the literature, and it appears that it has anti-steroidogenic effect. Yoneda et al. [16] reported a case of a 41 year old man who had a left sided APA. The plasma renin activity (PRA) was 0.6 ng/ml/h and the plasma aldosterone concentration (PAC) was 362 pg/ml in the supine position. CT showed a 5 mm left sided nodule and AVS indices showed left lateralization. The patient received spironolactone 75 mg OD daily for 5 years and 50 mg for another 4–5 years. At 10 year follow up after discontinuation of spironolactone, the patient's blood pressure, serum potassium level, and plasma aldosterone concentration remained in the normal range. Although the left adrenal gland tumor was still present on computed tomography after treatment,

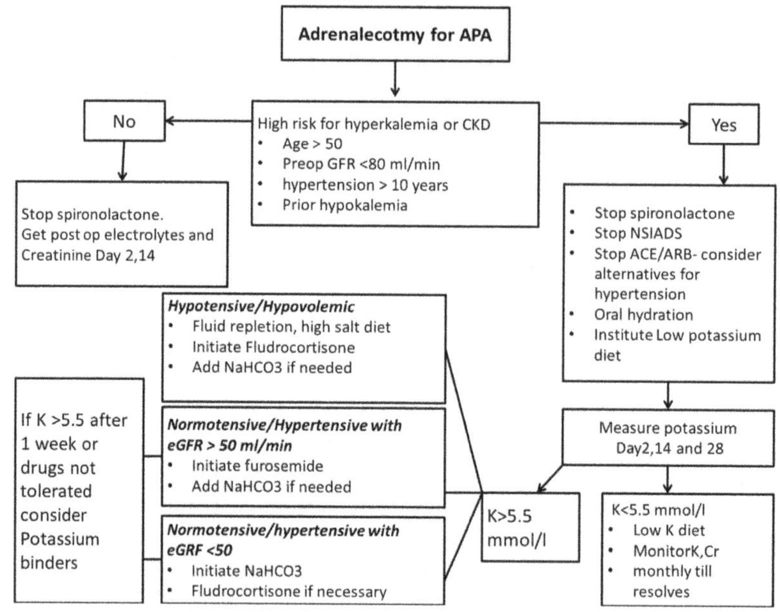

Fig. 1 Post-adrenalectomy hyperkalemia- prediction, monitoring and treatment algorithm

a furosemide and upright posture test, a captopril challenge test, and a saline loading test produced no evidence of PA. Adrenal vein sampling demonstrated no sign of lateralization.

Demura et al. [17] have shown that the aldosterone synthetic enzyme, CYP11B2, is influenced by epigenetic factors. Long-term treatment with spironolactone may influence the epigenetic modulation of CYP11B2. SP (spironolactone) not only is an MR antagonist, but also forms SP body inclusions in cells after long-term treatment. Histological examination of SP body-containing cells demonstrates enhanced but abortive steroidogenic activity [18]. These observations suggest that MR antagonists, at long exposure times, may actually impair aldosterone production, something that may explain or aggravate the post adrenalectomy hypoaldosterone state.

Park et al. [5] found that out of 124 patients, 93 were treated with spironolactone at a mean dose of 88 mg for mean duration of 45 days. The proportion of MR antagonist users was not significantly different between subjects with persistent hyperkalemia, transient hyperkalemia and normokalemia. Preoperative treatment with MR antagonists did not influence the incidence of hypoaldosteronism and hyperkalemia.

Table 2 Known risk factors increasing likelihood of post-operative hyperkalemia

Risk Factors
1. Older age
2. Long duration of hypertension
3. Impaired pre-operative GFR
4. Impaired post-operative GFR
5. Higher per-operative aldosterone level

These clinical reports do not yet confirm the role of pre-operative MR antagonists in the development of post-operative hyperkalemia but at the very least should emphasize the importance of immediate post-operative discontinuation of such medications.

Management of hyperkalemia post adrenalectomy

Post adrenalectomy hyperkalemia can be severe and life threatening, sometimes requiring emergency treatment. Preventative strategies in high risk patients would include restricting dietary potassium intake and a useful patient-oriented website (http://www.kidney.ca/document.doc?id=945. https://www.kidney.org/atoz/content/potassium) may help with patient dietary education. Reversible causes should be addressed in all patients such as hypovolemia, urinary tract obstruction and non-steroidal anti-inflammatory drugs and renin-angiotensin-aldosterone-system inhibitors which can all cause aggravate hyperkalemia in these patients, usually by further decreasing an already impaired GFR. Pharmacological therapies work mainly by potassium removal either by binding it in gut or excreting it through kidneys.

There are several agents which promote renal excretion of potassium. Fludrocortisone is traditionally the obvious choice for hypo-aldosteronism. However, it can be challenging to treat with fludrocortisone in the long term on account of the risk of hypertension and peripheral edema and potentially worsening heart failure in patients with underlying cardiac disease. An alternate

Table 3 Pros and cons of different drugs used to treat hyperkalemia

Drugs	Pros	Cons
Fludrocortisone	1. Effective and quick resolution of hyperkalemia 2. Easy titration of dosing 3. Can be used early post operatively	1. Can cause/worsen hypertension 2. Can mask underlying renal disease 3. Can worsen edema, heart failure
Sodium bicarbonate	1. Can be used safely in CKD 2. Can be used early post operatively	1. Unfamiliarity with the drug 2. Not much data available regarding dosing regimen
Loop diuretics	1. Effective and familiar drug 2. Can be used in hypertensive population	1. Can worsen kidney disease by dehydration
Potassium binders	1. Can be used in CKD 2. Does not interfere with blood pressure	1. Can cause complications in post-operative and constipated patients

approach would use furosemide and oral sodium bicarbonate to increase renal potassium (K) excretion. Studies on the mechanism of distal K secretion have highlighted the importance of renal outer-medullary K (ROMK) and maxi-K channels in distal nephron [19]. Flow dependant K secretion works via apical membrane stretch in the distal nephron, which activates calcium channels, increasing intracellular calcium and activation of maxi-k and ROMK channels to facilitate potassium excretion [20]. Distal Na delivery is however indispensable for K secretion as it provides the electro-chemical gradient driving for K efflux via maxi-K and ROMK. Therefore, an alternative solution to replacing mineralocorticoid is to increase distal nephron flow and sodium delivery via increased Na intake (ideally with NaHCO3), increased water intake and/or loop diuretics or carbonic anhydrase inhibitors. Potassium binders are used to excrete potassium mainly through binding in the gut. A major concern with binders especially sodium polystyrene sulfonate is the development of intestinal necrosis involving colon and ileum [21]. It is a rare event, on the order of 0.2 to 0.3 %. Binders should be avoided in patients with ileus, opiate use and recent abdominal surgery [22]. Therefore these agents are not recommended in the immediate post-adrenalectomy state.

Clinical approach to management

Since there are no formal studies or guidelines to inform the best practices in treating hyperkalemia post-adrenalectomy, we propose following prediction, monitoring and treatment strategy outlined in Fig. 1. Vigilance and early intervention with careful follow up testing is the cornerstone of the clinical approach.

Conclusion

Post APA resection severe hyperkalemia may be a common entity and screening should be actively considered in high risk patients. Older age, longer duration of hypertension, impaired pre-op and post-op GFR and higher levels of pre-op aldosterone and are all risk factors which predict the likelihood of developing post-operative hyperkalemia (see Table 2). Treatment choice should be tailored to patient characteristics including fluid status, blood pressure and serum creatinine (Table 3).

The long term cure of primary aldosterone excess and hypertension is expected to yield renal benefits but development of irreversible post adrenalectomy renal impairment after a long duration of hypertension may argue for earlier consideration of a PA diagnosis in hypertensive populations. With increasing numbers patients diagnosed with PA and submitted to adrenalectomy, endocrinologists will need to become familiar with the factors that predict severe hyperkalemia and adopt an aggressive approach to prevent life threatening hyperkalemic complications.

Abbreviations

APA, aldosterone producing adenoma; ARR, aldosterone to renin ratio; BAH, bilateral adrenal hyperplasia; MR, mineralocorticoid receptor; PA, primary aldosteronism; TTKG, trans tubular potassium gradient

Acknowledgements

We do not have someone to acknowledge to.

Funding

We do not have funding source to disclose.

Authors' contributions

GK and KM conceived the study helped to draft the manuscript. AT did the literature review and helped drafting the manuscript. All authors read and approved the manuscript.

Competing interests

The authors declare that they have no competing interests.

Author details

[1]Department of Internal Medicine, Cummings School of Medicine- University of Calgary, Alberta, Canada. [2]Department of Nephrology, Cummings School of Medicine- University of Calgary, Alberta, Canada. [3]Department of Endocrinology, Cummings School of Medicine- University of Calgary, Alberta, Canada.

References

1. Funder JW, Carey RM, Fardella C, Gomez-Sanchez CE, Mantero F, Stowasser M, Young Jr WF, Montori VM. Case detection, diagnosis, and treatment of patients with primary aldosteronism: an endocrine society clinical practice guideline Endocrine Society. J Clin Endocrinol Metab. 2008;93(9):3266–81. doi:10.1210/jc.2008-0104. Epub 2008 Jun 13.
2. Rossi GP, Bernini G, Caliumi C, Desideri G, Fabris B, Ferri C, Ganzaroli C, Giacchetti G, Letizia C, Maccario M, Mallamaci F, Mannelli M, Mattarello MJ, Moretti A, Palumbo G, Parenti G, Porteri E, Semplicini A, Rizzoni D, Rossi E, Boscaro M, Pessina AC, Mantero F; PAPY Study Investigators. A prospective study of the prevalence of primary aldosteronism in 1,125 hypertensive patients. J Am Coll Cardiol. 2006;48(11):2293–300. Epub 2006 Nov 13.
3. Chiang WF, Cheng CJ, Wu ST, Sun GH, Lin MY, Sung CC, Lin SH. Incidence and factors of post-adrenalectomy hyperkalemia in patients with aldosterone producing adenoma. Clin Chim Acta. 2013;424:114–8. doi:10.1016/j.cca.2013.05.017. Epub 2013 May 28.
4. Fischer E, Hanslik G, Pallauf A, Degenhart C, Linsenmaier U, Beuschlein F, Bidlingmaier M, Mussack T, Ladurner R, Hallfeldt K, Quinkler M, Reincke M. Prolonged zona glomerulosa insufficiency causing hyperkalemia in primary aldosteronism after adrenalectomy. J Clin Endocrinol Metab. 2012;97(11):3965–73. doi:10.1210/jc.2012-2234. Epub 2012 Aug 14.
5. Park KS, Kim JH, Ku EJ, Hong AR, Moon MK, Choi SH, Shin CS, Kim SW, Kim SY. Clinical risk factors of postoperative hyperkalemia after adrenalectomy in patients with aldosterone-producing adenoma. Eur J Endocrinol. 2015;172(6):725–31. doi:10.1530/EJE-15-0074. Epub 2015 Mar 12.
6. Iwakura Y, Morimoto R, Kudo M, Ono Y, Takase K, Seiji K, Arai Y, Nakamura Y, Sasano H, Ito S, Satoh F. Predictors of decreasing glomerular filtration rate and prevalence of chronic kidney disease after treatment of primary aldosteronism: renal outcome of 213 cases. J Clin Endocrinol Metab. 2014;99(5):1593–8. doi:10.1210/jc.2013-2180. Epub 2013 Nov 27.
7. Ribstein J, Du Cailar G, Fesler P, Mimran A. Relative glomerular hyperfiltration in primary aldosteronism. J Am Soc Nephrol. 2005;16(5):1320–5. Epub 2005 Mar 30.
8. Tanase-Nakao K, Naruse M, Nanba K, Tsuiki M, Tagami T, Usui T, Okuno H, Shimatsu A, Hashimoto S, Katabami T, Ogo A, Okumura A, Umakoshi H, Suzuki T. Chronic kidney disease score for predicting postoperative masked renal insufficiency in patients with primary aldosteronism. Clin Endocrinol (Oxf). 2014;81(5):665–70. doi:10.1111/cen.12497. Epub 2014 Jun 12.
9. Reincke M, Rump LC, Quinkler M, Hahner S, Diederich S, Lorenz R, Seufert J, Schirpenbach C, Beuschlein F, Bidlingmaier M, Meisinger C, Holle R, Endres S; Participants of German Conn's Registry. Risk factors associated with a low glomerular filtration rate in primary aldosteronism. J Clin Endocrinol Metab. 2009;94(3):869–75. doi:10.1210/jc.2008-1851. Epub 2008 Dec 30.
10. Sechi LA, Novello M, Lapenna R, Baroselli S, Nadalini E, Colussi GL, Catena C. Long-term renal outcomes in patients with primary aldosteronism. JAMA. 2006;295(22):2638–45.
11. Alistair Connell & Mark Cohen. A case of severe hypoaldosteronism following unilateral adrenalectomy for Conn's syndrome. Endocrine Abstracts (2013) 31 P82 | doi: 10.1530/endoabs.31.P82.
12. Gadallah MF, Kayyas Y, Boules F. Reversible suppression of the renin-aldosterone axis after unilateral adrenalectomy for adrenal adenoma. Am J Kidney Dis. 1998;32(1):160–3.
13. Kamel KS, Ethier JH, Richardson RM, Bear RA, Halperin ML. Urine electrolytes and osmolality: when and how to use them. Am J Nephrol. 1990;10(2):89–102.
14. Choi MJ1, Ziyadeh FN. The utility of the transtubular potassium gradient in the evaluation of hyperkalemia. J Am Soc Nephrol. 2008 Mar; 19(3):424–6. doi: 10.1681/ASN.2007091017. Epub 2008 Jan 23.
15. Taniguchi R, Koshiyama H, Yamauchi M, Tanaka S, Inoue D, Sato Y, Sugawa A, Muramatsu Y, Sasano H. A Case of Aldosterone-Producing Adenoma with Severe Postoperative Hyperkalemia. Tohoku J Exp Med. 1998;186(3):215–23.
16. Yoneda T, Demura M, Takata H, Kometani M, Karashima S, Yamagishi M, Takeda Y. Unilateral primary aldosteronism with spontaneous remission after long-term spironolactone therapy. J Clin Endocrinol Metab. 2012;97(4):1109–13. doi:10.1210/jc.2011-2563. Epub 2012 Feb 15.
17. Demura M, Wang F, Yoneda T, Karashima S, Mori S, Oe M, Kometani M, Sawamura T, Cheng Y, Maeda Y, Namiki M, Ino H, Fujino N, Uchiyama K, Tsubokawa T, Yamagishi M, Nakamura Y, Ono K, Sasano H, Demura Y, Takeda Y. Multiple noncoding exons 1 of nuclear receptors NR4A family (nerve growth factor-induced clone B, Nur-related factor 1 and neuron-derived orphan receptor 1) and NR5A1 (steroidogenic factor 1) in human cardiovascular and adrenal tissues. J Hypertens. 2011;29(6):1185–95. doi:10.1097/HJH.0b013e32834626bb.
18. Conn JW, Hinerman DL. Spironolactone-induced inhibition of aldosterone biosynthesis in primary aldosteronism: morphological and functional studies. Metabolism. 1977;26(12):1293–307.
19. Rodan AR, Huang CL. Distal potassium handling based on flow modulation of maxi-K channel activity. Curr Opin Nephrol Hypertens. 2009;18(4):350–5. doi:10.1097/MNH.0b013e32832c75d8.
20. Liu W, Xu S, Woda C, Kim P, Weinbaum S, Satlin LM. Effect of flow and stretch on the [Ca2+]i response of principal and intercalated cells in cortical collecting duct. Am J Physiol Renal Physiol. 2003;285(5):F998–F1012. Epub 2003 Jul 1.
21. McGowan CE, Saha S, Chu G, Resnick MB, Moss SF. Intestinal necrosis due to sodium polystyrene sulfonate (Kayexalate) in sorbitol. South Med J. 2009;102(5):493–7. doi:10.1097/SMJ.0b013e31819e8978.
22. Watson M, Abbott KC, Yuan CM. Damned if you do, damned if you don't: potassium binding resins in hyperkalemia. Clin J Am Soc Nephrol. 2010;5(10):1723–6. doi:10.2215/CJN.03700410. Epub 2010 Aug 26.

22

Subclinical and clinical hypothyroidism and non-alcoholic fatty liver disease: a cross-sectional study of a random population sample aged 18 to 65 years

Ulla Ludwig[1†], Daniela Holzner[1†], Christian Denzer[2], Artur Greinert[1], Mark Martin Haenle[1], Suemeyra Oeztuerk[1], Wolfgang Koenig[3,4,5], Bernhard Otto Boehm[6,7], Richard Andrew Mason[8], Wolfgang Kratzer[1*], Tilmann Graeter[9] and the EMIL-Study

Abstract

Background: Non-alcoholic fatty liver disease (NAFLD) is one of the most common disorders of the liver worldwide. Recently, a correlation between thyroid dysfunction and NAFLD has been discussed. Objective of the present study was to investigate the association between thyroid dysfunction and hepatic steatosis.

Methods: Data from 2,445 subjects (51.7 % females) aged 18 to 65 years participating in a population-based cross-sectional study were assessed based on a standardized questionnaire and documentation of physical, biochemical and ultrasonographic findings. After application of exclusion criteria, a total of 1,276 subjects were included in the study collective. The influence of potential factors on the development of hepatic steatosis was assessed using multivariate logistic regression.

Results: The prevalence of hepatic steatosis in the study collective was 27.4 % (n = 349). The serum thyroxin (TT4) concentration in subjects with hepatic steatosis was reduced (p = 0.0004). Adjusting for age, or BMI, there was an increased prevalence of hepatic steatosis in subjects with reduced TT4 concentrations (p = 0.0143; p = <.0001).

Conclusions: The findings of the present study confirm an association between both subclinical and clinical hypothyroidism and hepatic steatosis

Keywords: NAFLD, Thyroid, Hypothyroidism, NASH, Cross-sectional studies

Background

Non-alcoholic fatty liver disease (NAFLD) represents one of the most common chronic disorders of the liver in the Western industrialized nations [1–4]. Its prevalence worldwide is estimated at 20 % -30 % [5–7]. NAFLD subsumes a variety of entities ranging from simple fatty liver or hepatic steatosis, to non-alcoholic steatohepatitis (NASH) and cirrhosis of the liver [8–10] and is associated with the risk of malignant degeneration to hepatocellular carcinoma (HCC) and the increased necessity of liver transplantation [11, 12]. A central role in the development of NAFLD has been ascribed to the metabolic syndrome, whose main characteristics, such as obesity, insulin resistance and/or type-2 diabetes mellitus and dyslipidemia are closely associated to NAFLD [8]. Not surprisingly, there is also an association between NAFLD and cardiovascular disorders [1, 2].

Increasingly, a correlation between thyroid dysfunction, especially clinical or subclinical hypothyroidism, and NAFLD has been discussed [6, 13–16]. Hormones synthesized in the thyroid gland play an important role in the regulation of diverse metabolic processes. Disturbances in thyroid hormone concentrations may promote hyperlipidemia and obesity, thus contributing to NAFLD [13, 17]. Early identification of at-risk patients is important since treatment of the hypothyroidism may reduce the risk of NAFLD and potential complications [18]. It

* Correspondence: wolfgang.kratzer@uniklinik-ulm.de
†Equal contributors
[1]Department of Internal Medicine I, Center for Internal Medicine, University Medical Center Ulm, Albert-Einstein-Allee 23, 89081 Ulm, Germany
Full list of author information is available at the end of the article

was the objective of the present study to investigate the association between thyroid dysfunction and hepatic steatosis in an epidemiological cross-sectional study in a random population-based sample of subjects aged 18 to 65 years.

Methods

Study population

A cross-sectional survey assessing the prevalence of *Echinococcus Multilocularis Infection and other medical disorders in Leutkirch* (EMIL-Study), was conducted in Leutkirch, Germany in 2002. Initially, 4,000 of the total 12,475 residents were randomly selected by the staff of the municipal registry office from the roster of inhabitants. Out of these 4,000 persons, 107 were excluded because their address was unknown or they had not given their informed consent. A total of 2,445 individuals finally participated in the study, corresponding to a participation rate of 62.8 % [19]. Following exclusion of subjects less than 18 years (n = 258) and subjects with incomplete laboratory results (n = 230), those with past or present hepatitis B or hepatitis C virus infections (n = 146), hemochromatosis (n = 1) or elevated alcohol consumption (>40 g/day in males and > 20 g/day in females; n = 69), intake of iodone (n = 344), antithyroid agents (n = 2) or thyroid hormones (n = 437), missing ultrasonographic data on hepatic steatosis (n = 16), missing data on BMI (n = 11) or metabolic syndrome (n = 77), a total of 1,276 subjects were finally included in the present analysis (Fig. 1). This study collective was then divided, based on the diagnosis of NAFLD, into an NAFLD group (n = 349) and a healthy control group (n = 927).

The study was conducted in accordance with the principles of good clinical practice and the Declaration of Helsinki. It was approved by the ethics committee of the Medical Association of Baden-Württemberg. All participants provided written informed consent.

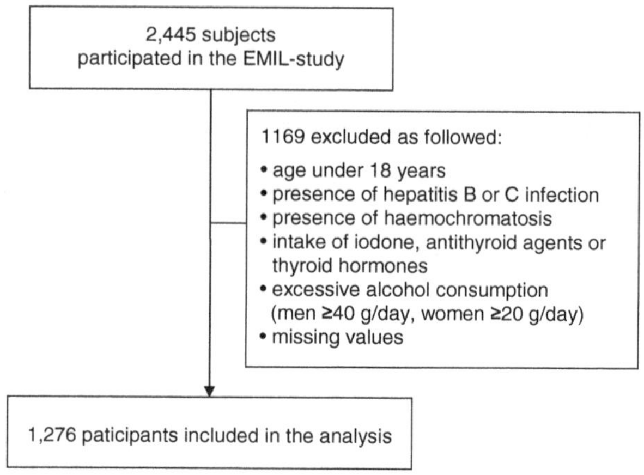

Fig. 1 Flow of the subjects across the study. The base collective for the present study consisted of the 2,445 subjects of the EMIL study. Of these, 258 subjects were excluded due to age < 18 years; 69 due to excessive alcohol consumption (>40 g/day in males and > 20 g/day in females); 146 due to past or current hepatitis B or hepatitis C infections;intake of iodone (n = 344), antithyroid agents (n = 2) or thyroid hormones (n = 437); and 1 due to hemochromatosis. Incomplete data, laboratory values or other data were also exclusion criteria. Each box represents an exclusion criterion and contains the corresponding number of subjects in relation to the total collective. An individual subject may meet multiple exclusion criteria. For the present study, the resulting collective consisted of 1,276 individuals

Examination methods and anthropometric data

Patient history, including demographics, leisure activities, past medical history, family medical history, medication history as well as nicotine and alcohol use and nutritional habits were compiled and documented using a standardized interview. Body height, body weight, hip, and waist circumference were measured. The body-mass index (BMI) and the waist-to-hip ratio (WHR) were calculated according to recommendations of the World Health Organization (WHO).

Laboratory testing

About 25 ml of whole blood was obtained from each study participant through phlebotomy of the cubital vein. Random glucose, alanine aminotransferase (ALT), aspartate aminotransferase (AST), γ-glutamyl transferase (GGT), alkaline phosphatase (AP), C-reactive protein (CRP), albumin, cholesterol, high density lipoprotein (HDL), transferrin and ferritin were measured using the Dimension XL unit (Dade Behring Inc., Newark, DE 19714, USA). Fibrinogen and coeruloplasmin were measured using the Siemens Dade Behring BII Nephelometer (Siemens Healthcare Diagnostics GmbH; Ludwig-Erhard-Straße 12; 65760 Eschborn, Germany). The concentration of low density lipoprotein (LDL) was calculated using the Friedewald formula: LDL cholesterol = total cholesterol–HDL–(triglycerides*0.45). Thyroid-stimulating hormone (TSH), triiodothyronine (TT3), thyroxine (TT4) and anti-thyroid autoantibodies (Anti-TPO) were measured using an Elecsys® 2010 Disk & Rack Analyzers (Roche Diagnostics, 9115 Hague Road, Indianapolis, USA). Each parameter was measured twice. All assays were performed according to the manufacturer's recommendations. Regular precision controls were performed to assure proper functioning of all laboratory equipment.

Criteria for thyroid dysfunction and metabolic syndrome

The diagnosis of *subclinical* hypothyroidism was made in subjects with TSH concentrations ≥ 34 IU/ml and normal thyroid hormone concentrations (TT4: 12.8-20.4 pmol/l; TT3: 3.92-6.74 pmol/l). The diagnosis of clinically manifest hypothyroidism required reduced TT4 concentrations (<12.8 pmol/) and elevated TSH levels (TSH ≥ 34 IU/ml).

Metabolic syndrome was defined according to modified U.S. National Cholesterol Education Program Adult Treatment Panel III criteria (ATP III), whereby at least three of the following criteria had to be met: waist circumference >102 cm in males or >88 cm females; serum triglyceride (TG) concentration ≥ 1.7 mmol/l; serum HDL cholesterol ≤ 1.28 mmol/l (males, 1.0 mmol/l; females, 1.3 mmol/l); history of hypertension and random blood glucose ≥ 160 mg/dl (fasting glucose ≥ 110 mg/dl) or confirmed diabetes mellitus [20].

Ultrasound examination and criteria for hepatic steatosis

The ultrasound examinations were performed under standardized conditions by specially trained examiners using four identical HDI 5000 diagnostic ultrasound units (ALTATL Ultrasound, Philips Medical Systems, P.O. Box 3003, Bothell, WA, USA). Unclear or pathological findings were reviewed by an experienced supervisor (>4,000 ultrasonographic examinations per year). As far as possible, identical settings were maintained for all units. Findings were documented using a standardized recording questionnaire. Examinations included assessment of the liver, gallbladder, kidneys and spleen. The liver was assessed with respect to size, the presence of focal lesions, and the presence of hepatic steatosis. The diagnosis of hepatic steatosis was made based on the basis of criteria established by Saverymuttu *et al.* [21], Hamaguchi *et al.* [22] and Charatcharoenwitthaya *et al.* [23]. The hepatic parenchyma was compared with the renal parenchyma under consideration of the dorsal echo attenuation, visualization of the diaphragm and ability to assess the intrahepatic vessels. The degree of steatosis was assigned to classes of "none" (grade 0), "mild" (grade I), "moderate" (grade II) and "severe" (grade III).

Statistical analysis

Statistical calculations were performed using the SAS 9.2 statistics software package (SAS Institute Inc., Cary, North Carolina, USA). Data were first analyzed descriptively. Mean and standard deviation were determined for continuous variables. Categorical data were presented with absolute and relative frequencies. In order to detect differences between subjects with and without hepatic steatosis, the Wilcoxon rank-sum test was used for continuous variables, while, for categorical variables, the χ^2 test or, when the number of cases was too small, Fisher's exact test were used. In order to identify possible correlations between thyroid hormone levels and demographic, anthropometric and biochemical parameters, we calculated the Spearman rank correlation. In a further analytic step, subjects were divided into four equal groups (quartiles) on the basis of thyroid hormone concentrations (TSH, TT4, TT3; Table 1). The Kruskal-Wallis test was used to identify differences between the four groups. Bivariate and multivariate logistic regression served to identify correlations with hepatic steatosis and other potential risk factors. All tests were two-tailed. A *P* value of less than 0.05 was considered statistically significant.

Table 1 Breakdown of thyroid hormone parameters in quartiles in the present study

	Quartile 1	Quartile 2	Quartile 3	Quartile 4
TSH	<1.0	1.01-1.49	1.50-2.18	>2.19
TT4	<74.5	74.6-83.9	84.0-94.2	>94.3
TT3	<1.40	1.41-1.57	1.58-1.81	>1.82

Results

Hepatic steatosis

The study collective included 1,276 subjects (47.2 %, females; 52.8 %, males), whose mean age stood at 40.7 ± 12.7 years (40.0 ± 12.7 years, women; 41.3 ± 12.6 years, men). The characteristics of the study population are presented in Table 2. A diagnosis of hepatic steatosis was made in 349 subjects. The prevalence of ultrasonographically diagnosed hepatic steatosis was significantly higher in males (70.8 %; n = 247) than in females (29.2 %; n = 102; Table 2). The NAFLD group was characterized by a higher BMI, WHR, arterial hypertension and higher prevalence of metabolic syndrome according

Table 2 Characteristics of study subjects with and without NAFLD

Variables	Subjects with NAFLD (n = 349) Mean ± SD	Subjects without NAFLD (n = 927) Mean ± SD	*P* value
Gender, *n (%)*			
female	102 (29.2)	500 (53.7)	<.0001
male	247 (70.8)	427 (46.1)	
Age	47.7 ± 11.5	38.0 ± 12.1	<.0001
BMI	29.7 ± 4.7	24.0 ± 3.7	<.0001
WHR	0.9 ± 0.1	0.8 ± 0.1	<.0001
ALT	20.9 ± 10.3	13.5 ± 5.8	<.0001
AST	11.2 ± 5.1	9.0 ± 2.6	<.0001
GGT	20.5 ± 20.6	11.0 ± 10.5	<.0001
TSH (μU/ml)	1.8 ± 1.4	1.8 ± 3.5	0.6381
TT3 (nmol/l)	1.6 ± 0.3	1.6 ± 0.3	0.3293
TT4 (nmol/l)	83.2 ± 15.6	92.0 ± 17.4	0.0004
Anti-TPO (IU/ml)	23.9 ± 72.1	23.9 ± 74.0	0.4063
Diabetes, n (%)	22 (6.3)	8 (0.9)	<.0001
Metabolic syndrome, n (%)	65 (18.6)	15 (1.6)	<.0001
Hypertension, n (%)	99 (28.4)	67 (7.2)	<.0001

BMI = body-mass-index; WHR = waist to hip ratio; ALT = Alanine transaminase; AST = Aspartate transaminase; GGT = Gamma-glutamyl transferase; TSH = thyroid-stimulating hormone; TT3 = triiodothyronine; TT4 = thyroxine; Anti-TPO = anti-thyroid autoantibodies

to ATPIII criteria ($p < 0.001$). The biochemical parameters ALT, AST, GGT were also significantly higher in the group with hepatic steatosis (Table 2).

Association of NAFLD with thyroid hormone concentrations

Hypothyroidism was diagnosed in 4.1 % ($n = 52$) subjects. Of these, 34 subjects met criteria for subclinical, 18 for clinically manifest hypothyroidism. In the subgroup with hepatic steatosis, 1.3 % of subjects ($n = 16$; 7 females, 9 males) exhibited thyroid hormone levels consistent with hypothyroidism. Of these, eight subjects (0.6 %) met criteria for subclinical, eight (0.6 %) for clinically manifest hypothyroidism (Table 2). Among subjects with both hepatic steatosis *and* elevated serum transaminases ($n = 125$), six (4.8 %) exhibited thyroid hormone levels consistent with hypothyroidism. Of these, five subjects met criteria for subclinical, one for clinically manifest hypothyroidism. By comparison, in the control group, 46 subjects (25 females, 21 males) exhibited reduced thyroid hormone concentrations. Of these, 29 subjects met criteria for subclinical, 17 for clinically manifest hypothyroidism. With respect to the thyroid hormone concentrations, there was a significant difference only for TT4 levels ($p = 0.0.0004$; Table 2). The mean values for TSH, TT3 and Anti-TPO did not differ significantly between the groups.

In order to assess the prevalence of NAFLD, the findings for TSH, TT3 and TT4 were broken down into quartiles (Table 1) and the individual subjects analyzed. Fig. 2 displays a downward trend in the prevalence rate of hepatic steatosis with increasing TT4 values. By contrast, except in the first quartile, the prevalence rate for hepatic steatosis showed an upward trend with increasing TSH concentrations.

Association of NAFLD with other variables

Males had a 2.8-fold increased risk of NAFLD compared with females (OR = 2.836; CI = 2.177-3.694). There was a significant correlation between NAFLD and age ($p < 0.0001$). Furthermore, NAFLD shows a significant association with BMI ($p < 0.0001$) and WHR ($p < 0.0001$). There was also a significant correlation between the presence of NAFLD and both metabolic syndrome (OR = 13.913; 95 % -CI 7.813 24.773; $p = 0.0001$) and diabetes mellitus (OR = 7.727; 95 % -CI = 3.407-17.525; $p < 0.0001$).

Association of NAFLD with thyroid hormones

In the univariate analysis, TSH and TT3 show no significant association with hepatic steatosis ($p = 0.7453$; $p = 0.1142$). For TT4 a significant correlation with NAFLD was shown ($p = 0.008$; OR = 0.987; 95 % -CI = 0.979-0.995). After adjusting for age or BMI, a significant association could be shown for TT4 and hepatic steatosis. Adjusted for WHR or gender, no significant association could detected (Table 3).

Discussion

Over the past decade, beginning with a study by Liangpunsakul and Chalasani in 2003 [14], the association between thyroid dysfunction and non-alcoholic fatty liver disease (NAFLD) has increasingly become a focus of research. After some controversial reports [24, 25], numerous studies have confirmed an association between thyroid function and NAFLD [13, 15, 26, 27]. Unfortunately, most studies have been characterized by either a relatively small or selected study collective, or by a gender imbalance [6, 14, 15, 28–30]. In addition, study subjects were in many cases patients rather than being a collective representative of the general population [14, 29, 30]. By contrast, the present study, like those of Chung *et al.*, Ittermann *et al.* und Zhang *et al.*, is characterized by a balanced gender distribution and its large study collective representative of the general population [13, 27, 31]. In addition, with a mean age of 40.7 ± 12.7 years, our collective is one of the younger populations studied, and includes the age group with the highest prevalence of NAFLD [5, 6].

The findings of the present study agree in general with those reported from the cross-sectional study of Ittermann *et al.* In both studies, a significant inverse association between the FT4 concentration of NAFLD could be demonstrated, while no significant association could be identified for TT3 or TSH [31]. This underscores the importance of the TT4 or FT4 concentration as a marker for hepatic steatosis in the general population. By contrast, the TT3 concentration, both in the present study and in those of Ittermann *et al.* and Xu *et al.*, had no identified value as a marker [6, 31]. This finding could related to an inhibition of the conversion of TT4 to TT3, possibly explaining the subordinate diagnostic role of the TT3 or FT3. Even the study of Chung *et al.*, which presented clear evidence of the association between hypothyroidism and NAFLD, did not ascribe any diagnostic value to the TT3 concentration [13].

Beside the inverse association with FT4, Chung *et al.* and Xu *et al.* identified a positive association between NAFLD and TSH [6, 13]. This association was observed in other studies [28, 29]. The difference between these studies and the present investigation may be the result of a divergent classification of study subjects regarding thyroid function or differences in recruitment of subjects from population-based sources or from a patient collective. Data reported by Carulli *et al.* and Pagadala *et al.* suggest, in addition, that the TSH concentration is associated with the severity of the hepatic steatosis [15, 28].

The above observations point to a possible correlation between thyroid dysfunction and NAFLD. This correlation may be explained, on the one hand, by a significant

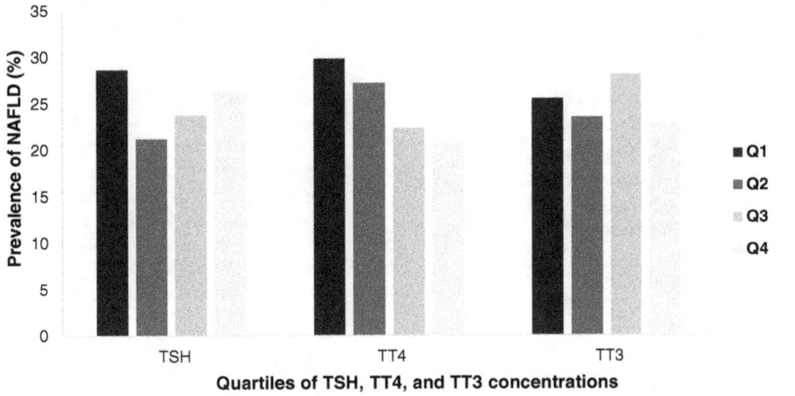

Fig. 2 Prevalence of non-alcoholic fatty liver disease (NAFLD) in relation to thyroid function in the present study. The figure plots the thyroid hormone concentrations in their respective quartiles (*x*-axis) against NAFLD prevalence rates in percent (*y*-axis). NAFLD prevalence rates show a downward trend with increasing TT4 concentrations. In addition, a positive trend is also seen for NAFLD prevalence rates with increasing TSH levels in the first quartile

association between thyroid dysfunction, a hypothyroid metabolic state and the metabolic syndrome [28, 32, 33]. Metabolic syndrome, in turn, is associated with NAFLD [1, 7, 9] and would point indirectly to a possible correlation between thyroid dysfunction and NAFLD. On the other hand, the correlation may be grounded in the association of reduced TT4 levels with hypertriglyceridemia and overweight. Beside studies which confirm the association between thyroid dysfunction, especially the hypothyroid metabolic state, and metabolic syndrome, there are studies with controversial findings [34, 35]. These studies highlight the correlation between NAFLD and thyroid dysfunction. For example, the study by Roos *et al.* shows a correlation between the FT4 level and triglycerides [33]. Our study would confirm this finding, as our data show a significant association between the TT4 level and triglycerides ($p = 0.0027$). These observations agree with the findings of other studies that suggest a correlation between hypothyroidism and hyperlipidemia [33, 36]. The increase in triglycerides in patients with hypothyroidism is explained by the reduced hepatic activity of triglyceride lipase [32, 33] and increased fatty acid oxidation. Loria *et al.* come to the conclusion that hepatic steatosis may develop from hypothyroidism-induced hyperlipidemia and overweight [17]. The development of hepatic steatosis may be explained by an increase influx of triglycerides and an imbalance between the in- and outflow of other lipids in the liver.

Because thyroid dysfunction, especially the hypothyroid metabolic state, affects the overall metabolism and may contribute to the development of hepatic steatosis and more serious forms of NAFLD, future interventional studies, similar to that of Ineck *et al.* should focus on treatment of thyroid dysfunction [18].

The present study has some limitations. Because of the choice of study design, it was possible to investigate associations but not causalities. While liver biopsy represents the gold standard for diagnosis of NAFLD [1], the diagnosis of hepatic steatosis in our study was made using ultrasonography. Also, because serum insulin levels were not determined in fasting subjects and thus could not be used, insulin resistance was not assessed in this study as a possible factor impacting the association between thyroid dysfunction and NAFLD.

Table 3 Association of hepatic steatosis with thyroid hormone

	OR (95 % -CI)	p-value
bivariate		
TSH	0.992 (0.945-1.042)	0.7453
TT3	0.738 (0.506-1.076)	0.1142
TT4	0.987 (0.979-0.995)	0.0008
multivariate		
TT4 *adjusted for age*	0.990 (0.982-0.998)	0.0143
TT4 *adjusted for BMI*	0.988 (0.979-0.997)	<.0001
TT4 *adjusted for WHR*	0.997 (0.987-1.006)	0.5048
TT4 Adjusted for gender	0.994 (0.985-1.002)	0.1172
TT4 *Adjusted for BMI, age, WHR, gender*	0.994 (0.984-1.005)	0.2959

TSH = thyroid-stimulating hormone; TT3 = triiodothyronine; TT4 = thyroxine; BMI = body-mass-index; WHR = waist to hip ratio

Conclusions

In summary, the results of the present study agree in many points with the findings of numerous publications and confirm a correlation between low TT4 concentrations and hepatic steatosis in a study collective representative of the general population. The prevalence of hepatic steatosis rises significantly with reductions in TT4 concentrations. A low TT4 concentration appears to be an independent risk factor for hepatic steatosis. Future studies should further elucidate the impact of thyroid hormone parameters on NAFLD. This could serve to clarify the underlying pathogenetic mechanisms and provide potentially important data for therapeutic and preventive measures.

Abbreviations

ALT: Alanine Aminotransferase; Anti-TPO: Anti-Thyroid Peroxidase antibodies; AST: Aspartate Aminotransferase; ATP III: Adult Treatment Panel III; BMI: Body-Mass Index; FT3: Free Triiodthyronin; FT4: Free Thyroxin; GGT: γ-Glutamyl transferase; NAFLD: Non-Alcoholic Fatty Liver Disease; NASH: Non-Alcoholic Steatohepatitis; nmol: Nanomol; SD: Standard Deviation; TT3: Triiodthyronin; TT4: Thyroxin; TSH: Thyroid-Stimulating Hormone; WHO: World Health Organization; WHR: Waist-to-Hip-Ratio.

Competing interests

The authors declare that they have no competing interests.

Authors' contributions

UL and DH wrote the manuscript. MMH, SO, WKoe, BOB, WK were involved in the design and conduction of the study. MMH, SO, WKoe, BOB and TG collected and analysed the data. AG, CD, WK were involved in data interpretation and manuscript writing. All authors read and approved the final manuscript.

Acknowledgements

Members of the EMIL-Study-Group (in alphabetical order)
Adler G, Armsen A, Banzhaf H-M, Bauerdick M, Bertling U, Boehm BO, Brandner BO, Brockmann SO, Deckert M, Dingler C, Eggink S, Fuchs M, Gaus W, Goussis H, Gruenert A, Haenle MM, Hampl W, Haug C, Hay B, Huetter M-L, Imhof A, Kern P, Kimmig P, Kirch A, Klass D, Koenig W, Kratzer W, Kron M, Manfras B, Meitinger K, Mertens T, Oehme R, Pfaff G, Piechotowski I, Reuter S, Romig T, von Schmiesing AFA, Steinbach G, Tourbier M, Voegtle A, Walcher T, Wolff S.

Author details

[1]Department of Internal Medicine I, Center for Internal Medicine, University Medical Center Ulm, Albert-Einstein-Allee 23, 89081 Ulm, Germany. [2]Department of Pediatrics and Adolescent Medicine, University Medical Center Ulm, Eythstr. 24, 89075 Ulm, Germany. [3]Department of Internal Medicine II, Center for Internal Medicine, University Medical Center Ulm, Albert-Einstein-Allee 23, 89081 Ulm, Germany. [4]Deutsches Herzzentrum München, Technische Universität München, Munich, Germany. [5]DZHK (German Centre for Cardiovascular Research), partner site Munich Heart Alliance, Munich, Germany. [6]Lee Kong Chian School of Medicine, Nanyang Technological University, Singapore, Singapore. [7]Imperial College London, London, UK. [8]Louis Stokes Cleveland Department of Veterans Affairs Medical Center, 10701 East Boulevard, Cleveland, OH 44106, USA. [9]Department of Diagnostic and Interventional Radiology, University Medical Center Ulm, Albert-Einstein-Allee 23, 89081 Ulm, Germany.

References

1. Musso G, Gambino R, Cassader M. Non-alcoholic fatty liver disease from pathogenesis to management: an update. Obes Rev. 2010;11:430–45.
2. Oh HJ, Kim TH, Sohn YW, Kim YS, Oh YR, Cho EY, et al. Association of serum alanine aminotransferase and gamma-glutamyltransferase levels within the reference range with metabolic syndrome and nonalcoholic fatty liver disease. Korean J Hepatol. 2011;17:27–36.
3. Starley BQ, Calcagno CJ, Harrison SA. Nonalcoholic fatty liver disease and hepatocellular carcinoma: a weighty connection. Hepatology. 2010;51:1820–32.
4. Vuppalanchi R, Chalasani N. Nonalcoholic fatty liver disease and nonalcoholic steatohepatitis: Selected practical issues in their evaluation and management. Hepatology. 2009;49:306–17.
5. Frith J, Day CP, Henderson E, Burt AD, Newton JL. Non-alcoholic fatty liver disease in older people. Gerontology. 2009;55:607–13.
6. Xu C, Xu L, Yu C, Miao M, Li Y. Association between thyroid function and nonalcoholic fatty liver disease in euthyroid elderly Chinese. Clin Endocrinol (Oxf). 2011;75:240–6.
7. Zelber-Sagi S, Nitzan-Kaluski D, Halpern Z, Oren R. Prevalence of primary non-alcoholic fatty liver disease in a population-based study and its association with biochemical and anthropometric measures. Liver Int. 2006;26:856–63.
8. Anstee QM, McPherson S, Day CP. How big a problem is non-alcoholic fatty liver disease? BMJ. 2011;343:d3897.
9. Bookman ID, Pham J, Guindi M, Heathcote EJ. Distinguishing nonalcoholic steatohepatitis from fatty liver: serum-free fatty acids, insulin resistance, and serum lipoproteins. Liver Int. 2006;26:566–71.
10. Papandreou D, Rousso I, Mavromichalis I. Update on non-alcoholic fatty liver disease in children. Clin Nutr. 2007;26:409–15.
11. Angulo P. Non-alcoholic fatty liver disease. N Engl J Med. 2002;346:1221–31.
12. Kotronen A, Yki-Järvinen H. Fatty liver: a novel component of the metabolic syndrome. Arterioscler Thromb Vasc Biol. 2008;28:27–38.
13. Chung GE, Kim D, Kim W, Yim JY, Park MJ, Kim YJ, et al. Non-alcoholic fatty liver disease across the spectrum of hypothyroidism. J Hepatol. 2012;57:150–6.
14. Liangpunsakul S, Chalasani N. Is hypothyroidism a risk factor for non-alcoholic steatohepatitis? J Clin Gastroenterol. 2003;37:340–3.
15. Pagadala MR, Zein CO, Dasarathy S, Yerian LM, Lopez R, McCullough AJ. Prevalence of hypothyroidism in nonalcoholic fatty liver disease. Dig Dis Sci. 2012;57:528–34.
16. Xu L, Ma H, Miao M, Li Y. Impact of subclinical hypothyroidism on the development of non-alcoholic fatty liver disease: A prospective case–control study. J Hepato. 2012;57:1153–4.
17. Loria P, Carulli L, Bertolotti M, Lonardo A. Endocrine and liver interaction: the role of endocrine pathways in NASH. Nat Rev Gastroenterol Hepatol. 2009;6:236–47.
18. Ineck BA, Ng TM. Effects of subclinical hypothyroidism and its treatment on serum lipids. Ann Pharmacother. 2003;37:725–30.
19. Haenle MM, Brockmann SO, Kron M, Bertling U, Mason RA, Steinbach G, et al. Overweight, physical activity, tobacco and alcohol consumption in a cross-sectional random sample of German adults. BMC Public Health. 2006;6:233.
20. Expert Panel on Detection. Evaluation, and treatment of high blood cholesterol in adults: executive summary of the third report of the national cholesterol education program (NCEP) (2001) expert panel on detection, evaluation, and treatment of high blood cholesterol in adults (adult treatment panel III). JAMA. 2001;285:2486–97.
21. Saverymuttu SH, Joseph AE, Maxwell JD. Ultrasound scanning in the detection of hepatic fibrosis and steatosis. Br Med J (Clin Res Ed). 1986;292:13–5.
22. Hamaguchi M, Kojima T, Itoh Y, Harano Y, Fujii K, Nakajima T, et al. The severity of ultrasonographic findings in nonalcoholic fatty liver disease reflects the metabolic syndrome and visceral fat accumulation. Am J Gastroenterol. 2003;102:2708–15.
23. Charatcharoenwitthaya P, Lindor KD. Role of radiologic modalities in the management of non-alcoholic steatohepatitis. Clin Liver. 2007;11:37–54.
24. Eshraghian A, Dabbaghmanesh MH, Eshraghian H, Fattahi MR, Omrani GR. Nonalcoholic fatty liver disease in a cluster of Iranian population: thyroid status and metabolic risk factors. Arch Iran Med. 2013;16:584–9.
25. Mazo DF, Lima VM, Stefano JT, Rabelo F, Faintuch J, Oliveira CP. Gluco-lipidic indices in treated hypothyroidism associated with nonalcoholic fatty liver disease. Arq Gastroenterol. 2011;48:186–9.
26. Gardner CJ, Richardson P, Wong C, Polavarapu N, Kemp GJ, Cuthbertson DJ. Hypothyroidism in a patient with non-alcoholic fatty liver disease. BMJ. 2011;342:c7199.
27. Zhang Y, Chang Y, Ryu S, Cho J, Lee WY, Rhee EJ, et al. Thyroid hormones and mortality risk in euthyroid individuals: the Kangbuk Samsung health study. J Clin Endocrinol Metab. 2014;99:2467–76.
28. Carulli L, Ballestri S, Lonardo A, Lami F, Violi E, Losi L, et al. Is nonalcoholic steatohepatitis associated with a high-though-normal thyroid stimulating hormone level and lower cholesterol levels? Intern Emerg Med. 2013;8:297–305.
29. Moustafa AH, Ali EM, Mohamed TM, Abdou HI. Oxidative stress and thyroid hormones in patients with liver diseases. Eur J Intern Med. 2009;20:703–8.
30. Silveira MG1, Mendes FD, Diehl NN, Enders FT, Lindor KD. Thyroid dysfunction in primary biliary cirrhosis, primary sclerosing cholangitis and non-alcoholic fatty liver disease. Liver Int. 2009;29:1094–100.
31. Ittermann T, Haring R, Wallaschofski H, Baumeister SE, Nauck M, Dörr M, et al. Inverse association between serum free thyroxine levels and hepatic steatosis: results from the Study of Health in Pomerania. Thyroid. 2012;22:568–74.
32. Park HT, Cho GJ, Ahn KH, Shin JH, Hong SC, Kim T, et al. Thyroid stimulating hormone is associated with metabolic syndrome in euthyroid postmenopausal women. Maturitas. 2009;62:301–5.

33. Roos A, Bakker SJ, Links TP, Gans RO, Wolffenbuttel BH. Thyroid function is associated with components of the metabolic syndrome in euthyroid subjects. J Clin Endocrinol Metab. 2007;92:491–6.
34. Garduño-Garcia Jde J, Alvirde-Garcia U, López-Carrasco G, Padilla Mendoza ME, Mehta R, Arellano-Campos O, et al. TSH and free thyroxine concentrations are associated with differing metabolic markers in euthyroid subjects. Eur J Endocrinol. 2010;163:273–8.
35. Liu C, Scherbaum WA, Schott M, Schinner S. Subclinical hypothyroidism and the prevalence of the metabolic syndrome. Horm Metab Res. 2011;43:417–21.
36. Tagami T, Kimura H, Ohtani S, Tanaka T, Tanaka T, Hata S, et al. PHPH study group: multi-center study on the prevalence of hypothyroidism in patients with hypercholesterolemia. Endocr J. 2011;58:449–57.

Impaired lung function is associated with non-alcoholic fatty liver disease independently of metabolic syndrome features in middle-aged and elderly Chinese

Li Qin[1,2†], Weiwei Zhang[1,2†], Zhen Yang[1,2*], Yixin Niu[1,2], Xiaoyong Li[1,2], Shuai Lu[1], Yin Xing[1], Ning Lin[1,2], Hongmei Zhang[1,2], Guang Ning[3], Jiangao Fan[4] and Qing Su[1,2*]

Abstract

Background: Associations between lung function and non-alcoholic fatty liver disease (NAFLD) have been reported. However, evidence from large-scale populations about the relationship is scarce. The objective of the study was to evaluate the relationship between lung function and NAFLD in middle-aged and elderly Chinese.

Methods: A total of 1842 participants aged 40 years or older were recruited from Chongming District, Shanghai, China. Lung function, evaluated by forced vital capacity (FVC) and forced expiratory volume in one second (FEV1) was measured with standard spirometry. The NAFLD was evaluated by ultrasonography.

Results: The subjects with NAFLD had lower FVC (% predicted) (0.85 ± 0.26 vs. 0.90 ± 0.28, $p < 0.001$) and FEV1 (% predicted) (0.93 ± 0.29 vs. 0.98 ± 0.34, $p < 0.001$) than non-NAFLD. After adjusting for potential risk factors, the lowest quartile of FVC (% predicted) and FEV1 (% predicted) was associated with increased prevalence of NAFLD, with the fully adjusted odds ratio of 1.37 and 1.24 (95% confidence interval [CI] 1.18–1.97, $p < 0.001$, 95% CI 1.11–1.87, $p = 0.009$), respectively.

Conclusions: Impaired lung function is associated with non-alcoholic fatty liver disease, independent of conventional metabolic risk factors.

Keywords: Lung function, Non-alcoholic fatty liver disease, Chinese, Metabolic risk factors

Background

Nonalcoholic fatty liver disease (NAFLD) is characterized by excessive hepatic fat accumulation of patients who have no history of alcohol abuse [1]. Recently, the combination of overnutrition condition and less physical activity have made NAFLD become the most common disease of chronic liver damage, with increased prevalence of obesity, diabetes, and metabolic syndrome in developed and developing counties [2]. The traditional risk factors of NAFLD, such as central obesity, insulin resistance, systemic inflammation, current smoking, diabetes, and oxidative stress, contribute to, but cannot fully explain the increased risk of NAFLD in the general population [3–5].

Recently, lung function parameters, estimated by forced vital capacity (FVC) and forced expiratory volume in one second (FEV1) were proved to be well associated with the development of diabetes, cardiovascular disease, inflammation process and metabolic syndrome [6–25]. NAFLD has been considered as a hepatic manifestation of the metabolic syndrome and is associated with various metabolic abnormalities, including hyperlipidemia, central obesity, and type 2 diabetes [1, 26, 27]. So, reduced

* Correspondence: yangzhen1020@hotmail.com; suqingxinhua@163.com
†Equal contributors
1Department of Endocrinology, Xinhua Hospital Chongming Branch, Shanghai Jiao Tong University School of Medicine, Shanghai, China
Full list of author information is available at the end of the article

lung function may link to an increased risk of NAFLD. In a previous study, association of reduced lung function with NAFLD was detected among men in a health examination program [28]. However, evidence from large-scale populations about the relationship between reduced lung function and NAFLD is scarce. In addition, it is unclear whether the association can be observed in Chinese population.

For this purpose, the aims of this study were to test the hypotheses that reduced lung function is independently associated with NAFLD in a cross-sectional population study of 1,842 middle-aged and older Chinese subjects.

Methods

Study population

In 2011, China launched a national survey of Risk Evaluation of cAncers in Chinese diabeTic Individuals: a lONgitudinal (REACTION) study, which was conducted among 259,657 adults, aged 40 years and older in 25 communities across mainland China, from 2011 to 2012 [29]. The data presented in this article are based on the baseline survey of subsamples from Shanghai in eastern China [30, 31]. All studied individuals came from the Chongming District in Shanghai, China. There were 9930 participants who had complete information about age; sex; smoking and alcohol consumption habits; and a medical history including the use of medications, BMI, and a hepatic ultrasonic examination. Participants meeting the following criteria were excluded: 1) those with a history of known liver diseases such as hepatitis, cirrhosis, or malignancy; 2) those with alcohol consumption greater than 140 g/wk for men and 70 g/wk for women. Thus, a total of 8850 participants were eventually included in this analysis. Of these, two communities participants received lung function test. 1,842 participants were eventually included in the analysis. The protocol was approved by the Institutional Review Board of Xinhua Hospital affiliated with Shanghai Jiao-Tong University School of Medicine.

Data collection

A standardized questionnaire was used by trained physicians to collect information such as age; sex; current smoking (yes/no); current drinker (yes/no). Physical activity level was classified as low, moderate, or high according to the International Physical Activity Questionnaire scoring protocol. According to participants' responses to the corresponding questions, family history of diabetes was classified as yes or no.

The details of anthropometric measurements including height, weight, waist circumference, hip circumference were carried by trained physicians. Blood pressure was measured at the right arm with an automated electronic device (OMRON Model1 Plus; Omron Company, Kyoto, Japan) three times consecutively with 1 min intervals after at least 5 min rest in the seated position; the three readings were averaged for analysis. Body mass index (BMI) was calculated as weight in kilograms divided by the square of height in meters.

All subjects were assessed after overnight fasting for at least 10 h, Overnight fasting and 2 h OGTT (Oral Glucose Tolerance Test) 75 g glucose blood samples were collected in tubes containing EDTA and were centrifuged at 4 °C and stored at−80 °C until analysis. The fasting glucose, glucose 2 h after oral glucose tolerance test, total cholesterol (TC), triglycerides, low-density lipoprotein (LDL) cholesterol and high-density lipoprotein (HDL) cholesterol were measured on an automatic analyzer (Hitachi 7080; Tokyo, Japan). Fasting insulin was determined by RIA (Linco Research, St. Charles, MO). The homeostasis model assessment of insulin resistance (HOMA-IR) was calculated according to the equation described by Matthews et al. [32].

Definition of NAFLD

Hepatic ultrasonic examination was performed on all participants by two trained ultrasonographists who were blinded to the clinical and laboratory data, using a high-resolution B-mode tomographic ultrasound system (Esaote Biomedica SpA, Italy) with a 3.5-MHz probe. Diagnosis of fatty liver by ultrasonography was defined by the presence of at least two of three abnormal

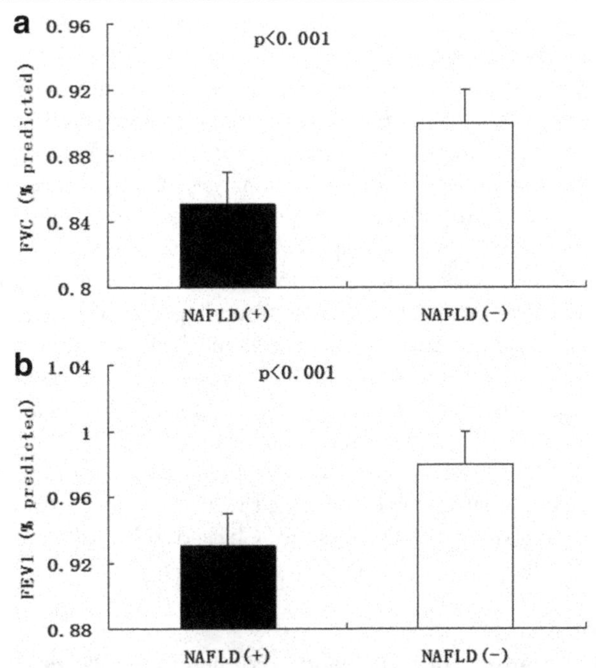

Fig. 1 The levels of FVC (% pred) and FEV1 (% pred) in subjects with NAFLD and without NAFLD. Data are shown as means ± SE after adjustment for age and sex. (A for FVC and B for FEV1)

findings: diffusely increased echogenicity of the liver relative to the kidney, ultrasound beam attenuation, and poor visualization of intrahepatic structures. NAFLD was diagnosed by hepatic ultrasound after the exclusion of alcohol abuse and other liver diseases.

Lung function measurements

Lung function tests including FVC and FEV1 were conducted by a trained physician using Electronic Spirometer (Model BF-II, Jintan, China). Each participant received at least two tests (with acceptable maneuvers) at a seated position and with nose clips in place. The predicted values for FVC and FEV1 were calculated from the following equations obtained in a representative sample of Chinese population [25].

Predicted FVC of man = −4.33058–(0.01326× age [years]) + (0.04669× height [cm]) + (0.01664× weight [kg]).

Predicted FVC of woman = −4.79287– (0.01326× age [years]) + (0.04669× height [cm]) + (0.01664× weight [kg]).

Predicted FEV1 of man = −3.65523– (0.01850× age [years]) + (0.04283× height [cm]) + (0.009228832× weight [kg]).

Predicted FEV1 of woman = −4.04947– (0.01850× age [years]) + (0.04283× height [cm]) + (0.009228832× weight [kg]).

The percentage of predicted values for FEV1, FEV1 (% pred), equals to FEV1 devided by the predicted values of FEV1. The percentage of predicted values for FVC, FVC (% pred), equals to FVC divided by the predicted values of FVC. The ratio of FEV1 to FVC was calculated.

Statistical analysis

Normally distributed data were expressed as means ± SD, whereas variables with a skewed distribution were reported as median (interquartile range) and log transformed to approximate normality before analysis. Comparisons of means and proportions were performed with the standard normal z and $\chi 2$ tests, respectively. Multivariate logistic regression models were used to estimate the odds ratios (ORs) for NAFLD. Potential confounding variables including age, gender, current smoking, family history of diabetes, systolic blood pressure, diastolic blood pressure, fasting plasma glucose, 2 h OGTT plasma glucose, hemoglobin A1c, waist circumference, BMI, HOMA-IR, TG, TC, LDL-c and HDL-c were controlled in the regression models. All statistical analysis were performed with the SPSS Statistical Package (version 13.0; SPSS Inc., Chicago, IL). $P < 0.05$ was considered statistically significant.

Results

Characteristics of participants according to FVC (% pred) or FEV1 (% pred) quartile

Mean values of FVC (% pred), FEV1 (% pred) in subjects with NAFLD were significantly lower than in those without (0.85 ± 0.26 vs. 0.90 ± 0.28, 0.93 ± 0.29 vs. 0.98 ± 0.34; both $p < 0.001$) (Fig. 1). Individuals with NAFLD were elder, more likely to be metabolic syndrome, current drinker, and heavy smoking, and had higher levels of BMI, SBP, DBP, waist circumference, hip circumference, waist-hip ratio, fasting plasma glucose FPG, postprandial 2-h plasma glucose, A1C, HOMA-IR, TG, TC, LDL-c, AST, ALT and GGT (all p values < 0.001), and had lower levels of HDL-c ($p < 0.001$) (Table 1).

When analyzed by quartiles of FVC (% pred) or FEV1 (% pred) levels, as summarized in Tables 2 and 3, the subjects with lower FVC (% pred) or FEV1 (% pred) were more likely to be more metabolic syndrome ($p < 0.001$), more smoker ($p < 0.001$), more drinker ($p < 0.001$), more aged ($p < 0.001$), With respect to metabolic parameters, the subjects in the higher FVC (% pred) or FEV1 (% pred) quartiles exhibited low er levels of LDL cholesterol

Table 1 Baseline characteristics of the study participants, grouped according to NAFLD status

	Without NAFLD (*n* = 1164)	With NAFLD (*n* = 678)	*P* value
ATPIII-defined metabolic syndrome n(%)	433(37.21)	526(77.64)	<0.001
Sex n (% men)	376(32.3)	213(31.4)	0.38
Age (years)[b]	55.38 ± 8.10	56.97 ± 7.55	<0.001
BMI (kg/m2)	23.32 ± 2.95	26.47 ± 6.33	<0.001
Currents smokers n (%)	275(23.63)	178(26.30)	<0.001
SBP (mmHg)	127.49 ± 20.64	133.10 ± 20.98	<0.001
DBP (mmHg)	78.99 ± 10.53	81.77 ± 10.34	<0.001
Waist circumference (cm)	81.18 ± 10.46	89.42 ± 8.70	<0.001
Hip circumference (cm)	94.12 ± 6.06	99.05 ± 6.95	<0.001
Waist-hip ratio	0.86 ± 0.14	0.90 ± 0.07	<0.001
Fasting plasma glucose (mmol/l)	6.02 ± 1.45	6.65 ± 1.93	<0.001
2 h PG (mmol/L)	7.87 ± 3.40	9.17 ± 4.22	<0.001
A1C(%)	5.82 ± 0.86	6.25 ± 1.14	<0.001
HOMA-IR	1.47 (1.13–1.92)	2.36 (1.63–3.27)	<0.001
Triglycerides (mmol/l)	1.38 ± 0.95	2.16 ± 1.54	<0.001
HDL-cholesterol (mmol/l)	1.29 ± 0.33	1.15 ± 0.28	<0.001
LDL-cholesterol (mmol/l)	2.55 ± 0.74	2.70 ± 0.80	<0.001
AST(units/l)	15.92 ± 8.67	22.29 ± 12.54	<0.001
ALT(units/l)	14.15 ± 10.03	21.19 ± 15.87	<0.001
GGT(units/l)	24.09 ± 28.30	38.61 ± 48.45	<0.001

SBP systolic blood pressure, *DBP* diastolic blood pressure, *BMI* body mass index; *2hPG* postprandial 2-h plasma glucose, *HbA1C* Glycated hemoglobin, *LDL* Low-density lipoprotein, *HDL* high-density lipoprotein, *ALT* Alanine aminotransferase, *AST* aspartate aminotransferase, GGT γ-glutamyltransferase
[a]Data are presented as mean ± SD, median (interquartile range), or number (percent); *P* value was calculated after adjustment for age, gender
[b]Not adjusted for itself
[c]This variables was log transformed before analysis

Table 2 Characteristic according to quartiles of FVC (% predicted)[a]

	Quartile 1 ($n = 450$)	Quartile 2 ($n = 471$)	Quartile 3 ($n = 460$)	Quartile 4 ($n = 471$)	P value
FVC (% predicted)	0.63 ± 0.09	0.77 ± 0.25	0.87 ± 0.03	1.22 ± 0.28	<0.001
FEV1 (% predicted)	0.70 ± 0.18	0.86 ± 0.15	1.01 ± 0.26	1.27 ± 0.31	<0.001
FEV1/FVC ratio	0.77 ± 0.22	0.77 ± 0.22	0.76 ± 0.23	0.74 ± 0.24	<0.001
MS (n, %)	294(65.33)	271(57.53)	253(55.00)	232(49.26)	<0.001
NAFLD (n, %)	193(42.89)	188(39.92)	160(34.78)	137(29.09)	<0.001
Age (years)[b]	56.64 ± 8.23	55.65 ± 7.87	55.37 ± 7.48	56.31 ± 7.91	0.007
Male (n, %)	45(10.00)	78 (16.56)	168(36.52)	384(81.53)	<0.001
Current smoking (n, %)	51(11.33)	66(14.01)	87(18.91)	166(35.24)	<0.001
Current drinker (n, %)	61(13.56)	88(18.68)	86(18.70)	183(38.85)	<0.001
Regular exerciser (n, %)	265(58.89)	282(59.87)	275(59.78)	284(60.29)	0.978
BMI (kg/m^2)	24.82 ± 3.97	25.09 ± 3.59	24.48 ± 3.27	24.73 ± 3.34	0.102
SBP (mmHg)	137.56 ± 19.42	134.32 ± 18.82	131.51 ± 19.15	135.78 ± 18.95	<0.001
DBP (mmHg)	82.40 ± 10.44	82.16 ± 10.87	80.98 ± 9.98	82.53 ± 10.57	<0.001
WC (cm)	86.54 ± 11.48	85.76 ± 11.11	83.93 ± 10.31	84.73 ± 10.45	0.002
FPG (mmol/L)	6.54 ± 1.87	6.65 ± 2.21	6.32 ± 1.75	6.31 ± 1.36	0.011
2 h PG (mmol/L)	9.42 ± 4.23	9.43 ± 4.57	8.70 ± 4.01	8.38 ± 3.61	<0.001
A1C (%)	5.90 ± 1.10	5.94 ± 1.23	5.75 ± 1.01	5.67 ± 0.83	<0.001
HOMA-IRc	2.32(1.44–3.31)	1.84 (1.30–2.68)	1.75(1.22–2.50)	1.66(1.18–2.32)	0.029
eGFR	124.75 ± 25.25	122.57 ± 21.90	120.30 ± 19.95	114.73 ± 21.85	<0.001
Triglycerides (mmol/L)[c]	1.88 ± 1.27	1.76 ± 1.30	1.63 ± 1.05	1.89 ± 1.65	0.009
TC (mmol/L)	5.14 ± 0.96	5.07 ± 0.88	4.87 ± 0.85	4.86 ± 0.88	<0.001
HDL-c (mmol/L)	1.34 ± 0.32	1.36 ± 0.31	1.31 ± 0.32	1.29 ± 0.33	0.004
LDL-c (mmol/L)	2.84 ± 0.75	2.81 ± 0.74	2.73 ± 0.70	2.71 ± 0.72	<0.001
ALT (units/l)	21.37 ± 17.36	21.08 ± 15.98	19.78 ± 14.06	17.82 ± 11.15	<0.001
AST (units/l)	25.35 ± 13.05	24.28 ± 12.53	24.13 ± 10.75	22.14 ± 7.31	<0.001
GGT (units/l)	42.19 ± 42.29	36.22 ± 51.10	30.96 ± 33.42	29.91 ± 37.36	<0.001

SBP systolic blood pressure, *DBP* diastolic blood pressure, *BMI* body mass index, *OGTT* Oral Glucose Tolerance Test, *FPG* Fasting Plasma Glucose, *2 h PG* postprandial 2-h Plasma Glucose, *HbA1C* Glycated hemoglobin, *LDL* Low-density lipoprotein, *HDL* high-density lipoprotein, *ALT* Alanine aminotransferase, *AST* aspartate aminotransferase, *GGT* γ-glutamyltransferase

[a]Data are presented as mean ± SD, median (interquartile range), or number (percent); *P* value was calculated after adjustment for age, gender

[b]Not adjusted for itself

[c]This variables was log transformed before analysis

($p < 0.001$). However, elevated FVC (% pred) or FEV1 (% pred) levels showed no association with the regular exerciser ($p > 0.05$).

Association between quartiles of FVC (% pred) and FEV1 (% pred) and NAFLD

As shown in Table 4, the lowest quartile of FVC (% pred) and FEV1 (% pred) was associated with increased odds of NAFLD, with age- and sex-adjusted odds ratio (OR) of 1.82 and 1.74, respectively (95% confidential interval (CI), 1.38–2.39 and 95% CI, 1.32–2.28; both $p < 0.001$). Further adjustments for current smoking, family history of diabetes systolic blood pressure, diastolic blood pressure, fasting plasma glucose, 2 h OGTT plasma glucose, Hemoglobin A1c, waist circumference, BMI, HOMA-IR, TG, TC, LDL-c and HDL-c did not eliminate the associations (OR, 1.37, 95% CI, 1.18–1.97, $p < 0.001$ and OR,1.24, 95% CI, 1.11–1.87, $p = 0.009$).

Discussion

In the present study, we found that impaired lung function as measured by FVC and FEV1 was significantly and inversely associated with prevalence of NAFLD in a middle-aged and elderly population without chronic pulmonary diseases after adjustment for a wide range of variables including age, gender, current smoking, family history of diabetes, systolic blood pressure, diastolic blood pressure, fasting plasma glucose, 2 h OGTT plasma glucose, hemoglobin A1c, waist circumference, BMI, HOMA-IR and lipid profile.

Our results are consistent with previous study that restrictive lung function (reduced FVC and FEV1) but not

Table 3 Characteristic according to quartiles of FEV1 (% predicted)[a]

	Quartile 1 ($n = 454$)	Quartile 2 ($n = 467$)	Quartile 3 ($n = 464$)	Quartile 4 ($n = 467$)	*P* value
FEV1 (%)	0.66 ± 0.11	0.83 ± 0.03	0.95 ± 0.05	1.42 ± 0.26	<0.001
FVC (%)	0.66 ± 0.14	0.79 ± 0.12	0.92 ± 0.20	1.13 ± 0.30	<0.001
FEV1/FVC ratio	73.21 ± 22.91	77.23 ± 22.01	76.63 ± 22.81	78.02 ± 22.61	<0.001
MS (n, %)	282(62.11)	273(58.46)	255(54.96)	240(51.39)	<0.001
NAFLD (n, %)	200(44.05)	171(36.62)	162(34.91)	145(30.79)	<0.001
Age (years)[b]	56.37 ± 8.22	55.51 ± 7.72	55.17 ± 8.12	56.68 ± 7.50	0.004
Male (n, %)	47(10.35)	82(17.56)	164(35.34)	382(81.80)	<0.001
Current smoking (n, %)	55(12.11)	68(14.56)	87(18.75)	159(34.05)	<0.001
Current drinker (n, %)	64(14.10)	90(19.27)	89(19.18)	175(37.47)	<0.001
Regular exerciser (n, %)	263(57.93)	285(61.03)	272(58.62)	287(61.46)	0.872
BMI (kg/m^2)	24.81 ± 3.93	24.76 ± 3.64	25.05 ± 3.42	24.74 ± 3.32	0.556
SBP (mmHg)	136.28 ± 19.26	135.84 ± 19.25	134.38 ± 18.12	133.54 ± 20.55	0.002
DBP (mmHg)	82.50 ± 10.43	82.12 ± 10.49	82.06 ± 10.36	81.90 ± 10.81	<0.001
WC (cm)	86.04 ± 11.68	85.06 ± 11.34	86.05 ± 10.27	84.70 ± 10.29	0.015
FPG (mmol/L)	6.55 ± 1.88	6.50 ± 3.64	6.48 ± 1.90	6.36 ± 1.49	0.004
2 h PG (mmol/L)	9.30 ± 4.20	9.10 ± 4.39	9.03 ± 4.09	8.47 ± 3.79	0.017
A1C(%)	5.88 ± 1.07	5.88 ± 1.14	5.83 ± 1.11	5.70 ± 0.93	0.035
HOMA-IR[c]	2.30(1.42–3.33)	1.79(1.28–2.63)	1.70(1.23–2.52)	1.64(1.15–2.31)	0.025
eGFR	124.85 ± 25.05	121.73 ± 21.24	119.85 ± 21.90	115.14 ± 21.27	<0.001
Triglycerides (mmol/L)	1.86 ± 1.26	1.73 ± 1.35	1.80 ± 1.38	1.77 ± 1.42	0.035
TC (mmol/L)	5.06 ± 0.93	4.95 ± 1.02	4.98 ± 0.84	4.92 ± 0.82	0.125
HDL-c (mmol/L)	1.33 ± 0.32	1.32 ± 0.30	1.32 ± 0.31	1.32 ± 0.31	0.031
LDL-c (mmol/L)	2.83 ± 0.75	2.79 ± 0.79	2.70 ± 0.67	2.69 ± 0.68	0.007
ALT(units/l)	21.22 ± 14.07	21.15 ± 14.28	19.94 ± 13.53	18.17 ± 13.09	<0.001
AST(units/l)	24.97 ± 12.85	24.31 ± 12.66	24.03 ± 11.49	22.47 ± 10.29	<0.001
GGT(units/l)	41.25 ± 37.73	38.07 ± 43.25	31.24 ± 34.71	28.99 ± 36.52	<0.001

SBP systolic blood pressure, *DBP* diastolic blood pressure, *BMI* body mass index, *OGTT* Oral Glucose Tolerance Test, *FPG* Fasting Plasma Glucose, *2 h PG* postprandial 2-h Plasma Glucose, *HbA1C HbA1C* hemoglobin A1C, *eGFR* estimate the glomerular filtration rate, *LDL* Low-density lipoprotein, *HDL* high-density lipoprotein, *ALT* Alanine aminotransferase, *AST* aspartate aminotransferase, *GGT* γ-glutamyltransferase

[a]Data are presented as mean ± SD, median (interquartile range), or number (percent); *P* value was calculated after adjustment for age, gender

[b]Not adjusted for itself

[c]This variables was log transformed before analysis

Table 4 Odds ratio for the non-alcoholic fatty liver disease according to quartiles of FVC (% pred) or FEV1 (% pred)

	FVC(% pred)				
	Quartile 1	Quartile 2	Quartile 3	Quartile 4	*P* value
Model 1	1.82(1.38–2.39)	1.60(1.23–2.12)	1.29(0.97–1.70)	1	<0.001
Model 2	1.65(1.27–2.24)	1.39(1.18–2.01)	1.12(0.87–1.52)	1	<0.001
Model 3	1.37(1.18–1.97)	1.19(1.08–1.82)	1.04(0.79–1.28)	1	<0.001
	FEV1(% pred)				
	Quartile 1	Quartile 2	Quartile 3	Quartile 4	*P* value
Model 1	1.74(1.32–2.28)	1.27(0.96–1.67)	1.18(0.90–1.55)	1	<0.001
Model 2	1.48(1.24–2.12)	1.13(0.89–1.48)	1.09(0.81–1.39)	1	0.004
Model 3	1.24(1.11–1.87)	1.07(0.76–1.21)	1.03(0.72–1.19)	1	0.009

Model 1, adjusted for age and sex; model 2, further adjusted for current smoking, family history of diabetes systolic blood pressure and diastolic blood pressure; model 3, further adjusted for fasting plasma glucose, 2 h OGTT plasma glucose, Hemoglobin A1c, waist circumference, BMI, HOMA-IR, TG, TC, LDL-c and HDL-c

obstructive pulmonary function (FEV1-to-FVC ratio) is associated with the development of NAFLD [28]. The underlying mechanisms relating reduced lung function to this type of metabolic disorder remain unclear; integration of inflammatory process and metabolic pathways in NAFLD patients may be a pivotal underlying mechanism link between reduced pulmonary function and incident NAFLD. Previous studies have demonstrated that a strong association between both restrictive and obstructive lung patterns and inflammatory markers [33, 34]. As we best known, low-grade systemic inflammation play a causal role in the development of NAFLD. Thus, the inflammatory process may contribute to the association between reduced lung function and NAFLD. However, the measurement of inflammatory markers was absent, limiting the ability to access the role of this factor in the association in the present study.

In our study, we observed that the positive association of FVC (% pred) in particular and FEV1 (% pred) with metabolic abnormalities and components of the insulin resistance syndrome, which is consistent with several previous studies that have reported associations between restrictive lung patterns with glucose metabolism and metabolic syndrome [6–23]. Moreover, our study also demonstrated that FVC (% pred) and FEV1 (% pred) were associated with insulin sensitivity as measured by the HOMA-IR. It has been well demonstrated that insulin resistance plays a key role in the development of NAFLD [35, 36]. Metabolic risk factors closely associated with insulin resistance (BMI, glucose, waist circumference, blood pressure, triglycerides, and HDL cholesterol) may affect the association of FVC (% pred), FEV1 (% pred) and NAFLD. However, our further analysis indicated that the effects of reduced lung function on NAFLD were independent of metabolic syndrome features.

The strengths of this study include the community-based sample, standardized spirometric techniques, extensive data on potential confounders, and a large sample size that increased precision and permitted multiple statistical adjustments. However, several limitations of our study have to be addressed. First, due to the cross-sectional nature of the current study, no causal inference can be drawn. Prospective studies are needed to clarify their precise interrelationship. Also, it has yet to be seen whether our results in middle-aged and older Chinese subjects can be generalized to younger populations or other ethnic groups. Secondly, liver biopsies, the best diagnostic tool for confirming NAFLD, were not available in our participants. The diagnosis of NAFLD was based on ultrasonic examination, which is not sensitive enough to detect mild steatosis. However, this method is the most widely used noninvasive technique to detect fatty infiltration of the liver in clinical practice and epidemiological studies, and it has been reported to have a sensitivity of 89% and specificity of 93% for the identification of fatty liver [37]. Third, the lack of inflammatory markers, which precluded more detailed investigations of the causal pathway. Furthermore, sleep duration/quality and symptoms of sleep apnea which was related to both insulin resistance and lung function may affect the association of impaired lung function and NAFLD, however, due to study design defect, we couldn't further analyze the effect in this study.

Conclusions

We have found that impaired lung function was associated with NAFLD in middle-aged and elderly Chinese population. These findings suggest the need to screen impaired of lung function in people without respiratory disease for the presence of NAFLD.

Abbreviations

ALT: Alanine aminotransferase; AST: Aspartate aminotransferase; BMI: Body mass index; FEV1: Forced expiratory volume in one second; FVC: Forced vital capacity; GGT: γ-glutamyltransferase; HDL: High-density lipoprotein cholesterol; HOMA-IR: Homeostasis model assessment of insulin resistance; LDL: Low-density lipoprotein cholesterol; NAFLD: Nonalcoholic fatty liver disease; Ors: Odds ratios.; TC: Total cholesterol

Acknowledgements

Not applicable.

Funding

This work was supported by National Natural Science Foundation of China (81370953, 81300667, 81370935), Shanghai Health System Outstanding Young Talents Training Program (XYQ2013098), Shanghai Science and Technology Commission (15411953200, 10411956600, 14ZR1427400), Shanghai Education Committee Key Program (14zz110), National Clinical Research Center for Metabolic Diseases (2013BAI09B13), National Key New Drug Creation and Manufacturing Program of Ministry of Science and Technology (2012ZX09303006-001) and State Key Development Program for Basic Research of China (2012CB517501). We thank the field workers for their contribution and the participants for their cooperation.

Authors' contributions

Conceived and designed the experiments: ZY and QS. Analyzed the data: LQ, WWZ, ZY, YXN, SL, YX, NL, HMZ, QS. Contributed reagents/materials/analysis tools: LQ, WWZ, ZY, GN, JGF,QS. Wrote the paper: LQ, WWZ, ZY, QS. All authors read and approved the final manuscript.

Competing interest

The authors declare that they have no competing interests.

Author details

[1]Department of Endocrinology, Xinhua Hospital Chongming Branch, Shanghai Jiao Tong University School of Medicine, Shanghai, China. [2]Department of Endocrinology, Xinhua Hospital, Shanghai Jiao Tong University School of Medicine, 1665 Kongjiang Road, Shanghai, China. [3]Department of Endocrinology and Metabolism, Key Laboratory for Endocrine and Metabolic Diseases of Ministry of Health, RuiJin Hospital, Shanghai Jiao Tong University School of Medicine, E-Institute of Shanghai Universities, Shanghai, China. [4]Department of Gastroenterology, Shanghai Key Laboratory of Children's Digestion and Nutrition, Xinhua Hospital, Shanghai Jiaotong University School of Medicine, Shanghai, China.

References

1. Fan JG, Farrell GC. Epidemiology of non-alcoholic fatty liver disease in China. J Hepatol. 2009;50:204–10.
2. Gaggini M, Morelli M, Buzzigoli E, DeFronzo RA, Bugianesi E, Gastaldelli A. Non-alcoholic fatty liver disease (NAFLD) and its connection with insulin resistance, dyslipidemia, atherosclerosis and coronary heart disease. Nutrients. 2013;5:1544–60.
3. Anstee QM, McPherson S, Day CP. How big a problem is non-alcoholic fatty liver disease? BMJ. 2011;343:d3897.
4. Williamson RM, Price JF, Glancy S, Perry E, Nee LD, Hayes PC, et al. Prevalence of and risk factors for hepatic steatosis and nonalcoholic Fatty liver disease in people with type 2 diabetes: the Edinburgh Type 2 Diabetes Study. Diabetes Care. 2011;34:1139–44.
5. Leung TM, Nieto N. CYP2E1 and oxidant stress in alcoholic and non-alcoholic fatty liver disease. J Hepatol. 2013;58:395–8.
6. Hickson DA, Burchfiel CM, Liu J, Petrini MF, Harrison K, White WB, et al. Diabetes, impaired glucose tolerance, and metabolic biomarkers in individuals with normal glucose tolerance are inversely associated with lung function: the Jackson Heart Study. Lung. 2011;189:311–21.
7. Ubhi BK, Riley JH, Shaw PA, Lomas DA, Tal-Singer R, MacNee W, et al. Metabolic profiling detects biomarkers of protein degradation in COPD patients. Eur Respir J. 2012;40:345–55.
8. Walter RE, Beiser A, Givelber RJ, O'Connor GT, Gottlieb DJ. Association between glycemic state and lung function: the Framingham Heart Study. Am J Respir Crit Care Med. 2003;167:911–6.
9. McKeever TM, Weston PJ, Hubbard R, Fogarty A. Lung function and glucose metabolism: an analysis of data from the Third National Health and Nutrition Examination Survey. Am J Epidemiol. 2005;161:546–56.
10. Davis WA, Knuiman M, Kendall P, Grange V, Davis TM. Fremantle Diabetes Study. Glycemic exposure is associated with reduced pulmonary function in type 2 diabetes: the Fremantle Diabetes Study. Diabetes Care. 2004;27:752–7.
11. Nakajima K, Ebata M, Saito M. The relationship between low vital capacity and impaired glucose metabolism in men. Diabet Med. 2010;27:1460–1.
12. Klein OL, Krishnan JA, Glick S, Smith LJ. Systematic review of the association between lung function and Type 2 diabetes mellitus. Diabet Med. 2010;27:977–87.
13. van den Borst B, Gosker HR, Zeegers MP, Schols AM. Pulmonary function in diabetes: a meta-analysis. Chest. 2010;138:393–406.
14. Heianza Y, Arase Y, Tsuji H, Saito K, Amakawa K, Hsieh SD, et al. Low lung function and risk of type 2 diabetes in Japanese men: the Toranomon Hospital Health Management Center Study 9 (TOPICS 9). Mayo Clin Proc. 2012;87:853–61.
15. Kwon CH, Rhee EJ, Song JU, Kim JT, Kwag HJ, Sung KC. Reduced lung function is independently associated with increased risk of type 2 diabetes in Korean men. Cardiovasc Diabetol. 2012;11:38.
16. Engstrom G, Janzon L. Risk of developing diabetes is inversely related to lung function: a population-based cohort study. Diabet Med. 2002;19:167–70.
17. Ford ES, Mannino DM. National Health and Nutrition Examination Survey Epidemiologic Follow-up Study. Prospective association between lung function and the incidence of diabetes: findings from the National Health and Nutrition Examination Survey Epidemiologic Follow-up Study. Diabetes Care. 2004;27:2966–70.
18. Rana JS, Mittleman MA, Sheikh J, Hu FB, Manson JE, Colditz GA, et al. Chronic obstructive pulmonary disease, asthma, and risk of type 2 diabetes in women. Diabetes Care. 2004;27:2478–84.
19. Yeh HC, Punjabi NM, Wang NY, Pankow JS, Duncan BB, Brancati FL. Vital capacity as a predictor of incident type 2 diabetes: the Atherosclerosis Risk in Communities study. Diabetes Care. 2005;28:1472–9.
20. Song Y, Klevak A, Manson JE, Buring JE, Liu S. Asthma, chronic obstructive pulmonary disease, and type 2 diabetes in the Women's Health Study. Diabetes Res Clin Pract. 2010;90:365–71.
21. Yeh HC, Punjabi NM, Wang NY, Pankow JS, Duncan BB, Cox CE, et al. Cross-sectional and prospective study of lung function in adults with type 2 diabetes: the Atherosclerosis Risk in Communities (ARIC) study. Diabetes Care. 2008;31:741–6.
22. Wannamethee SG, Shaper AG, Rumley A, Sattar N, Whincup PH, Thomas MC, et al. Lung function and risk of type 2 diabetes and fatal and nonfatal major coronary heart disease events: possible associations with inflammation. Diabetes Care. 2010;33:1990–6.
23. Engstrom G, Hedblad B, Nilsson P, Wollmer P, Berglund G, Janzon L. Lung function, insulin resistance and incidence of cardiovascular disease: a longitudinal cohort study. J Intern Med. 2003;253:574–81.
24. Engström G, Lind P, Hedblad B, Wollmer P, Stavenow L, Janzon L, et al. Lung function and cardiovascular risk: relationship with inflammation-sensitive plasma proteins. Circulation. 2002;106:2555–60.
25. Ma Z, Liu Y, Xu Y, Huang Y, Xu M, Zhu X, et al. Impaired lung function is associated with increased carotid intima-media thickness in middle-aged and elderly Chinese. PLoS One. 2013;8:e53153.
26. Marchesini G, Bugianesi E, Forlani G, Cerrelli F, Lenzi M, Manini R, et al. Nonalcoholic fatty liver, steatohepatitis, and the metabolic syndrome. Hepatology. 2003;37:917–23.
27. Marchesini G, Brizi M, Bianchi G, Tomassetti S, Bugianesi E, Lenzi M, et al. Nonalcoholic fatty liver disease: a feature of the metabolic syndrome. Diabetes. 2001;50:1844–50.
28. Jung DH, Shim JY, Lee HR, Moon BS, Park BJ, Lee YJ. Relationship between non-alcoholic fatty liver disease and pulmonary function. Intern Med J. 2012;42(5):541–6.
29. Ning G, Reaction Study Group. Risk Evaluation of cAncers in Chinese diabeTic Individuals: a lONgitudinal (REACTION) study. J Diabetes. 2012;4:172–3.
30. Yang Z, Zhang H, Niu Y, Zhang W, Zhu L, Li X, et al. Circulating periostin in relation to insulin resistance and nonalcoholic fatty liver disease among overweight and obese subjects. Sci Rep. 2016;6:37886.
31. Yang Z, Yan C, Liu G, Niu Y, Zhang W, Lu S, et al. Plasma selenium levels and nonalcoholic fatty liver disease in Chinese adults: a cross-sectional analysis. Sci Rep. 2016;6:37288.
32. Matthews DR, Hosker JP, Rudenski AS, Naylor BA, Treacher DF, Turner RC. Homeostasis model assessment: insulin resistance and beta-cell function from fasting plasma glucose and insulin concentrations in man. Diabetologia. 1985;28(7):412–9.
33. Gan WQ, Man SF, Senthilselvan A, Sin DD. Association between chronic obstructive pulmonary disease and systemic inflammation: a systematic review and a meta-analysis. Thorax. 2004;59:574–80.
34. Qin L, Yang Z, Zhang W, Gu H, Lu S, Shi Q, et al. Association between metabolic syndrome and lung function in middle-aged and elderly Chinese individuals. Diabetes Res Clin Pract. 2015;108:e46-8.
35. Gariani K, Philippe J, Jornayvaz FR. Non-alcoholic fatty liver disease and insulin resistance: from bench to bedside. Diabetes Metab. 2013;39:16–26.
36. Takamura T, Misu H, Ota T, Kaneko S. Fatty liver as a consequence and cause of insulin resistance: lessons from type 2 diabetic liver. Endocr J. 2012;59:745–63.
37. Joseph AE, Saverymuttu SH, Al-Sam S, Cook MG, Maxwell JD. Comparison of liver histology with ultrasonography in assessing diffuse parenchymal liver disease. Clin Radiol. 1991;43:26–31.

24

Association of blood glucose level and hypertension in Elderly Chinese Subjects

Qun Yan[1†], Dongmei Sun[1,2†], Xu Li[1], Guoliang Chen[2], Qinghu Zheng[2], Lun Li[2], Chenhong Gu[2] and Bo Feng[1*]

Abstract

Background: There is a scarcity of epidemiological researches examining the relationship between blood pressure (BP) and glucose level among older adults. The objective of the current study was to investigate the association of high BP and glucose level in elderly Chinese.

Methods: A cross-sectional study of a population of 2092 Chinese individuals aged over 65 years was conducted. Multiple logistic analysis was used to explore the association between hypertension and hyperglycemia. Independent risk factors for systolic and diastolic BP were analyzed using stepwise linear regression.

Results: Subjects in impaired fasting glucose group (IFG) ($n = 144$) and diabetes ($n = 346$), as compared with normal fasting glucose (NFG) ($n = 1277$), had a significant higher risk for hypertension, with odds ratios (ORs) of 1.81 (95 % CI, 1.39–2.35) ($P = 0.000$) and 1.40 (95 % CI, 1.09–1.80) ($P = 0.009$), respectively. Higher fasting plasma glucose (FPG) levels in the normal range were still significantly associated with a higher prevalence of hypertension in both genders, with ORs of 1.24 (95 % CI, 0.85–1.80), $R^2 = 0.114$, $P = 0.023$ in men and 1.61 (95 % CI, 1.12–2.30), $R^2 = 0.082$, $P = 0.010$ in women, respectively, when compared with lower FPG. Linear regression analysis revealed FPG was an independent factor of systolic and diastolic BP.

Conclusions: Our findings suggest that hyperglycemia as well as higher FPG within the normal range is associated with a higher prevalence of hypertension independent of other cardiovascular risk factors in elderly Chinese. Further studies are needed to explore the relationship between hyperglycemia and hypertension in a longitudinal setting.

Keywords: Fasting plasma glucose, Diabetes, Hypertension, Cross-sectional study

Background

Metabolic syndrome is defined as the occurrence of 3 of any of the 5 following factors: abdominal obesity, elevated triglyceride (TG), low high-density lipoprotein cholesterol (HDL-c), elevated blood pressure (BP) and elevated fasting glucose level [1]. It is well known that metabolic syndrome increases the risk for morbidity and mortality from cardiovascular diseases [2, 3]. Actually, the coexistence of hypertension and diabetes alone confers 2–3 times the risk for cardiovascular morbidity and mortality as for people without diabetes [4, 5]. Epidemiological research established that hypertension is more common in subjects with diabetes mellitus (DM) than in the general population [6, 7]. On the other hand, higher BP is associated with increased risk of diabetes [8–12], even in individuals with normotension [7]. However, current studies evaluating the relationship of BP with blood glucose level were limited to age of younger [8–10], or from across the age spectrum [6, 7, 13], did not separate out the data of elderly subjects. Furthermore, referral-based samples in most were mainly with hyperglycemia and hypertension [6, 7, 11, 12]. Some studies relied on self-reported DM or BP [8–10].

Considering the influence of hypertension or hyperglycemia on vascular disease and mortality are age-specific [13], we therefore conducted a cross-sectional survey study in a well-characterized community-based sample of individuals in East China aged over 65 to assess

* Correspondence: fengbo@medmail.com.cn
†Equal contributors
[1]Department of Endocrinology, Shanghai East Hospital, Tongji University School of Medicine, 150 Jimo Road, Shanghai 200120, China
Full list of author information is available at the end of the article

whether higher fasting plasma glucose (FPG) is independently associated with a higher prevalence of hypertension, and conversely, whether higher BP is associated with a higher prevalence of hyperglycemia in elder people.

Methods

Population

A cross-sectional study was conducted in Shanghai Pudong New Area between January 2012 and March 2012. Residents who had lived here over 5 years were recruited. Among the 2777 individuals who were aged over 65 year, 2250 subjects participated in the current study.

Inclusion criteria were: (i) men or women aged over 65 year; (ii) with no severe chronic disease or systemic disease; (iii) willing and able to give informed consent; and (iv) with complete data on key research variables. Subjects with medical diseases such as cardiac disease (heart failure), chronic liver and kidney dysfunction (including serum alanine aminotransferase > 120 IU/l, and aspartate aminotransaminase >80 IU/l, and serum creatinine > 2.0 mg/dl), acute infection, severe systemic diseases (e.g., cancer) or Acquired Immune Deficiency Syndrome (AIDS) as well as patients who had secondary hypertension were excluded ($n = 89$). Those with incomplete data on key research variables were also excluded ($n = 69$). Subsequently, 2092 individuals (971 men and 1121 women) were included in the current analysis (Fig. 1).

All participants were screened with regard to medical history (i.e., smoking, alcohol consumption, and medical treatments). Current smokers were defined as those who currently smoke every day or some days and who reported having smoked over 100 cigarettes during their lifetimes. Alcohol consumption was defined as having up to 20–30 g of ethanol per day for men and up to 10–20 g of ethanol per day for women. Details of this survey have been reported previously [14]. Written informed consent was obtained from all participants.

BP Measurements

BP was measured using a mercury sphygmomanometer by an experienced physician. Subjects were in a seated position with an arm flexed at the level of the heart. After the cuff was wrapped around the upper arm with the cuff's lower edge one inch above the antecubital fossa, the cuff was rapidly inflated to 180 mmHg. Then air was released from the cuff at a rate of 3 mm/s. During this period, the physician listened carefully with a stethoscope while simultaneously observing the sphygmomanometer. The first knocking sound (Korotkoff) was the subject's systolic pressure. When the knocking sound disappeared, that was the diastolic pressure. BP was measured in either the right upper or left upper arm after each subject had been seated for at least 10 min. The arm with the higher blood pressure would be measured twice. The average was used for analysis. If the difference of SBP or DBP between the twice was over 5 mmHg, it would be measured for the third time, and then the average of three times was used for analysis.

Hypertension was defined as systolic blood pressure (SBP) ≥140 mmHg and/or diastolic blood pressure (DBP) ≥90 mmHg or reported receiving antihypertensive medication. Participants who were diagnosed hypertensive for the first time during this survey were called new-onset

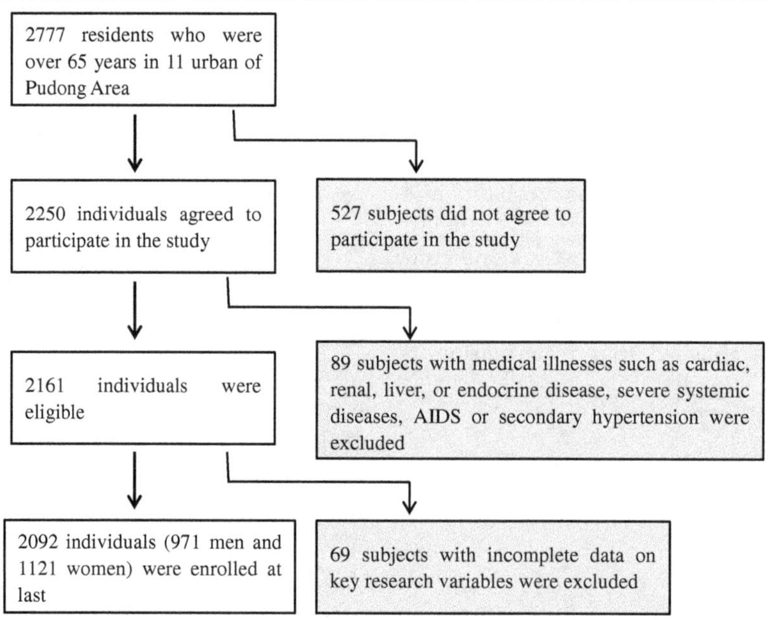

Fig. 1 Study design and participant flow diagram for the present study

hypertension; participants who had a history of hypertension were called previously-diagnosed hypertension. High-normal BP was defined as not having hypertension, and with SBP 120–139 mmHg or DBP 80–90 mmHg; normal BP included SBP < 120 mmHg and DBP < 80 mmHg and with no antihypertensive treatment [15].

DM Ascertainment

Participants were considered to have DM if fasting blood glucose ≥ 7.0 mmol/L or reported using insulin or oral hypoglycemic medication. Participants who were diagnosed DM for the first time during this survey were called new-onset DM, participants who had a history of DM were called previously-diagnosed DM. Normal fasting glucose (NFG) was defined as FPG < 6.1 mmol/L. Impaired fasting glucose (IFG) was defined as FPG ≥ 6.1 mmol/L but <7.0 mmol/L according to WHO criteria, 1999 [16].

Covariates

Height and weight of all subjects were measured in light clothes with no shoes. Waist circumference was measured at the level midway between the lower rib margin and the iliac crest. Body mass index (BMI) was calculated as weight (kg) divided by the square of height (m).

Blood samples were collected from venous blood after overnight fasting, and FPG, total cholesterol and triglyceride were measured. Glucose measurement was done in a central lab in Shanghai East Hospital. Plasma fasting glucose level was determined in NaF preserved plasma using the glucose oxidase method by automatic analyzer, Accurizer Autochem 400 (Affinitech, China).

Statistical analysis

Continuous data were summarized by the mean ± SD or median, and categorical data by number (percentages). All of the continuous data had skewed distribution even after logarithmically transformed. Mann–Whitney test (for data that was not normally distributed) and Chi-square test (for data that were categorical variables) were used to compare the differences between the Men and Women groups.

The participants were divided into 4 groups according to FPG levels: NFG (n = 1277), IFG (n = 144), New-onset DM (n = 325), and previously-diagnosed DM (n = 346). Binary logistic analysis was used to examine the association of hyperglycemia status with hypertension. Then NFG group was further divided into two subgroups according to the median FPG level by sex. Multiple logistic analyses were used to explore the associations between hypertension and hyperglycemia. Independent risk factors for systolic and diastolic pressure were analyzed using stepwise linear regression.

Results

Clinical characteristics

The baseline characteristics of the study population by sex were shown in Table 1. The study population consisted of 2092 (971 men and 1121 women, mean age 72.8 and 73.6 years, respectively). The prevalence of total DM in men and women were 23.1 % and 23.7 %, respectively (P = 0.381). The prevalence of hypertension in men and women were 45.3 % and 48.5 %, respectively (P = 0.077). There were no significant differences in the prevalence of IFG and high-normal BP between the sexes. Other metabolic and anthropometric variables, except for BMI and FPG, were significantly different between the sexes (all P < 0.05).

Association of FPG and risk of hypertension

After adjusting for sex, age, smoking, alcohol using, BMI, TG and TC levels, subjects in IFG and previously-diagnosed DM, as compared with NFG (<6.1 mmol/L), had a significant higher risk for hypertension in whole sample, with odds ratios (OR) of 1.81 (95 % CI, 1.39–2.35) (P = 0.000) and 1.40 (95 % CI, 1.09–1.80) (P = 0.009), respectively. Subjects in the IFG group were also associated with an increased OR of new-onset hypertension (OR 1.68 [95 % CI, 1.18–2.41], P = 0.004) when comparing with NFG. Of note, there were strong

Table 1 Baseline characteristics by sex

Parameters	Men	Women	*P* value
Number	971	1121	
Age(y)	72.8 ± 6.4	73.6 ± 7.0	0.027
Current smoker n (%)	215(22.1 %)	27(2.4 %)	0.000
Alcohol consumption n (%)	143(14.7 %)	17(1.5 %)	0.000
T2DM n (%)	224(23.1 %)	266(23.7)	0.381
IFG n (%)	142(14.6 %)	167(14.9 %)	0.455
Hypertension n (%)	440(45.3 %)	544(48.5 %)	0.077
High-normal BP n (%)	427(44.0 %)	489(43.6 %)	0.453
BMI(kg/m^2)	23.7 ± 3.3	23.9 ± 3.8	0.316
WC(cm)	87.9 ± 9.1	85.4 ± 10.3	0.000
SBP (mmHg)	133.7 ± 16.1	135.4 ± 15.8	0.013
DBP (mmHg)	78.6 ± 8.9	77.4 ± 8.6	0.002
FPG (mmol/L, Mean)	6.2 ± 1.6	6.3 ± 1.8	0.268
FPG (mmol/L, Median) [a]	5.45	5.51	0.268
TG (mmol/L)	1.5 ± 0.9	1.6 ± 0.9	0.000
TC (mmol/L)	5.2 ± 1.0	5.8 ± 1.0	0.000

Categorical data were described as n (%) and continuous data were described as means ± SD

BMI body mass index, *WC* waist circumference, *SBP* systolic blood pressure, *DBP* diastolic blood pressure, *FPG* fasting plasma glucose, *TG* triglyceride, *TC* total cholesterol

[a]The median of FPG in subjects with normal fasting glucose level (<6.1 mmol/L)

P values < 0.05 were considered significant

associations of hyperglycemic status with SBP and but not DBP (Table 2).

The median of FPG was 5.45 mmol/L in men, and 5.51 mmol/L in women respectively in NFG group (Table 3). NFG group was further divided into two subgroups according to the median FPG level by sex. Even in the normal range of FPG, using below the median level of FPG as the reference, when adjusting for age, smoking and alcohol consumption (Model 1), higher FPG above the median was still significantly associated with a higher prevalence of hypertension in both gender, with OR of 1.93 (95 % CI, 1.60–2.34) ($R^2 = 0.028$, $P =$ 0.000) in men and 1.96 (95 % CI, 1.51–2.54) ($R^2 = 0.033$, $P = 0.000$) in women respectively. After further adjusting for BMI, WC, TG and TC (Model 2), the association between higher FPG and the prevalence of hypertension was attenuated but remained statistically significant (OR 1.24 [95 % CI, 0.85–1.80], $R^2 = 0.114$, $P = 0.023$ in men and 1.61 [95 % CI, 1.12–2.30], $R^2 = 0.082$, $P = 0.010$ in women respectively). Similar associations were found between higher FPG levels and higher SBP in both genders. However, we did not find any association between higher FPG and higher DBP in both genders in Model 2.

Table 4 showed the independent risk factors for SBP and DBP in whole sample and in individuals without hypoglycemic nor antihypertensive drugs ($n = 924$) by stepwise linear regression analysis. After adjusting for sex, age, smoking, alcohol consumption, BMI, WC, TC, and TG, FPG levels were significantly associated with SBP in both samples ($\beta = 0.10$, $R^2 = 0.013$, $P < 0.01$ in whole sample and $\beta = 0.12$, $R^2 = 0.013$, $P < 0.01$ in individuals without hypoglycemic or antihypertensive drugs respectively). As for DBP, FPG levels were also associated with DBP in individuals without hypoglycemic or antihypertensive drugs ($\beta = 0.08$, $R^2 = 0.006$, $P < 0.05$).

Association of BP and risk of hyperglycemia

We explored the possible effect of high-normal BP and hypertension on the risk of IFG and DM by using multiple logistic regression analysis (Table 5). After adjusting for age, sex, smoking and alcohol consumption, when compared with the normal BP group, hypertensives had a significantly higher prevalence of IFG (OR 3.92 [95 % CI, 2.17–7.10], $P < 0.01$), and DM (2.83 [95 % CI, 1.83–4.38], $P < 0.01$) respectively, and subjects with high-normal BP had a similarly increased prevelance in IFG and DM (OR 2.07 [95 % CI, 1.13–3.78], $P < 0.05$, and OR 1.78 [95 % CI, 1.14–2.76], $P < 0.05$, respectively) (Table 5, Model 1). When further adjusting for BMI, WC, TG, and TC, the associations between hypertension and IFG and DM remained statistically significant, though attenuated (OR 3.17 [95 % CI, 1.70–5.68], $P < 0.01$, and 1.93 [95 % CI, 1.22–3.04], $P < 0.01$, respectively). Similar associations were also seen between high-normal BP and IFG, but not DM (Table 5, Model 2).

Discussion

The close relationship between diabetes and hypertension has been recognized since the 1980s [6, 10], but how much this effect varies by race-ethnicity, age or levels of traditional risk factors is uncertain. The extent to which glucose concentration is associated with elevated blood pressure is also uncertain. The data for pure elders in China is more limited. In our present study, we aimed to explore the association of diabetes and FPG concentration with hypertension or high-normal BP in a select groups of elderly subjects in China. We found that, compared with subjects with NFG, subjects with IFG and previously-diagnosed DM had a higher prevalence of hypertension. Even among the subjects with NFG, higher FPG was still associated with a higher prevalence of hypertension after adjusting for covariates such as age, smoking, alcohol consumption, BMI, WC, TG, and TC level. FPG was an independent factor of systolic and diastolic BP. Conversely, multiple analyses revealed that subjects with hypertension also had a higher prevalence of IFG and DM.

Our study is comply with other studies that have indicated an increased risk for hypertension and other cardiovascular risk factors in diabetic individuals as well as in impaired glucose regulation than those with NFG [6, 7, 17, 18]. Our study extends this observation by illustrating that a high but normal FPG level was also a risk factor for hypertension in elderly Chinese subjects,

Table 2 Logistic regression analysis of association of hyperglycemia status with risk of hypertension[a]

	SBP ≥ 140 mmHg		DBP ≥ 90 mmHg		Total Hypertension		New-onset Hypertension	
	OR (95 % CI)	*P* value	OR (95 % CI)	*P* value	OR (95 % CI)	*P* value	OR (95 % CI)	*P* value
NFG	1	-	1	-	1	-	1	-
IFG	1.89(1.46–2.45)	0.000	1.31(0.94–1.84)	0.111	1.81(1.39–2.35)	0.000	1.68(1.18–2.41)	0.004
New-onset DM	1.44(0.99–1.65)	0.053	1.23(0.78–1.95)	0.375	1.35(0.93–1.94)	0.115	1.49(0.91–2.42)	0.113
Previously-diagnosed DM	1.46(1.13–1.87)	0.003	1.02(0.72–1.44)	0.913	1.40(1.09–1.80)	0.009	0.90(0.61–1.33)	0.592

NFG normal fasting glucose, *IFG* impaired fasting glucose, New-onset DM, newly diagnosed diabetes mellitus; Previously-Diagnosed DM, previously diagnosed diabetes mellitus; New-onset hypertension, newly diagnosed hypertension; OR (95 % CI), odds ratio (95 % confidence index); other abbreviations see Table 1
[a]Adjusted for sex, age, smoking, alcohol consumption, BMI, TG and TC level
P values < 0.05 were considered significant

Table 3 Logistic regression analysis of risk of hypertension in subjects with NFG (above vs. below the median fasting glucose level [a])

	Men			Women		
	OR (95 % CI, below vs above the median $)	*P* value#	Adjusted R^2	OR (95 % CI, below vs above the median $)	*P* value#	Adjusted R^2
Total Hypertension						
Model 1	1.93(1.60–2.34)	0.000	0.028	1.96(1.51–2.54)	0.000	0.033
Model 2	1.24(0.85–1.80)	0.023	0.114	1.61(1.12–2.30)	0.010	0.082
SBP ≥ 140 mmHg						
Model 1	2.04(1.54–2.70)	0.000	0.022	2.03(1.56–2.65)	0.000	0.026
Model 2	1.50(1.07–2.10)	0.019	0.058	1.27(0.93–1.74)	0.013	0.071
DBP ≥ 90 mmHg						
Model 1	1.21(0.84–1.75)	0.301	0.022	1.67(1.12–2.67)	0.011	0.063
Model 2	0.72(0.46–1.15)	0.167	0.048	1.35(0.85–2.12)	0.201	0.015

Abbreviations see Tables 1 and 2
Model 1, adjusted for age, smoking and alcohol using
Model 2, adjusted for age, smoking, alchol using, BMI, WC, TG and TC level
[a]The median fasting glucose level was 5.45 mmol/L in men and 5.51 mmol/L in women respectively
P values < 0.05 were considered significant

and this relation was independent of other traditional cardiovascular risk factors. What's more, we found that elevated FPG was independently associated with an increased risk of SBP and DBP. This is also in line with two recent studies [19, 20]. In Di Bonito P's study among Southern European Caucasian children and adolescents (age 6–16 years), they found that subjects with high-normal FPG (83–99 mg/dL) had 1.57–2.23 times the risk for hypertension when compared with subjects with low-normal FPG (≤82 mg/dL) independent of BMI [19]. In a cohort study of a Japanese population (age 20–80 years), Y Heianza found that elevated concentration of FPG in normal range (<4.9 mmol/L vs. 4.9–5.6 mmol/L) was associated with higher risk of developing hypertension (OR 1.35–1.39) during a 5-year follow-up after adjusting for age and gender [20].

Our data also matches with other epidemiological data demonstrating that basal BP and BP progression are strong and independent predictors of incident hyperglycemia [7, 10–12, 18], and is also consistent with clinical trial data demonstrating that lower BP are associated with lower risk of cardiovascular diseases [13]. In the Women's Health Study in the USA by David Conen et al, a baseline BP of 130-139/85-89 mmHg and hypertension will increase risk of incident Type 2 diabetes in the following 10 years by 1.45–2.03 times [7]. In a recent study of Chinese subjects in Hong Kong aged over 18 years, Sau NF found that subjects with IFG were

Table 4 Stepwise linear regression analysis of risk factors for SBP and DBP

	All subjects (*n* = 2092)				Subjects without hypoglycemic or antihypertensive drugs (*n* = 924)			
	SBP		DBP		SBP		DBP	
	β	R^2	β	R^2	β	R^2	β	R^2
BMI (kg/m^2)	0.15**	0.034	0.13**	0.032	0.15**	0.028	0.42	-
FPG (mmol/L)	0.10**	0.013	0.022	-	0.12**	0.013	0.08*	0.006
Age (years)	0.09**	0.008	-0.16**	0.019	0.07*	0.004	-0.17**	0.026
Smoking (yes/no)	−0.07	-	−0.03	-	−0.13*	0.012	−0.23	-
Alcohol consumption (yes/no)	0.06**	0.003	0.021	-	0.07*	0.004	0.026	-
TC (mmol/L)	0.05*	0.003	0.09**	0.005	0.04	-	0.061	-
TG (mmol/L)	0.07**	0.002	0.05*	0.007	0.01	-	-0.34	-
Male (vs.Female)	0.02	-	−0.09	-	0.03	-	0.109	-
WC(mmol/L)	0.57	-	0.61	-	0.09	-	0.14**	0.021

Abbreviations see Table 1
* *P* value < 0.05; ***P* value < 0.01

Table 5 Multiple logistic regression analysis of risk of IFG and DM

	IFG		DM	
	OR (95 % CI)	Adjusted R^2	OR (95 % CI)	Adjusted R^2
Model 1 [a]		0.045		0.028
Age (years)	1.01(0.99–1.03)		1.00(0.99–1.02)	
Male (vs. female)	0.95(0.73–1.25)		0.99(0.78–1.24)	
Smoking(yes/no)	0.92(0.68–1.08)		1.01(0.85–1.21)	
Alcohol consumption (yes/no)	1.06(0.84–1.43)		0.93(0.76–1.41)	
High-normal BP (vs. normal BP)	2.07(1.13–3.78)*		1.78(1.14–2.76)*	
Hypertension (vs. normal BP)	3.92(2.17–7.10)**		2.83(1.83–4.38)**	
Model 2 [b]		0.095		0.140
Age (years)	1.01(0.99–1.03)		1.01(0.99–1.03)	
Male (vs. female)	0.96(0.71–1.30)		0.97(0.81–1.18)	
Smoking(yes/no)	0.83(0.65–1.05)		0.92(0.74–1.14)	
Alcohol consumption (yes/no)	1.09(0.86–1.39)		0.99(0.77–1.28)	
BMI (kg/m^2)	1.02(0.95–1.09)		1.04(0.99–1.10)**	
WC(mmol/L)	1.03(1.00–1.06)*		1.04(1.02–1.06)**	
TG (mmol/L)	1.42(1.22–1.66)**		1.55(1.36–1.77)**	
TC (mmol/L)	0.96(0.84–1.10)		0.95(0.85–1.06)	
High-normal BP (vs. normal BP)	1.87(1.03–3.44)*		1.46(0.94–2.31)	
Hypertension (vs. normal BP)	3.17(1.70–5.68)**		1.93(1.22–3.04)**	

Abbreviations see Tables 1 and 2
Normal BP, SBP < 120 mmHg and DBP < 80 mmHg and not using antihypertensive medication; high-normal BP, SBP 120–139 mmHg or DBP 80–90 mmHg; hypertension, SBP ≥ 140 mmHg and/or DBP ≥ 90 mmHg or using antihypertensive medication
[a]Model 1: Logistic regression analysis with IFG and DM as dependent variable respectively, and age, male (vs. female), smoking, alcohol consumption, and high-normal BP (vs. normal BP) and hypertension (vs. normal BP) as independent variables
[b]Model 2: Model 1 + BMI, WC, TG and TC
* *P* value < 0.05; ***P* value < 0.01

more likely to develop diabetes within 5 years if they were hypertensive (aHR = 1.44) [11]. A large Japanese cohort study also showed that having both high-normal BP and hypertension in middle age was associated with increased risk of developing diabetes [9]. In our present study, we also found high-normal BP associated with risk of IFG after adjusting for conventional risk factors.

Although the association between hypertension and hyperglycemia has long been discussed, the underlying biological basis mediating this clinical association remains unclear. Hyperinsulinemia, an important component of the metabolic syndrome, may be one of the main factors [21]. Insulin resistance, which further contributes to hyperinsulinemia, often progresses to Type 2 diabetes [22]. In addition, the resistance in the hemodynamic properties of insulin may impair the blood flow in peripheral tissues, which indirectly contributes to the development of the atherogenic dysglycemia and dyslipidemia [23]. Hyperinsulinemia may directly contribute to elevation of blood pressure by increasing renal sodium retention [24] and enhancing sympathetic nervous system activity [25], whereas chronic sympathetic nervous system overactivity may contribute to a further increase of insulin resistance creating a vicious circle that may lead to the development of hypertension and diabetes. In addition, insulin resistance is also associated with a decreased vasodilatory response to insulin in peripheral tissue [26, 27] and an increased vasoconstrictor response to various vasopressors [28, 29], which mainly results the increase of systolic blood pressure. The pathophysiological mechanism linking insulin and hypertension is complex and still needs to be fully elucidated.

Our present study adds to the literature by demonstrating that hyperglycemia is closely correlated with hypertension in a population of the elderly. We were able to explore the associations between blood glucose levels and BP in a relative large, well-defined cohort. However, several potential limitations of the study merit discussion. First, because of the observational nature of the study, we cannot infer causality from our present data. Second, lack of evaluation of postprandial blood glucose level and repeated FPG measurement should underestimate the prevalence of diabetes in this population. As this was a survey based on the elderly population, postprandial blood glucose measurement may pose certain problems for the elderly, as they would need to wait 2 h for venous draw blood after a meal. Third, although multiple potential confounders have been adjusted for, we cannot completely rule out the residual confounders attributed to the inaccurate measurement of confounders, or some unmeasured confounders.

Conclusions

Our study suggests that hyperglycemia as well as a high but normal FPG level was associated with a higher prevalence of hypertension independent of other cardiovascular risk factors among elderly Chinese. On the other hand, hypertension, even high-normal BP, was also associated with a higher prevalence of hyperglycemia. Further studies are needed to explore the relationship between hyperglycemia and hypertension in a longitudinal setting.

Abbreviations

BP, blood pressure; TG, triglyceride; HDL-c, high-density lipoprotein cholesterol; DM, diabetes mellitus; FPG, fasting plasma glucose; AIDS, acquired immune deficiency syndrome; SBP, systolic blood pressure; DBP, diastolic blood pressure; NFG, normal fasting glucose; IFG, impaired fasting glucose; BMI, body mass index; TC, total cholesterol

Acknowledgments

We were grateful to the participants, physicians and nurses in the Department of endocrinology of Shanghai East hospital and Shanghai Puxing Community Health-Care Center for taking part in this study.

Funding

This study was funded by Key Disciplines Group Construction Project of Pudong Health Bureau of Shanghai (Grant No.PWZxkq2010-04), Key Specialty Construction Project of Pudong Health and Family Planning Commission of Shanghai (Grant No.PWZz2013-04) and Project of Science and Technology of Pudong Health and Family Planning Commission of Shanghai (Grant No.PW2013c-11).

Authors' contributions

BF was the principal investigator (PI). He designed the study and oversaw the project implementation, participated in data collection, analyses and interpretation and writing publications. QY and DS participated in study design and participated in data collection, data analyses and interpretation and writing publications. XL participated in the design of the study and performed the statistical analysis. GC, QZ, LL and CG conceived of the study, and participated in its coordination and helped to draft the manuscript. All authors read and approved the final manuscript.

Authors' information

Professor Bo Feng, the Ph.D supervisor, the member of the Chinese Diabetes Society; the Vice Chairman of Shanghai Diabetes Association; the member of Shanghai Diabetes Rehabilitation Association; the Director of the Committee of Endocrinology, Shanghai Pudong New District.

Competing interests

The authors declare that they have no conflict of interest to declare.

Author details

[1]Department of Endocrinology, Shanghai East Hospital, Tongji University School of Medicine, 150 Jimo Road, Shanghai 200120, China. [2]Puxing Community Health-Care Center, Pudong New District, 250 GuiChang Road, Shanghai 200136, China.

References

1. Grundy SM, Cleeman JI, Daniels SR, Donato KA, Eckel RH, Franklin BA, et al. Diagnosis and management of the metabolic syndrome: an American Heart Association/NationalHeart, Lung, and Blood Institute scientific statement. Circulation. 2005;112:2735–52.
2. Lakka HM, Laaksonen DE, Lakka TA, Niskanen LK, Kumpusalo E, Tuomilehto J, et al. The metabolic syndrome and total and cardiovascular disease mortality in middle-aged men. JAMA. 2002;288:2709–16.
3. Isomaa B, Almgren P, Tuomi T, Forsén B, Lahti K, Nissén M, et al. Cardiovascular morbidity and mortality associated with the metabolic syndrome. Diabetes Care. 2001;24:683–9.
4. Emerging Risk Factors Collaboration, Sarwar N, Gao P, Seshasai SR, Gobin R, Kaptoge S, et al. Diabetes mellitus, fasting blood glucose concentration, and risk of vascular disease: a collaborative meta-analysis of 102 prospective studies. Lancet. 2010;375:2215–22.
5. Stamler J, Vaccaro O, Neaton JD, Wentworth D. Diabetes, other risk factors, and 12-yr cardiovascular mortality for men screened in the Multiple Risk Factor Intervention Trial. Diabetes Care. 1993;16:434–4.
6. Hypertension in Diabetes Study (HDS): I. Prevalence of hypertension in newly presenting type 2 diabetic patients and the association with risk factors for cardiovascular and diabetic complications. J Hypertens. 1993;11:309-17.
7. Yang Z, Xing X, Xiao J, Lu J, Weng J, Jia W, et al. Prevalence of cardiovascular disease and risk factors in the Chinese population with impaired glucose regulation: the 2007-2008 China national diabetes and metabolic disorders study. Exp Clin Endocrinol Diabetes. 2013;121:372–74.
8. Conen D, Ridker PM, Mora S, Buring JE, Glynn RJ, et al. Blood pressure and risk of developing type 2 diabetes mellitus: the Women's Health Study. Eur Heart J. 2007;28:2937–43.
9. Golden SH, Wang NY, Klag MJ, Meoni LA, Brancati FL. Blood pressure in young adulthood and the risk of type 2 diabetes in middle age. Diabetes Care. 2003;26:1110–5.
10. Hayashi T, Tsumura K, Suematsu C, Endo G, Fujii S, Okada K. High normal blood pressure, hypertension, and the risk of type 2 diabetes in Japanese men. The Osaka Health Survey. Diabetes Care. 1999;22:1683–87.
11. Wei GS, Coady SA, Goff Jr DC, Brancati FL, Levy D, Selvin E, et al. Blood pressure and the risk of developing diabetes in African Americans and whites: ARIC, CARDIA, and the Framingham heart study. Diabetes Care. 2011;34:873–9.
12. Fu SN, Luk W, Wong CK, Cheung KL. Progression from impaired fasting glucose to type 2 diabetes mellitus among Chinese subjects with and without hypertension in a primary care setting. J Diabetes. 2014;6:438–46.
13. Lewington S, Clarke R, Qizilbash N, Peto R, Collins R, Prospective Studies Collaboration. Age-specific relevance of usual blood pressure to vascular mortality: a meta-analysis of individual data for one million adults in 61 prospective studies. Lancet. 2002;360:1903–13.
14. Yan Q, Sun D, Li X, Zheng Q, Li L, Gu C, Feng B. Neck circumference is a valuable tool for identifying metabolic syndrome and obesity in Chinese elder subjects: a community-based study. Diabetes Metab Res Rev. 2014;30:69–76.
15. Chobanian AV, Bakris GL, Black HR, Cushman WC, Green LA, Izzo JL, et al. Seventh report of the Joint National Committee on prevention, detection, evaluation, and treatment of high blood pressure. Hypertension. 2003;42:1206–52.

16. Alberti KG, Zimmet PZ. Definition, diagnosis and classification of diabetes mellitus and its complications. Part 1: diagnosis and classification of diabetes mellitus provisional report of a WHO consultation. Diabet Med. 1998;15:539–53.
17. Williams DE, Cadwell BL, Cheng YJ, Cowie CC, Gregg EW, Geiss LS, et al. Prevalence of impaired fasting glucose and its relationship with cardiovascular disease risk factors in US adolescents, 1999-2000. Pediatrics. 2005;116:1122–6.
18. Chen G, McAlister FA, Walker RL, Hemmelgarn BR, Campbell NR. Cardiovascular outcomes in Framingham participants with diabetes: the importance of blood pressure. Hypertension. 2011;57:891–7.
19. Di Bonito P, Sanguigno E, Forziato C, Saitta F, Iardino MR, Capaldo B. Fasting plasma glucose and clustering of cardiometabolic risk factors in normoglycemic outpatient children and adolescents. Diabetes Care. 2011;34:1412–14.
20. Heianza Y, Arase Y, Kodama S, Hsieh SD, Tsuji H, Saito K, et al. Fasting glucose and HbA1C levels as risk factors for the development of hypertension in Japanese individuals: Toranomon hospital heath management center study 16(TOPICS 16). J Hum Hypertens. 2015;29:254–9.
21. Lambert GW, Straznicky NE, Lambert EA, Dixon JB, Schlaich MP. Sympathetic nervous activation in obesity and the metabolic syndrome--causes, consequences and therapeutic implications. Pharmacol Ther. 2010;126:159–72.
22. Dimitriadis G, Mitrou P, Lambadiari V, Maratou E, Raptis SA. Insulin effects inmuscle and adipose tissue. Diabetes Res Clin Pract. 2011;93 Suppl 1:S52–9.
23. Lambadiari V, Triantafyllou K, Dimitriadis GD. Insulin action in muscle and adipose tissue in type 2 diabetes: The significance of blood flow. World J Diabetes. 2015;6:626–33.
24. Chávez-Canales M, Arroyo JP, Ko B, Vázquez N, Bautista R, Castañeda-Bueno M, et al. Insulin increases the functional activity of the renal NaCl cotransporter. J Hypertens. 2013;31:303–11.
25. Reaven GM. Role of insulin resistance in human disease. Diabetes. 1988;37:1595–607.
26. Doronzo G, Russo I, Mattiello L, Anfossi G, Bosia A, Trovati M. Insulin activates vascular endothelial growth factor in vascular smooth muscle cells: influence of nitric oxide and of insulin resistance. Eur J Clin Invest. 2004;34:664–73.
27. Anfossi G, Russo I, Doronzo G, Trovati M. Contribution of insulin resistance to vascular dysfunction. Arch Physiol Biochem. 2009;115:199–217.
28. Jia G, DeMarco VG, Sowers JR. Insulin resistance and hyperinsulinaemia in diabetic cardiomyopathy. Nat Rev Endocrinol. 2016;12:144–53.
29. Zhou MS, Liu C, Tian R, Nishiyama A, Raij L. Skeletal muscle insulin resistance in salt-sensitive hypertension: role of angiotensin II activation of NFkB. Cardiovasc Diabetol. 2015;14:45.

Mortality in children with classic congenital adrenal hyperplasia and 21-hydroxylase deficiency (CAH) in Germany

Helmuth G. Dörr[1*], Hartmut A. Wollmann[2], Berthold P. Hauffa[3], Joachim Woelfle[4] and on behalf of the German Society of Pediatric Endocrinology and Diabetology

Abstract

Background: Adrenal crises in children with classic congenital adrenal hyperplasia due to 21-hydroxylase deficiency (CAH) are life-threatening and have the potential to death.

Methods: A survey was performed among Paediatric Endocrinologists in Germany to report on deceased children with CAH. Our survey covered the whole of Germany.

Results: The participating centres reported 14 cases of death (9 female, 5 male) from 1973 until 2004, but no deaths thereafter. 11 children had the SW form and 3 the simple virilizing (SV) form. All patients were on glucocorticoid replacement, and the SW forms additionally on mineralocorticoid replacement. The age at death varied between 6 weeks and 16.5 years. Seven children died before introduction of general neonatal screening, and 7 children thereafter. Before death, the clinical signs of impending crisis were nonspecific. Five patients developed hypoglycaemia and convulsions with cerebral oedema. Half of the deceased patients died at home. The hydrocortisone dosage was only doubled in two of the 14 cases.

Conclusions: According to the assessments by the attending centres, almost all deaths could be related to an inadequate administration of stress doses of hydrocortisone. Since no deceased CAH children were reported in Germany from 2005 on, we assume the effectiveness of educational programs over the past years.

Keywords: Adrenal crisis, CYP21A2, 21-hydroxylase deficiency, Mortality

Background

Congenital adrenal hyperplasia (CAH) comprises a group of autosomal recessively inherited disorders of cortisol biosynthesis in the adrenal cortex. More than 95% of the disorders are based on a defect of CYP21A2 (21-hydroxylase). The classic defect of CYP21A2 occurs in two forms: CAH with salt wasting (SW) and simple virilizing CAH [1–4]. The reported disease incidence varies between 1:15,000 and 1:16,000 in Europe and North America and 1:19,000 in Japan [5–7]. The treatment of choice is lifelong glucocorticoid replacement and, additionally, mineralocorticoid replacement in the SW-form of the disease [8–13]. Adrenal crisis occurring within the scope of stress situations is especially feared and a major cause of morbidity and mortality in children [14]. In adults with classic CAH, the frequency of adrenal crises was 5.8 per 100 patient years [15], and Falhammer et al. reported on an increased mortality in adults with SW-CAH [16]. Reports on mortality of children with CAH vary between 3 and 13% [17–19].

The aim of our study was to collect data from deceased CAH children in Germany and to review the cases in an attempt to determine the factors that may have contributed to their death.

Methods

Our survey covered the whole of Germany, i.e. also the situation before reunification of East and West Germany in 1990. All members of the German Society of Paediatric

* Correspondence: helmuth-guenther.doerr@uk-erlangen.de
[1]Paediatric Endocrinology, Department Paediatrics, University Hospital of Erlangen, Erlangen, Germany
Full list of author information is available at the end of the article

Endocrinology and Diabetology in Germany participated and were asked to report on deceased children with classical CAH. The first survey was conducted between September 2001 and September 2002, the second survey was conducted in 2015. Overall 88 centres including all Paediatric University Hospitals in Germany responded, and 11 centres reported 14 cases of death (9 females, 5 males). Additionally, three deaths in adults between 21 and 32 years of age were reported, but the data were not included in our analysis. General newborn screening for CAH was introduced in Germany in 1999. The reported cases of deaths occurred during the period from 1973 to 2004; 7 cases (5 females) before screening, and 7 cases (4 females) thereafter.

A questionnaire with common questions regarding clinical background data of the deceased patients (see Additional file 1) was sent to the 11 clinics, but the questionnaire was not always fully completed because the records on file in the hospitals concerning the circumstances or cause of death were incomplete.

There is no accredited registry in Germany for children with CAH. In 1997, the AQUAPE CAH initiative (AQUAPE: Arbeitsgemeinschaft für Qualitätssicherung in der pädiatrischen Endokrinologie) was installed for prospective documentation of clinical follow-up data in patients with CAH. The database does not mirror the real situation in Germany since the participation is voluntarily and therefore not all centres provide data. Cases of deceased children are not reported in this database.

Our survey was conducted upon approval of the German Society of Paediatric Endocrinology and Diabetology (DGKED). Consent was obtained from the paediatric endocrinologists that completed the questionnaire, and the data of the deceased children was collected anonymously by a questionnaire in accordance with the Declaration of Helsinki. The study was approved by the local ethics committee of the Dept. Paediatrics of Erlangen.

Results

Of the 14 CAH patients who died, 11 patients were clinically characterized with the salt-wasting (SW) form, and three female children with the simple virilizing (SV) form. All patients were born in Germany and received regular replacement of glucocorticoids. The patients with the SW form also received mineralocorticoids (Table 1). Molecular genetic classification of the severity of CAH according to Krone et al. [20]. The genotype Group "Null" included patients with biallelic mutations that resulted in completely inactive enzymes (e.g. gene deletions), and Group "A" included patients with homozygous I2G or heterozygous I2G in trans with a null mutation. The genetic classification was only possible in 8 cases, because 6 children were not analysed. The genotype Null was found in 5 children, and genotype A in 3 children, i.e., all these children had a severe form of CAH. The number of girls with CAH who died before newborn screening was slightly higher ($n = 5$) than the number of girls ($n = 4$) who died after screening. The sex ratio (female to male) was 2.5 before screening and 1.3 after screening. Two children died at 6 weeks and 10 months of age, whereas most children died as toddlers ($n = 9$) between 1 and 5 years of age. This group

Table 1 Clinical data of children with CAH who died between 1973 and 2004 in Germany

Cases	CAH Form	Sex	Age at Death	Symptoms	Place of death	Comments
1	SW	F	6 wks.	fever, vomiting	at home	no GC increase
2 [a]	SW	M	2.5 yrs.	fever, respiratory infection	at home	cerebral oedema
3	SW	M	3.5 yrs.	fever, seizure	tertiary centre	cerebral oedema
4 [a]	SV	F	5.0 yrs.	fever, seizure	tertiary centre	cerebral oedema
5	SW	F	2.5 yrs.	fever, vomiting	at home	no GC increase
6	SV	F	16 yrs.	gastroenteritis, salmonella	at home	no GC increase
7	SW	F	1 yr.	fever, dehydration	secondary centre	no GC increase
8	SW	M	13 yrs.	fever, vomiting, seizure	secondary centre	no GC increase
9 [a]	SW	F	10 mo.	fever, MCAD deficiency	at home	unclear?, SIDS?
10 [a]	SW	F	3 yrs.	fever, gastroenteritis, diarrhoea	secondary centre	cerebral oedema
11	SW	M	7 yrs.	fever, seizure	tertiary centre	no GC increase cerebral oedema
12	SW	M	16.5 yrs.	fever, chicken pox	at home	no GC increase
13	SW	F	2.5 yrs.	fever, vomiting	tertiary centre	no GC increase
14	SV	F	1.5 yrs.	fever, vomiting	at home	no GC increase

Autopsy[a]; performed on 4 children

Case 8: Addisonian crisis at the age of 18 months; since that event: persistent vegetative state (children's home)

Case 9: MCAD = Medium-Chain-Acyl-CoA-Dehydrogenase

Abbreviations: *SW* salt wasting, *SV* simple virilizing, *GC* glucocorticoid dose, *SIDS* sudden infant death syndrome

also includes a boy who was in a persistent vegetative state in connection with an Addisonian crisis at the age of 1 ½ years and lived in a home for severely handicapped children for years before he died of pneumonia at the age of 13. One boy died at school age (7 years). Moreover, two adolescents died at the age of 16. Almost all deceased patients had German parents ($n = 12$); in one case, the parents were from Turkey, and in another case, the parents were not married (German mother, Turkish father). The attending resident physicians included 10 paediatricians and 4 general practitioners.

Almost all deceased CAH children ($n = 13$) were besides their family doctor or paediatrician also under the care of a centre with a paediatric endocrinologist. Laboratory controls were performed regularly, and the three females classified as CAH-SV patients who were detected at birth by ambiguous genitalia had normal serum electrolytes and plasma renin activity (PRA) until the event that caused their death. The boy in the persistent vegetative state (case No. 8) was treated by the head physician of a county hospital. The centres rated the cooperation of the parents/patients as good in 9 cases and as poor in 5 cases. For 9 patients, information was provided on the date when they last presented as outpatients at the relevant centres. One patient presented as an outpatient and was released after being examined the day before he died (case No. 3), whereas the last outpatient examination of case No. 12 at a centre dated back to more than a year prior to his death. Half of the children died at home. Three children died in the hospital where they had also been treated as outpatients in the specialized outpatient department. Three children died immediately after admission to an external hospital. One child died of pneumonia in a home for severely handicapped children, where the boy (case No. 8) had been treated for apallic syndrome for 11 years. The event leading to the persistent vegetative state had occurred at the age of 1½ years. All children received treatment with hydrocortisone, with a mean dosage of 14.8 mg/m^2 /day (range: 8.2–20 mg/m^2 /day). Information on the fludrocortisone dosage was only provided in 9 cases, and the mean dosage was 163 µg/day (range: 100–375 µg/day).

Immediately before their deaths, 13 patients suffered from a high fever along with vomiting ($n = 4$), convulsions (n = 4), gastroenteritis with diarrhoea ($n = 2$), dyspnoea and/or upper respiratory tract infection (n = 2), and varicella ($n = 1$). One patient additionally suffered from a metabolic defect (MCAD defect). Considering the measures taken by the parents at home by themselves or upon consultation with the attending physicians, treatment of the children with elevated body temperature always focused on lowering the fever. In two cases, the parents also used antiemetic suppositories. The hydrocortisone dosage was doubled in 2 cases. No symptomatic or specific treatment was provided in 7 cases.

According to the assessments by the attending centres, the cause of death in these patients was a lack or inadequate adaptation of glucocorticoid dosage to the acute stress situation. Five patients developed hypoglycaemia and severe convulsions with cerebral oedema. In case No. 9, the centre did not find any correlation with CAH and specified "sudden infant death syndrome" as the cause of death. The cause of death certified on the death certificate by the reporting physicians was "death of natural causes" in 11 cases, "death of non-natural causes" in 2 cases, and "not clarified" in one case. An autopsy was only performed in 4 of the 14 cases of death. The pathologist/forensic medical expert found severe cerebral oedema in 3 cases. The autopsy did not yield any new findings in one case.

Discussion

Deaths in patients with classic CAH in the context of an acute adrenal crisis (Addisonian crisis) are described in the literature. Mortality in CAH children is generally considered higher and assumed to be between 2 and 13% [17–19, 21].

Studies on mortality in CAH patients from Finland and the United Kingdom performed before the introduction of newborn screening for CAH report 7 deaths in 108 CAH patients in Finland [22] and 8 deaths (7 girls) in 333 patients (219 female) in the UK [21].

In the UK, the mortality rate was 3 times higher than that in the general population, and primarily toddlers between 1 and 4 years of age died. Our data strongly confirm the published results. In the UK, most affected children descended from Indian immigrant families [21], whereas in Germany, only one child had an immigrant background. Almost all deceased children in the UK had been under the care of specialized centres, and a similar situation was found in Germany.

In the UK, the high portion of deceased girls is explained by the high portion of girls in the cohort analysed. In Germany, the number of deceased girls was also slightly higher than that of boys, but the number of girls who died before newborn screening was almost equal to the number of girls who died after screening. It has to be kept in mind that half of the CAH children died after the introduction of newborn screening. In Japan, 12 deaths in CAH children were reported 12 years after the introduction of a newborn screening program [23]. Two of these children died during the newborn period at the ages of 13 and 23 days, whereas 10 children died under replacement therapy. In Hungary, 19 of 235 CAH patients died, including 17 with the SW-form of CAH (8 boys, 9 girls) and 2 boys with the SV-form of the disease. Sixteen of 17 CAH patients with the SW-form of the disease died within their first year of life. The mortality rate in CAH children with SW was 11.3% in the first year of life and thus significantly higher than the rate of 2.29% found in the Hungarian population [24].

It is known that in the presence of feverish infections and/or other acute stress situations, CAH children can be affected by an adrenal crisis at any stage of life. A study from the UK defines an adrenal crisis as an acute event that affects a patient's health and requires i.v. glucocorticoid treatment and inpatient care. In this study, a survey was performed in 122 adults with CAH, and the medical records of the adult patients were analysed from the time of diagnosis until the date when they last presented as outpatients. The incidence of adrenal crises was highest in the first 10 years of life (70%), but crises were also observed in adults [15]. The data from Germany is highly consistent with these results.

In CAH patients, both adrenocortical and adrenomedullary dysfunction can result in severe hyponatremia, hyperkalemia and hypoglycemia due to impaired production of cortisol, aldosterone and epinephrine secretion [25–27]. Data extracted from a population-based prospective long-term follow-up study of 102 children with classic CAH detected in neonatal screening in Bavaria show that 22 children experienced a salt wasting adrenal crises (seven also with low blood glucose) and 16 children hypoglycemic episodes during the first 6 years of life [14].

Although the causes of death and/or the concomitant circumstances resulting in death have not been clarified in some of our cases, we assume that inadequate adaptation of the glucocorticoid dosage is likely in most cases. Glucocorticoid deficiency results in failure of the body's compensation mechanisms. The most common form of shock in childhood is hypovolemic shock, which occurs due to constant fluid loss, e.g., within the scope of gastroenteritis. Cardiac output decreases before the onset of arterial hypotension. Therefore, therapy for shock in children must be started before the onset of hypotension [28]. CAH children seem to have a markedly elevated risk of acute adrenal crisis in the presence of acute gastroenteritis due to dehydration and/or lack of drug uptake during diarrhoea and/or vomiting. In our survey, two children died while suffering from gastroenteritis, including one case in which salmonella was detected.

Altogether, acute adrenal insufficiency is very rare in childhood. Most physicians only know the symptoms from textbooks, and only a few paediatricians have specific experience in the treatment of adrenal crisis. Well-known symptoms include hyponatremia, vomiting, diarrhoea, hypoglycaemia, dysrhythmia due to hyperkalaemia and increasing disorientation. In a recent study, it was noted that, in contrast to hyperkalaemia, hyponatremia is a constant laboratory finding in children with primary adrenal insufficiency [29].

It was also reported that the symptoms and the neuro-radiologic findings can include severe cerebral oedema [30]. In our survey, autopsies in three deceased CAH children provided evidence of cerebral oedema. The occurrence of cerebral oedema and/or water intoxication has been associated with CAH since the 1930s from animal experiments following adrenalectomy and/or in patients with Addison's disease [31–33]. The secretion of antidiuretic hormone is increased in these situations, and the mere supply of volume without adequate adaptation of the glucocorticoid dosage can result in water intoxication [34, 35].

According to calculations performed in Japan, one in 25–80 affected CAH children dies in childhood [23]. The mortality is 1 in 12 CAH patients in Hungary [24], 1 in 15 CAH patients in Finland [22], and 1 in 24 CAH patients in the UK [21]. The data available in Germany do not allow calculating mortality rates.

Half of the deceased patients died at home. The hydrocortisone dosage was only doubled in two of the 14 cases. Therefore, delayed timing and/or lack of administration of life-saving emergency medication and/or inadequate dosage adaptation to the acute stress situation might have triggered the adrenal crisis and could be the underlying cause of almost all deaths.

The medical care of a child with CAH requires a close cooperation between all involved parties e.g. general practitioner, paediatrician, and parents or other caregiver as well as a confidence in the recommendations given by the paediatric endocrinologist. Already in 1977, it was recommended in the first German Textbook of Paediatric Endocrinology, to increase the hydrocortisone dose 3–5 times in all CAH children with febrile infections, surgery or after an accident [30]. The current recommendations in Germany correspond to the standards published by the Endocrine Society [31].

From 2005 on, there was no report of a deceased CAH patient in Germany. This result is very encouraging and shows the effectiveness of programs which have been conducted over the past years to educate and train parents, patients, caregivers and practitioners in realizing and managing adrenal crisis situations [36]. Emphasis should be placed on communication and training, even in case of emergency, and the knowledge of caregivers of affected children should be checked at regular intervals.

Conclusions

There were some limitations to our study. The data were obtained by a survey and covered a period from 1973 to 2015. Our survey covered the whole of Germany, but it is not certain whether all cases of deceased CAH patients were reported. We speculate that most patients who died between 1973 and 2004 had an inadequate stress dosing of glucocorticoids. We assume that the quality of adrenal crisis management had improved over the past years since no deceased CAH children were reported from 2005 on.

Abbreviations
CAH: Congenital adrenal hyperplasia; SW: Salt wasting

Acknowledgements
The authors are indebted to all members of the German Society of Pediatric Endocrinology and Diabetology.

Authors' contributions
HGD, HAW, BPH and JW contributed to the design of the work, acquisition, analysis and interpretation of data, drafting the work and final approval of the version to be published.

Competing interests
The authors declare that they have no conflict of interest.

Author details
[1]Paediatric Endocrinology, Department Paediatrics, University Hospital of Erlangen, Erlangen, Germany. [2]Department Paediatrics, University Hospital of Tübingen, Tübingen, Germany. [3]Paediatric Endocrinology, Department Paediatrics, University Hospital of Essen, Essen, Germany. [4]Paediatric Endocrinology, Department Paediatrics, University Hospital of Bonn, Bonn, Germany.

References

1. Forest MG. Recent advances in the diagnosis and management of congenital adrenal hyperplasia due to 21-hydroxylase deficiency. Hum Reprod Update. 2004;10(6):469–85.
2. Miller WL, Auchus RJ. The molecular biology, biochemistry, and physiology of human steroidogenesis and its disorders. Endocr Rev. 2011;32(1):81–151.
3. New MI. An update of congenital adrenal hyperplasia. Ann N Y Acad Sci. 2004;1038:14–43.
4. Speiser PW, White PC. Congenital adrenal hyperplasia. N Engl J Med. 2003; 349(8):776–88.
5. Tajima T, Fujikura K, Fukushi M, Hotsubo T, Mitsuhashi Y. Neonatal screening for congenital adrenal hyperplasia in Japan. Pediatr Endocrinol Rev. 2012; 10(Suppl 1):72–8.
6. van der Kamp HJ, Wit JM. Neonatal screening for congenital adrenal hyperplasia. Eur J Endocrinol. 2004;151(Suppl 3):U71–5.
7. White PC. Neonatal screening for congenital adrenal hyperplasia. Nat Rev Endocrinol. 2009;5(9):490–8.
8. Trapp CM, Speiser PW, Oberfield SE. Congenital adrenal hyperplasia: an update in children. Curr Opin Endocrinol Diabetes Obes. 2011;18(3):166–70.
9. Speiser PW. Medical treatment of classic and nonclassic congenital adrenal hyperplasia. Adv Exp Med Biol. 2011;707:41–5.
10. Riepe FG. Adrenal gland: congenital adrenal hyperplasia: new treatment guidelines. Nat Rev Endocrinol. 2011;7(1):6–8.
11. Padidela R, Hindmarsh PC. Mineralocorticoid deficiency and treatment in congenital adrenal hyperplasia. Int J Pediatr Endocrinol. 2010;2010:656925.
12. Hindmarsh PC. Management of the child with congenital adrenal hyperplasia. Best Pract Res Clin Endocrinol Metab. 2009;23(2):193–208.
13. Claahsen-van der Grinten HL, Stikkelbroeck NM, Otten BJ, Hermus AR. Congenital adrenal hyperplasia–pharmacologic interventions from the prenatal phase to adulthood. Pharmacol Ther. 2011;132(1):1–14.
14. Odenwald B, Nennstiel-Ratzel U, Dorr HG, Schmidt H, Wildner M, Bonfig W. Children with classic congenital adrenal hyperplasia experience salt loss and hypoglycemia: evaluation of adrenal crises during the first 6 years of life. Eur J Endocrinol. 2016;174(2):177–86.
15. Reisch N, Willige M, Kohn D, Schwarz HP, Allolio B, Reincke M, Quinkler M, Hahner S, Beuschlein F. Frequency and causes of adrenal crises over lifetime in patients with 21-hydroxylase deficiency. Eur J Endocrinol. 2012;167:35–42.
16. Falhammar H, Frisen L, Norrby C, Hirschberg AL, Almqvist C, Nordenskjold A, Nordenstrom A. Increased mortality in patients with congenital adrenal hyperplasia due to 21-hydroxylase deficiency. J Clin Endocrinol Metab. 2014; 99(12):E2715–21.
17. Cleveland WW, Green OC, Wilkins L. Deaths in congenital adrenal hyperplasia. Pediatrics. 1962;29:3–17.
18. Lim YJ, Batch JA, Warne GL. Adrenal 21-hydroxylase deficiency in childhood: 25 years' experience. J Paediatr Child Health. 1995;31(3):222–7.
19. Thilen A, Larsson A. Congenital adrenal hyperplasia in Sweden 1969-1986. Prevalence, symptoms and age at diagnosis. Acta Paediatr Scand. 1990; 79(2):168–75.
20. Krone N, Roscher AA, Schwarz HP, Braun A. Comprehensive analytical strategy for mutation screening in 21-hydroxylase deficiency. Clin Chem. 1998;44(10):2075–82.
21. Swerdlow AJ, Higgins CD, Brook CG, Dunger DB, Hindmarsh PC, Price DA, Savage MO. Mortality in patients with congenital adrenal hyperplasia: a cohort study. J Pediatr. 1998;133(4):516–20.
22. Jaaskelainen VR. Long-term outcome of classical 21-hydroxylase deficiency: diagnosis, complications and quality of life. *Acta Paediatr.* 2000;89(2):183–7.
23. Ogawa E, Fujieda K, Tachibana K, Inomata H, Kinoshita E, Kusuda S, Nishi Y, Okada T, Saisho S, Tajima T, et al. Mortaility in patients with congenital 21-. Hydroxylase deficiency diagnosed after the introduction of a newborn screening program in Japan. Clin Pediatr Endocrinology. 2003;12(1):19–23.
24. Kovacs J, Votava F, Heinze G, Solyom J, Lebl J, Pribilincova Z, Frisch H, Battelino T, Waldhauser F. Lessons from 30 years of clinical diagnosis and treatment of congenital adrenal hyperplasia in five middle European countries. J Clin Endocrinol Metab. 2001;86(7):2958–64.
25. Merke DP, Chrousos GP, Eisenhofer G, Weise M, Keil MF, Rogol AD, Van Wyk JJ, Bornstein SR. Adrenomedullary dysplasia and hypofunction in patients with classic 21-hydroxylase deficiency. N Engl J Med. 2000;343(19):1362–8.
26. Tutunculer F, Saka N, Arkaya SC, Abbasoglu S, Bas F. Evaluation of adrenomedullary function in patients with congenital adrenal hyperplasia. Horm Res. 2009;72(6):331–6.
27. Green-Golan L, Yates C, Drinkard B, Van Ryzin C, Eisenhofer G, Weise M, Merke DP. Patients with classic congenital adrenal hyperplasia have decreased epinephrine reserve and defective glycemic control during prolonged moderate-intensity exercise. J Clin Endocrinol Metab. 2007;92(8):3019–24.
28. Meyburg J, Bernhard M, Hoffmann GF, Motsch J. Principles of pediatric emergency care. Deutsches Arzteblatt Int. 2009;106(45):739–47. quiz 748
29. Hsieh S, White PC. Presentation of primary adrenal insufficiency in childhood. J Clin Endocrinol Metab. 2011;96(6):E925–8.
30. Von Petrykowski W, Abel M, Brämswig J: Schweres Hirnödem - eine wenig bekannte Manifestation des Glukokortikoidmangels. Pädiatrische Praxis 1986/87, 34:5.
31. Walsh FB. Papilledema associated with increased intracranial pressure in Addison's disease. *AMA*. Arch Ophthalmol. 1952;47(1):86.
32. Swingle WW, Pfiffner JJ, Vars HM, Bott PA, Parkins WM. The function of the adrenal cortical hormone and the cause of death from adrenal insufficiency. Science. 1933;77(1985):58–64.
33. Swingle WW, Swingle AJ. Effect of adrenal steroids upon plasma volume of intact and Adrenalectomized dogs. Proc Soc Exp Biol Med. 1965;119:452–5.
34. Salpietro V, Polizzi A, Di Rosa G, Romeo AC, Dipasquale V, Morabito P, Chirico V, Arrigo T, Ruggieri M. Adrenal disorders and the paediatric brain: pathophysiological considerations and clinical implications. Int J Endocrinol 2014. 2014:282489. https://doi.org/10.1155/2014/282489.
35. Zieg J. Pathophysiology of hyponatremia in children. Frontiers in Pediatr. 2017;5:213.
36. Fleming L, Knafl K, Knafl G, Van Riper M. Parental management of adrenal crisis in children with congenital adrenal hyperplasia. J Spec Pediatr Nurs. 2017. https://doi.org/10.1111/jspn.12190.

Effects of an eight-week supervised, structured lifestyle modification programme on anthropometric, metabolic and cardiovascular risk factors in severely obese adults

Catherine Crowe[1], Irene Gibson[2], Katie Cunningham[1,2], Claire Kerins[2], Caroline Costello[2], Jane Windle[2], Paula M. O'Shea[3], Mary Hynes[1,4], Brian McGuire[4], Katriona Kilkelly[1], Helena Griffin[1], Tim O'Brien[1,5], Jenni Jones[5,6] and Francis M Finucane[1,5*]

Abstract

Background: Lifestyle modification is fundamental to obesity treatment, but few studies have described the effects of structured lifestyle programmes specifically in bariatric patients. We sought to describe changes in anthropometric and metabolic characteristics in a cohort of bariatric patients after participation in a nurse-led, structured lifestyle programme.

Methods: We conducted a retrospective, observational cohort study of adults with a body mass index (BMI) ≥40 kgm^{-2} (or ≥35 kgm^{-2} with significant co-morbidity) who were attending a regional bariatric service and who completed a single centre, 8-week, nurse-led multidisciplinary lifestyle modification programme. Weight, height, waist circumference, blood pressure, HbA1c, fasting glucose and lipid profiles as well as functional capacity (Incremental Shuttle Walk Test) and questionnaire-based anxiety and depression scores before and after the programme were compared in per-protocol analyses.

Results: Of 183 bariatric patients enrolled, 150 (81.9 %) completed the programme. Mean age of completers was 47.9 ± 11.2 years. 34.7 % were male. There were statistically significant reductions in weight (129.6 ± 25.9 v 126.9 ± 26.1 kg, $p < 0.001$), BMI (46.3 ± 8.3 v 44.9 ± 9.0 kgm^{-2}, $p < 0.001$), waist circumference (133.0 ± 17.1 v 129.3 ± 17.5 cm in women and 143.8 ± 19.0 v 135.1 ± 17.9 cm in men, both $p < 0.001$) as well as anxiety and depression scores, total- and LDL-cholesterol and triglyceride levels, with an increase in functional capacity (5.9 ± 1.7 v 6.8 ± 2.1 metabolic equivalents of thermogenesis (METS), $p < 0.001$) in completers at the end of the programme compared to the start. Blood pressure improved, with reductions in systolic and diastolic blood pressure from 135 ± 16.2 to 131.6 ± 17.1 ($p = 0.009$) and 84.7 ± 10.2 to 81.4 ± 10.9 mmHg ($p < 0.001$), respectively. The proportion of patients achieving target blood pressure increased from 50.3 to 59.3 % ($p = 0.04$). The proportion of patients with diabetes achieving HbA1c <53 mmol/mol increased from 28.6 to 42.9 %, $p = 0.02$.

(Continued on next page)

* Correspondence: francis.finucane@hse.ie
[1]Bariatric Medicine Service, Galway Diabetes Research Centre, HRB Clinical Research Facility, Galway University Hospital, Galway, Ireland
[5]Discipline of Health Promotion, National University of Ireland, Galway, Ireland
Full list of author information is available at the end of the article

(Continued from previous page)

Conclusions: Bariatric patients completing an 8 week, nurse-led structured lifestyle programme had improved adiposity, fitness, lipid profiles, psychosocial health, blood pressure and glycaemia. Further assessment of this programme in a pragmatic randomised controlled trial seems warranted.

Keywords: Bariatric, Structured lifestyle modification, Cardiovascular risk, CLANN (Changing Lifestyle with Activity and Nutrition) Programme, Nurse-led, Diabetes

Background

Consistent with global trends, the prevalence of overweight and obesity has increased steadily in Ireland over the past three decades [1, 2]. This is a public health concern because of the associated morbidity and mortality from diseases like type 2 diabetes, for which the population attributable risk from obesity is 50 to 80 % [3, 4]. There is also a significant health economic burden associated with obesity, which accounts for €1.1 billion of public spending per annum in Ireland [5]. Public health strategies to reduce calorie intake and increase physical activity have not been successful to date. The population shift in body mass index (BMI) has led to a particularly dramatic rise in the prevalence of severe obesity [6]. For these individuals (conventionally defined as those with a BMI ≥40 kg m^{-2} or ≥35 kg m^{-2} with co-morbidities such as type 2 diabetes), relatively intensive "bariatric" interventions need to be adopted [7]. These include intensive dietary restriction [8] and bariatric surgery [9]. In a US cohort of bariatric surgical patients, the prevalence of hypertension was 49 %, type 2 diabetes was 28 % and dyslipidaemia was 46 % at baseline, which was reduced or resolved by 68, 75 and 71 % respectively after a mean post-surgical follow up of 34 months, with a 40 % relative reduction in cardiovascular risk in that time [10]. While bariatric surgical interventions are efficacious and cost effective [11], they are also invasive, expensive and unsuitable for a significant proportion of bariatric patients.

Lifestyle modification is the cornerstone of the therapeutic approach to the obese patient. Several studies have confirmed the benefits of structured lifestyle interventions in different patient subgroups, including those with non-diabetic hyperglycaemia [12–14], prevalent cardiovascular disease [15] or established type 2 diabetes [16]. However, studies of such interventions in bariatric patients are limited and often include meal replacement regimes, which can be very effective in the short term but are not designed to induce sustained dietary changes and are associated with low retention rates [17]. In one US study of 130 bariatric patients undergoing a twelve-month diet and physical activity programme, weight loss at 1 year was 11 kg, with significant reductions in waist circumference, visceral and hepatic fat, blood pressure and insulin resistance, with a study retention rate of 78 % [18]. However, there was still a meal replacement component to this trial and to our knowledge, no previous study has examined the effects of a multidisciplinary lifestyle modification programme that does not include a prescribed diet or meal replacement regimen in bariatric patients.

As part of the recent establishment of a regional bariatric service in the West of Ireland, we have adopted an 8 week structured lifestyle modification programme known as the CLANN (Changing Lifestyle with Activity and Nutrition) for patients with severe obesity. This programme incorporates some key principles which have already been associated with successful reduction in anthropometric and metabolic cardiovascular risk factors in adults with prevalent cardiovascular disease [19, 20]. Our objective in this study was to measure the effect of this programme on relevant cardiovascular outcomes. In achieving that objective, we hope to facilitate the more robust design of a randomised controlled trial to determine the programme's effectiveness in bariatric patients.

Methods

The study population included bariatric patients ≥18 years old with a BMI ≥40 kg m^{-2} (or ≥35 with co-morbidity) who were willing to attend a community-based facility where the CLANN programme is delivered for 2 h per week for 8 weeks. Each patient was referred after careful assessment for suitability by the hospital-based, multidisciplinary bariatric team. Patients with poorly controlled diabetes or hypertension, symptoms suggestive of untreated ischaemic heart disease, an inability to walk 10 m or those deemed unlikely to attend for the full programme (e.g. frequent clinic non-attendance) were excluded from the programme.

The 8-week programme focused on weight management as part of a comprehensive cardiovascular risk reduction strategy. The main emphasis of the programme is on lifestyle modification, namely healthy food choices, weight reduction, physical activity and smoking cessation. We based our definition of "healthy food choices" on the European guidelines on healthy eating for cardiovascular disease prevention [21]. Specifically, these stipulate saturated fatty acids <10 % of total daily energy intake, trans-unsaturated fatty acids <1 % of total daily energy intake, salt consumption <5 g/ day, fibre intake 30–45 g/ day, fruit >200 g/ day (2–3 servings), vegetables >200 g/

day (2–3 servings), fish at least twice per week, (one "oily") and alcohol consumption <20 g/ day for men and <10 g/ day for women. The Irish "Food Pyramid" (published by the Irish Government's Department of Health in 2012) was used as a visual tool to encourage the adoption of these dietary guidelines and to describe portion sizes to the participants. We sought to encourage a cardioprotective diet and to achieve an energy deficit of 600 kcal/ day, in order to achieve a target weekly weight loss of 0.5 kg.

Initially, all patients received an individualised assessment by the multidisciplinary team (nurse, dietitian, physiotherapist, physical activity specialist). This included recording use of cardioprotective medications such as antihypertensive and antiplatelet agents and statins. The assessment also sought to identify individual priorities and needs and to explore beliefs, barriers and motivators to change. Following this assessment, patients attended the 8-week programme, consisting of a group-based exercise programme combined with educational workshops, lasting 2 h each week. Effective exercise and physical activity strategies which were specific, measurable, achievable, realistic and timed were also emphasised. These were initiated in the programme without specialist gym equipment with the objective of the patient maintaining these behaviours in the longer term after completion of the programme. While the exercise sessions were group-based for maximum efficiency, each patient had an individualised programme based on an assessment of their needs by the physiotherapist and exercise physiologist. The curriculum of eight theory-based health promotion workshops incorporated a module on "understanding cardiovascular disease", two modules on "eating for a healthy shape" (emphasising dietary modification techniques such as carbohydrate counting, food label interpretation and portion size calculation) and a module each on "exercising for life", "reading and understanding food labels", "stress management", "dealing with the psychological issues of obesity" (including mindfulness) and "maintaining a healthy lifestyle".

Individualised goal setting occurred at the initial assessment and then continued throughout the programme. Motivational interviewing was used to support patients in progressing through the stages of behaviour change, by enhancing intrinsic motivation, autonomy and self-efficacy. All patients were given a personal record card which they were encouraged to use on a weekly basis to record their goals and track their progress in relation to weight, BMI, blood pressure, lipid profile and for patients with diabetes, HbA1c and glucose levels.

At initial assessment, dietary habits, physical activity levels (7-day physical activity recall), functional capacity (Incremental Shuttle Walk Test [22], (ISWT) from which a Heart Rate Walking Speed Index (HRWSI) was derived) and psychosocial measures (questionnaire-based anxiety and depression scores) were recorded. Specifically, the Hospital Anxiety and Depression Scale (HADS) [23], EQVAS (European Quality of Life Questionnaire, Visual Analogue Scale) [24] and Dartmouth COOP [25] questionnaires were administered. Weight was measured using a Seca® 877 scale and height with a Seca® Leicester stadiometer. Blood pressure was measured with an Omron® 705IT oscillometric device in both arms after the patient was sitting comfortably for five minutes. All of these measures were repeated following completion of the programme. The outcome targets were based on the 2012 European Society of Cardiology (ESC) prevention guidelines [21]. Specifically, the blood pressure target was 140/ 90 mmHg (140/ 85 in patients with type 2 diabetes) while the lipid targets were total cholesterol <5 mmol/l, LDL cholesterol <3 mmol/l and triglycerides <1.7 mmol/l. The study was approved by the Galway Clinical Research Ethics Committee (the ethics committee for Galway University Hospitals). Patients signed written informed consent for their data to be used in the study.

Laboratory analysis

All blood samples were analysed locally in the Galway University Hospitals' Department of Clinical Biochemistry (certified to ISO 15189 2007 accreditation standard). HbA1c was measured with HPLC (Menarini® HA8160 auto-analyzer). Total cholesterol was measured using the CHOP-PAP method. High density lipoprotein (HDL)-cholesterol and triglycerides were measured using the enzymatic and the GPO-PAP methods, respectively (Roche COBAS® 8000 modular analyzer). Low density lipoprotein (LDL)-Cholesterol was derived with the Friedewald equation [26].

Statistical analysis

Differences between outcomes at the start and the end of the programme for patients who completed the programme were assessed using the paired exact test for categorical variables, the paired *t*-test for normally distributed continuous variables and the Wilcoxon matched pairs test for non-normally distributed continuous variables. All analyses were performed using SPSS version 21.

Results

Of 183 patients enrolled, 150 (81.9 %) completed the programme. Their baseline socio-demographic characteristics are shown in Table 1. Mean age was 47.9 ± 11.3 years. 57 (31 %) had type 2 diabetes at baseline. Overall, of 136 (92.7 %) of participants who provided information about their employment status, 78 (57.4 %) were unemployed. Most participants were "White Irish", though 51 (34 %) did not provide information about their ethnicity. Similarly, 47 participants (31.3 %) did not provide information about their educational background.

Table 1 Baseline socio-demographic characteristics of 150 severely obese adults completing the Croi CLANN programme

	N	Proportion (%)
Demographic variables		
Female	98/ 150	65.3
Current smoker	18/ 150	12
Living with partner	91/ 144	60.7
Prevalent diabetes	53/ 148	35.8
Employment status ($N = 136$)		
Employed full time	38	27.9
Employed part time	13	9.6
Self-employed full time	6	4.4
Self-employed part time	1	0.7
Retired	17	12.5
Unemployed	25	18.4
Looking after family	20	14.7
Student	9	6.6
Permanently sick	2	1.5
Temporarily sick	2	1.5
Other	3	2.2
Ethnicity ($N = 99$)		
White / White Irish	98	99
Other ethnicity	1	1
Education level ($N = 103$)		
Primary	23	22.3
Secondary	38	36.9
College / University	42	40.8

Proportions are expressed as a percentage of the total number of participants for which data were available for that variable

The baseline and follow-up anthropometric and metabolic characteristics of programme completers are presented in Table 2. Patients who completed the programme had statistically significant reductions in weight, BMI, waist circumference and blood pressure. Changes in blood pressure were greater in those who had suboptimal blood pressure at baseline, defined as >140/85 and >140/ 90 mmHg in patients with and without type 2 diabetes, respectively [27]. The proportion of patients with blood pressure readings at target increased from 50.3 % at baseline to 59.3 % at follow-up, $p = 0.04$. There were reductions also in self-reported depression and anxiety levels and some, but not all components of the lipid profile. HbA1c decreased slightly in the whole group, with greater reductions in those with type 2 diabetes. The proportion of patients with type 2 diabetes achieving optimal control (HbA1c <53 mmol/mol or 7 %) increased from 28.6 % at baseline to 42.9 % at follow-up, $p = 0.02$. The proportion of patients achieving targets for moderate intensity aerobic activity of 30 min five times per week [28] increased from 4.0 % at baseline to 38.4 % at follow-up, $p < 0.001$. There were significant increases in various indices of aerobic fitness and functional status, as shown in Table 1. Lastly, changes in medication usage were minimised to the greatest extent possible (Table 2). One patient stopped their calcium channel blocker and one patient started an ACE inhibitor, otherwise no changes were made to these medications.

In order to determine whether the response to the intervention was different for men and women, we used regression modelling with the follow-up measure of the variable of interest being the outcome and sex as the exposure, adjusting for the baseline measure of that variable. Overall, there were differential responses for only a small number of outcomes. Specifically, men had a greater reduction in waist circumference than women (−3.4 [−6.0, −0.8] cm, $p = 0.009$). Men had statistically significantly greater improvements in some but not all indices of aerobic fitness. Their reduction in heart rate walking speed index (HRWSI) was greater (−1.0 [−1.8, −0.2], $p = 0.02$) and their increase in estimated MET max was greater (0.6 [0.1, 1.0] METs, $p = 0.02$), though changes in metres scored on ISWT and METs achieved were not statistically significantly different by sex. After adjusting for baseline values, triglycerides were 12 % lower in men than in women at follow up ($p = 0.02$). Conversely the reduction in systolic blood pressure was lower for men than for women, such that the decrease in women was 6.6 [1.8, 11.4] mmHg ($p = 0.007$) more than for men.

We also sought to determine whether there were any differences at baseline in patients who completed the programme compared to those who dropped out and did not attend for follow-up assessment. Compared to non-completers, completers were older (47.9 ± 11.2 versus 40.7 ± 12.9 years, $p = 0.003$), were more likely to be men (34.7 versus 10.3 %, $p = 0.008$) and were more likely to have diabetes (35.8 versus 13.8 %, $p = 0.03$). There were no differences in smoking, employment, ethnicity or educational status, nor were there differences in anthropometric measures such as weight, BMI, waist circumference or blood pressure. As anticipated given the above differences, HbA1c was higher in completers than non-completers at baseline (47.9 ± 15.5 versus 39.7 ± 5.1 mmol/mol, $p = 0.02$) and HDL cholesterol was lower (1.15 ± 0.28 versus 1.29 ± 0.38, $p = 0.03$), though there was no difference in other components of the lipid profile. Also, medication usage was higher at baseline in completers, for statins (33.6 versus 11.1 %, $p = 0.02$), antiplatelets (27.9 versus 3.6 %, $p = 0.004$), ACEI/ ARBs (38.9 versus 15.4 %, $p = 0.03$) and calcium channel blockers (22.5 versus 0 %, $p = 0.03$) but not for betablockers (7.4 versus 17.5 %, $p = 0.26$). Completers had less self-reported anxiety at baseline (7 [5, 11] versus

Table 2 Baseline and follow-up anthropometric and metabolic characteristics of 150 severely obese adults completing the Croi CLANN programme

Variable	N	Baseline	Follow-up	Difference		P-value
		Mean ± SD	Mean ± SD	Mean	95 % Confidence Interval	
Weight (kg)	150	129.6 ± 29.5	126.9 ± 26.1	−2.7	[−3.4, −2.0]	<0.001
BMI (kg/m^2)	150	46.3 ± 8.3	44.9 ± 9.0	−1.4	[−2.1, −0.7]	<0.001
Waist (cm) - women	93	133.3 ± 17.1	129.3 ± 17.5	−3.7	[−4.9, −2.4]	<0.001
Waist (cm) – men	50	143.8 ± 19.0	135.1 ± 17.9	−8.0	[−10.5, −5.4]	<0.001
SBP (mmHg)	144	135.0 ± 16.2	131.6 ± 17.1	−3.3	[−5.8, −0.8]	0.009
DBP (mmHg)	144	84.7 ± 10.2	81.4 ± 10.9	−3.2	[−4.9, −1.6]	<0.001
SBP (mmHg) [a]	71	145.5 ± 14.8	138.2 ± 17.3	−7.3	[−11.3, −3.3]	<0.001
DBP (mmHg)[a]	71	91.7 ± 8.0	85.7 ± 11.3	−6.0	[−8.5, −3.5]	<0.001
HbA1c (mmol/mol)	114	42 (37, 60)	41 (37, 53)	0	[−2, 0]	0.007
HbA1c (mmol/mol)[b]	51	61 (49, 71)	59 (45, 66)	−3	[−5, 0]	0.006
Total Cholesterol (mmol/L)	145	4.7 ± 1.1	4.5 ± 1.0	−0.2	[−0.3, −0.1]	0.001
LDL Cholesterol (mmol/L)	138	2.7 ± 1.0	2.6 ± 0.9	−0.1	[−0.2, 0.0]	0.05
HDL Cholesterol (mmol/L)	145	1.2 ± 0.3	1.1 ± 0.3	−0.02	[−0.04, 0.01]	0.16
Triglycerides (mmol/L)	145	1.6 (1.1, 2.2)	1.4 (1.0, 1.9)	−0.1	[−0.2, −0.01]	<0.001
Total Cholesterol (mmol/L) [c]	62	5.8 ± 0.8	5.2 ± 0.9	−0.6	[−0.8, −0.4]	<0.001
LDL Cholesterol (mmol/L) [c]	62	3.8 ± 0.8	3.4 ± 0.7	−0.4	[−0.6, −0.2]	<0.001
Triglycerides (mmol/L)[c]	62	2.2 (1.9, 2.8)	1.9 (1.4, 2.8)	−0.4	[−0.6, −0.03]	<0.001
Metres scored on ISWT (m)	133	295 ± 130	350 ± 153	53	[41, 66]	<0.001
METs achieved on ISWT (MET)	133	3.5 ± 0.9	3.8 ± 1.3	0.4	[0.3, 0.6]	<0.001
Estimated MET max (MET)	133	5.9 ± 1.7	6.8 ± 2.1	0.9	[0.6, 1.1]	<0.001
HRWSI	133	16.9 ± 4.3	15.5 ± 3.6	−1.4	[−1.9, −0.9]	<0.001
Functional limitations score	83	20.5 ± 5.5	22.5 ± 5.3	2.0	[1.1, 2.9]	<0.001
Anxiety score	110	7 (5, 11)	7 (4, 10)	−1	[−2, 0]	<0.001
Depression score	110	8 (5, 11)	4 (2, 7)	−2	[−3, −1]	<0.001
Dartmouth Coop score	110	26 ± 6	23 ± 7	−3	[−4, −2]	<0.001
EQ-VAS	110	53 ± 22	60 ± 20	8	[4, 11]	<0.001
Antiplatelet agents (%)	150	27.4	27.4	0	[−0.7, 0.7]	1.0
Statins (%)	150	34.3	34.3	0	[−0.7, 0.7]	1.0
ACEI/ ARB (%)	150	38.5	39.2	0.7	[−2.4, 3.8]	1.0
Betablockers (%)	150	17.6	17.6	0	[−0.7, 0.7]	1.0
Calcium channel blockers (%)	150	22.6	21.9	−0.7	[−2.7, 1.3]	1.0

Data are presented as mean ± standard deviation or as median (interquartile range)
[a]Denotes subgroup with elevated blood pressure at baseline assessment (>140/85 mmHg with diabetes or >140/90 with no diabetes)
[b]Denotes subgroup with prevalent type 2 diabetes at baseline
[c]Denotes subgroup not meeting that specific lipid subtype target at baseline [21]

9 [6, 12], $p = 0.04$), though other psychometric measures were not different. They achieved a shorter distance on the incremental shuttle walk test (295 ± 130 versus 364 ± 106, $p = 0.01$), though there were no differences in other measures of fitness. We sought also to determine whether the response to the programme was different according to diabetes status. Compared to non-diabetic patients, patients with diabetes who completed the programme had a greater reduction in waist circumference (−3.2 [−5.6, −0.7] cm, $p = 0.01$), though changes in weight and BMI were not different. There was a trend to a greater reduction in systolic blood pressure in those without diabetes of 4.8 mmHg [0.0, 9.6], $p = 0.05$, but not in diastolic blood pressure, lipid profile or any measures of fitness. Changes in psychometric scores were no different by diabetes status (data not shown).

Discussion

These findings confirm that a structured lifestyle modification programme for carefully selected bariatric patients is feasible and safe and leads to statistically significant improvements in several cardiovascular risk-related outcomes. The retention rate of 81.9 % compares favourably with similar lifestyle intervention studies in this patient group [17, 18]. While the overall effect size of the programme in completers was relatively modest, the reduction in BMI of 1.4 kgm^{-2} is identical to that seen in cardiovascular patients attending the Croi "MyAction" programme at the same facility [19]. We anticipated that blood pressure and lipid profiles might not change to the same extent in "Clann" as in "MyAction", because we sought to minimise any changes in medications during this programme to the greatest extent possible, whereas in the Croi "MyAction" programme the proportions of patients on antiplatelets, renin-angiotensin related antihypertensives and calcium channel blockers increased by 4.6, 4.9 and 5.6 %, respectively while the proportion on statins increased from 40.3 to 65.1 %. The improvements we have observed in the "Clann" programme have not arisen because of increased prescribing of medications which lower cardiovascular risk and are likely therefore to have been driven by the programme itself.

The relatively small changes in body weight and BMI, particularly in the context of the very abnormal level of adiposity these patients have, might be seen as an indicator that the overall impact on health of this programme is not strong enough. While pervading dogma suggests that any weight loss is good, recent guidelines state that bariatric patients need to lose 15 % or more of their body weight to have a meaningful improvement in their health [29]. However, favourable changes in body composition such as reduced fat mass with concurrent increases in lean mass are unlikely to be identified through changes in weight or BMI, so important and meaningful improvements may still have occurred [30]. Moreover, fitness is a far more relevant index of overall wellness and cardiovascular risk than fatness [31, 32]. The mean increase of 15 % in aerobic capacity (estimated MET max) of completers was a strong indicator that the programme is in fact effective and if sustained, might lead to a substantial reduction in mortality [33, 34]. The improvements in depression scores and components of the lipid profile are also clearly relevant and important.

This study has a number of limitations. Firstly, it is a retrospective, post-hoc cohort analysis without a pre-specified primary outcome or a control group, so while the findings provide a useful indication for effect size of this programme on various outcomes, we cannot determine its effectiveness. Out of necessity we have only measured changes in outcomes in patients who attended for follow-up assessments. These are likely to represent a more motivated subgroup than non-completers, which would lead to an overestimation of the potential benefits of the intervention compared to an analysis which included data from patients who did not complete the intervention. Completers were older, more likely to be male and have diabetes, were taking more medications and may have been less fit, but we don't believe these differences with non-completers account exclusively for the changes we have observed after participation in the programme. It is difficult to refine a target population for recruitment to the programme on the basis of results reported herein, but larger scale studies might help to identify patients who are likely to remain in the intervention and benefit from it. Notwithstanding the differences in the response to the intervention for some outcomes by sex and diabetes status, these weren't strong or consistent enough to suggest that the intervention should be limited to specified subgroups of patients.

There may have been a Hawthorne effect, whereby outcomes were different by virtue of the fact that they were being measured twice [35]. For example patients may have felt it polite to report that they were feeling less depressed or may have made more of an effort on their ISWT at the second attempt. However, objective improvements in the HRWSI, several metabolic variables and validated questionnaires are unlikely to be due entirely to measurement effect, we believe. As these patients were carefully selected for inclusion by a hospital-based regional bariatric multidisciplinary team, the results may not be generalisable to the broader population of adults with severe obesity. For some variables, there was a relatively high proportion of missing data. For example, the functional limitations score was measured before and after the programme in only 55 % of completers, while 73 % completed questionnaires and 76 % had HbA1c measured at both visits. This may have introduced bias to the results. A prospectively designed pragmatic randomised controlled trial, with blinded assessment, would address many of these limitations. The study has a number of strengths in addition to the high patient retention rate. The programme was delivered in a consistent way to all patients by experienced staff. Adherence to a predefined curriculum of teaching objectives during the health-promotion workshops is likely to have enhanced the integrity of the programme. Similarly, the assessments were comprehensive and were completed according to standardised protocols. Medication usage for hypertension, dyslipidaemia and diabetes was recorded carefully at the start and end of the programme.

Conclusions

In a well-defined cohort of predominantly white adult bariatric patients attending a regional obesity referral centre who were identified as highly motivated and suitable for a nurse-led structured lifestyle modification programme, the programme led to significant improvements in anthropometric, metabolic and cardiovascular risk variables over 10 weeks. Given that the programme appears feasible, safe and acceptable to patients, with a high retention rate and equivalent improvements to similar interventions in other cohorts of high risk individuals, future studies assessing the impact of structured lifestyle modification in bariatric patients could use it as a framework. The paucity of effective therapeutic strategies apart from bariatric surgery and meal replacement diets for these patients justify the formal assessment of this programme in a randomised controlled trial. Future studies might include more detailed patient phenotyping to determine changes not just in weight and BMI but in fat- and lean- mass and other indices of body composition. Additionally, future studies might examine proximal metabolic outcomes such as insulin sensitivity which are linked to cardiovascular risk. These studies will need to focus on more complete acquisition of socio-demographic and functional limitation questionnaire data.

Abbreviations

ACEI: Angiotensin converting enzyme inhibitor; ARB: Angiotensin receptor blocker; BMI: Body mass index; CLANN: Changing lifestyle with activity and nutrition; DBP: Diastolic blood pressure; EQ-VAS: European quality of life questionnaire, visual analogue scale; HDL: High density lipoprotein cholesterol; HRWSI: Heart rate walking speed index; ISWT: Incremental shuttle walk test; LDL: Low density lipoprotein cholesterol; METS: Metabolic Equivalents (of Thermogenesis); SBP: Systolic blood pressure.

Competing interests

The authors declare that they have no competing interests.

Authors' contributions

CC contributed to data analysis and interpretation and to writing the manuscript. IG led the design and implementation of the programme, assisted with data analysis and interpretation and writing the manuscript. KC helped to deliver the programme, acquire the data and write the manuscript. CK helped to deliver the programme, acquire the data and write the manuscript. CC helped to deliver the programme, acquire the data and write the manuscript. JW helped to deliver the programme, acquire the data and write the manuscript. POS supervised the analyses of laboratory samples and helped to write the manuscript. MH contributed to patient educational sessions during the programme and helped to write the manuscript. BMG helped with interpretation of the data and drafting the manuscript. KK helped with interpretation of the data and drafting the manuscript. HG helped with patient enrolment and follow-up and drafting the manuscript. TOB helped with patient enrolment, interpretation of the data and drafting the manuscript. JJ helped to design and implement the programme, assisted the analysis and interpretation of the data and helped to draft the manuscript. FF contributed to funding the programme, helped to design it, provided clinical oversight and governance for the programme, helped with data acquisition, analysis and interpretation and supervised the writing of the manuscript. All authors read and approved the final manuscript.

Acknowledgments

The authors would like to thank the patients attending the Bariatric Medicine Service at Galway University Hospital and the clinical staff who provide care to these patients. The programme was designed by and delivered at the Croi (West of Ireland Cardiac Foundation) Heart and Stroke Centre, Newcastle, Galway, Ireland. We are grateful to Paul Bassett for help with statistical analyses. This programme was funded by a project grant from the Health Service Executive, Ireland.

Author details

[1]Bariatric Medicine Service, Galway Diabetes Research Centre, HRB Clinical Research Facility, Galway University Hospital, Galway, Ireland. [2]Croi, the West of Ireland Cardiac Foundation, Heart and Stroke Centre, Moyola Lane, Newcastle, Galway, Ireland. [3]Department of Clinical Biochemistry, Galway University Hospitals, Galway, Ireland. [4]School of Psychology, National University of Ireland, Galway, Ireland. [5]Discipline of Health Promotion, National University of Ireland, Galway, Ireland. [6]National Institute of Preventive Cardiology, Galway, Ireland.

References

1. Stevens GA, Singh GM, Lu Y, Danaei G, Lin JK, Finucane MM, et al. National, regional, and global trends in adult overweight and obesity prevalences. Popul Health Metrics. 2012;10(1):22. doi:10.1186/1478-7954-10-22.
2. Harrington J, Perry I, Lutomski J, Morgan K, McGee H, Shelley E. SLAN 2007: Survey of Lifestyle, Attitudes and Nutrition in Ireland. In: Dietary Habits of the Irish Population. Ireland: Department of Health and Children Dublin: The Stationery Office; 2008.
3. Laaksonen MA, Knekt P, Rissanen H, Harkanen T, Virtala E, Marniemi J, et al. The relative importance of modifiable potential risk factors of type 2 diabetes: a meta-analysis of two cohorts. Eur J Epidemiol. 2010;25(2):115–24. doi:10.1007/s10654-009-9405-0.
4. Jiang Y, Chen Y, Mao Y. The contribution of excess weight to prevalent diabetes in Canadian adults. Public Health. 2008;122(3):271–6. doi:10.1016/j.puhe.2007.06.002.
5. Perry I. The cost of overweight and obesity on the Island of Ireland. University College Cork: Department of Epidemiology and Public Health; 2012.
6. Sturm R. Increases in morbid obesity in the USA: 2000–2005. Public Health. 2007;121(7):492–6. doi:10.1016/j.puhe.2007.01.006.
7. NICE. Clinical Guideline CG43- Obesity: guidance on the prevention, identification, assessment and management of overweight and obesity in adults and children. 2006.
8. Lean M. VLED and formula LED in the management of type 2 diabetes: defining the clinical need and research requirements. Obesity: Clinical; 2011.
9. Schauer PR, Bhatt DL, Kirwan JP, Wolski K, Brethauer SA, Navaneethan SD, et al. Bariatric surgery versus intensive medical therapy for diabetes - 3-Year outcomes. N Engl J Med. 2014;370(21):2002–13. doi:10.1056/NEJMoa1401329.
10. Heneghan HM, Meron-Eldar S, Brethauer SA, Schauer PR, Young JB. Effect of bariatric surgery on cardiovascular risk profile. Am J Cardiol. 2011;108(10):1499–507. doi:10.1016/j.amjcard.2011.06.076.
11. Office of Health Economics U. Shedding the Pounds: Obesity Management, NICE Guidance and Bariatric Surgery in England. 2010.
12. Li G, Zhang P, Wang J, Gregg EW, Yang W, Gong Q, et al. The long-term effect of lifestyle interventions to prevent diabetes in the China Da Qing Diabetes Prevention Study: a 20-year follow-up study. Lancet. 2008;371(9626):1783–9.
13. Lindstrom J, Ilanne-Parikka P, Peltonen M, Aunola S, Eriksson JG, Hemio K, et al. Sustained reduction in the incidence of type 2 diabetes by lifestyle intervention: follow-up of the Finnish Diabetes Prevention Study. Lancet. 2006;368(9548):1673–9.
14. Knowler WC, Barrett-Connor E, Fowler SE, Hamman RF, Lachin JM, Walker EA, et al. Reduction in the incidence of type 2 diabetes with lifestyle intervention or metformin. N Engl J Med. 2002;346(6):393–403.
15. Clark AM, Hartling L, Vandermeer B, McAlister FA. Meta-analysis: secondary prevention programs for patients with coronary artery disease. Ann Intern Med. 2005;143(9):659–72.
16. Wing RR, Bolin P, Brancati FL, Bray GA, Clark JM, Coday M, et al. Cardiovascular effects of intensive lifestyle intervention in type 2 diabetes. N Engl J Med. 2013;369(2):145–54. doi:10.1056/NEJMoa1212914.
17. Ryan DH, Johnson WD, Myers VH, Prather TL, McGlone MM, Rood J, et al. Nonsurgical weight loss for extreme obesity in primary care settings: results of the Louisiana Obese Subjects Study. Arch Intern Med. 2010;170(2):146–54. doi:10.1001/archinternmed.2009.508.
18. Goodpaster BH, Delany JP, Otto AD, Kuller L, Vockley J, South-Paul JE, et al. Effects of diet and physical activity interventions on weight loss and

cardiometabolic risk factors in severely obese adults: a randomized trial. JAMA. 2010;304(16):1795–802. doi:10.1001/jama.2010.1505.
19. Gibson I, Flaherty G, Cormican S, Jones J, Kerins C, Walsh AM, et al. Translating guidelines to practice: findings from a multidisciplinary preventive cardiology programme in the west of Ireland. Eur J Prev Cardiol. 2014;21(3):366–76. doi:10.1177/2047487313498831.
20. Wood DA, Kotseva K, Connolly S, Jennings C, Mead A, Jones J, et al. Nurse-coordinated multidisciplinary, family-based cardiovascular disease prevention programme (EUROACTION) for patients with coronary heart disease and asymptomatic individuals at high risk of cardiovascular disease: a paired, cluster-randomised controlled trial. Lancet. 2008;371(9629):1999–2012. doi:10.1016/S0140-6736(08)60868-5.
21. Perk J, De Backer G, Gohlke H, Graham I, Reiner Z, Verschuren M, et al. European Guidelines on cardiovascular disease prevention in clinical practice (version 2012). The Fifth Joint Task Force of the European Society of Cardiology and Other Societies on Cardiovascular Disease Prevention in Clinical Practice (constituted by representatives of nine societies and by invited experts). Eur Heart J. 2012;33(13):1635–701. doi:10.1093/eurheartj/ehs092.
22. Singh SJ, Morgan MD, Scott S, Walters D, Hardman AE. Development of a shuttle walking test of disability in patients with chronic airways obstruction. Thorax. 1992;47(12):1019–24.
23. Snaith RP. The hospital anxiety and depression scale. Health Qual Life Outcomes. 2003;1:29. doi:10.1186/1477-7525-1-29.
24. Dolan P. Modeling valuations for EuroQol health states. Med Care. 1997;35(11):1095–108.
25. Bentsen BG, Natvig B, Winnem M. Questions you didn't ask? COOP/WONCA Charts in clinical work and research. World Organization of Colleges, Academies and Academic Associations of General Practitioners/Family Physicists. Fam Pract. 1999;16(2):190–5.
26. Friedewald WT, Levy RI, Fredrickson DS. Estimation of the concentration of low-density lipoprotein cholesterol in plasma, without use of the preparative ultracentrifuge. Clin Chem. 1972;18(6):499–502.
27. Mancia G, Fagard R, Narkiewicz K, Redon J, Zanchetti A, Bohm M, et al. 2013 ESH/ESC guidelines for the management of arterial hypertension: the Task Force for the Management of Arterial Hypertension of the European Society of Hypertension (ESH) and of the European Society of Cardiology (ESC). Eur Heart J. 2013;34(28):2159–219. doi:10.1093/eurheartj/eht151.
28. Haskell WL, Lee IM, Pate RR, Powell KE, Blair SN, Franklin BA, et al. Physical activity and public health: updated recommendation for adults from the American College of Sports Medicine and the American Heart Association. Circulation. 2007;116(9):1081–93. doi:10.1161/CIRCULATIONAHA.107.185649.
29. SIGN. Scottish Intercollegiate Guidelines Network- Guideline 115: Management of obesity. 2010.
30. Cruz P, Johnson BD, Karpinski SC, Limoges KA, Warren BA, Olsen KD, et al. Validity of Weight loss to estimate improvement in body composition in individuals attending a wellness center. Obesity (Silver Spring). 2011;19(11):2274–9. doi:10.1038/oby.2011.102.
31. McAuley PA, Artero EG, Sui X, Lavie CJ, Almeida MJ, Blair SN. Fitness, fatness, and survival in adults with prediabetes. Diabetes Care. 2014;37(2):529–36. doi:10.2337/dc13-1347.
32. Wei M, Kampert JB, Barlow CE, Nichaman MZ, Gibbons LW, Paffenbarger Jr RS, et al. Relationship between low cardiorespiratory fitness and mortality in normal-weight, overweight, and obese men. JAMA. 1999;282(16):1547–53.
33. Gulati M, Pandey DK, Arnsdorf MF, Lauderdale DS, Thisted RA, Wicklund RH, et al. Exercise capacity and the risk of death in women: the St James Women Take Heart Project. Circulation. 2003;108(13):1554–9. doi:10.1161/01.CIR.0000091080.57509.E9.
34. Myers J, Prakash M, Froelicher V, Do D, Partington S, Atwood JE. Exercise capacity and mortality among men referred for exercise testing. N Engl J Med. 2002;346(11):793–801. doi:10.1056/NEJMoa011858.
35. Gale EA. The Hawthorne studies-a fable for our times? QJM. 2004;97(7):439–49.

27

A rare case of juvenile hypertension: coexistence of type 2 multiple endocrine neoplasia-related bilateral pheochromocytoma and reninoma in a young patient with ACE gene polymorphism

Rosa Maria Paragliola[1], Ettore Capoluongo[2], Francesco Torino[3], Angelo Minucci[2], Giulia Canu[2], Alessandro Prete[1], Alfredo Pontecorvi[1] and Salvatore Maria Corsello[1*]

Abstract

Background: Pheochromocytoma and reninoma represent two rare diseases causing hypertension. We here reported a rare case of association between type 2 multiple endocrine neoplasia related bilateral pheochromocytoma and reninoma. Moreover, polymorphism of ACE gene, which is known to be related to an increase of cardiovascular risk, has been found in the same patient.

Case presentation: A 24 year old Caucasian man came to our attention for severe hypertension, resistant to anti-hypertensive polytherapy. At the age of twenty he had undergone total thyroidectomy with lymphadenectomy for medullary carcinoma. Genetic testing showed a *RET* mutation of codon 918 (exon 16) not documented in other family members. During the follow-up, a progressive increase of urinary metanephrines and catecholamines was recorded. Our evaluation confirmed the presence of severe hypertension (220/140 mmHg) and a severe increase of urinary catecholamines and metanephrines. Due to the presence of hypokalemia, other causes of hypertension were researched leading to the discovery of hyperreninemia (236 μUI/ml) with mild hyperaldosteronism, and a mild increase of the renal artery resistance at ultrasound. An abdominal MRI showed multiple adrenal masses and a right kidney nodular lesion of about 2 cm.
The patient underwent bilateral adrenalectomy and right nephrectomy, and histology confirmed the presence of bilateral pheochromocytoma and right reninoma. The post-surgery laboratory evaluation showed a rapid reduction of the urinary metanephrines while plasma renin level remained low in spite of the bilateral adrenalectomy without any mineralocorticoid supplementation. To further investigate these unusual feature, we performed genetic testing for the ACE gene, which revealed the presence of ACE I/D polymorphism.

Conclusion: This unique report describes the association between two rare causes of hypertension in the same patient. Furthermore, the absence of requirement of mineralocorticoid supplementation in spite of bilateral adrenalectomy, represent an uncommon and interest finding.

Keywords: Pheochromocytoma, Reninoma, MEN2B, ACE polymorphism, Hypertension

* Correspondence: corsello.sm@mclink.it
[1]Endocrinology Unit, Università Cattolica del Sacro Cuore, Largo Agostino Gemelli 8, 00168 Rome, Italy
Full list of author information is available at the end of the article

Background

Pheochromocytoma (PHEO) and reninoma both represent two rare causes of juvenile hypertension. PHEO is a neural crest-derived tumor, which produces and secretes catecholamines and which is related to the classical clinical symptoms associated with the inappropriate catecholamines secretion, such as are paroxysmal hypertension, tachycardia, palpitations, headaches and sweating [1]. Even if PHEO is a rare disease (less than 0.2% of patients with hypertension [2]) the related cardiovascular symptoms have a significant morbidity and even mortality. PHEO can occur sporadically or as hereditary form related to genetic background. In particular, type 2 multiple endocrine neoplasia (MEN2) is an autosomal dominant inherited endocrine malignancy syndrome, due to germline mutations in the REarranged during Transfection (*RET*) proto-oncogene, which encodes a tyrosine kinase receptor involved in cell growth, differentiation and survival. MEN syndrome includes the following three subtypes: MEN2A (association between medullary thyroid carcinoma [MTC], PHEO and primary hyperparathyroidism); familial medullary thyroid cancer and MEN2B. The latter represents a less common but more aggressive form and it is characterized by the association between MTC and PHEO with other particular features such as mucosal neuromas, intestinal ganglioneuromas, and marfanoid habitus with skeletal deformations and joint laxity [3].

Reninoma is a rare juxtaglomerular cell tumor causing renin-mediated hypertension. This condition is usually diagnosed in adolescents and young adults and is typically characterized by sustained hypertension well responding to antihypertensive treatment targeting the renin-angiotensin-aldosterone (RAA) system [4].

We here described a unique case of association between bilateral MEN2B related PHEO in whom also a reninoma causing secondary hyperaldosteronism was diagnosed.

Case presentation

Case report

In March 2010 a 24 year old Caucasian man with marphanoid habitus (height: 175 cm; weight: 65 Kg) was referred to us for severe hypertension that was resistant to beta blockers, angiotensin converting enzyme (ACE) inhibitors, and diuretics. Four years earlier he had undergone total thyroidectomy with lymphadenectomy due to MTC (pT4N+; stage III UICC 2009). The preoperative diagnostic workup had excluded PHEO, and his family history was negative for MEN2B-related tumors. Genetic testing for germline mutations in *RET* proto-oncogene was not done. However, after his thyroid surgery a progressive increase of the urinary metanephrines and catecholamines was noted, with absence of abnormal findings at the magnetic resonance imaging (MRI) and metaiodobenzylguanidine (MIBG) scan.

At our clinical examination, a severe systo-diastolic hypertension (220/140 mmHg) was observed, and mucosal neuromas of the tongue were found. Laboratory findings included severe hypokaliemia (potassium 2.5 mEq/L), hyperreninemia and mild hyperaldosteronism. Urinary catecholamines were also increased, as well as urinary metanephrines and vanil-mandelic acid. Inappropriate cortisol secretion was ruled out on the basis of the presence of normal serum and urinary free cortisol and detectable adrenocorticotropic hormone (ACTH) levels (Table 1). An ultrasound of the kidneys revealed a mass of approximately 2 cm at the right kidney with an increased artery resistance (0.88; normal value < 0.7). Furthermore, an enlargement of both adrenal glands was detected.

The genetic test for *RET* germline mutations showed the substitution of methionine for threonine in exon 16 at codon 918 (p.M918T) which was not present in other family members (father, mother and sister). A recurrence of MTC was excluded through assessment of serum markers, showing undetectable levels of serum calcitonin and normal carcinoembryonic antigen (CEA) levels, and an ultrasound of the neck which was negative. Replacement therapy with levothyroxine (150 mcg/day) appeared to be adequate and post-surgical hypoparathyroidism was well controlled with calcitriol (0.5 mcg/day).

An abdominal MRI confirmed the presence of adrenal bilateral hyperplasia with multiple adrenal masses (16 and 18 mm in the right gland, and 10 and 15 mm in the left gland), and the right kidney nodular lesion of 20 x 20 mm, hyperintensive in T2-weighted sequences. MIBG scintigraphy showed bilateral adrenal uptake, strongly suggestive for bilateral PHEO. Thus, the patient started anti-hypertensive therapy with phenoxybenzamine 20 mg four-times daily, nifedipine slow release 30 mg twice-daily, and atenolol 50 mg once-daily. Blood pressure control eventually improved. An ecocardiography showed dilated cardiomyopathy and moderate systolic dysfunction (ejection fraction 46 %). One month later the patient underwent bilateral adrenalectomy and right nephrectomy. No hypertensive crisis occurred during the surgery. The tumors were soft brown-red well-circumscribed masses without cystic degeneration. Histology of the adrenal glands confirmed the presence of bilateral and multifocal adrenal PHEO. No vascular or capsular invasion was noted; mitotic figures were less than 3/10 high power field and no atypical mitoses were present. The Ki 67 index was 2 % and immunoistrochemistry was positive for chromogranin A and synaptophysin. The histology of the right kidney mass revealed a capsulated neoplasm with nests and diffused sheets of tumor cells interrupted by abundant vascularity in the form of capillary channels and sinusoids, which were suggestive for reninoma.

Table 1 Laboratory evaluation performed preoperatively, post-operatively and after 3 years of follow-up

	Preoperative value	Postoperative value	Value after 3 years of follow-up	Normal range
Reninemia (clinostatism)	236 μUI/ml	10 μUI/ml	25 μUI/ml	2.8–40 μUI/ml
Aldosterone (clinostatism)	536 pmol/L	267 pmol/L	186 pmol/L	55–415 pmol/L
Epinephrine	145 nmol/d	65 nmol/d	43 nmol/d	11–120 nmol/d
Norepinephrine	708 nmol/d	265 nmol/d	218 nmol/d	71–507 nmol/d
Metanephrine	15,681 nmol/d	310 nmol/d	225 nmol/d	253–1,720 nmol/d
Normetanephrine	6,932 nmol/d	479 nmol/d	615 nmol/d	491–2,430 nmol/d
Vanil-mandelic acid	15 mg/d	2 mg/d	3.6 mg/d	<7 mg/d
ACTH	7 pmol/L	16 pmol/L	21 pmol/L	2.2–12.2 pmol/L
Serum cortisol	370 nmol/L	<14 nmol/L	<14 nmol/L	221–607 nmol/L
Urinary free cortisol	185 nmol/d	Not performed	Not performed	102–375 nmol/d

ACTH: adrenocorticotropic hormone; d: 24 h

After surgery, glucocorticoid replacement therapy with hydrocortisone was immediately started together with adequate hydration. Anti-hypertensive therapy was withdrawn and blood pressure was low to normal. Laboratory evaluation showed a sudden reduction of urinary metanephrines and catecholamines. Serum ACTH levels increased accordingly to post-surgical hypoadrenalism while serum cortisol was undetectable, but renin levels were normal-low (10 μUI/ml), in the absence of mineralocorticoid supplementation. Currently, 3 years after surgery, the patient is tumor-free. During this follow-up, the patient has been treated with replacement therapy comprised of hydrocortisone 30 mg, levothyroxine 150 mcg, and calcitriol 0.5 mcg.

Because of the persistence of normal renin values and serum electrolytes (Table 1) and normal blood pressure values mineralocorticoid substitutive therapy was not proposed. Surprisingly, aldosterone serum levels were detectable in spite of bilateral adrenalectomy (Table 1). MRI evaluation performed during follow-up failed to reveal adrenal remnants which could justify these clinical and biochemical findings. Moreover, undetectable serum cortisol performed about 18 h after the last hydrocortisone administration, was extremely suggestive for the absence of adrenal remnants or for the presence of ectopic functioning adrenal tissue. To further investigate this unusual feature, we hypothesized that it could be due to a dysregulation of RAA axis. After obtaining the informed consent, we searched for ACE polymorphisms. Genetic test revealed ACE I/D polymorphism.

Gene analysis

After obtaining informed consent, genomic DNA was isolated from peripheral blood by a manual method (Roche Diagnostics, Basel, Switzerland, http://www.roche.com/index.htm), while spectral analysis was performed spectrophotometrically in order to determine DNA concentration and purity (NanoPhotometer™, Implen, München Germany, http://www.implen.de). Mutation analysis of the *RET* gene was performed by sequencing of coding region and exon-intron boundaries of the exons 2, 5, 8, 10, 11, 13–16. Primers used and the respective annealing temperatures are reported in Table 2. PCR products were sequenced using the Big Dye Terminator v1.1 Cycle Sequencing kit (Applied Biosystems, Foster City, CA, USA, http://www.appliedbiosystems.com/absite/us/en/home.html) in an automated sequencer ABI Prism 3500 Genetic Analyzer (Applied Biosystems).

Finally, using the SeqScape® Software v2.5, sequences were aligned to the reference sequence NG_007489.1.

For detecting *ACE I/D* polymorphism we followed the molecular method reported in literature [5].

Discussion

We describe the unusual association between two very rare conditions causing juvenile hypertension, bilateral PHEO and reninoma, in a patient affected by MEN2B and ACE-polymorphism. The coexistence of PHEO and hyperreninemia secondary to renal artery stenosis has been previously reported [6], while only a paper, which described a 18 years follow-up in a family affected by MEN 2 B, found the association between adrenal medullary hyperplasia and renin-secreting juxtaglomerular tumor [7]. Furthermore, we discovered in this patient the presence of ACE gene I/D polymorphism which is known to be associated with cardiovascular risk.

The estimated incidence of cathecolamine secreting tumors is 2–8 per million, with the peak age of occurrence in the third to fifth decade of life [8]. Recent population based studies suggest that up to 32 % of patients have a germline mutation in one of the known common susceptibility genes [9]. In particular, mutations of *VHL*, *NF1* and *RET* cause well characterized cancer susceptibility syndrome

Table 2 Primers used for *RET* amplification and sequencing

Oligo Name	Sequence (5′ → 3′)	Annealing Temperature (Ta) [°C]
RET-2 F	GCT TCC CCT GTT TCC TTT TC	
RET-2R	AGT GTC AGC GGC TGT GAT AA	
RET-5 F	CGT GCA GCA TTC TAA GGT CTC	
RET-5R	CAT GTC TGT AGG GTG CTG CT	
RET-8 F	TGC TCC TGG CAC TGT CTT	
RET-8R	TGG GGA CCA ATC ACT GTA CTC	
RET-10 F	GGA CAC TGC CCT GGA AAT A	
RET-10R	ACT CGC CTC CCA GCA ATT T	
RET-11 F	ATA CGC AGC CTG TAC CCA CT	
RET-11R	AAA TGG GGG CAG AAC ACA	58
RET-13 F	CCA TCC TGA CCT GGT ATG GT	
RET-13R	AAA CAG GGC AGG AGC AGT AG	
RET-14 F	GTC CAC CCC CTT ACT CAT TG	
RET-14R	GTG GTG AGC CAT AGC ATG G	
RET-15 F	CCC CCG GCC CAG GTC TC	
RET-15R	GCT CCA CTA ATC TTC GGT ATC TTT	
RET-16 F	TCT CCT TTA CCC CTC CTT CC	
RET-16R	CAG TGA GGG GGT CAT TGC	

(von Hippel Lindau, Neurofibromatosis Type 1 and MEN2, respectively).

These patients usually have other clinical characteristics of the associated syndrome at time of presentation.

Moreover, mutations of mitochondrial succinate dehydrogenase (SDH) complex subunits genes (SDHA, SDHB, SDHC, and SDHD) and one complex cofactor (SDHAF2) have been reported in head and neck and abdominal paragangliomas. Recently, other genes (TME M127, MAX, HIF2A, EGLN1, KIF1B, H-RAS) have been added to the group of susceptibility genes involved in the development of paragangliomas/PHEO [10].

In our case, the association between MTC and PHEO, which was diagnosed about 4 years after the diagnosis of MTC, in addition to specific clinical features, was strongly suggestive for MEN2B. Germline mutations in *RET* codon 918 (M918T) were found to be related to the classic MEN2B phenotype in 95 % of cases [11] but patients often lack a family history of MTC and harbor a *de novo* mutation [12]. MEN 2B is the most severe form of MEN 2: in normal conditions, activation of the RET receptor involves interaction with different ligands which triggers RET dimerization and determinates tyrosine kinase activation. The M918T mutation can both induce a conformational change in the kinase catalytic core leading to the activation of RET without dimerization enhancing the intrinsic kinase activity and alter the substrate specificity of RET [13].

Genetic test performed in our patient showed the presence of M918T mutation (exon 16) confirming the diagnosis of MEN 2B, while screening performed in other family members was negative. This mutation of *RET* protoncogene was described as strongly associated with the onset of PHEO [14].

In this patient both the presence of a syndrome predisposing to catecholamine-secreting tumors and the onset of a severe juvenile hypertension, led to a work-up for PHEO. Biochemical evaluation for the diagnosis of cathecolamine secreting tumors is based on the measurements of fractionated metanephrines and cathecolamines in urine or plasma, the latter not available in our Institution. Urinary fractionated metanephrines and cathecolamines show high sensitivity (97 and 86 % respectively) and good specificity (69 and 88 % respectively) in the diagnosis of cathecolamine secreting tumors, while vanil-mandelic acid provides superior specificity (95 %) but lower sensitivity (64 %) [15].

About tumor localization, either computed tomography (CT) or MRI are recommended and can identify more than 95 % of tumors. However, the higher specificity in detecting PHEO is guaranteed by nuclear medicine techniques, which provides functional imaging. ^{123}I-MIBG is a guanethidine analogue resembling norepinephrine. For this reason, MIBG scintigraphy is very useful and extremely specific for the diagnostic localization of PHEO [16]. In our patient a bilateral tumor, which can occur in about one third of MEN2 related PHEO, was found. However, the patient was also evaluated for all other possible causes of secondary hypertension, thus discovering renin-dependent hyperaldosteronism. Eventually a reninoma, suspected on the basis of biochemical evaluation and radiological findings, was confirmed by post-operative histology. Furthermore, a very particular finding in this case is the occurrence of ACE gene polymorphism detected post-operatively, which may represent an additional cause of cardiovascular risk.

ACE induces the catalytic conversion of angiotensin I to angiotensin II which represents a crucial step in the regulation of the RAA axis in turn involved in the regulation of blood pressure and serum electrolytes. However, ACE can cleave other many substrates, including bradykinin and substance P [17], and is probably responsible of other effects. ACE is widely distributed throughout the body, including central nervous system, surface of vascular endothelium and epithelium of the renal proximal tubule [17, 18]. This raises the question about a possible local effect of ACE in these sites. In fact, the multiple activities of ACE are demonstrated by the phenotype exhibited by ACE knock-out mice, which have profound hypotension, hypoplastic renal medulla, but also some other abnormalities (such as infertility) which are not present in knock-out mice for other components of RAA system [19].

ACE polymorphism, first described in 1990, seems to be one of the major factors influencing ACE levels. In their report, Rigat et al. [20] reported a 287 base pair Alu repeat in 16th intron of *ACE* (17q23), which was termed I (insert) allele. Conversely, the lack of the repeat is D (deletion) allele. It has been demonstrated that subjects with D/D genotype have the highest serum ACE levels (50 % more relative to I/I), heterozygous individuals (genotype I/D) have intermediate ACE levels (25 % more relative to I/I) while homozygous I/I have the lowest ACE levels [21]. The D/D genotype was found more frequently in patients with myocardial infarction than in control subjects [22], but other studies showed no correlation with coronary disease or stroke [23]. The I/D genotype, which has been detected in our patient, is described in association with several condition as diabetic peripheral neuropathy [24], risk of recurrent miscarriage [25] as well as hypertension and cardiovascular disease.

A very important point, in our opinion, is the association between *ACE* polymorphism, MEN2B-related PHEO and reninoma, which can all contribute, through different pathways, to severe juvenile hypertension.

To our knowledge, there are not data available in the Literature to affirm the possibility of a common genetic background which could justify this association. In particular, the possibility that reninoma could represent another possible disorder in MEN 2 B syndrome can only be supposed in consideration of the reported cases. However, these findings do not justify the screening of hyperaldosteronism in all patients affected by MEN 2 B, unless severe concomitant hypokaliemia is present, as in our case.

Moreover, this patient represents a unique model of ACE I/D polymorphism in post-surgical hypoadrenalism, condition in which aldosterone secreting tissue is "virtually" absent. The absence of adrenal remnants or ectopic functioning adrenal tissue is supported by undetectable serum cortisol values after adequate pharmacological wash-out. Furthermore, postoperative radiological imaging excluded the presence of adrenal remnants. As well known, in patients who have undergone bilateral adrenalectomy, an increase of ACTH and renin levels is expected, and subjects need both glucocorticoid and mineralocorticoid replacement. In our patient, in spite of the predictable increase of ACTH values, renin levels were unexpectedly normal, while serum aldosterone remained detectable. The low-normal renin levels that were seen immediately after the removal of the reninoma may have been due to the persistent suppression of the normal renin secretion by the reninoma, overriding the stimulation due to the reduction of aldosterone. Surprisingly, the renin levels remained low-normal long after the removal of both adrenal glands and the reninoma and the patient did not need mineralocorticoid replacement therapy and did not experience hypotension or hyperkaliemia, as expected in a condition of mineralocorticoid defect. We can try to explain this particular phenomenon by considering a possible extra-adrenal aldosterone production. In fact, the existence of extra-adrenal sites of aldosterone synthesis, such as heart or brain, has been clearly demonstrated [26] and an endogenous corticosteroid biosynthesis after bilateral adrenalectomy has been described [27], even if the contribution of these sources to the circulating hormone levels is not completely known. In fact, while mRNA levels of aldosterone synthase (CYP11B2) are about 100 to 10,000 times lower in the normal human heart than in the human adrenal gland [28], the aldosterone synthase expression has been found to be elevated in patient with heart failure. It is well known that both inappropriate cathecolamine [29] and aldosterone [28] secretion *per se* cause cardiac remodeling, similarly to what has been found in our patient who developed dilated cardiomyopathy and impaired systolic function. While we cannot exclude that the heart failure may have resulted in an increase in aldosterone synthase expression, on the other hand it is difficult to determine whether the presence of the ACE I/D polymorphism may have played a contributing role in this setting, except that it likely worsened the degree of hypertension and reduced the response to ACE-inhibitors which had been used for several years to treat the patient.

A possible hypothesis involving the role of ACE I/D polymorphism in explaining this particular biochemical finding, is an increase of ACE activity in extra-adrenal aldosterone biosynthesis. In fact, tissue expressing a "local angiotensin-aldosterone axis", such as kidneys, heart and blood vessels, can generate angiotensin II independently from systemic renin-angiotensin-aldosterone axis [30].

We cannot exclude that ACE I/D polymorphism can enhance the synthesis of angiotensin II in "local angiotensin-aldosterone axis".

Conclusion

In conclusion, we describe a unique association of 3 independent causes of hypertension. The most interesting points (other than the association between two rare causes of hypertension such as reninoma and bilateral MEN2B-related PHEO) are the persistence of detectable aldosterone levels in spite of bilateral adrenalectomy and the detection of ACE I/D polymorphism. We cannot confirm whether these two findings are related or randomly associated. Although the data seem to suggest the potential for an additional source of ectopic adrenal aldosterone production that could justify the presence of normal renin values and detectable aldosterone levels, the exact role of the concomitant ACE I/D polymorphism and its impact on the clinical features of this case are not known.

Abbreviations
PHEO: Pheochromocytoma; MEN2: type 2 multiple endocrine neoplasia; RET: REarranged during Transfection; MTC: Medullary thyroid carcinoma; RAA: Renin-angiotensin-aldosterone; ACE: Angiotensin converting enzyme; MRI: Magnetic resonance imaging; MIBG: Metaiodobenzylguanidine; CEA: Carcinoembryonic antigen; ACTH: Adrenocorticotropic hormone.

Competing interest
The authors declare that they have no competing interests

Authors' contributions
RMP, FT, SMC, AP and AP participated in the design of the study and drafted the manuscript. EC, AM and GC carried out the molecular genetic studied and helped to draft the manuscript. All authors read and approved the final manuscript.

Acknowledgements
None.

Funding
Authors declare that no funding has been received for the preparation of this manuscript.

Author details
[1]Endocrinology Unit, Università Cattolica del Sacro Cuore, Largo Agostino Gemelli 8, 00168 Rome, Italy. [2]Biochemistry and Clinical Biochemistry Unit, Università Cattolica del Sacro Cuore, Rome, Italy. [3]Department of Systems Medicine, Università degli Studi Tor Vergata, Rome, Italy.

References
1. Plouin PF, Amar L, Lepoutre C. Phaeochromocytomas and functional paragangliomas: clinical management. Best Pract Res Clin Endocrinol Metab. 2010;24:933–41.
2. Pacak K, Linehan WM, Eisenhofer G, Walther MM, Goldstein DS. Recent advances in genetics, diagnosis, localization, and treatment of pheochromocytoma. Ann Intern Med. 2001;134:315–29.
3. Torino F, Paragliola RM, Barnabei A, Corsello SM. Medullary thyroid cancer: a promising model for targeted therapy. Curr Mol Med. 2010;10:608–25.
4. Trnka P, Orellana L, Walsh M, Pool L, Borzi P. Reninoma: an uncommon cause of renin-mediated hypertension. Front Pediatr. 2014;2:89.
5. Minucci A, Canu G, Concolino P, Guarino D, Boccia S, Ficarra S, et al. DNA from buccal swab is suitable for rapid genotyping of angiotensin-converting enzyme insertion/deletion (I/D) polymorphism. Clin Chim Acta. 2014;431:125–30.
6. Kota SK, Kota SK, Meher LK, Tripathy PR, Sruti J, Modi KD. Pheochromocytoma with renal artery stenosis: a case-based review of literature. J Cardiovasc Dis Res. 2012;3:36–9.
7. Sizemore GW, Carney JA, Gharib H, Capen CC. Multiple endocrine neoplasia type 2B: eighteen-year follow-up of a four-generation family. Henry Ford Hosp Med J. 1992;40:236–44.
8. DeLellis RA, Lloyd RV, Heitz PU, Eng C. World health organization classification of tumours. Pathology and genetics of tumours of endocrine organs. Lyon, France: IARC Press; 2004.
9. Mannelli M, Castellano M, Schiavi F, Filetti S, Giacchè M, Mori L, et al. Clinically guided genetic screening in a large cohort of italian patients with pheochromocytomas and/or functional or nonfunctional paragangliomas. J Clin Endocrinolol Metab. 2009;94:1541–7.
10. Martins R, Bugalho MJ. Paragangliomas/pheochromocytomas: clinically oriented genetic testing. Int J Endocrinol. 2014;2014:794187.
11. Machens A, Ukkat J, Brauckhoff M, Gimm O, Dralle H. Advances in the management of hereditary medullary thyroid cancer. J Intern Med. 2005;257:50–9.
12. Raue F, Frank-Raue K. Genotype-phenotype relationship in multiple endocrine neoplasia type 2. Implications for clinical management. Hormones. 2009;8:23–8.
13. Gujral TS, Singh VK, Jia Z, Mulligan LM. Molecular mechanisms of RET receptor-mediated oncogenesis in multiple endocrine neoplasia 2B. Cancer Res. 2006;66:10741–9.
14. Eng C, Clayton D, Schuffenecker I, Lenoir G, Cote G, Gagel RF. The relationship between specific RET proto-oncogene mutations and disease phenotype in multiple endocrine neoplasia type 2. International RET mutation consortium analysis. JAMA. 1996;276:1575–9.
15. Zelinka T, Eisenhofer G, Pacak K. Pheochromocytoma as a catecholamine producing tumor: implications for clinical practice. Stress. 2007;10:195–203.
16. Vaidyanathan G. Meta-iodobenzylguanidine and analogues: chemistry and biology. Q J Nucl Med Mol Imaging. 2008;52:351–68.
17. Erdos EG, Skidgel RA. The angiotensin I-converting enzyme. Lab Invest. 1987;56:345–8.
18. Alhenc-Gelas F, Baussant T, Hubert C, Soubrier F, Corvol P. The angiotensin converting enzyme in the kidney. J Hypertens Suppl. 1989; 7:S9–S13 (discussion S14).
19. Esther Jr CR, Howard TE, Marino EM, Goddard JM, Capecchi MR, Bernstein KE. Mice lacking angiotensin-converting enzyme have low blood pressure, renal pathology, and reduced male fertility. Lab Invest. 1996;74:953–65.
20. Rigat B, Hubert C, Alhenc-Gelas F, Cambien F, Corvol P, Soubrier F. An insertion/deletion polymorphism in the angiotensin I-converting enzyme gene accounting for half the variance of serum enzyme levels. J Clin Invest. 1990;86:1343–6.
21. Danser AH, Deinum J, Osterop AP, Admiraal PJ, Schalekamp MA. Angiotensin I to angiotensin II conversion in the human forearm and leg. Effect of the angiotensin converting enzyme gene insertion/deletion polymorphism. J Hypertens. 1999;17:1867–72.
22. Cambien F, Poirier O, Lecerf L, Evans A, Cambou JP, Arveiler D, et al. Deletion polymorphism in the gene for angiotensin-converting enzyme is a potent risk factor for myocardial infarction. Nature. 1992;359:641–4.
23. Agerholm-Larsen B, Nordestgaard BG, Tybjaerg-Hansen A. ACE gene polymorphism in cardiovascular disease: meta-analyses of small and large studies in whites. Arterioscler Thromb Vasc Biol. 2000;20:484–92.
24. Inanir A, Basol N, Karakus N, Yigit S. The importance of association between angiotensin-converting enzyme (ACE) I/D polymorphism and diabetic peripheral neuropathy. Gene. 2013;530:253–6.
25. Wang Z, Wang P, Wang X, He X, Wang Z, Xu D, et al. Significant association between angiotensin-converting enzyme gene insertion/deletion polymorphism and risk of recurrent miscarriage: A systematic review and meta-analysis. Metabolism. 2013;62:1227–38.
26. MacKenzie SM, Connell JM, Davies E. Non-adrenal synthesis of aldosterone: a reality check. Mol Cell Endocrinol. 2012;350:163–7.
27. Freel EM, Bernhardt R, Ingram M, Wallace AM, Fraser R, Davies E, et al. Endogenous corticosteroid biosynthesis in subjects after bilateral adrenalectomy. Clin Endocrinol (Oxf). 2007;66:659–65.
28. Essick EE, Sam F. Cardiac hypertrophy and fibrosis in the metabolic syndrome: a role for aldosterone and the mineralocorticoid receptor. Int J Hypertens. 2011;346985.
29. Prejbisz A, Lenders JW, Eisenhofer G, Januszewicz A. Cardiovascular manifestations of phaeochromocytoma. J Hypertens. 2011;29:2049–60.
30. MacKenzie SM, Fraser R, Connell JM, Davies E. Local renin-angiotensin systems and their interactions with extra-adrenal corticosteroid production. J Renin Angiotensin Aldosterone Syst. 2002;3:214–21.

Screening for vitamin D deficiency in a tropical area: results of a sun exposure questionnaire

Fernanda Barros Bittar, Charlles H. M. Castro* and Vera Lúcia Szejnfeld

Abstract

Background: Vitamin D deficiency is pandemic while resources available to measure 25-hydroxyvitamin D (25OHD) are limited. The present study aimed to verify whether sun exposure measured by a structured questionnaire could predict serum 25OHD concentrations in healthy Caucasian individuals living in a tropical area.

Methods: A cross-sectional study was carried out in subjects living in the greater São Paulo area, Brazil. Two groups of 50 young (20 to 40 years old) and 50 older (60 to 80 years old) subjects ($N = 200$) answered a structured questionnaire on sun exposure and had blood samples drawn for serum 25OHD concentration measurement during both summer and winter. Anthropometric data were also recorded. Correlation between the questionnaire variables (duration of sun exposure, amount of exposed skin, total sun exposure score - TSES and other data) and serum 25OHD concentration was evaluated.

Results: Mean serum 25OHD concentration was 17.60 ± 7.3 ng/mL with no difference between age groups ($p = 0.293$). TSES weakly correlated with serum 25OHD levels ($r = 0.264$; $p < 0.001$). Separate analyzes by age groups demonstrated that TSES correlated significantly with serum 25OHD concentration only in the older subjects during summer ($r = 0.322$; $p = 0.023$). Using linear regression analyses, TSES and body mass index (BMI) were significantly associated with serum 25OHD levels. On the other hand, Receiver operating characteristic (ROC) analysis for TSES showed no significance as a screening tool for vitamin D deficiency ($p = 0.172$).

Conclusion: Sun exposure questionnaire associated with BMI correlates with serum 25OHD concentration with very low accuracy. The use of the questionnaire does not discriminate between vitamin D sufficient and deficient individuals.

Keywords: Questionnaire, Sun exposure, Vitamin D, Young, And elderly, Summer, Winter

Background

Vitamin D is important for calcium and phosphorus homeostasis, with a fundamental participation in bone mineralization and remodeling [1]. It has been demonstrated that vitamin D plays an important role in bone development in children, maintenance of bone in adults and prevention of osteoporosis in the elderly [2, 3]. In humans the main source for vitamin D comes from the conversion of 7-dehydrocholesterol precursors in the skin through interaction with ultraviolet B (UVB) radiation. 7-dehydrocholesterol UVB-induced conversion to cholecalciferol is dependent on latitude, time of the day, season, duration of exposure and amount of exposed skin, as well as age and cutaneous pigmentation [4]. Vitamin D synthesis in the skin under UVB radiation is significantly limited at latitudes > 33°, including North America and Europe. In those locations the sun is only an effective source of vitamin D during the summertime [5]. Dietary sources of vitamin D are limited and predominantly comprise fatty fish and nuts [6].

Vitamin D deficiency is currently one of the most common and neglected medical conditions, affecting a large part of the world population [1, 7]. The increasing concern about the high prevalence of vitamin D deficiency and its skeletal consequences especially among the elderly has led to a large increase in the demand for

* Correspondence: cheldan@uol.com.br
Rheumatology Division, Universidade Federal de São Paulo - Escola Paulista de Medicina (UNIFESP-EPM), Rua Botucatu, 740 – 3° andar – Vila Clementino, CEP, São Paulo, SP 04023-900, Brazil

serum 25OHD measurements, currently the best marker of vitamin D status [8]. Simple and low-cost methods that allow for direct measurement of 25OHD in patients who are at risk of deficiency are needed [9, 10]. The economical impact of such strategies would be rather strong among developing countries with no solid initiatives for public health care [11].

We have recently reported a very high prevalence of vitamin D deficiency among Brazilian men and women [12]. Vitamin D deficiency is pandemic and can be observed even in a sunny country like Brazil where excessive sunlight exposure related outcomes such as non-melanoma skin cancer are highly prevalent [13, 14].

The variables that may affect 25OHD status are relatively well defined [4, 7]. On the other hand, only a few studies have designed indirect tools to predict serum 25OHD concentrations and identify individuals who may be at risk of vitamin D deficiency [15]. The use of specific tools to rationally indicate 25OHD testing would be welcome in our current scenario where extensive screening for vitamin D deficiency is not recommended [16]. In the present study we hypothesize that sun exposure assessment by a structured questionnaire [17] may correlate with serum 25OHD measurement and thus could be helpful as an indicator for 25OHD testing in adults with suspected vitamin D deficiency.

Methods

Participants

A total of 200 healthy Caucasian men and women living in the greater São Paulo area, Brazil, were invited to participate. Participants were divided into 4 groups: 50 young participants aged 20 to 40 years old during summer, 50 young participants during winter, 50 older participants aged 60 to 80 years old during summer and 50 older participants during winter. All participants were Caucasian with Fitzpatrick skin phototype I to III [18]. Exclusion criteria were: Non-Caucasian individuals and Fitzpatrick skin phototype IV and higher, age outside the study bands, conditions that could impair 25OHD metabolism and use of vitamin D supplementation. Vitamin D supplements were defined as all oral supplements containing vitamin D other than food. The use of sunscreen was also an exclusion criterion. Sunscreen use was defined as the use of any sunscreen products within 3 months prior to the study regardless of the frequency. Participants were volunteers and gave written informed consent before entering the study. UNIFESP/EPM's Ethics and Research Committee approved the present study (reference number 464.939).

Data collection

The study was conducted between December 2013 and February 2014 (summer in the south hemisphere) and between June 2014 and August 2014 (winter). Blood samples were collected in photoprotected tubes and stored at − 70 °C until serum 25OHD was measured. Serum 25OHD measurements were performed using chemiluminescence technique with a coefficient of variation of 11.7% [19]. Vitamin D status was classified as normal when serum 25OHD concentration was ≥20 ng/mL and deficient when < 20 ng/mL, according to the recommendation from the American Institute of Medicine (IOM) [6]. The Endocrine Society definition criteria for vitamin D deficiency were also evaluated [9].

Simultaneously with blood collection all the participants answered a questionnaire on daily sun exposure correspondent to the previous week, as formerly published [17]. Sun exposure between 9:00 AM and 4:00 PM was recorded. Scores in the questionnaire are based on the duration of sun exposure (Time in sun: less than 5 min = 0, between 5 and 30 min = 1 and greater than 30 min = 2) and in the amount of exposed skin surface (Skin Exposure: face and hands = 1; face, hands and arms = 2; face, hands and legs = 3; bathing suit = 4). Scores were calculated for each day of the previous week. A final score to estimate the mean amount of sun exposure was calculated as the product of the amount of time by the amount of exposed skin. This final score was calculated for each day to reflect the Daily Sun Exposure Score (minimum = 0, maximum = 8). All seven Daily Sun Exposure Scores were summed to generate the Total Sun Exposure Score (TSES) for the entire week (minimum = 0, maximum = 56). We also considered the Weekly Time of Exposure Score and the Weekly Skin Amount Score, which were calculated by adding the scores corresponding to each day of the week (minimum = 0 and maximum = 14; minimum = 7 and maximum = 28, respectively). Body weight was measured (after removal of shoes and heavy outer clothing) using a balance beam scale. Height was measured (after removal of shoes) using a Filizola® stadiometer. Height and weight were used to calculate the body mass index (BMI; kg/m^2).

Statistical analyzes

All statistical analysis was performed using SPSS 19.0 software package (SPSS Inc., Chicago, IL). Mann-Whitney test was used to analyze the anthropometric data between independent groups. Student's *t*-test was used to compare TSES as well as mean serum 25OHD concentrations between groups. A linear regression model was used to identify variables associated with serum 25OHD measurements while logistic regression models were used to identify anthropometric and questionnaire variables that were associated with vitamin D deficiency. Receiver operating characteristic (ROC) curve analysis was performed to determine the performance of

TSES to predict vitamin D deficiency (serum 25OHD concentration below 20 ng/mL). Significance level was set as $p < 0.05$.

Results

Table 1 shows anthropometric data and vitamin D status for the study participants. Using the IOM definition criteria [6] we observed a very high prevalence of vitamin D deficiency. A total of 133 subjects (66.5%) had serum 25OHD concentration below 20 ng/mL. Mean serum 25OHD concentrations did not differ significantly between young and old subjects (18.27 ± 7.13 ng/mL and 16.93 ± 7.45 ng/mL, respectively, $p = 0.29$). Significant effect of seasonality on 25OHD measurement was detected in young participants. For this age group mean serum 25OHD concentration was significantly higher in the summer than that measured in the winter (21.58 ± 6.08 ng/mL and 14.95 ± 6.58 ng/mL, respectively, $p = 0.003$). The same was not observed in the older participants.

The overall mean TSES was 14.9 ± 9.58 (maximum was 28). Young participants had TSES significantly higher than those observed for the older group ($p < 0.001$). As expected, TSES were higher in the summer as compared to the winter in both age groups ($p = 0.005$).

We observed modest although statistically significant correlation between TSES and serum 25OHD concentration ($r = 0.264$, $p < 0.001$), as shown in Fig. 1. This association was particularly confirmed when the older participants were analyzed separately. In this age group, a weak but significant correlation was found between TSES, Weekly Time of Exposure Score and serum 25OHD concentrations only in the summer ($r = 0.322$, $p = 0.023$ and $r = 0.433$, $p = 0.002$, respectively). For the young age group, none of the variables of the questionnaire correlated significantly with serum 25OHD concentration neither in the summer nor in the winter.

Multiple linear regression analyses demonstrated that TSES and BMI were significantly associated with serum 25OHD measurements, as shown in Table 2. The equation was significant ($R = 0.297$), however the analyzed variables explained only 8.8% of the variability of serum 25OHD measurements ($R^2 = 0.088$).

Using logistic regression analysis, an inverse correlation was found between BMI and 25OHD status (OR = 0.926, $p = 0.027$). Multiple logistic regression analysis demonstrated that BMI and TSES were the main variables associated with vitamin D deficiency (serum 25OHD below 20 ng/mL), as shown in Table 2. The performance of TSES to predict vitamin D deficiency (25OHD < 20 ng/mL) was considered poor with a non-significant area under the curve (AUC) ($p = 0.172$) (Additional file 1: Figure S1). Similar results were found when vitamin D deficiency was defined according to the Endocrine Society cut off value (25OHD < 30 ng/mL) [9].

Discussion

Our results demonstrated that the sun exposure questionnaire proposed by Hanwell et al. [17] was not able to discriminate vitamin D sufficient from deficient individuals when applied to healthy young and old Caucasian subjects living in a tropical area in Brazil. TSES estimated by the questionnaire showed a significant but weak correlation with serum 25OHD concentration. The questionnaire thus did not hold as a reliable tool to guide or indicate serum 25OHD concentration measurement. Separate analyses by age group (young and older) or season (summer and winter) did not hold significance. As expected, TSES and BMI were significantly associated with serum 25OHD concentration but were able to explain just a minimal amount of its variability.

In Brazil, 99.3% of 2040 subjects evaluated in the population-based BRAZOS study had vitamin D intake below recommendation [7]. Likewise, a high prevalence of vitamin D deficiency has been systematically observed in several samples of our population [8–11]. The prevalence of vitamin D deficiency depends upon the definition criteria used [6, 9]. In our present study mean serum 25OHD measurements in the subgroups evaluated (with the exception of young subjects measured during winter) were greater than 16 ng/mL (with the exception of wintertime in young patients), level that covers the requirements of approximately half the population, according to the IOM [6].

Table 1 Anthropometric data and serum 25-hydroxyvitamin D concentration in young (20 to 40 years old) and old (60 to 80 years old) healthy Caucasian individuals living in São Paulo, Brazil

	All ($N = 200$)	Young ($N = 100$)	Old ($N = 100$)	p^a
Age (years, mean ± SD)	49.6 ± 19.4	31.5 ± 7.0	67.8 ± 6.4	–
Sex (Men: Women, N)	52: 148	19: 81	33: 67	0.02
BMI (kg/m^2, mean ± SD)	26.44 ± 4.76	25.85 ± 3.57	27.04 ± 4.62	0.05
25OHD (ng/mL, mean ± SD)	17.6 ± 7.3	18.27 ± 7.13	16.93 ± 7.45	0.29
25OHD < 20 ng/mL (N, %)	133 (66.5%)	66 (66%)	67 (67%)	0.36

25OHD 25-hydroxyvitamin D, *BMI* body mass index
[a]Chi-squared or Mann-Whitney

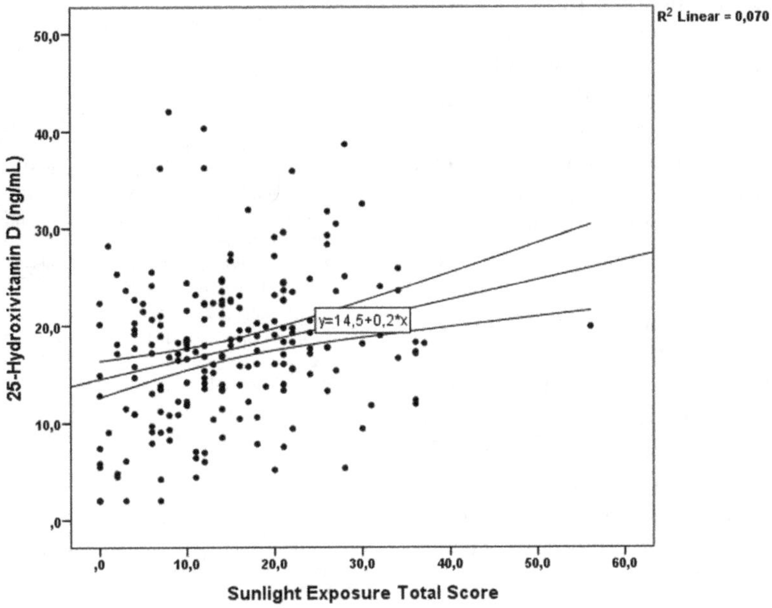

Fig. 1 Linear regression between serum 25-hydroxyvitamin D concentrations and total sun exposure score in 200 healthy Caucasian Brazilian individuals

The questionnaire we used in the present study is very easy to be applied and has shown satisfactory results in another Caucasian population with strong correlation with serum 25OHD levels (Spearman's rho = 0.59) [17]. On the other hand, there was no significant association between TSES and serum 25OHD levels in a Canadian cohort [20]. Mean TSES in our sample (14.9) are low and could underscore a current trend of an indoor lifestyle. On the other hand, the moderate to low sun exposure measured by the questionnaire is not in agreement with the evidence about sun exposure in Brazil. Due to our tropical and subtropical climate, geographic characteristics and a culturally low frequency of photo protection, Brazilians are among the populations with the highest annual sun exposure [13]. The lack of association in our study and in the Canadian cohort [20] between sun exposure measured by the questionnaire and serum 25OHD concentration may, at least in part, reflect the poor accuracy of the questionnaire to measure sun exposure. Based on subjects' recall of sun exposure in the previous week, the questionnaire may lack internal validity. The high level of atmospheric pollution in the greater São Paulo area [21] might have affected our current results since it reduces the ability of UVB radiation to induce vitamin D synthesis [22]. As expected, mean sun exposure was higher among young people as opposed to the elderly and also in the summer as compared to the winter.

Table 2 Multiple linear regression analyses for serum 25-hydroxyvitamin D concentration in healthy Caucasian Brazilian individuals living in São Paulo, Brazil

	B (95% confidence interval)	Standard error	*p*
25OHD	20.052 [14.238/25.866]	2.948	< 0.001
TSES	0.206 [0.102/0.310]	0.053	< 0.001
BMI	- 0.211 [−0.420/− 0.001]	0.106	0.048

25OHD 25-hydroxyvitamin D, *TSES* total sun exposure score, *BMI* body mass index

It could sound unrealistic to hypothesize that a sun exposure questionnaire would give us an insight into the circulating 25OHD concentrations. Multiple reasons would certainly work against that hypothesis including time of day of exposure, season, skin phototype and area of sun exposure, use of sunscreen and other barrier factors. The study tried to take that into account and only recruited Caucasian individuals with light phototypes (I to III). Skin area of exposure was also calculated. The fact that sun exposure was recorded from 9 AM up to 4 PM can have a dramatic effect on the cutaneous synthesis of vitamin D: very early (between 9 and 10 AM) and late hours (3 to 4 PM) certainly are associated with significantly less vitamin D synthesis when compared to peak hours from 11 AM to 1 PM. Unfortunately the questionnaire used does not consider those observations and that might have had an effect on our results.

It has been now well established that obesity can contribute to hypovitaminosis D. Significant inverse correlation between BMI and serum 25OHD concentration seen in our sample has been described [15, 23, 24]. It is estimated that for every 10% increase in BMI there will be a 4.2% decrease in serum 25OHD concentration [23]. About 57% of our participants had BMI above 25 kg/m^2 and 14% above 30 kg/m^2.

Important limitations of the present study need to be pointed out. As other variables such as photo protection methods other than sunscreen, diet and physical activity were not considered, it could be inferred that such information could have also affected the relationship between the questionnaire variables and serum 25OHD concentration. More complex questionnaires including a number of other variables might have improved performance to identify individual at risk of vitamin D deficiency [25]. The questionnaire was tested in healthy Caucasian subjects with no clear recommendation for screening for vitamin D deficiency. Even though the prevalence of vitamin D deficiency in the study population was significantly high, using the questionnaire in patients with osteoporosis or at a higher risk for vitamin D deficiency might lead to different results. The cross sectional nature of the study design precludes us from establishing a cause effect relationship between the variables in analysis. Continuous follow-up of the same individuals at two seasons could reduce the differences depending on the individual characteristics, minimizing the variability of the data.

Conclusion

In conclusion, in spite of being simple to use, the studied sun exposure questionnaire has very low accuracy to estimate serum 25OHD concentration. The questionnaire does not allow discriminating between vitamin D sufficient and deficient individuals in a tropical area. There remains the need of reliable tools to better indicate 25OHD testing and reduce costs of diagnosis and management of vitamin D deficiency.

Abbreviations

25OHD: 25-hydroxyvitamin D; AUC: Area under the curve; BMI: Body mass index; IOM: Institute of Medicine; ROC: Receiver operating characteristic; TSES: Total sun exposure score; UVB: Ultraviolet B

Authors' contributions

FBB performed all individuals' selection and data collection, being responsible for analyzing and interpreting the data. CHMC performed all serum 25OHD measurements, and was a major contributor in writing the manuscript. VLS was responsible for the study conception and data interpretation. All authors read and approved the final manuscript.

Competing interests

The authors declare that they have no competing interests.

References

1. Holick MF. The vitamin D deficiency pandemic: approaches for diagnosis, treatment and prevention. Rev Endocr Metab Disord. 2017;18(2):153–65.
2. Abrahamsen B, Harvey NC. The role of vitamin D supplementation in patients with rheumatic diseases. Nat Rev Rheumatol. 2013;9(7):411–22.
3. Christakos S, DeLuca HF. Minireview: vitamin D: is there a role in extraskeletal health? Endocrinology. 2011;152(8):2930–6.
4. Holick MF. Environmental factors that influence the cutaneous production of vitamin D. Am J Clin Nutr. 1995;61(3 Suppl):638S–45S.
5. Brouwer-Brolsma EM, Bischoff-Ferrari HA, Bouillon R, Feskens EJ, Gallagher CJ, Hypponen E, Llewellyn DJ, Stoecklin E, Dierkes J, Kies AK, et al. Vitamin D: do we get enough? A discussion between vitamin D experts in order to make a step towards the harmonisation of dietary reference intakes for vitamin D across Europe. Osteoporos Int. 2013;24(5):1567–77.
6. Ross AC, Manson JE, Abrams SA, Aloia JF, Brannon PM, Clinton SK, Durazo-Arvizu RA, Gallagher JC, Gallo RL, Jones G, et al. The 2011 report on dietary reference intakes for calcium and vitamin D from the Institute of Medicine: what clinicians need to know. J Clin Endocrinol Metab. 2011;96(1):53–8.
7. Holick MF. Vitamin D deficiency. N Engl J Med. 2007;357(3):266–81.
8. DeLuca HF. Overview of general physiologic features and functions of vitamin D. Am J Clin Nutr. 2004;80(6 Suppl):1689S–96S.
9. Holick MF, Binkley NC, Bischoff-Ferrari HA, Gordon CM, Hanley DA, Heaney RP, Murad MH, Weaver CM. Evaluation, treatment, and prevention of vitamin D deficiency: an Endocrine Society clinical practice guideline. J Clin Endocrinol Metab. 2011;96(7):1911–30.
10. Maeda SS, Borba VZ, Camargo MB, Silva DM, Borges JL, Bandeira F, Lazaretti-Castro M. Recommendations of the Brazilian Society of Endocrinology and Metabology (SBEM) for the diagnosis and treatment of hypovitaminosis D. Arquivos brasileiros de endocrinologia e metabologia. 2014;58(5):411–33.
11. Rautiainen S, Manson JE, Lichtenstein AH, Sesso HD. Dietary supplements and disease prevention - a global overview. Nat Rev Endocrinol. 2016;12(7):407–20.
12. Eloi M, Horvath DV, Szejnfeld VL, Ortega JC, Rocha DA, Szejnfeld J, Castro CH. Vitamin D deficiency and seasonal variation over the years in Sao Paulo, Brazil. Osteoporos Int. 2016;27(12):3449–56.
13. Schalka S, Steiner D, Ravelli FN, Steiner T, Terena AC, Marcon CR, Ayres EL, Addor FA, Miot HA, Ponzio H, et al. Brazilian consensus on photoprotection. An Bras Dermatol. 2014;89(6 Suppl 1):1–74.
14. Correa Mde P. Solar ultraviolet radiation: properties, characteristics and amounts observed in Brazil and South America. An Bras Dermatol. 2015; 90(3):297–313.
15. Nabak AC, Johnson RE, Keuler NS, Hansen KE. Can a questionnaire predict vitamin D status in postmenopausal women? Public Health Nutr. 2014;17(4):739–46.
16. Summaries for patients. Screening for vitamin D deficiency in adults: US preventive services task force recommendation statement. Ann Intern Med. 2015;162(2):I–28.
17. Hanwell HE, Vieth R, Cole DE, Scillitani A, Modoni S, Frusciante V, Ritrovato G, Chiodini I, Minisola S, Carnevale V. Sun exposure questionnaire predicts circulating 25-hydroxyvitamin D concentrations in Caucasian hospital workers in southern Italy. J Steroid Biochem Mol Biol. 2010;121(1–2):334–7.
18. Fitzpatrick TB. The validity and practicality of sun-reactive skin types I through VI. Arch Dermatol. 1988;124(6):869–71.
19. Eloi M, Horvath DV, Ortega JC, Prado MS, Andrade LE, Szejnfeld VL, de Moura Castro CH. 25-Hydroxivitamin D serum concentration, not free and bioavailable vitamin D, is associated with disease activity in systemic lupus erythematosus patients. PLoS One. 2017;12(1):e0170323.
20. Sham L, Yeh EA, Magalhaes S, Parra EJ, Gozdzik A, Banwell B, Hanwell HE. Evaluation of fall sun exposure score in predicting vitamin D status in young Canadian adults, and the influence of ancestry. J Photochem Photobiol B. 2015;145:25–9.
21. Maeda SS, Saraiva GL, Hayashi LF, Cendoroglo MS, Ramos LR, Correa Mde P, Henrique de Mesquita C, Lazaretti-Castro M. Seasonal variation in the serum 25-hydroxyvitamin D levels of young and elderly active and inactive adults in Sao Paulo, Brazil: The Sao PAulo Vitamin D Evaluation Study (SPADES). Dermatoendocrinol. 2013;5(1):211–7.
22. Feizabad E, Hossein-Nezhad A, Maghbooli Z, Ramezani M, Hashemian R, Moattari S. Impact of air pollution on vitamin D deficiency and bone health in adolescents. Arch Osteoporos. 2017;12(1):34.
23. Vimaleswaran KS, Berry DJ, Lu C, Tikkanen E, Pilz S, Hiraki LT, Cooper JD, Dastani Z, Li R, Houston DK, et al. Causal relationship between obesity and vitamin D status: bi-directional Mendelian randomization analysis of multiple cohorts. PLoS Med. 2013;10(2):e1001383.
24. Daly RM, Gagnon C, Lu ZX, Magliano DJ, Dunstan DW, Sikaris KA, Zimmet PZ, Ebeling PR, Shaw JE. Prevalence of vitamin D deficiency and its determinants in Australian adults aged 25 years and older: a national, population-based study. Clin Endocrinol. 2012;77(1):26–35.
25. Bolek-Berquist J, Elliott ME, Gangnon RE, Gemar D, Engelke J, Lawrence SJ, Hansen KE. Use of a questionnaire to assess vitamin D status in young adults. Public Health Nutr. 2009;12(2):236–43.

Cost-effectiveness of tolvaptan for the treatment of hyponatraemia secondary to syndrome of inappropriate antidiuretic hormone secretion in Sweden

Clare Jamookeeah[2], Paul Robinson[2], Karl O'Reilly[2*], Johan Lundberg[3], Martin Gisby[2], Michael Ländin[3], Jakob Skov[4] and David Trueman[1]

Abstract

Background: Tolvaptan is the only vasopressin V_2 receptor antagonist licensed by the European Medicines Agency for the treatment of hyponatraemia (HN) secondary to the syndrome of inappropriate antidiuretic hormone secretion (SIADH). We have investigated the cost-effectiveness of tolvaptan versus no active treatment (NAT) in adult patients within the licensed indication who have either failed to respond to fluid restriction or for whom the use of fluid restriction is not suitable, from the societal perspective in Sweden.

Methods: A cost-utility analysis, considering a 'general SIADH' population and two subpopulations of patients (small-cell lung cancer [SCLC] and pneumonia) to broadly represent the complex clinical pathway of SIADH, was performed. A discrete event simulation was developed to model the progression of individuals through inpatient admissions over a 30-day time horizon (180 days for the SCLC cohort). Clinical data were derived from tolvaptan trials and observational data sources. All costs are given in Swedish kronor (SEK).

Results: In the 'general SIADH' population, tolvaptan was associated with reduced costs (SEK 5,779 per patient [€624]) and increased quality-adjusted life-years (QALYs) (0.0019) compared with NAT and was therefore the dominant treatment strategy. Tolvaptan was also associated with reduced costs and increased QALYs in the SCLC and pneumonia subpopulations. The most influential variables in our analysis were reduction in hospital length of stay, duration of treatment and long term treatment with tolvaptan in SCLC patients.

Conclusions: Tolvaptan represents a cost-effective treatment option in Sweden for hospitalised patients with HN secondary to SIADH who have either failed to respond to or are unsuitable for fluid restriction.

Keywords: Hyponatraemia, Tolvaptan, Cost-effectiveness, Cost-utility, Discrete event simulation, SIADH

Background

Hyponatraemia (HN) is the most common electrolyte disturbance in clinical practice, occurring in approximately 15–30 % of hospitalised patients [1, 2]. It is commonly defined as a serum sodium concentration ($[Na^+]$) <135 mmol/L [2–5], with severe HN defined as <125 mmol/L [2]. Hyponatraemia is associated with increased mortality, morbidity and length of hospital stay [2].

Hyponatraemia can be euvolaemic (i.e. without an associated change in body fluid volume), hypervolaemic (i.e. body fluid volume is increased), or hypovolaemic (body fluid volume is decreased). These three types of HN have different sets of possible aetiologies. The most common cause of euvolaemic HN is the syndrome of inappropriate antidiuretic hormone secretion (SIADH) [3, 6], which is the focus of our analysis. In SIADH water retention is caused by inappropriate increased release of, or responsiveness to, antidiuretic hormone (ADH) [7]. This can be due to malignancy, pneumonia, central nervous system disorders or certain drugs [7].

* Correspondence: KO'Reilly@otsuka-europe.com
[2]Otsuka Pharmaceutical Europe Ltd., Gallions, Wexham Springs, Framewood Road, Wexham SL3 6PJ, UK
Full list of author information is available at the end of the article

Although SIADH can be associated with many different types of malignancy, it is most commonly observed with small cell lung cancer (SCLC) and studies have shown a higher mortality rate in SCLC patients with HN than in those without [8, 9]. Drug-induced SIADH usually resolves upon discontinuation of the medication [7].

Swedish guidelines for HN, published by the Swedish Endocrine Society and the Swedish Association for Anaesthesiology and Intensive Care [1], recommend resolution of the underlying condition as the primary treatment strategy in patients with SIADH. If symptoms are mild, HN secondary to SIADH may be treated with fluid restriction. Diagnosis and treatment should be re-evaluated if the patient does not respond within 12–24 h. If the symptoms are more pronounced the patient will require treatment in intensive care [1]. In patients who do not respond to or cannot be treated with fluid restriction, symptoms may exacerbate and patient outcomes may be signficiantly affected. For patients in whom fluid restriction has been unsuccessful or is unsuitable, vasopressin receptor antagonists (i.e., tolvaptan) are recommended [1]. In clinical practice, subjects with HN, especially if it is associated with no or mild symptoms, or if initial treatment was unsuccessful, may often not receive treatment [10].

Tolvaptan, an oral vasopressin V_2 receptor antagonist, is the only vaptan approved by the European Medicines Agency (EMA) for the treatment of adult patients with HN secondary to SIADH in 2009 [11]. Tolvaptan blocks binding of ADH to the V_2 receptor which induces electrolyte-free water excretion. The result is a reduction in body water without loss of body electrolytes, which leads to an increase in serum [Na^+] [4, 5].

The cost-effectiveness of tolvaptan for the treatment of HN secondary to SIADH has never been studied in a European setting. Worldwide, three studies have previously evaluated the potential cost impact of tolvaptan in HN [12–14]; however, one of these was performed in a different indication (heart failure) (14). Of the remaining two studies, Dasta et al. [13] considered a US hospital population with HN secondary to SIADH and observed a total cost offset, including the acquisition cost of tolvaptan, of $694 per admission. The authors estimated that tolvaptan would be cost-neutral with duration of therapy of ≥6.78 days. In a South Korean analysis, Lee et al. [14] found that, in patients hospitalised for treatment and monitoring of euvolaemic and hypervolaemic HN, tolvaptan treatment was less costly and more efficacious compared with placebo.

We have performed an economic evaluation, from a Swedish societal perspective, to determine the cost-effectiveness of tolvaptan, compared with no active treatment (NAT) for HN secondary to SIADH in adult patients who have either failed to respond to fluid restriction or for whom the use of fluid restriction is not suitable.

Methods

Design of the economic evaluation

A cost-utility analysis was conducted. The primary outcome was the incremental cost-effectiveness ratio (ICER) expressed as a cost per quality-adjusted life-year (QALY) in line with Tandvårds- och läkemedelsförmånsverket (The Dental and Pharmaceutical Benefits Agency [TLV]) guidance at the time of analysis [15]. The base case used a societal perspective, also in line with TLV guidance.

Tolvaptan was compared with NAT. This choice was based on advice from clinicians and evidence from the HN registry, a multi-centre, prospective, observational study. The HN registry showed that, of patients provided with fluid restriction as a first therapy, 56 % experienced a total increase of [Na^+] of ≤5 mEq/L and of these patients, 56 % were not provided a second therapy [10]. This suggests that NAT is a relevant option widely used in clinical practice, despite being inappropriate in many cases.

The economic evaluation considered a hypothetical cohort of individuals with HN secondary to SIADH who had either failed to respond to or were unsuitable for fluid restriction. This population was chosen in line with current Swedish guidance and clinical practice [1, 16]. For the purpose of the economic evaluation, HN is defined as [Na^+] <135 mmol/L and sodium correction is defined as [Na^+] ≥135 mmol/L, consistent with the tolvaptan clinical trial programme [4, 5].

Three clinically relevant patient populations were evaluated in the analysis: all patients with HN secondary to SIADH ('general SIADH'); the subgroup of patients with SCLC and HN secondary to SIADH (SCLC cohort); the subgroup of patients with pneumonia and HN secondary to SIADH (pneumonia cohort). The SCLC and pneumonia populations were selected as examples of two highly relevant subpopulations, for which the clinical and patient pathways are very different. They were chosen to broadly represent the complex clinical pathway of SIADH.

A 30-day time horizon was chosen in the base case analysis for the 'general SIADH' population, reflecting the relatively short duration of treatment for HN secondary to SIADH and the duration of the tolvaptan Phase III clinical studies [4, 5]. The 30-day time horizon is also thought to capture all relevant consequences for most patients in this population. Similarly, a 30-day time horizon was also deemed appropriate for the pneumonia subgroup, due to the short duration of treatment for HN secondary to SIADH in this population. However, based on clinical expert opinion, a 180-day time horizon was assumed for the SCLC population.

Future costs and benefits are discounted at a rate of 3.0 % per annum, in line with current TLV guidance, but due to the short time horizon of the analysis this is mainly applicable to scenario analyses [15].

Outline of the model

An individual-level model (specifically, a discrete event simulation [DES]), which simulates multiple clinical outcomes over time was developed to model the progression of individuals, one at a time, through multiple inpatient admissions over the defined time horizon. The DES approach was adopted in preference to a cohort model (which is more commonly seen in this type of analysis) due to the ability to easily incorporate time dependency. For example, many economic and clinical aspects of HN secondary to SIADH may occur at rates that change over time (time to hospital discharge; time to mortality; time to hospital readmission; time to discontinuation of tolvaptan).

The flow of hypothetical individuals through the model and the order in which events may occur are depicted in Fig. 1. In summary:

1. An individual is admitted to hospital and is diagnosed with HN secondary to SIADH
2. The individual undergoes active treatment or receives NAT for HN secondary to SIADH
3. The individual may undergo further treatment for their underlying condition (such as chemotherapy) before being discharged
   a. In the base case, all individuals are assumed to be discharged to home
   b. Individuals are assumed to have their underlying condition resolved ('general SIADH' and pneumonia) or not (SCLC) at discharge and this affects quality of life (QoL) between admissions
4. The individual may die, either during hospitalisation or following discharge
5. The individual may be readmitted at a later date and will flow through the model again
6. The individual leaves the model at the end of the set time horizon, or at death, whichever occurs first, and a new patient is selected.

The DES was run for 100,000 hypothetical patients to arrive at a set of outputs representative of a cohort in each subpopulation, both with and without tolvaptan treatment. Comparative modelled outputs, other than QALYs, included hospital length of stay (LOS), readmissions, and mortality.

Data sources

The economic evaluation relies on evidence from several sources, listed below. A summary of how these sources inform the required clinical parameters, across the three base case analyses, is presented in Table 1.

- The Study of Ascending Levels of Tolvaptan in Hyponatremia I and II (SALT I and SALT II) are both randomised, placebo-controlled, double-blind trials examining the effect of tolvaptan on hypervolaemic and euvolaemic HN of different aetiologies [4, 5].
- The Assessment of epidemiology, patient characteristics and outcomes Related To patients with HN/SIADH in Sweden: a population-based register study (ART) is a retrospective cohort study conducted using the compulsory population-based health registers governed by the National Board of Health and Welfare [17].
- The HN Registry is a global, multicentre (US and European), prospective, observational study of current treatment approaches for hospitalised patients with euvolaemic or hypervolaemic HN [10].

Model inputs

A summary of base case inputs is presented in Table 2. Health-related QoL (HRQL, in the form of health state utilities) for the 'general SIADH' population were obtained by mapping SF-12 (12-Item Short Form Health Survey) responses from SALT I and II to EQ-5D (a standardised health outcome questionnaire) [18] using a mapping algorithm developed by Gray et al. [19]. Simulated EQ-5D scores were then used to estimate changes in EQ-5D from baseline at Day 30 using ordinary least squares regression as a function of baseline characteristics, treatment arm and achievement of [Na^+] correction at Day 4 (≥135 mmol/L) (i.e. the definition of sodium correction, in line with a predefined endpoint in SALT I & II [4]). Literature sources were sought to estimate the baseline utility scores for the

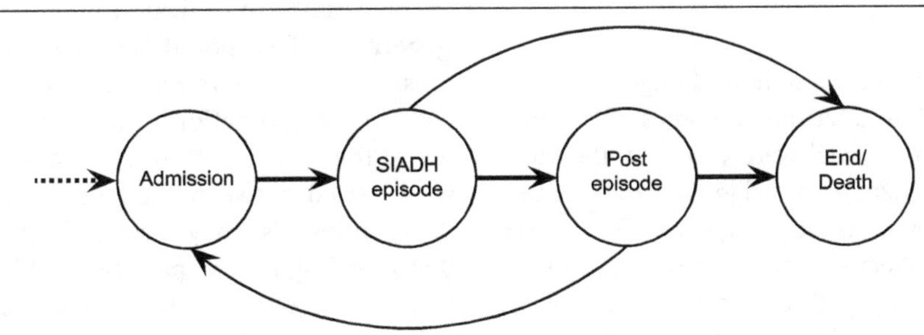

Fig. 1 Event graph depicting flow of patients in model

Table 1 Application of clinical data sources in the model base cases

Parameter	Population modelled General SIADH	SCLC	Pneumonia
Population characteristics	HN Registry and ART	HN Registry and ART	HN Registry and ART
[Na^{+}] correction	HN Registry and SALT I & II	HN Registry and SALT I & II	HN Registry and SALT I & II
Duration of tolvaptan treatment	HN Registry	Expert clinical opinion	Expert clinical opinion
HRQL change	SALT I & II	SALT I & II	SALT I & II
Length of inpatient stay	SALT I & II	SALT I & II	SALT I & II
Inpatient mortality	ART	ART	ART
Readmission	ART	ART	ART
Long-term mortality	Swedish life-tables	ART	Swedish life-tables

Abbreviations: ART the Assessment of epidemiology, patient characteristics and outcomes Related To patients with hyponatraemia/SIADH in Sweden, *HN* hyponatraemia, *HRQL* health related quality of life, *SALT* the Study of Ascending Levels of Tolvaptan in Hyponatremia, *SCLC* small cell lung cancer, *SIADH* syndrome of inappropriate antidiuretic hormone secretion

SCLC and pneumonia populations [20, 21]. Unit costs were collected from a number of different sources including hospital price lists [22], TLV official price database [23] and Statistics Sweden [24]. The reference year of the costs was 2013, and costs are given in Swedish kronor (SEK). Additional details are provided in the Additional file 1.

Key assumptions

Assumptions had to be made where no suitable data sources could be identified. Key assumptions concerned the benefit of correction of HN, which was conservatively assumed not to affect rates of hospital readmission, inpatient mortality or long-term mortality. An overview of other assumptions can be found in the Additional file 1.

Scenario analyses

A number of alternative scenarios were analysed. These included alternative time horizons of 60, 90 and 180 days and 1 year for all subpopulations in the model. Alternative durations of tolvaptan treatment were also analysed, as well as removing the early discontinuation of treatment rule and different hospital LOS. An SCLC population receiving tolvaptan for extended periods, typically to increase QoL in a palliative care setting, was also considered as a scenario analysis. The alternative scenarios tested are described in the Additional file 1.

Sensitivity analysis

Sensitivity analysis is used to explore how changes in model parameters and assumptions alter the outcomes of the analysis. All parameters in the model were varied by the 95 % CI around the mean or, where unavailable, by ±15 %. A tornado diagram, visually representing the results (Fig. 2), was generated, in which the effect on the net monetary benefit (NMB) at a willingness-to-pay threshold SEK 1.2 million was plotted, with variables ordered by the magnitude of their effect. The NMB applies a monetary value to QALYs and is calculated by rearranging the cost-effectiveness decision rule to $\lambda \cdot \Delta E - \Delta C > 0$ (λ, willingness to pay threshold; ΔE, change in effect; ΔC, change in cost) [25]. This approach was preferred to plotting changes to ICERs directly to ensure appropriate values were presented in the presence of negative ICERs.

Results

Base case results for the three different populations, based on cohorts of 100,000 individually modelled patients, are presented in Table 3. Detailed results are provided in the Additional file 1. Tolvaptan was associated with reduced per patient costs (savings of SEK 2,678 to SEK 8,411[€289 to €908]) and increased incremental QALYs (0.0018 to 0.0028) versus NAT. Tolvaptan was therefore considered to be the dominant (i.e. both cost-saving and resulting in a QALY gain) strategy in all three populations.

The results from the scenario analyses are presented in the Additional file 1. The most important determinants of cost-effectiveness in our model were reduction in hospital LOS associated with tolvaptan (removal of this benefit resulting in ICERs of SEK >1.4 million), duration of treatment with tolvaptan (an increase in treatment duration resulting in a considerable ICER increase in the 'all SIADH', but not change in the SCLC and pneumonia populations) and long term treatment with tolvaptan in SCLC patients (SEK 2.9 million).

The results of univariate sensitivity analyses for the 'general SIADH' population are presented in Fig. 2. The most influential parameters were two of the coefficients used in the estimation of the duration of tolvaptan treatment; the constant term and baseline [Na^{+}]. When these were varied between their upper and lower 95 % confidence intervals, they were able to generate NMB < SEK 0 at a willingness-to-pay threshold of SEK 1.2 million. A recent review of the literature around the value of a statistical life in Sweden suggests a willingness-to-pay threshold of SEK 1.2 million per QALY [26].

Table 2 Base case inputs by population (data value or type; source)

Model element	General SIADH	SCLC	Pneumonia
Clinical parameters			
Mean age (years)	70; ART (with SIADH)[a]	64; ART (SCLC with SIADH)[a]	69; ART (pneumonia with SIADH)[a]
% Male	33 %; ART (with SIADH)[a]	31 %; ART (SCLC with SIADH)[a]	43 %; ART (pneumonia with SIADH)[a]
Baseline [Na^+]	125; HN Registry[b]	123; HN Registry [38]	125; HN Registry[b]
Baseline probability [Na^+] correction (≥135 mmol/L)	Binary logistic regression; HN Registry (SIADH)[b]	Binary logistic regression; HN Registry (SIADH)[b]	Binary logistic regression; HN Registry (SIADH)[b]
Odds ratio normalisation tolvaptan vs. NAT	11.50; SALT I & II [4]	11.50; SALT I & II [4]	11.50; SALT I & II [4]
Duration of tolvaptan treatment	Mean 3 days; Lognormal survival distribution; HN Registry (SIADH)[b]	Mean 4 days; Petereit et al. [28]	Mean 3 days; clinical opinion
Early tolvaptan treatment discontinuation rule	2 days	2 days	2 days
Mean hospital LOS NAT	8.00; SALT I & II (SIADH with [Na^+] <130 mmol/L) [4]	8.00; SALT I & II (SIADH with [Na^+] <130 mmol/L) [4]	8.00; SALT I & II (SIADH with [Na^+] <130 mmol/L) [4]
Percentage reduction hospital LOS with tolvaptan	20.0 %; SALT I & II (SIADH with [Na^+] <130 mmol/L)[c]	20.0 %; SALT I & II (SIADH with [Na^+] <130 mmol/L)[c]	20.0 %; SALT I & II (SIADH with [Na^+] <130 mmol/L)[c]
Probability inpatient mortality	2.2 %; ART (with SIADH)[a]	4.4 %; ART (SCLC with SIADH)[a]	6.2 %; ART (pneumonia with SIADH)[a]
Long-term survival	Based on age; Swedish life-tables [24]	Based on disease; Gompertz distribution from ART (SCLC with SIADH)	Based on age; Swedish life-tables [24]
Time to readmission	Weibull distribution; ART (with SIADH)[a]	Weibull distribution; ART (SCLC with SIADH)[a]	Weibull distribution; ART (pneumonia with SIADH)[a]
Probability of SIADH (and HN) resolution at end of inpatient admission	100 %; assumption	88 %; List et al. [39]	100 %; assumption
Time to resolution[d]	NA in base case	NA in base case	NA in base case
Costs			
Tolvaptan dosing/cost assumption	15/30 mg once daily[e]	15/30 mg once daily[e]	15/30 mg once daily[e]
Care setting for admission	Internal medicine clinic	Oncology clinic	Pulmonary care clinic
Discharge location	Home	Home	Home
Palliative care costs	None	Applied for a maximum of 84 days (3 months)	None
Chemotherapy costs	None	Applied once per inpatient stay	None
Percentage patients in work between readmissions	17 %; [40]	0 %; Assumption	17 %; [40]
HRQL			
Baseline utility	0.58; SALT I & II [41]	0.61; Loveman et al. [20] with HN reduction from SALT I & II [41]	0.73; Schuetz et al. [21] with HN reduction from SALT I & II [41]
Treatment-specific change in EQ-5D at Day 4	Absolute change in simulated EQ-5D at Day 30 from SALT I & II [41]	Absolute change in simulated EQ-5D at Day 30 from SALT I & II [41]	Absolute change in simulated EQ-5D at Day 30 from SALT I & II [41]
Model structure			
Time horizon	30 days	180 days	30 days

Abbreviations: ART The Assessment of epidemiology, patient characteristics and outcomes Related To patients with hyponatraemia/SIADH in Sweden: a population-based register study, *HN* hyponatraemia, *HRQL* health-related quality of life, *LOS* length of stay, *NA* not applicable, *NAT* no alternative treatment, *SALT* study of ascending levels of Tolvaptan in Hyponatremia, *SCLC* small cell lung cancer, *SIADH* syndrome of inappropriate antidiuretic hormone secretion

[a]Based on data from ART (unpublished observations)

[b]Analysis of HN registry data

[c]post-hoc analysis of SALT1 and SALT-2

[d]If resolution did not occur as an inpatient

[e]15/30 mg daily associated with equal cost

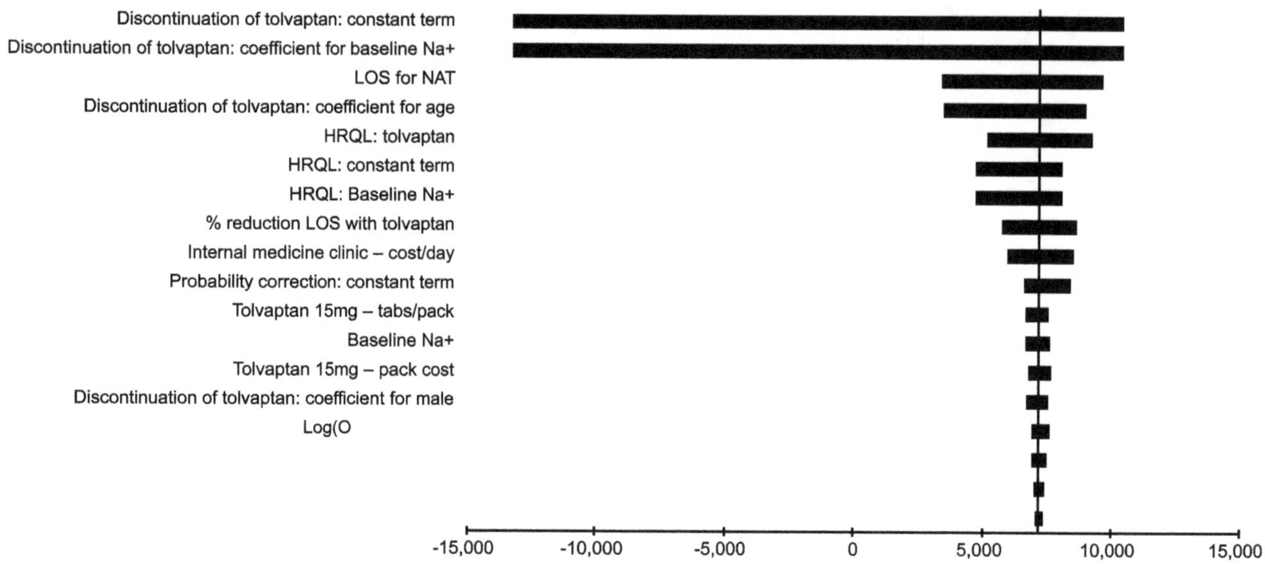

Fig. 2 Tornado diagram showing effect of varying parameters on NMB (threshold = SEK 1.2 m). Abbreviations: HRQL, health-related quality of life; LOS, length of stay; NAT, no active treatment; NMB, net monetary benefit; OR, odds ratio; SEK, Swedish kronor

Discussion

The present analysis assessed the cost-effectiveness of tolvaptan in three populations of patients with HN secondary to SIADH for whom the alternative treatment option is NAT. In the base case for the 'general SIADH' population, tolvaptan was the dominant strategy compared with NAT, as it was associated with a reduction in cost and an incremental QALY gain. Cost savings are predicted based on reductions in LOS, whilst QALY gains are a consequence of associated improvements in HRQL. Compared with NAT, tolvaptan was also the dominant strategy in the SCLC and pneumonia populations, associated with incremental cost savings and an incremental QALY gain. The results were sensitive to assumptions relating to the duration of tolvaptan treatment, LOS associated with NAT and the reduction in LOS associated with tolvaptan treatment.

Table 3 Base case results (per patient)

	NAT	Tolvaptan	Incremental
General SIADH			
Total costs	SEK 45,462	SEK 39,683	-SEK 5,779
QALYs	0.05381	0.05567	0.00186
ICER			Tolvaptan dominates
SCLC			
Total costs	SEK 372,717	SEK 364,306	-SEK 8,411
QALYs	0.21817	0.22101	0.00284
ICER			Tolvaptan dominates
Pneumonia			
Total costs	SEK 26,541	SEK 23,863	-SEK 2,678
QALYs	0.05689	0.05868	0.00179
ICER			Tolvaptan dominates

Abbreviations: HRQL health-related quality-of-life, *ICER* incremental cost-effectiveness ratio, *NAT* no active treatment, *QALY* quality-adjusted life-year, *SCLC* small-cell lung cancer, *SIADH* syndrome of inappropriate antidiuretic hormone secretion

The data used to calculate LOS and HRQL was obtained from the SALT I and SALT II clinical trials [4, 5]. The patients in the trials were treatment-naïve, whereas patients in the model had either failed to respond to fluid restriction or the use of fluid restriction was not suitable. Patients that fail to respond to fluid restriction may have more severe forms of SIADH and may be unable to excrete electrolyte-free water [27]. Therefore, they may respond differently to tolvaptan compared with the patients in SALT I and SALT II. Although the assumed positioning of tolvaptan in the model may be considered a limitation of the analysis, the positioning was based on Swedish guidelines for HN [1]. Furthermore, there are indications, from small case series [28, 29] that tolvaptan quickly restores serum [Na^+] concentrations in a population consistent with that modelled (i.e. in patients with HN secondary to SIADH who have failed fluid restriction or for whom fluid restriction is unsuitable).

The model assumes a reduction in LOS of 20 % based on the overall reduction observed in patients receiving tolvaptan compared with patients receiving placebo in the SIADH population of the SALT trials [4]. This reduction was not statistically significant, and the studies were not powered to demonstrate a difference in reduction of LOS. However, a subgroup analysis of euvolaemic patients with HN in the investigator-diagnosed SIADH group, combined with patients classified as 'other' (all patients not meeting clinical criteria for diagnosis of heart failure or cirrhosis), demonstrated a significantly shortened LOS favouring tolvaptan (4.70 ± 3.89 versus 8.40 ± 9.67 days; $p = 0.045$; a reduction of 44 %) [4]. These preliminary findings should ideally be confirmed by clinical trials designed to evaluate this outcome. A reduction of LOS, as demonstrated in the SALT trials, is supported by preliminary data from the HN registry [30] showing that the median LOS from the start of treatment was shortest for tolvaptan (3 days) and longest for no treatment (6 days). Published data in HN relevant to the current analysis are limited, not least due to the complexity of the condition and the clinical pathway. Every effort was made to identify the most relevant data for the model, using real word data sources where possible. Sweden-specific data were used where available.

Basing model LOS data in the SCLC and pneumonia populations on evidence from the SALT trials may be considered a source of uncertainty, as the percentage of patients in the study population with SCLC or pneumonia is not known. The patients enrolled in these studies had either euvolaemic or hypervolaemic HN associated with chronic heart failure, cirrhosis or SIADH (with no condition affecting >50 % of patients) [5]. Our approach is also supported by other studies, which suggest that the mean LOS assumed for the NAT arm of the model (8 days) is reasonable for the pneumonia population [31–33]. Data for the SCLC population are scarce; Salahudeen et al. [34] report mean (SD) LOS of 10.3 (10.0) for patients with HN in a mixed US oncology population.

Patient baseline characteristics were derived from the ART study, which identifies HN patients using ICD-9/10 codes. This method of identifying patients has high specificity, but low sensitivity [35]. However, the data are specific to Sweden and include patients from all three populations modelled. The ART study is therefore the most relevant source of patient characteristics data for this analysis.

It remains unclear to what extent [Na^+] correction or improvement is associated with improved long-term outcomes. There is some evidence that HN in hospitalised patients is associated with increased mortality (5-year data are available), with mild HN showing similar mortality rates to severe HN [36]. The model assumes no mortality benefit associated with [Na^+] correction and does not explicitly include the benefits of treatments which may be administered to achieve [Na^+] correction. The model assumes no residual HRQL or cost benefits associated with tolvaptan following discontinuation, and other longer-term benefits, such as any benefits of [Na^+] correction on readmissions, are ignored by the model, and therefore cost-effectivness may be underestimated.

Another possible factor not considered in our analysis, due to the lack of data, is the possibility of overcorrection, which may occur due to unexpected diuresis after resolution of the cause of the original water retention. Overcorrection of HN can have severe neurological consequences due to demyelination occurring in the brain [37].

In modelling this condition, there was dissociation between the treatment effect (e.g. changes in [Na^+] and HRQL. HRQL is based on reported QoL at Day 30 of SALT I and II. Transient adverse events could therefore have been missed, which would lead to an underestimation of HRQL losses. Although the assumption that 100 % of the 'general SIADH' population resolve their underlying condition following discharge is an over-simplification, the effect on incremental cost-effectiveness is likely to be minimal (please see Section 1.1.6 of the Additional file 1 for the underlying reasoning). Modelling HN secondary to SIADH without building several disease-specific models required a high degree of generalisation.

Published data relevant to the current analysis are limited but the best available data have been utilised from the randomised SALT trials. The main costs and benefits associated with short-term tolvaptan use are included in the model, but data limitations could lead to additional benefits not being accounted for, resulting in a possible under-estimation of cost-effectiveness. Despite a possible underestimation of cost-effectiveness, due to data limitations, the current analysis shows that tolvaptan treatment is associated with cost savings. The results of our analysis will be helpful to clinicians in the field of HN in establishing appropriate treatment strategies for patients with euvolaemic HN in the hospital setting.

Conclusion

This is the first cost-utility analysis of tolvaptan for the treatment of HN secondary to SIADH in a European setting. Treatment with tolvaptan was associated with reduced costs and better health outcomes (measured as QALYs) compared with NAT in the 'general SIADH', SCLC and pneumonia populations considered in this economic evaluation. Based on the assumptions within this evaluation, tolvaptan therefore represents a cost-effective treatment option for patients with HN secondary to SIADH who have either failed to response to fluid restriction or for whom the use of fluid restriction is not suitable.

Abbreviations

ADH: antidiuretic hormone; DES: discrete event simulation; HN: hyponatraemia; HRQoL: health related quality of life; ICER: incremental cost-effectiveness ratio; LOS: length of stay; NAT: no active treatment; QALYs: quality-adjusted life-years; QoL: quality of life; SCLC: small-cell lung cancer; SEK: Swedish kronor; SIADH: syndrome of inappropriate antidiuretic hormone secretion; TLV: the dental and pharmaceutical benefits agency.

Competing interests

Dr. Jacob Skov has received honorarium for his contribution to the writing of this manuscript from Otsuka Pharmaceuticals Europe Ltd. The authors declare that they have no competing interests.

Authors' contributions

DT, MG, PR designed and developed the economic model. CJ, KO, JL, ML and JS provided expert health economic and clinical input throughout the model and writing stages of the manuscript. DT drafted the manuscript. All authors read and approved the final manuscript.

Acknowledgements

We thank Sue Blokage for statistical support and Peter Dale for his health economic expertise during the initial manuscript development.

Funding

This study was funded by Otsuka Pharmaceuticals Europe Ltd. No other funding sources were provided throughout the conduct of the study. Medical writing and editorial support for the preparation of this manuscript was provided by Abacus International and funded by Otsuka Pharmaceuticals Europe Ltd.

Author details

[1]Abacus International, Bicester, Oxfordshire, UK. [2]Otsuka Pharmaceutical Europe Ltd., Gallions, Wexham Springs, Framewood Road, Wexham SL3 6PJ, UK. [3]Otsuka Pharma Scandinavia AB, Stockholm, Sweden. [4]Department of Medicine, Karlstad Central Hospital, Karlstad, Sweden.

References

1. Swedish Endocrine Society. Svenskt vardprogram for hyponatremi. 2012. Available from: http://endokrinologforeningen.se/documents/Svenskt%20vardprogram%20for%20hyponatremi_120120.pdf [Accessed 10 Aug 2015]
2. Spasovski G, Vanholder R, Allolio B, Annane D, Ball S, Bichet D, et al. Clinical practice guideline on diagnosis and treatment of hyponatraemia. Eur J Endocrinol. 2014;170(3):G1–47. doi:10.1530/EJE-13-1020.
3. Anderson RJ, Chung HM, Kluge R, Schrier RW. Hyponatremia: a prospective analysis of its epidemiology and the pathogenetic role of vasopressin. Ann Intern Med. 1985;102(2):164–8. ISSN: 0003–4819.
4. Verbalis JG, Adler S, Schrier RW, Berl T, Zhao Q, Czerwiec FS. Efficacy and safety of oral tolvaptan therapy in patients with the syndrome of inappropriate antidiuretic hormone secretion. Eur J Endocrinol Suppl. 2011; 164(5):725–32. doi:10.1530/EJE-10-1078.
5. Schrier RW, Gross P, Gheorghiade M, Berl T, Verbalis JG, Czerwiec FS, et al. Salt Investigators: Tolvaptan, a selective oral vasopressin V2-receptor antagonist, for hyponatremia. N Engl J Med. 2006;355(20):2099–112. doi:10.1056/NEJMoa065181.
6. Munger MA. New agents for managing hyponatremia in hospitalized patients. Am J Health Syst Pharm. 2007;64(3):253–65. doi:10.2146/060101.
7. BMJ best practice. Syndrome of inappropriate antidiuretic hormone. 2014. Available from: http://bestpractice.bmj.com/best-practice/monograph/196/basics/aetiology.html [Accessed 20 Jan 2015]
8. Rosner MH, Dalkin AC. Electrolyte disorders associated with cancer. Adv Chronic Kidney Dis. 2014;21(1):7–17. doi:10.1053/j.ackd.2013.05.005.
9. Gross AJ, Steinberg SM, Reilly JG, Bliss Jr DP, Brennan J, Le PT, et al. Atrial natriuretic factor and arginine vasopressin production in tumor cell lines from patients with lung cancer and their relationship to serum sodium. Cancer Res. 1993;53(1):67–74. ISSN: 0008–5472.
10. Greenberg A, Verbalis JG, Amin AN, Burst VR, Chiodo 3rd JA, Chiong JR, et al. Current treatment practice and outcomes. Report of the hyponatremia registry. Kidney Int. 2015;88(1):167–77. doi:10.1038/ki.2015.4.
11. European Medicines Agency. Samsca, tolvaptan, EPAR summary for the public. 2009. Available from: http://www.ema.europa.eu/docs/en_GB/document_library/EPAR_-_Summary_for_the_public/human/000980/WC500048713.pdf [Accessed 5 Mar 2014]
12. Chiong JR, Kim S, Lin J, Christian R, Dasta JF. Evaluation of costs associated with tolvaptan-mediated length-of-stay reduction among heart failure patients with hyponatremia in the US, based on the EVEREST trial. J Med Econ. 2012;15(2):276–84. doi:10.3111/13696998.2011.643329.
13. Dasta JF, Chiong JR, Christian R, Lin J. Evaluation of costs associated with tolvaptan-mediated hospital length of stay reduction among US patients with the syndrome of inappropriate antidiuretic hormone secretion, based on SALT-1 and SALT-2 trials. Hospital practice (1995). 2012;40(1):7–14. ISSN: 2154–8331.
14. Lee MY, Kang HJ, Park SY, Kim HL, Han E, Lee EK. Cost-effectiveness of tolvaptan for euvolemic or hypervolemic hyponatremia. Clin Ther. 2014; 36(9):1183–94. doi:10.1016/j.clinthera.2014.07.010.
15. Tandvårds- och läkemedelsförmånsverket (TLV). General guidelines for economic evaluations from the Pharmaceutical Benefits Board (LFNAR 2003:2). 2003. Available from: http://www.tlv.se/Upload/English/Guidelines-for-economic-evaluations-LFNAR-2003-2.pdf [Accesssed 10 Aug 2015]
16. Olsson K, Ohlin B, Melander O. Epidemiology and characteristics of hyponatremia in the emergency department. Eur J Intern Med. 2013;24(2): 110–6. doi:10.1016/j.ejim.2012.10.014.
17. Gisby M, et al. The burden of illness in patients with hyponatraemia in Sweden: a population-based registry study. Int J Clin Pract. 2016;70:319–329.
18. Cyr PL, McInnis M, Slawsky K, Krasa H, Czerwiec F, Ouyang J, et al. Impact of tolvaptan on self-reported utility scores in hyponatremic patients. Value Health. 2009;12(7):A382. ISSN: 1098–3015.
19. Gray AM, Rivero-Arias O, Clarke PM. Estimating the association between SF-12 responses and EQ-5D utility values by response mapping. Med Decis Mak. 2006;26:18–29. doi:10.1177/0272989X05284108.
20. Loveman E, Jones J, Hartwell D, Bird A, Harris P, Welch K, et al. The clinical effectiveness and cost-effectiveness of topotecan for small cell lung cancer: a systematic review and economic evaluation. Health Technol Assess. 2010; 14(19):1–204. doi:10.3310/hta14190.
21. Schuetz P, Albrich W, Suter I, Hug B, Christ-Crain M, Holler T, Henzen C, Krause M, Schoenenberger R, Zimmerli W, et al. Quality of care delivered by fee-for-service and DRG hospitals in Switzerland in patients with community-acquired pneumonia. Swiss Medical Weekly 2011. Available from: www.smw.ch/scripts/stream_pdf.php?doi=smw-2011-13228 [Accessed 10 Aug 2015]
22. Southern region health board. Southern region price list. Available from: http://www.skanese/Upload/Webbplatser/Sodra%20regionvardsnamnden/prislista/2013/helaprislistan2013pdf [Accessed 10 Aug 2015]
23. Tandvårds- och läkemedelsförmånsverket (TLV). Periodens vara. Available from: http://www.tlvse/apotek/utbyte-av-lakemedel-pa-apotek/periodens-varor/[Accessed 20 Jan 2015]
24. Statistics Sweden. Life tables for 2012, divided into men and women. Available from: http://www.scb.se/en_/Finding-statistics/Statistics-by-subject-area/Population/Population-composition/Population-statistics/Aktuell-Pong/25795/[Accessed 10 Aug 2015]
25. Stinnett AA, Mullahy J. Net health benefits: a new framework for the analysis of uncertainty in cost-effectiveness analysis. Med Decis Making. 1998;18(2 Suppl):S68–80. ISSN: 0272-989X.
26. Hultkrantz L, Svensson M. The value of a statistical life in Sweden: a review of the empirical literature. Health Policy. 2012;108(2–3):302–10. doi:10.1016/j.healthpol.2012.09.007.
27. Furst H, Hallows KR, Post J, Chen S, Kotzker W, Goldfarb S, et al. The urine/plasma electrolyte ratio: a predictive guide to water restriction. Am J Med Sci. 2000;319(4):240–4. ISSN: 0002–9629.
28. Petereit C, Zaba O, Teber I, Luders H, Grohe C. A rapid and efficient way to manage hyponatremia in patients with SIADH and small cell lung cancer: treatment with tolvaptan. BMC Pulm Med. 2013;13:55. doi:10.1186/1471-2466-13-55.
29. Kenz S, Brabant G. Tolvaptan for the treatment of hyponatraemia secondary to SIADH in cancer patients. Endocr Abstr. 2012;28:P28.
30. Poch E, Greenberg A, Burst VR, Verbalis J, Chase S, Makin A. Hyponatraemia in the hospital setting: interim results from a prospective, observational, multicentre, global registry, Presented at the 49th Congress of the European Renal Association. Paris: France Poster number FP005 2012; 2012.
31. Nair V, Niederman MS, Masani N, Fishbane S. Hyponatremia in community-acquired pneumonia. Am J Nephrol. 2007;27(2):184–90. doi:10.1159/000100866.
32. Zilberberg MD, Exuzides A, Spalding J, Foreman A, Jones AG, Colby C, et al. Hyponatremia and hospital outcomes among patients with pneumonia: a retrospective cohort study. BMC Pulm Med. 2008;8:16. doi:10.1186/1471-2466-8-16.
33. Zilberberg MD, Exuzides A, Spalding J, Foreman A, Jones AG, Colby C, et al. Epidemiology, clinical and economic outcomes of admission hyponatremia among hospitalized patients. Curr Med Res Opin. 2008;24(6):1601–8. doi:10.1185/03007990802081675.

34. Salahudeen AK, Doshi SM, Shah P. The frequency, cost, and clinical outcomes of hypernatremia in patients hospitalized to a comprehensive cancer center. Support Care Cancer. 2013;21(7):1871–8. doi:10.1007/s00520-013-1734-6.
35. Holland-Bill L, Christiansen CF, Ulrichsen SP, Ring T, Jorgensen JO, Sorensen HT. Validity of the international classification of diseases, 10th revision discharge diagnosis codes for hyponatraemia in the danish national registry of patients. BMJ Open. 2014;4(4):e004956. doi:10.1136/bmjopen-2014-004956.
36. Waikar SS, Mount DB, Curhan GC. Mortality after hospitalization with mild, moderate, and severe hyponatremia. Am J Med. 2009;122(9):857–65. doi:10.1016/j.amjmed.2009.01.027.
37. Norenberg MD. Central pontine myelinolysis: historical and mechanistic considerations. Metab Brain Dis. 2010;25(1):97–106. doi:10.1007/s11011-010-9175-0.
38. Makin A, Verbalis J, Greenberg A, Grohe C. Small cell lung cancer and hyponatremia: interim results from a prospective, observational, global registry, Presented at the European Multidisciplinary Conference in Thoracic Oncology 2013; May 9–11, 2013; Lugano, Switzerland. 2013.
39. List AF, Hainsworth JD, Davis BW, Hande KR, Greco FA, Johnson DH. The syndrome of inappropriate secretion of antidiuretic hormone (SIADH) in small-cell lung cancer. J Clin Oncol. 1986;4(8):1191–8. ISSN: 0732-183X.
40. Statistics Sweden. Labour Force Survey October 2013. Available from: http://www.scbse/en_/Finding-statistics/Statistics-by-subject-area/Labour-market/Labour-force-surveys/Labour-Force-Survey-LFS/ [Accessed 10 Aug 2015]
41. Trueman D, Hancock E, Robinson P, Dale P, O'Reilly K, Gisby M. EQ-5D scores in patients receiving tolvaptan for the treatment of hyponatraemia secondary to the Syndrome of Inappropriate Antidiuretic Hormone Secretion. Amsterdam: Poster presented at ISPOR; 2014.

30

Mazabraud's syndrome and thyroid cancer, a very rare and confusing association

Doina Piciu[1,2], Elena Barbus[2], Andra Piciu[2,3*] and Bogdan Fetica[4]

Abstract

Background: Mazabraud's syndrome is defined as the association between fibrous dysplasia and intramuscular myxomas. The syndrome was first described in 1967 and, up until now, less than 100 cases have been reported worldwide. Here we report the association between this rare syndrome and thyroid cancer. When a malignant disease occurs in a patient affected by this syndrome, the differential diagnosis between benign and malignant bone lesions should be undertaken carefully.

Case presentation: We report the case of a 57-year-old Caucasian male, admitted for diffuse bone pain localized in the left leg and for the presence of an indolent, slow-growing mass in the left shoulder. The patient also presented with a thyroid nodule, highly suggestive of a malignancy. The radiologic examination showed multiple osteolytic lesions. The suspicion of multiple myeloma or bone metastases arising from a thyroid cancer was considered. Electrophoresis of proteins was negative and therefore excluded the diagnosis of multiple myeloma; the thyroid surgery was indicated. Thyroidectomy confirmed the papillary thyroid carcinoma, and the bone lesions were considered to be metastases from the thyroid cancer. After surgery, under thyroid-stimulated hormonal conditions, the patient underwent radioiodine therapy and a post-therapy radioiodine whole body scan. The lack of radioiodine uptake, both in the bone lesions and shoulder mass, suggested the possibility of less differentiated, non-avid radioiodine lesions, or the absence of any relation between pathologies. Considering the low level of the specific tumor marker, thyroglobulin, a bone biopsy and resection of the shoulder mass were indicated. The final diagnosis was intramuscular myxoma with polyostotic fibrous dysplasia in the deltoid muscle (Mazabraud's syndrome). A completely incidental cerebral tumor lesion was also discovered.

Conclusion: During the evolution of a malignant disease, Mazabraud's syndrome, known as the association of intramuscular myxoma with fibrous dysplasia, should be considered in the differential diagnosis of bone metastasis. This is the first report in the literature of Mazabraud's syndrome occurring in a patient with thyroid cancer.

Keywords: Mazabraud's syndrome, Bone dysplasia, Myxoma, Thyroid cancer

Background

In 1967, the French physician Mazabraud described the association of intramuscular myxoma with fibrous dysplasia for the first time, naming the syndrome after himself [1, 2]. Fibrous dysplasia is a benign lesion in intramedullary bone. It can be found in two forms: a polyostotic (disseminated bone lesions) and a monostotic form (unique bone lesion) [3]. Symptoms include localized tumoral and intermittent pain or even pathological fractures. The differential diagnosis includes neurofibromatosis, multiple myeloma, endochondromatosis, hyperparathyroidism and McCune–Albright syndrome [4]. Intramuscular myxomas represent benign mesenchymal tumors associated with the polyostotic form of fibrous dysplasia in most women.

The incidence of Mazabraud's syndrome is <1/1,000,000 [4–6], with only 68–80 cases reported in the medical literature worldwide [1, 2]. The official Orphanet report, published in July 2015 confirms the presence of 54 cases published in the literature (ORPHA number 57782) [5]. The molecular diagnosis involves mutations in the GNAS1 gene, which encodes for an alpha subunit of a G protein [7].

* Correspondence: piciuandra@gmail.com
[2]University of Medicine and Pharmacy "Iuliu Hatieganu" 6–8 V. Babes, 400012 Cluj-Napoca, Romania
[3]Department of Oncology, Institute of Oncology "Prof. Dr. Ion Chiricuta" 34–36 Republicii, 400015 Cluj-Napoca, Romania
Full list of author information is available at the end of the article

Treatment of Mazabraud's syndrome includes the specific treatment of the fibrous dysplasia when complications appear: pathological bone fractures treated using osteosynthesis, or when sarcoma transformation occurs, exceptionally, specific treatment for the malignant tumor. Intramuscular myxomas benefit from an excision and control of local and regional lesions.

We present the case of a 57-year-old Caucasian male with Mazabraud's syndrome that was associated with a papillary thyroid carcinoma [8, 9]. A papillary thyroid cancer has been described in the literature, although in association with the McCune-Albright syndrome [7].

Case presentation

A 57-year-old male was referred to the Institute of Oncology Cluj-Napoca for a second opinion, with suspicion of a multiple myeloma. The patient presented with diffuse post-traumatic pain in the left thorax and the left tibial diaphysis. The clinical exam revealed a tumor lesion localized in the left deltoid region and another one in the anterior cervical region, suggestive of thyroid nodules. Right lateral cervical enlarged lymph nodes were also described. Conventional radiological examination highlighted areas of osteolysis in the right IVth costal arch and areas of osteolysis with ballooning in the left IVth, Vth and VIIth costal arches, as well as deformation and erosion of the cortical area of the bone.

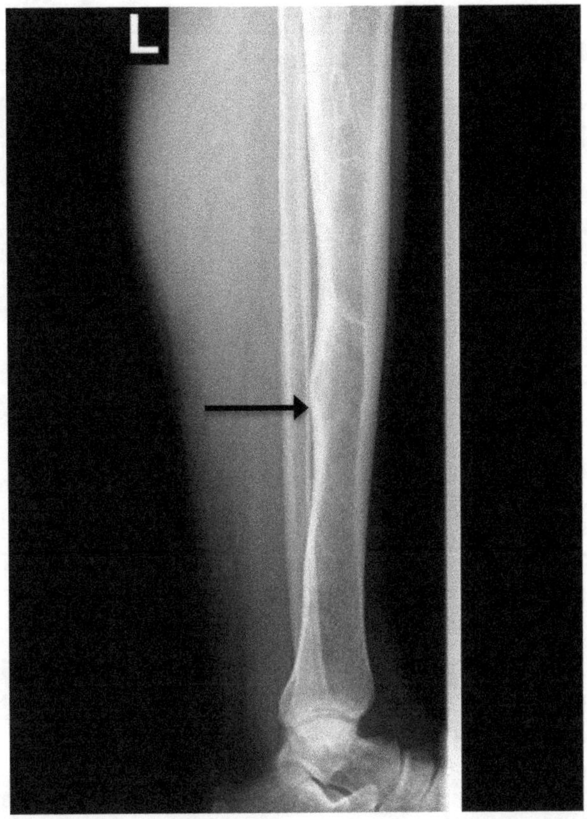

Fig. 1 Tibial radiograph showing bone dysplasia in the middle and distal parts of the diaphysis

Radiography of the tibia revealed a left tibia diaphysis with an irregular aspect of the compact bone (Fig. 1). Suspicion of a multiple myeloma or metastases in the bones with an undetermined origin was raised. Immunofixation electrophoresis of proteins was negative and therefore excluded a diagnosis of multiple myeloma. The patient was directed to the nuclear medicine department for a bone scintigraphy, which revealed the pathological uptake of tracer at the level of the costal arches and in the left diaphysis of the tibia (Fig. 2).

A blood sample was collected in order to determine the levels of tumor markers, which were at physiological normal levels: CA 19-9 = 25.2 U/mL (N.V. <27), CEA = 2.2 ng/mL (N.V. smokers <3.4; non-smokers <4.3), PSA = 1.31 ng/mL (N.V. <60 years old ≤3.1). Whole-body MRI showed multiple bone lesions localized at the level of the costal arches, left tibia, and left pubic branch, and an incidental tumor localized in the clivus that extended to the right sphenoid sinus (Fig. 3). In addition, there were multiple suspicious lymph nodes in the neck and in the right supraclavicular area and an inhomogeneous lesion in the right thyroid lobe (Fig. 4). The patient, at this point, was tentatively diagnosed to have thyroid cancer with bone and cutaneous metastases.

Blood samples were collected to determine thyroid stimulating hormone (TSH) and free-thyroxine-FT4 levels, which were found to be within normal limits. The thyroid peroxidase (TPO) test was also negative, thereby excluding a chronic lymphocytic thyroiditis. Calcium and parathyroid hormone (PTH) levels were also within normal limits, which excluded a parathyroid pathology, while a normal calcitonin level excluded a medullary thyroid carcinoma. Biopsy of one of the right cervical lymph nodes was performed and histology revealed a papillary thyroid cancer lymph node metastasis. Immunohistochemistry (IHC) of TTF-1 and thyroglobulin (TG) were positive in tumor cells. A total thyroidectomy and right selective lymphadenectomy were performed. This confirmed the diagnosis of a papillary thyroid carcinoma with lymph node metastasis (T3N1bMx stage IVA) (Fig. 5).

Radioiodine therapy was indicated and given at a total dose of 96 mCi (3.55 GBq). Figure 6 shows a whole body scan (WBS) at 48 h after the radioiodine cure and shows pathologic radioiodine uptake in the right thyroid bed, within the mediastinum area and in a left lateral cervical lymph node, but there was no uptake in the bone. There

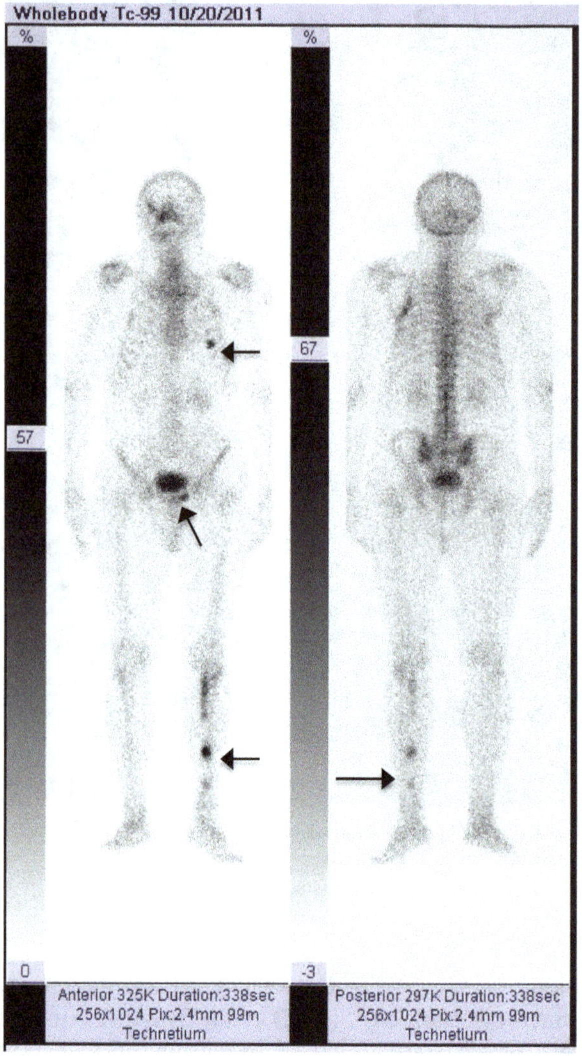

Fig. 2 Whole body bone scintigraphy using Tc-99m MDP, showing pathologic uptake of tracer in thorax, pelvic area and left tibia

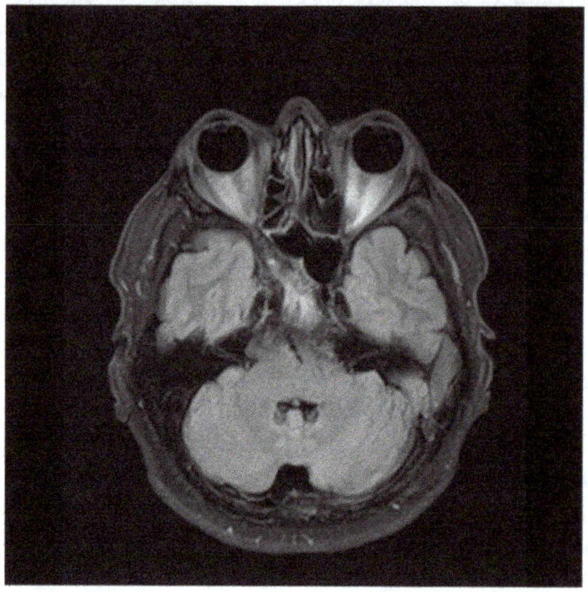

Fig. 3 Brain MRI showing a tumor in the clivus and involvement of sphenoid bone

were at least three possibilities as to what the bone lesions were: 1) a less differentiated thyroid tumor, confirmed by the relatively low level of the specific tumor marker, TG = 28 ng/mL (N.V. <0.04 ng/mL in cured thyroid cancer patients, and negative for anti-TG antibodies) determined under stimulated TSH; 2) non-avid radioiodine lesions, confirmed by the lack of radioiodine uptake, both in the bone lesions and in the shoulder mass; and 3) the absence of any relation between the bone, the muscle pathologies and the thyroid cancer.

A biopsy of the shoulder tumor lesion was taken from the left deltoid area and the histology exam revealed a macroscopic white-translucent specimen of 3.5/3/2 cm, and of gelatinous consistency, without any areas of necrosis. Microscopic examination revealed tumor proliferation consisting of fusocellular and star cells, without any nuclear atypia and mitosis in a myxoid stroma. Tumor proliferation infiltrated into the rib muscles and resected margins came in contact with proliferating tumor cells. IHC was negative for S100, actin and desmin; the histologic

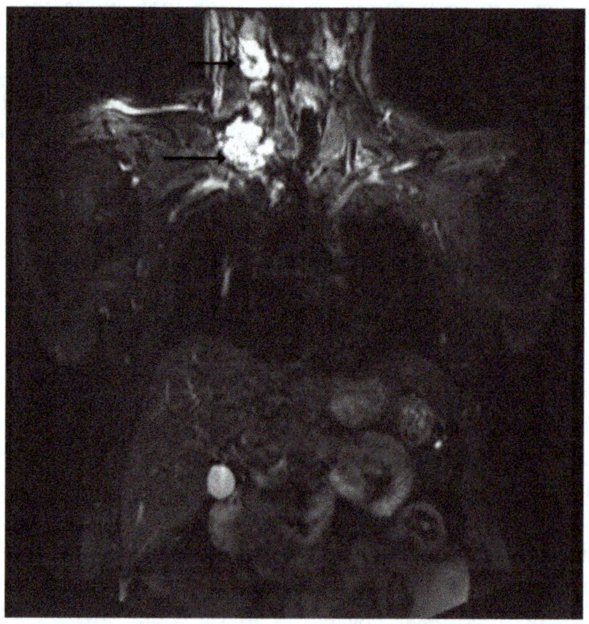

Fig. 4 MRI of the cervical region showing the right thyroid lobe with a nodular structure and right cervical lymph nodes highly suspicious for malignancy

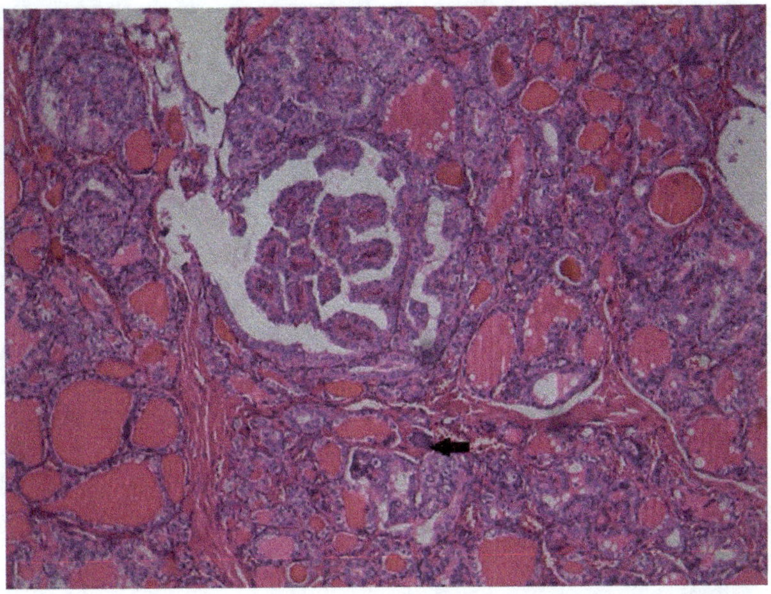

Fig. 5 Histopathology of the thyroid gland showing a papillary thyroid carcinoma (H&E staining, 100× magnification). Tumor cells have specific nuclear changes and form follicles and papillary structures. A small psammomatous body is visible (indicated by the black arrow)

aspect and IHC were specific for an intramuscular myxoma (Fig. 7). The association between the histology of the tumor and the bone lesions, with aspects of fibrous dysplasia, led to the diagnosis of Mazabraud's syndrome. Biopsy of the tibia confirmed the diagnosis.

At 2 years after surgery and irradiation, patient status revealed that: clinical tests and thyroid ultrasound were negative, antithyroglobulin (anti-TG) was <10 UI/mL (N.V. ≤115), TSH was 21.91 μUI/mL, TG was 0.82 ng/mL (N.V. athyroid patients <0.04) and I-131 WBS was negative (Fig. 8). The patient was therefore considered cured of his thyroid cancer and yearly follow-up was implemented; the bone lesions attributed to osseous dysplasia were stable.

During the follow-up at 3 years after the initial diagnosis of Mazabraud's syndrome a bone scintigraphy was performed and confirmed the bone tumor lesions already known, as well as a new lesion in the left ankle articulation, further corroborating the diagnosis of Mazabraud's syndrome (Fig. 9). No clinical signs of relapse were noted in the left deltoid area. No genetic testing for mutations in the GNAS1 gene was performed because it was not available nationally. The cerebral lesion described in the MRI was not biopsied, being refused by patient, and was therefore strictly monitored by the neurosurgery specialist.

Discussion

The medical case presented is typical of Mazabraud's syndrome, as described in the literature, however, the association with a malignant disease, seriously complicated the medical diagnosis and treatment.

Fibrous dysplasia has no predilection for the axial skeleton or the appendicular one. Statistics show that fibrous dysplasia has an incidence of 7 % of all benign bone lesions [9]. In the case presented, the polyostotic form was predominant, with lesions being situated in the diaphysis-metaphysis region, pelvis and the costal arches, which occurs with a frequency of 15 % of all lesions. The trigger for this type of lesion is a genetic mutation in the GNAS1 gene situated on chromosome 20q that encodes the alpha subunit of a G protein, which plays an important role in cell proliferation [8]. Fibrous dysplasia can also occur in the McCune–Albright syndrome, in which café-au-lait spots and endocrine disorders appear (nodular goiter, diabetes, early puberty and others) [4].

There are usually multiple intramuscular myxomas that occur in Mazabraud's syndrome that appear before any bone lesion [10]. The mean age at which Mazabraud's syndrome is diagnosed is 47 years, and the disease is predominant in the female population [8]. The most frequent pathologies associated with Mazabraud's syndrome are benign thyroid diseases and early puberty. When a malignant tumor such as thyroid cancer is suspected, the presence of any other tumors in the brain, bones or soft tissues should be considered as potential metastases, unless other pathologies are ruled out. In this particular case, although a possible association between the two entities of myxoma and osseous dysplasia in Mazabraud's syndrome is uncommon, it allowed the

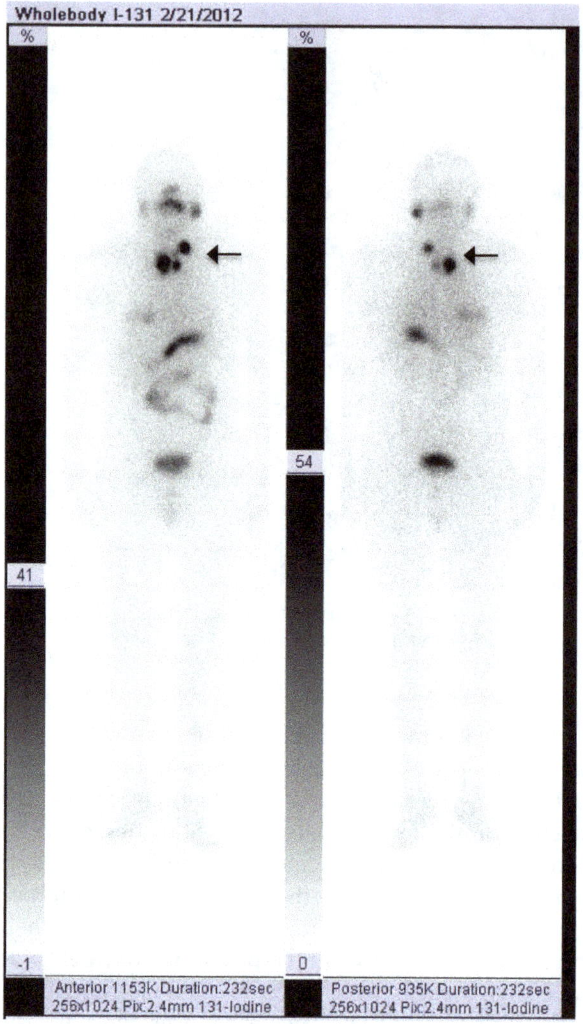

Fig. 6 Whole body scan (WBS) at 48 h after radioiodine I-131 therapy showing pathologic uptake in the thyroid bed and left cervical lymph nodes

clinician to select the correct radical therapeutic strategy to treat the thyroid pathology.

The imaging techniques used for the diagnosis of Mazabraud's syndrome involved conventional radiology to outline the bone lesions from the fibrous dysplasia using the "ground-glass" aspect and presenting areas of bone sclerosis [2]. Bone scintigraphy was indicated to outline the polyostotic form and the implication of multiple bone structures. MRI was used to detect muscle tumor lesions and to find new lesions that were not clinically evident [1]. Microscopy of the intramuscular myxoma was specific: hypocellularity, with a myxoid stroma, stellar aspect of the cells and the absence of nuclear atypia and of the necrosis [2].

There is no specific treatment for Mazabraud's syndrome. A follow-up of the bone pathology was indicated

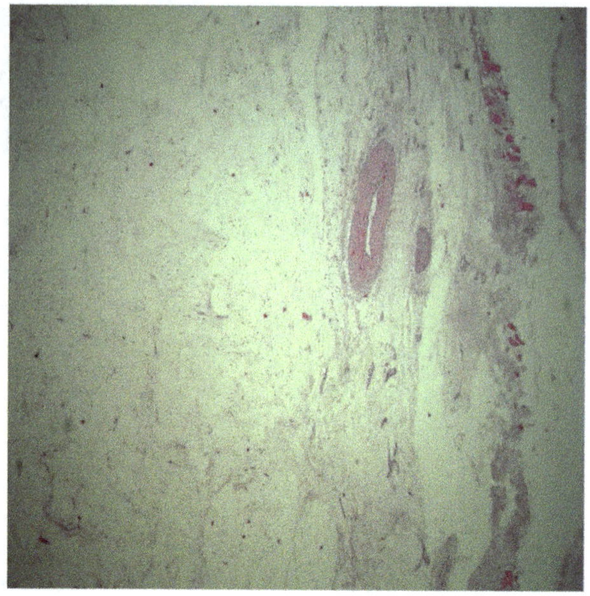

Fig. 7 Histopathology of an intramuscular myxoma from a deltoid tumor (H&E staining, 25× magnification). Paucicellular tumor with myofibroblasts and fibroblasts embedded in a myxoid stroma. Mitotic activity is inconspicuous. Skeletal muscle fibers can be seen on the right

in order to detect a possible malignant transformation. Intramuscular myxomas can be excised when they cause local pain [9]. The association with a malignant disease is very challenging, especially if the genetic test is missing.

In the present clinical case, the specific uptake of radioiodine into only normal and tumoral thyroid cells during the WBS was the main reason for understanding the non-thyroid origin of the bone lesions. The chance of this case was the good prognostic of the malignant disease, which was considered for radical treatment. The limited information about Mazabraud's syndrome and its low incidence might lead to the use of the wrong therapeutic strategy if other bone metastatic malignant diseases are involved.

Conclusions

Mazabraud's syndrome continues to be a very rare disease, with <100 cases worldwide. Therefore, in assessing a bone lesion associated with a malignant disease, we should be warned about its features, considering that the confusing clinical presentation might result in inappropriate staging and therapy for a cancer patient.

Competing interests
The authors declare that they have no competing interests.

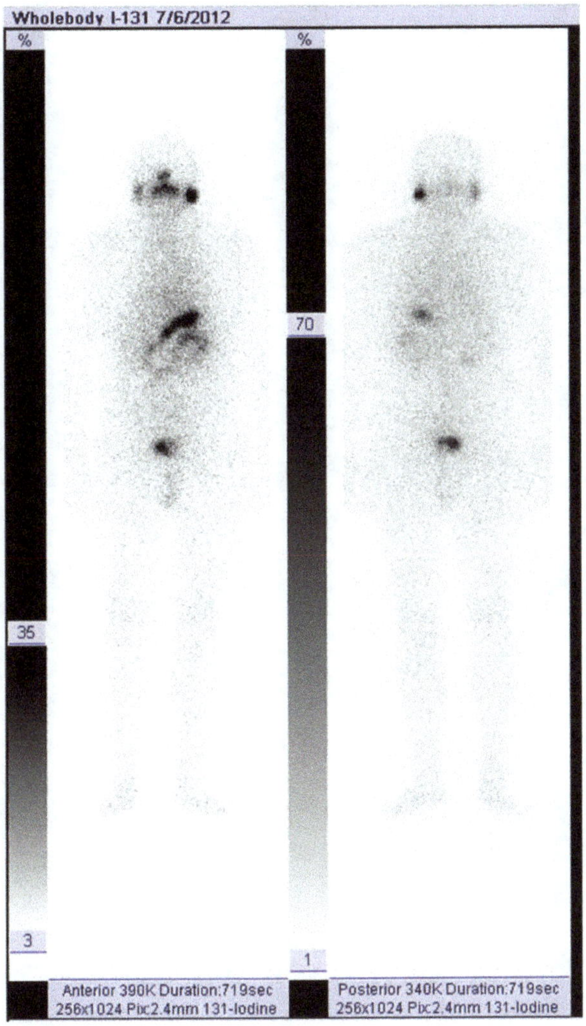

Fig. 8 Negative whole body scan (WBS) 24 h after radioiodine I-131 showing no pathologic radioiodine uptake, thus confirming that the patient was cured of his/her thyroid cancer

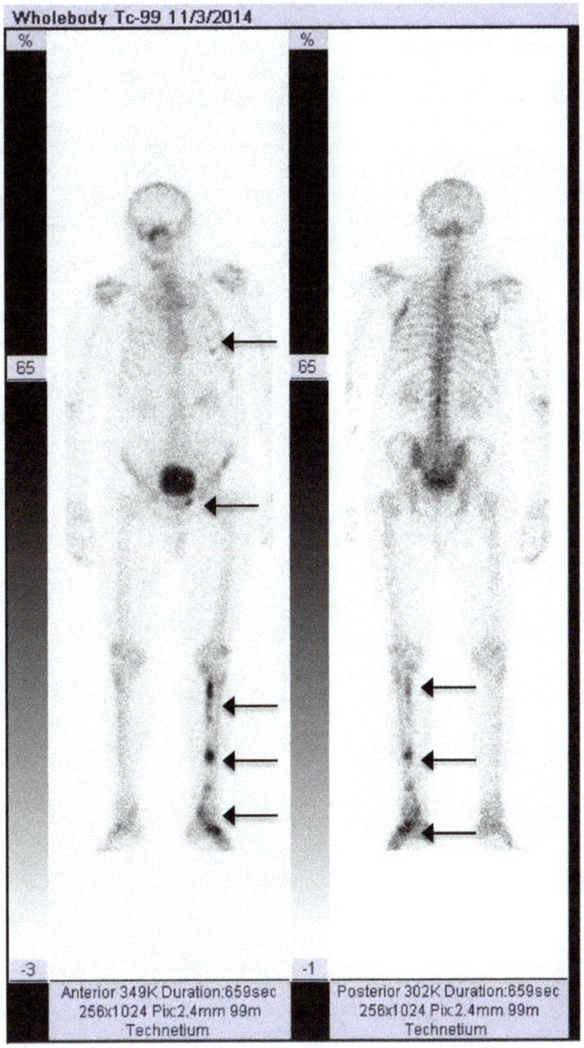

Fig. 9 Whole body bone scintigraphy with Tc-99m MDP at 3 years after the initial diagnosis, showing pathologic uptake of the tracer in thorax and left tibia, suggesting evolution of the disease in the left leg (indicated by arrows)

Authors' contributions

DP and EB treated the patient and drafted the article. BF performed the pathology exams. AP participated in the analysis and interpretation of data and together with DP and EB critically revised the manuscript. All authors read and approved the final manuscript.

Author details

[1]Department of Endocrinology and Nuclear Medicine, Institute of Oncology "Prof. Dr. Ion Chiricuta" 34–36 Republicii, 400015 Cluj-Napoca, Romania. [2]University of Medicine and Pharmacy "Iuliu Hatieganu" 6–8 V. Babes, 400012 Cluj-Napoca, Romania. [3]Department of Oncology, Institute of Oncology "Prof. Dr. Ion Chiricuta" 34–36 Republicii, 400015 Cluj-Napoca, Romania. [4]Department of Pathology, Institute of Oncology "Prof. Dr. Ion Chiricuta" 34–36 Republicii, 400015 Cluj-Napoca, Romania.

References

1. Dreizin D, Glen C, Jose J. Mazabraud syndrome. Am J Orthop (Belle Mead NJ). 2012;41:332–5.
2. Munksgaard PS, Salkus G, Iyer VV, Fisker RV. Mazabraud's syndrome: case report and literature review. Acta Radiol Short Reports. 2013;2:2047981613492532.
3. Van der Wal WA, Unal H, de Rooy JW, Flucke U, Veth RP. Fibrous dysplasia of bone associated with soft-tissue myxomas as well as an intra-osseous myxoma in a woman with Mazabraud's syndrome: a case report. J Med Case Rep. 2011;5:239.
4. Dumitrescu CE, Collins MT. McCune-Albright syndrome. Orphanet J Rare Dis. 2008;3:12.
5. Prevalence of rare diseases: bibliographic data, 2015, 1: http://www.orpha.net/consor/cgi-bin/Education_Home.php?lng=EN#REPORT_RARE_DISEASES. Accessed 4 Aug 2015.
6. Endo M, Kawai A, Kobayashi E, Morimoto Y, Yamaguchi U, Nakatani F, et al. Solitary intramuscular myxoma with monostotic fibrous dysplasia as a rare variant of Mazabraud's syndrome. Skeletal Radiol. 2007;36:523–9.

7. Collins MT, Sarlis NJ, Merino MJ, Monroe J, Crawford SE, Krakoff J, et al. Thyroid carcinoma in the McCune-Albright syndrome: contributory role of activating Gs alpha mutations. J Clin Endocrinol Metab. 2003;88:4413–7.
8. Zoccali C, Teori G, Prencipe U, Erba F. Mazabraud's syndrome: a new case and review of the literature. Int Orthop. 2009;33:605–10.
9. Muthusamy S, Subhawong T, Conway SA, Temple HT. Locally aggressive fibrous dysplasia mimicking malignancy: a report of four cases and review of the literature. Clin Orthop Relat Res. 2015;473:742–50.
10. Petscavage-Thomas JM, Walker EA, Logie CI, Clarke LE, Duryea DM, Murphey MD. Soft-tissue myxomatous lesions: review of salient imaging features with pathologic comparison. Radiographics. 2015;34:964–8.

Permissions

All chapters in this book were first published in ED, by BioMed Central; hereby published with permission under the Creative Commons Attribution License or equivalent. Every chapter published in this book has been scrutinized by our experts. Their significance has been extensively debated. The topics covered herein carry significant findings which will fuel the growth of the discipline. They may even be implemented as practical applications or may be referred to as a beginning point for another development.

The contributors of this book come from diverse backgrounds, making this book a truly international effort. This book will bring forth new frontiers with its revolutionizing research information and detailed analysis of the nascent developments around the world.

We would like to thank all the contributing authors for lending their expertise to make the book truly unique. They have played a crucial role in the development of this book. Without their invaluable contributions this book wouldn't have been possible. They have made vital efforts to compile up to date information on the varied aspects of this subject to make this book a valuable addition to the collection of many professionals and students.

This book was conceptualized with the vision of imparting up-to-date information and advanced data in this field. To ensure the same, a matchless editorial board was set up. Every individual on the board went through rigorous rounds of assessment to prove their worth. After which they invested a large part of their time researching and compiling the most relevant data for our readers.

The editorial board has been involved in producing this book since its inception. They have spent rigorous hours researching and exploring the diverse topics which have resulted in the successful publishing of this book. They have passed on their knowledge of decades through this book. To expedite this challenging task, the publisher supported the team at every step. A small team of assistant editors was also appointed to further simplify the editing procedure and attain best results for the readers.

Apart from the editorial board, the designing team has also invested a significant amount of their time in understanding the subject and creating the most relevant covers. They scrutinized every image to scout for the most suitable representation of the subject and create an appropriate cover for the book.

The publishing team has been an ardent support to the editorial, designing and production team. Their endless efforts to recruit the best for this project, has resulted in the accomplishment of this book. They are a veteran in the field of academics and their pool of knowledge is as vast as their experience in printing. Their expertise and guidance has proved useful at every step. Their uncompromising quality standards have made this book an exceptional effort. Their encouragement from time to time has been an inspiration for everyone.

The publisher and the editorial board hope that this book will prove to be a valuable piece of knowledge for researchers, students, practitioners and scholars across the globe.

List of Contributors

M Hassan Murad
Knowledge and Evaluation Research Unit, Mayo Clinic, Rochester, MN, USA
Division of Preventive Medicine, Mayo Clinic, Rochester, MN, USA

Ahmad Hazem
Knowledge and Evaluation Research Unit, Mayo Clinic, Rochester, MN, USA
Division of Preventive Medicine, Mayo Clinic, Rochester, MN, USA
Department of Internal Medicine, University of North Dakota, Fargo, ND, USA

Fernando Coto-Yglesias, Svitlana Dzyubak, Shabnum Gupta, Melanie A Lane, Patricia J Erwin and Tarig Elraiyah
Knowledge and Evaluation Research Unit, Mayo Clinic, Rochester, MN, USA

Lars Berglund
Davis and the VA Northern California Health Care System, University of California, Sacramento, USA

Irina Bancos and Victor M Montori
Knowledge and Evaluation Research Unit, Mayo Clinic, Rochester, MN, USA
Division of Endocrinology, Diabetes, Metabolism, Nutrition, Mayo Clinic, Rochester, MN, USA

Yolanda Ballestero, Marta Botran and Ana García
Pediatric Intensive Care Department, Hospital General Universitario Gregorio Marañón Complutense University of Madrid, Madrid, Spain

Jesús López-Herce, Rafael González, Maria José Solana, Jimena del Castillo and Javier Urbano
Pediatric Intensive Care Department, Hospital General Universitario Gregorio Marañón Complutense University of Madrid, Madrid, Spain
Instituto de Investigación biomédica del Hospital Gregorio Marañón, Madrid, Spain
Red de Salud Materno Infantil y del Desarrollo, Red SAMID II, Madrid, Spain

David Trueman
Abacus International, Bicester, Oxfordshire, UK

Nieves López
Laboratory Department, Hospital General Universitario Gregorio Marañón, Madrid, Spain

Jose María Bellón
Instituto de Investigación biomédica del Hospital Gregorio Marañón, Madrid, Spain

Chong-Gui Zhu, Qiu-Zi Zhang and Mei Zhu
Department of Endocrinology, Tianjin Medical University General Hospital, No 154 Anshan Road, Heping District, Tianjin 300052, China

Qiong-Li Zhai
Department of Pathology, Tianjin Medical University Cancer Hospital, Huan-Hu-Xi Road Tiyuanbei, Hexin District, Tianjin 300060, China

Xiao-Yu Liang
Department of Surgery, Tianjin Medical University General Hospital, No 154 Anshan Road, Heping District, Tianjin 300052, China

Zong-Hong Shao
Department of Hematology, Tianjin Medical University General Hospital, No 154 Anshan Road, Heping District, Tianjin 300052, China

Emily C Ver Hoeve and Hui-Qi Qu
Division of Epidemiology, Human Genetics and Environmental Sciences, University of Texas School of Public Health, 1200 Herman Pressler, Houston, Texas 77030, USA

Naji J Aljohani
Faculty of Medicine, King Saud bin Abdulaziz University for Health Sciences, King Fahad Medical City, Riyadh, Saudi Arabia
Prince Mutaib Chair for Biomarkers of Osteoporosis, King Saud University, Riyadh, Saudi Arabia

Nasser M Al-Daghri, Majed S Alokail, Sobhy Yakout and Shaun Sabico
Biochemistry Department, Biomarkers Research Program, College of Science, King Saud University, Riyadh, Saudi Arabia
Prince Mutaib Chair for Biomarkers of Osteoporosis, King Saud University, Riyadh, Saudi Arabia

Omar S Al-Attas
Biochemistry Department, Biomarkers Research Program, College of Science, King Saud University, Riyadh, Saudi Arabia
Prince Mutaib Chair for Biomarkers of Osteoporosis, King Saud University, Riyadh, Saudi Arabia
Center of Excellence in Biotechnology Research Center, King Saud University, Riyadh, Saudi Arabia

Khalid M Alkhrafy
Biochemistry Department, Biomarkers Research Program, College of Science, King Saud University, Riyadh, Saudi Arabia
Prince Mutaib Chair for Biomarkers of Osteoporosis, King Saud University, Riyadh, Saudi Arabia
Clinical Pharmacy Department, College of Pharmacy, King Saud University, Riyadh, Saudi Arabia

Abdulaziz Al-Othman
Biochemistry Department, Biomarkers Research Program, College of Science, King Saud University, Riyadh, Saudi Arabia
College of Applied Medical Sciences, King Saud University, Riyadh, KSA, Saudi Arabia

Abdulaziz F Alkabba, Ahmed S Al-Ghamdi, Mussa Almalki and Badurudeen Mahmood Buhary
Faculty of Medicine, King Saud bin Abdulaziz University for Health Sciences, King Fahad Medical City, Riyadh, Saudi Arabia

Lucia Gagliardi
Endocrine and Metabolic Unit, Royal Adelaide Hospital, North Terrace, Adelaide, SA 5000, Australia
Department of Genetics and Molecular Pathology, Centre for Cancer Biology, SA Pathology, Frome Road, Adelaide, SA 5000, Australia
School of Medicine, University of Adelaide, Adelaide, SA 5000, Australia

David J Torpy
Endocrine and Metabolic Unit, Royal Adelaide Hospital, North Terrace, Adelaide, SA 5000, Australia
School of Medicine, University of Adelaide, Adelaide, SA 5000, Australia

Jinghua Feng
Cancer Genomics Facility, Centre for Cancer Biology, SA Pathology, Adelaide, SA 5000, Australia School of Molecular and Biomedical Science, University of Adelaide, Adelaide, SA 5000, Australia

Hamish S Scott
Department of Genetics and Molecular Pathology, Centre for Cancer Biology, SA Pathology, Frome Road, Adelaide, SA 5000, Australia
School of Medicine, University of Adelaide, Adelaide, SA 5000, Australia
Cancer Genomics Facility, Centre for Cancer Biology, SA Pathology, Adelaide, SA 5000, Australia School of Molecular and Biomedical Science, University of Adelaide, Adelaide, SA 5000, Australia
Division of Health Sciences, School of Pharmacy and Medical Sciences, University of South Australia, Adelaide, SA 5000, Australia

M Forss and G Batcheller
DuoCort Pharma, Medicinaregatan 8A, 413 46, Gothenburg, Sweden

S Skrtic
Department of Clinical Pharmacology, Sahlgrenska Academy, University of Gothenburg, Gothenburg, Sweden

G Johannsson
Department of Endocrinology, Sahlgrenska Academy, University of Gothenburg, Gothenburg, Sweden

Elaine Hui, Kathryn CB Tan and Karen SL Lam
Department of Medicine, The University of Hong Kong, Queen Mary Hospital, Pokfulam Road, Pokfulam, Hong Kong

Matthew CW Yeung and Angel OK Chan
Department of Pathology, The University of Hong Kong, Queen Mary Hospital, Pokfulam Road, Pokfulam, Hong Kong

Pik To Cheung, Elaine Kwan and Louis Low
Department of Pediatrics and Adolescent Medicine, The University of Hong Kong, Queen Mary Hospital, Pokfulam Road, Pokfulam, Hong Kong

Jenifer M Brown, Kristina Secinaro, Jonathan S Williams and Anand Vaidya
Division of Endocrinology, Diabetes, and Hypertension, Brigham and Women's Hospital and Harvard Medical School, 221 Longwood Ave, RFB, Boston, MA 02115, USA

René Rodríguez-Gutiérrez, Maria Azucena Zapata-Rivera, Fernando Javier Lavalle-Gonzalez, José Gerardo González-González and Jesús Zacarías Villarreal-Pérez
Endocrinology Division, Internal Medicine Department, University Hospital "Dr. José E. González", Ave. Madero y Ave. Gonzalitos s/n, Colonia Mitras Centro, Monterrey, Nuevo León 64460, Mexico
Medical School of the Universidad Autónoma de Nuevo León, Ave. Madero y Ave. Gonzalitos s/n, Colonia Mitras Centro, Monterrey, Nuevo León 64460, Mexico

Dania Lizeth Quintanilla-Flores and Carlos Rodrigo Camara-Lemarroy
Medical School of the Universidad Autónoma de Nuevo León, Ave. Madero y Ave. Gonzalitos s/n, Colonia Mitras Centro, Monterrey, Nuevo León 64460, Mexico
Internal Medicine Department, University Hospital "Dr. José E. González", Monterrey, Nuevo León 64460, Mexico

Ángel Matute-Llorente, Germán Vicente-Rodríguez and José Antonio Casajús
GENUD (Growth, Exercise, Nutrition and Development) Research Group, University of Zaragoza, Ed. Cervantes Corona de Aragón St 42, 2nd floor, Zaragoza 50009, Spain
Faculty of Health and Sport Science, Department of Physiatry and Nursing, University of Zaragoza, Ronda Misericordia 5, Huesca 22001, Spain

Alejandro González-Agüero
GENUD (Growth, Exercise, Nutrition and Development) Research Group, University of Zaragoza, Ed. Cervantes Corona de Aragón St 42, 2nd floor, Zaragoza 50009, Spain
Department of Sport and Exercise Science, Aberystwyth University, Ceredigion, United Kingdom

Alba Gómez-Cabello
GENUD (Growth, Exercise, Nutrition and Development) Research Group, University of Zaragoza, Ed. Cervantes Corona de Aragón St 42, 2nd floor, Zaragoza 50009, Spain
Hospital Virgen del Valle, Complejo Hospitalario de Toledo, Toledo, Spain

Kristin Holvik
Division of Epidemiology, Norwegian Institute of Public Health, Oslo, Norway
Institute of Health and Society, University of Oslo, Oslo, Norway
Norwegian Institute of Public Health, Nydalen 0403 Oslo, Norway

Ahmed A Madar
Institute of Health and Society, University of Oslo, Oslo, Norway

Haakon E Meyer
Division of Epidemiology, Norwegian Institute of Public Health, Oslo, Norway
Institute of Health and Society, University of Oslo, Oslo, Norway

Cathrine M Lofthus
Department of Endocrinology, Oslo University Hospital, Oslo, Norway

Lars C Stene
Division of Epidemiology, Norwegian Institute of Public Health, Oslo, Norway

Giovanni Corona and Alessandra Sforza
Medical Department, Endocrinology Unit, Azienda USL Bologna, Maggiore-Bellaria Hospital, Bologna, Italy

Luigi Simonetti
Emergency Interventional Radiology and Neuroradiology Unit, Azienda USL Bologna, Maggiore-Bellaria Hospital, Bologna, Italy

Corinna Giuliani and Alessandro Peri
Department of Experimental and Clinical Biomedical Sciences, Endocrine Unit, University of Florence, Florence, Italy

Wen-Yu Lin
Jen-Ai Hospital, Taichung City 41265, Taiwan

Ting-Sung Liu, Zhi-Hong Jian, Pei-Chieh Ko and Jing-Yang Huang
Department of Public Health and Institute of Public Health, Chung Shan Medical University, Taichung City 40201, Taiwan

Chia-Chi Lung, Yi-Chen Chiang and Yung-Po Liaw
Department of Public Health and Institute of Public Health, Chung Shan Medical University, Taichung City 40201, Taiwan
Department of Family and Community Medicine, Chung Shan Medical University Hospital, Taichung City 40201, Taiwan

Chien-Chang Ho
Department of Health and Leisure Management, Yuanpei University, Hsinchu City 300, Taiwan

Shih-Chang Chen
Department of Leisure Industry and Health Promotion, National Ilan University, Yilan City 260, Taiwan

Ioana Rada Ilie, Ileana Duncea and Carmen Emanuela Pepene
Department of Endocrinology, University of Medicine and Pharmacy, 3-5 Louis Pasteur, 400349, Cluj-Napoca, Romania

Ioan Marian
Department of Internal Medicine-Cardiology, University of Medicine and Pharmacy, Cluj-Napoca, Romania

Teodora Mocan
Departmen of Physiology, University of Medicine and Pharmacy, Cluj-Napoca, Romania

Razvan Ilie
Department of Obstetrics and Gynecology, University of Medicine and Pharmacy, Cluj-Napoca, Romania

Lucian Mocan
3-rd Department of Surgery, University of Medicine and Pharmacy, Cluj-Napoca, Romania

Eun Sil Koh, Sungjin Chung and Yoon Sik Chang
Department of Internal Medicine, College of Medicine, The Catholic University of Korea, 222 Banpo-daero, Seoul 137-701, Republic of Korea
Division of Nephrology, The Catholic University of Korea Yeouido St. Mary's Hospital, 10, 63-ro, Yeongdeungpo-gu, Seoul 150-713, Republic of Korea

Sung Jun Kim, Hye Eun Yoon and Seok Joon Shin
Department of Internal Medicine, College of Medicine, The Catholic University of Korea, 222 Banpo-daero, Seoul 137-701, Republic of Korea
Division of Nephrology, The Catholic University of Korea Incheon St. Mary's Hospital, 56, Dongsu-ro, Bupyeong-gu, Incheon 403-720, Republic of Korea

Jong Hee Chung
Department of Statistics, The Graduate School of Ewha Womans University, 52, Ewhayeodae-gil, Seodaemun-gu, Seoul 120-750, Republic of Korea

Cheol Whee Park
Department of Internal Medicine, College of Medicine, The Catholic University of Korea, 222 Banpo-daero, Seoul 137-701, Republic of Korea
Division of Nephrology, The Catholic University of Korea Seoul St. Mary's Hospital, 222, Banpo-daero, Seoul 137-701, Republic of Korea

Siobhan Bacon, Ma Peyh Kyithar and Syed R Rizvi
Department of Diabetes, Mater Misericordiae University Hospital, Dublin 7, Ireland

Jasmin Schmid, Caroline Bonner and Jochen HM Prehn
Department of Physiology and Medical Physics, Centre for Systems Medicine, Royal College of Surgeons in Ireland, Dublin 2, Ireland

Rolf Graf
Department of Visceral and Transplantation Surgery, University Hospital Zurich, Zurich, Switzerland

Maria M Byrne
Department of Diabetes, Mater Misericordiae University Hospital, Dublin 7, Ireland
Department of Endocrinology, Mater Misericordiae University Hospital, 30 Eccles Street, Dublin 7, Ireland

Laura Lucaccioni
Paediatric Unit, Department of Medical and Surgical Sciences for the Children and Adults, University of Modena & Reggio Emilia, via del Pozzo n. 71, 41125 Modena, Italy
Paediatric Endocrinology Unit, Royal Hospital for Sick Children, Dalnair St, Yorkhill, G3 8SJ Glasgow, UK

Bernd C Schwahn
Metabolic Unit, Royal Hospital for Sick Children, Dalnair St, Yorkhill, G3 8SJ Glasgow, UK

Malcolm Donaldson
Paediatric Endocrinology Unit, Royal Hospital for Sick Children, Dalnair St, Yorkhill, G3 8SJ Glasgow, UK

Claudio Giacomozzi
Paediatric Endocrinology Unit, Royal Hospital for Sick Children, Dalnair St, Yorkhill, G3 8SJ Glasgow, UK
Dipartimento di Medicina Pediatrica, Bambino Gesù Children's Hospital, Piazza S. Onofiro 4, 00165 Rome, Italy

Ahmed Yusuf
Clinical Studies and Empirical Ethics Department, King Faisal Specialist Hospital and Research Center, Riyadh 11211, Saudi Arabia

Muhammad M. Hammami
Clinical Studies and Empirical Ethics Department, King Faisal Specialist Hospital and Research Center, Riyadh 11211, Saudi Arabia
Alfaisal University College of Medicine, Riyadh, Saudi Arabia

Stefano Stagi, Sabrina Becciani, Salvatore Seminara and Maurizio de Martino
Paediatric Endocrinology Unit, Health Sciences Department, University of Florence, Anna Meyer Children's University Hospital, Viale Pieraccini 24, 50139 Florence, Italy

Giovanna Traficante, Elisabetta Lapi and Marilena Pantaleo
Genetics and Molecular Medicine Unit, Anna Meyer Children's University Hospital, Florence, Italy

Marzia Mortilla
Radiology Unit, Anna Meyer Children's University Hospital, Florence, Italy

Pattaranatcha Charnwichai
Department of Bioscience, Faculty of Science, Chulalongkorn University, Bangkok 10330, Thailand
Excellence Center for Medical Genetics, Department of Pediatrics, Faculty of Medicine, Chulalongkorn University, Bangkok 10330, Thailand

Patra Yeetong
Excellence Center for Medical Genetics, Department of Pediatrics, Faculty of Medicine, Chulalongkorn University, Bangkok 10330, Thailand
Department of Botany, Faculty of Science, Chulalongkorn University, Bangkok 10330, Thailand

Kanya Suphapeetiporn and Vorasuk Shotelersuk
Excellence Center for Medical Genetics, Department of Pediatrics, Faculty of Medicine, Chulalongkorn University, Bangkok 10330, Thailand
Center of Excellence for Medical Genetics, King Chulalongkorn Memorial Hospital, Bangkok 10330, Thailand

Vichit Supornsilchai and Taninee Sahakitrungruang
Division of Pediatric Endocrinology, Department of Pediatrics, Faculty of Medicine, Chulalongkorn University, Bangkok 10330, Thailand

A. Tahir
Department of Internal Medicine, Cummings School of Medicine- University of Calgary, Alberta, Canada

K. McLaughlin
Department of Nephrology, Cummings School of Medicine- University of Calgary, Alberta, Canada

G. Kline
Department of Endocrinology, Cummings School of Medicine- University of Calgary, Alberta, Canada

Ulla Ludwig, Daniela Holzner, Artur Greinert, Mark Martin Haenle, Suemeyra Oeztuerk and Wolfgang Kratzer
Department of Internal Medicine I, Center for Internal Medicine, University Medical Center Ulm, Albert-Einstein-Allee 23, 89081 Ulm, Germany

Christian Denzer
Department of Pediatrics and Adolescent Medicine, University Medical Center Ulm, Eythstr. 24, 89075 Ulm, Germany

Wolfgang Koenig
Department of Internal Medicine II, Center for Internal Medicine, University Medical Center Ulm, Albert-Einstein-Allee 23, 89081 Ulm, Germany
Deutsches Herzzentrum München, Technische Universität München, Munich, Germany
DZHK (German Centre for Cardiovascular Research), partner site Munich Heart Alliance, Munich, Germany

Bernhard Otto Boehm
Lee Kong Chian School of Medicine, Nanyang Technological University, Singapore, Singapore
Imperial College London, London, UK

Richard Andrew Mason
Louis Stokes Cleveland Department of Veterans Affairs Medical Center, 10701 East Boulevard, Cleveland, OH 44106, USA

Tilmann Graeter
Department of Diagnostic and Interventional Radiology, University Medical Center Ulm, Albert-Einstein-Allee 23, 89081 Ulm, Germany

Li Qin, Weiwei Zhang, Zhen Yang, Yixin Niu, Xiaoyong Li, Ning Lin, Hongmei Zhang and Qing Su
Department of Endocrinology, Xinhua Hospital Chongming Branch, Shanghai Jiao Tong University School of Medicine, Shanghai, China
Department of Endocrinology, Xinhua Hospital, Shanghai Jiao Tong University School of Medicine, 1665 Kongjiang Road, Shanghai, China

Shuai Lu and Yin Xing
Department of Endocrinology, Xinhua Hospital Chongming Branch, Shanghai Jiao Tong University School of Medicine, Shanghai, China

Guang Ning
Department of Endocrinology and Metabolism, Key Laboratory for Endocrine and Metabolic Diseases of Ministry of Health, RuiJin Hospital, Shanghai Jiao Tong University School of Medicine, E-Institute of Shanghai Universities, Shanghai, China

Jiangao Fan
Department of Gastroenterology, Shanghai Key Laboratory of Children's Digestion and Nutrition, Xinhua Hospital, Shanghai Jiaotong University School of Medicine, Shanghai, China

Qun Yan, Xu Li and Bo Feng
Department of Endocrinology, Shanghai East Hospital, Tongji University School of Medicine, 150 Jimo Road, Shanghai 200120, China

Guoliang Chen, Qinghu Zheng, Lun Li and Chenhong Gu
Puxing Community Health-Care Center, Pudong New District, 250 GuiChang Road, Shanghai 200136, China

Dongmei Sun
Department of Endocrinology, Shanghai East Hospital, Tongji University School of Medicine, 150 Jimo Road, Shanghai 200120, China
Puxing Community Health-Care Center, Pudong New District, 250 GuiChang Road, Shanghai 200136, China

Helmuth G. Dörr
Paediatric Endocrinology, Department Paediatrics, University Hospital of Erlangen, Erlangen, Germany

Hartmut A. Wollmann
Department Paediatrics, University Hospital of Tübingen, Tübingen, Germany

Berthold P. Hauffa
Paediatric Endocrinology, Department Paediatrics, University Hospital of Essen, Essen, Germany

Joachim Woelfle
Paediatric Endocrinology, Department Paediatrics, University Hospital of Bonn, Bonn, Germany

Katie Cunningham
Bariatric Medicine Service, Galway Diabetes Research Centre, HRB Clinical Research Facility, Galway University Hospital, Galway, Ireland
Croi, the West of Ireland Cardiac Foundation, Heart and Stroke Centre, Moyola Lane, Newcastle, Galway, Ireland

Catherine Crowe, Katriona Kilkelly and Helena Griffin
Bariatric Medicine Service, Galway Diabetes Research Centre, HRB Clinical Research Facility, Galway University Hospital, Galway, Ireland

Irene Gibson, Claire Kerins, Caroline Costello and Jane Windle
Croi, the West of Ireland Cardiac Foundation, Heart and Stroke Centre, Moyola Lane, Newcastle, Galway, Ireland

Paula M. O'Shea
Department of Clinical Biochemistry, Galway University Hospitals, Galway, Ireland

Mary Hynes
Bariatric Medicine Service, Galway Diabetes Research Centre, HRB Clinical Research Facility, Galway University Hospital, Galway, Ireland
School of Psychology, National University of Ireland, Galway, Ireland

Brian McGuire
School of Psychology, National University of Ireland, Galway, Ireland

Tim O'Brien and Francis M Finucane
Bariatric Medicine Service, Galway Diabetes Research Centre, HRB Clinical Research Facility, Galway University Hospital, Galway, Ireland
Discipline of Health Promotion, National University of Ireland, Galway, Ireland

Jenni Jones
Discipline of Health Promotion, National University of Ireland, Galway, Ireland
National Institute of Preventive Cardiology, Galway, Ireland

Rosa Maria Paragliola, Alessandro Prete, Alfredo Pontecorvi and Salvatore Maria Corsello
Endocrinology Unit, Università Cattolica del Sacro Cuore, Largo Agostino Gemelli 8, 00168 Rome, Italy

Ettore Capoluongo, Angelo Minucci and Giulia Canu
Biochemistry and Clinical Biochemistry Unit, Università Cattolica del Sacro Cuore, Rome, Italy

Francesco Torino
Department of Systems Medicine, Università degli Studi Tor Vergata, Rome, Italy

Fernanda Barros Bittar, Charlles H. M. Castro and Vera Lúcia Szejnfeld
Rheumatology Division, Universidade Federal de São Paulo - Escola Paulista de Medicina (UNIFESP-EPM), Rua Botucatu, 740 - 3° andar - Vila Clementino, CEP, São Paulo, SP 04023-900, Brazil

Clare Jamookeeah, Paul Robinson, Karl O'Reilly and Martin Gisby
Otsuka Pharmaceutical Europe Ltd., Gallions, Wexham Springs, Framewood Road, Wexham SL3 6PJ, UK

Johan Lundberg and Michael Ländin
Otsuka Pharma Scandinavia AB, Stockholm, Sweden

Jakob Skov
Department of Medicine, Karlstad Central Hospital, Karlstad, Sweden

Doina Piciu
Department of Endocrinology and Nuclear Medicine, Institute of Oncology "Prof. Dr. Ion Chiricuta" 34-36 Republicii, 400015 Cluj-Napoca, Romania
University of Medicine and Pharmacy "Iuliu Hatieganu" 6-8 V. Babes, 400012 Cluj-Napoca, Romania

Elena Barbus
University of Medicine and Pharmacy "Iuliu Hatieganu" 6-8 V. Babes, 400012 Cluj-Napoca, Romania

Andra Piciu
University of Medicine and Pharmacy "Iuliu Hatieganu" 6-8 V. Babes, 400012 Cluj-Napoca, Romania
Department of Oncology, Institute of Oncology "Prof. Dr. Ion Chiricuta" 34-36 Republicii, 400015 Cluj-Napoca, Romania

Bogdan Fetica
Department of Pathology, Institute of Oncology "Prof. Dr. Ion Chiricuta" 34-36 Republicii, 400015 Cluj-Napoca, Romania

Index

www.ingramcontent.com/pod-product-compliance
Lightning Source LLC
LaVergne TN
LVHW080906210926
848485LV00004B/606